Cystic Fibrosis: A Genetic Disorder

Cystic Fibrosis: A Genetic Disorder

Editor: Marvin Ward

FOSTER ACADEMICS

www.fosteracademics.com

www.fosteracademics.com

FOSTER ACADEMICS

Cataloging-in-Publication Data

Cystic fibrosis : a genetic disorder / edited by Marvin Ward.
p. cm.
Includes bibliographical references and index.
ISBN 978-1-63242-660-4
1. Cystic fibrosis. 2. Genetic disorders. 3. Fibrosis. 4. Pancreas--Diseases.
I. Ward, Marvin.
RC858.C95 C97 2019
616.37--dc23

Foster Academics,
118-35 Queens Blvd., Suite 400,
Forest Hills, NY 11375, USA

ISBN 978-1-63242-660-4 (Hardback)

Printed and bound in China.

Contents

Preface

Cystic fibrosis (CF) is a genetic disorder affecting the lungs, liver, pancreas, kidneys and the intestine. It is characterized by frequent lung infections, which cause coughing up of mucus and difficulty in breathing. Other symptoms may consist of poor growth, sinus infections, clubbing of the fingers and toes, fatty stool, etc. Cystic fibrosis is usually caused due to the presence of mutations in both the copies of the gene responsible for the production of the cystic fibrosis transmembrane conductance regulator (CFTR) protein. An individual with a single working copy of the gene is a carrier of cystic fibrosis. It is diagnosed through genetic testing and a sweat test. There is no known cure for cystic fibrosis. Antibiotics are given for treating lung infections and for deteriorating lung condition. Lung transplantation may be recommended in some cases. This book is compiled in such a manner, that it will provide in-depth knowledge about cystic fibrosis. The topics covered herein deal with the core aspects of this genetic disorder. For all readers who are interested in cystic fibrosis, the case studies included in this book will serve as an excellent guide to develop a comprehensive understanding.

The researches compiled throughout the book are authentic and of high quality, combining several disciplines and from very diverse regions from around the world. Drawing on the contributions of many researchers from diverse countries, the book's objective is to provide the readers with the latest achievements in the area of research. This book will surely be a source of knowledge to all interested and researching the field.

In the end, I would like to express my deep sense of gratitude to all the authors for meeting the set deadlines in completing and submitting their research chapters. I would also like to thank the publisher for the support offered to us throughout the course of the book. Finally, I extend my sincere thanks to my family for being a constant source of inspiration and encouragement.

Editor

1

Hemoglobin Oxygen Affinity in Patients with Cystic Fibrosis

Dieter Böning[1]*, Angela Littschwager[1], Matthias Hütler[1], Ralph Beneke[1], Doris Staab[2]

1 Institut für Sportmedizin, Charité - Universitätsmedizin Berlin, Berlin, Germany, **2** Klinik für Pädiatrische Pneumologie und Immunologie, Charité - Universitätsmedizin Berlin, Berlin, Germany

Abstract

In patients with cystic fibrosis lung damages cause arterial hypoxia. As a typical compensatory reaction one might expect changes in oxygen affinity of hemoglobin. Therefore position (standard half saturation pressure P_{50}st) and slope (Hill's n) of the O_2 dissociation curve as well as the Bohr coefficients (BC) for CO_2 and lactic acid were determined in blood of 14 adult patients (8 males, 6 females) and 14 healthy controls (6 males, 8 females). While Hill's n amounted to approximately 2.6 in all subjects, P_{50}st was slightly increased by 1mmHg in both patient groups (controls male 26.7±0.2, controls female 27.0±0.1, patients male 27.7±0.5, patients female 28.0±0.3 mmHg; mean and standard error, overall $p<0.01$). Main cause was a rise of 1–2 µmol/g hemoglobin in erythrocytic 2,3-biphosphoglycerate concentration. One patient only, clearly identified as an outlier and with the mutation G551D, showed a reduction of both P_{50}st (24.5 mmHg) and [2,3-biphosphoglycerate] (9.8 µmol/g hemoglobin). There were no differences in $BCCO_2$, but small sex differences in the BC for lactic acid in the controls which were not detectable in the patients. Causes for the right shift of the O_2 dissociation curve might be hypoxic stimulation of erythrocytic glycolysis and an increased red cell turnover both causing increased [2,3-biphosphoglycerate]. However, for situations with additional hypercapnia as observed in exercising patients a left shift seems to be a more favourable adaptation in cystic fibrosis. Additionally when in vivo PO_2 values were corrected to the standard conditions they mostly lay left of the in vitro O_2 dissociation curve in both patients and controls. This hints to unknown fugitive factors influencing oxygen affinity.

Editor: Shree Ram Singh, National Cancer Institute, United States of America

Funding: Funding provided by the following Foundation: Christiane Herzog Stiftung für Mukoviszidose-Kranke, http://www.christianeherzogstiftung.de/. The funders had no role in study design, data collection and analysis, decision to publish, or preparation of the manuscript.

Competing Interests: The authors have declared that no competing interests exist.

* E-mail: dieter.boening@charite.de

Introduction

Cystic fibrosis (CF) is the most frequent genetic disease in Caucasians [1–3]. Mutations on chromosome 7 (location 7q31.2) reduce the effectiveness of the cystic fibrosis transmembrane conductance regulator (CFTR), which is essential for the secretion of chloride (Cl^-) and consequently water in many glands. The clinical manifestation with heaviest impact is the progressive pulmonary disease. Because of the resulting deteriorated lung function in patients with cystic fibrosis causing hypoxia and partly also hypercapnia one might expect compensatory reactions in concentration and oxygen affinity of hemoglobin (Hb) to secure oxygen loading in spite of the reduced oxygen pressure (PO_2) in pulmonary capillaries.

There are various strategies of defense against arterial hypoxia [4–8]. In addition to hyperventilation most healthy humans, except partly Tibetans and Ethiopeans [9–11], react to hypoxia with an increase in Hb concentration ([Hb]) which facilitates sufficient binding of oxygen at lowered PO_2 in the lungs. Furthermore a right shift of the oxygen dissociation curve (ODC) under standard conditions (pH 7.4, PCO_2 40 mmHg, 37°C) partly compensates for the reduced diffusion pressure in the tissues because of the low oxygen saturation (SO_2) in the capillaries; the shift is caused by more 2,3-biphosphoglyrate (BPG) in the red cells. In contrast typical altitude animals like llamas, guinea pigs and partly birds possess left-shifted ODCs securing oxygen loading in the lungs and rather low [Hb] reducing circulatory resistance. In addition small red blood cells and a dense capillary net in the tissues diminish the diffusion distance and thus compensate for the decreased capillary PO_2 [12]. The human fetus exists also at very low arterial PO_2 but the concentration of the high affinity fetal Hb (HbF) is increased. Recent in vivo determinations of the ODC in adults point to a possible left shift of its upper part at altitude [13,14].

Astonishingly few studies investigated the combined effect of hypoxia and hypercapnia. The fetal conditions with higher arterial PCO_2 than in maternal blood point to an advantage of a left shifted ODC. Moles living in earth holes with reduced air exchange inspire hypoxic/hypercapnic gas and possess also Hb with increased oxygen affinity [15]. Huckauf et al ([16]) describe a left shifted ODC in patients with chronic obstructive lung disease and in a review Morgan [17] mentions that [BPG] is often reduced in critically ill patients.

Patients with cystic fibrosis often show normal or even anemic [Hb] (e. g. [18–20]. Interestingly, however, they may possess an increased red cell volume masked by a concomitant rise in plasma volume [21,22]. Compensatory reactions of oxygen affinity in cystic fibrosis have been investigated rarely. Slight right shifts of the standard ODC, characterized by a rise of P_{50}st and caused by increased [BPG], were detected by some authors [18,23], while others found unchanged [BPG] or P_{50}st [19,24].

However, there are various additional mechanisms for the regulation of oxygen affinity. Besides phosphates other anions like lactate, chloride and glutathione (e. g. [25,26]) bind to Hb. Depending on the binding site these substances also influence the cooperativity of the subunits visible as change in the slope of the ODC (Hill's n); additionally they may modify the intraerythrocytic pH. The Bohr effect, which in the physiological pH range causes an increase of PO_2 at constant saturation by acidification (essential in working muscles), may vary depending on various factors like oxygen saturation [27,28], type of acid [27,28], substance concentrations and age of the erythrocytes (e. g. [29]); in altitude residents a tendency to lowered Bohr coefficients ($BC = \Delta logPO_2/\Delta pH$) has been observed [30,31]. Also sex differences in oxygen binding properties have been described: women [32–34] as well as children [35] tend to higher P_{50}st than men. Finally in vivo variations of the ODC in venous blood of anemic patients as well as of trained subjects have been observed during exercise which were no more detectable after in vitro equilibration of blood [36–38]. The underlying mechanisms are not yet clarified.

Previous studies on oxygen affinity in cystic fibrosis were performed on rather heterogeneous groups of patients. Differences in the severity of the illness are almost inevitable but possible effects of age and sex were not considered. Also control groups were small or not clearly defined or even lacking. To our knowledge neither cooperativity (Hill's n) nor the Bohr effect have ever been studied in cystic fibrosis.

Considering all these factors it seemed worthwhile to perform a systematic study of mechanisms influencing blood O_2 affinity as possible facilitation of oxygen uptake in cystic fibrosis.

Methods

Study Participants

Measurements were performed in 14 adult patients and 14 controls; anthropometric data are presented in Table 1. The patients (8 males, 6 females) showed severely reduced lung function but were in a stable clinical condition. One male subject was bearer of the Class III G551D mutation which is one of five mutations with a frequency >0.1% accounting for 2 to 3% mutations worldwide. It impairs CFTR-mediated Cl^- transport by limiting channel gating at the cell surface [3,39].

The patients were the members of a group with exercise therapy. They usually lived at home but were under continuous supervision by physicians of the pediatric clinic of the faculty. Twice a week they performed a disease status tailored exercise program addressing endurance, strength, coordination and flexibility supervised by staff of the Institute of Sports Medicine and received individual advice for additional daily exercises at home. Occasionally some patients used short term oxygen supplementation, but not on the test day. The nonsmoking controls (6 males, 8 females) were physically active but not specifically or regularly training staff members and students. One female was slightly anemic ([Hb] 11.2 g/dl), but all other measurements yielded clinically normal values within the range of the group. The study protocol was approved by the ethics committee of the faculty (Ethikkommission, Charité – Universitätsmedizin Berlin, Ethikausschuss CBF, No. ek.185-13b) and written informed consent was obtained from all participants.

Study Procedure

The subjects arrived at the laboratory between 9.00 and 10.00 a.m. Lung function (forced vital capacity FVC, forced expiratory

Table 1. Subjects.

		Age	Body mass	Height	BMI	FVC	FEV1	PEF
	n	years	kg	cm	kg/m^2	%	%	%
Controls male	6	28±3	80.4±3.2	185±4	24.2±1.2	93±2	92±3	102±8
Controls female	8	27±2	62.8±3.0	171±3	21.5±0.8	117±4	104±5	98±10
Patients male	8	28±2	59.0±3.0	177±4	18.8±0.6	59±7	38±6	57±5
Patients female	6	29±1	48.8±1.7	162±2	18.6±0.5	56±8	37±6	51±12

Means and standard errors (SE). BMI body mass index, FVC forced vital capacity, FEV1 forced expiratory volume during 1 s; PEF peak expiratory flow. % of expected values for age and sex [40] or of individual FVC. All anthropometrical and lung function values are significantly (P<0.001) reduced in the patients.

volume during 1 s FEV1, peak expiratory flow PEF) was measured with a spirometer system (Oxycon gamma, Mijnhardt, Bunnik, The Netherlands). Percent of expected values for age and sex [40] or of individual FVC are presented in Table 1. Blood was sampled in supine position. Acid base status at 37°C (ABL 500 or 510 with no systematic difference between apparatus, Radiometer Copenhagen, Denmark), oxygenation status (PO_2, SO_2, COHb, MetHb) and [Hb] (OSM 3; Radiometer Copenhagen, Denmark) were measured in heparinized blood samples taken from hyperemized ear-lobes. Values for PO_2 are slightly lower than in arterial blood [41], but this is of negligible importance for saturations above 90% in the flat part of the ODC. Fifty ml of venous blood were drawn without stasis using heparinized vaccutainers and stored in an ice-water mixture. Oxygenation status, [Hb], hematocrit (Hct, microhematocrit method) and [Cl^-] in plasma (EML 100, Radiometer Copenhagen) were determined immediately. Aliquots were deproteinized and stored at −20°C for duplicate measurements of ATP and BPG concentrations (enzymatic kits, Sigma Diagnostics) on the next day.

Five ml each were equilibrated 20 min in sphere tonometers at 37°C with air/CO_2 or nitrogen/CO_2 mixtures (3, 6 or 10% CO_2). Lactic acid (13.5 mmol/l blood) was added to an additional sample equilibrated thereafter with 6% CO_2 in air or N_2. After taking aliquots for additional ATP and BPG measurements 0.2 ml of oxygenated blood were successively added 8 to 10 times to 1 ml deoxygenated blood using 2 connected syringes and mixed. After measurement of SO_2, COHb, MetHb, [Hb], pH, PCO_2 and PO_2, ODCs were drawn in the Hill plot (log SO_2/100-SO_2) versus log PO_2).

Samples of native blood as well as of blood equilibrated with N_2/6% CO_2 and with air/6% CO_2 were centrifuged for 10 min (3500 rpm, 4°C). Part of the red cell sediment was hemolyzed by repeated freezing and thawing and used for measurement of pH and [Cl^-] in the erythrocytes.

Twelve patients (7 males, 5 females) performed an incremental test (initially 0.3 W/kg, plus 0.3 W/kg every 2 min) until exhaustion on a cycle ergometer (Lode Excalibur, The Netherlands) during exercise therapy. Blood gases and lactate concentration (Ebio plus, Eppendorf, Germany) were measured in ear lobe blood and used to calculate P_{50} at exhaustion.

Calculations

The slope n of the oxygen dissociation curves linearized in the Hill plot served as measure of cooperativity. For 5% steps of SO_2 between 15 and 90% logPO_2 values were calculated from the regression equations and the corresponding pH values obtained by interpolation. Comparison of the ODCs for 3 and 10% CO_2 yielded Bohr coefficients for CO_2 ($BCCO_2$), comparison of the 6% CO_2 and the 13.5 mmol/l lactic acid curves yielded Bohr coefficients for fixed acid (BCLa) at each saturation step. P_{50}st were calculated from the curves of blood equilibrated with 6% CO_2 by use of the corresponding individual $BCCO_2$. Mean cellular hemoglobin concentrations (MCHC) calculated from [Hb] and Hct were corrected for 2% trapped plasma. $[Cl^-]_{ery}$ were corrected for 10% in the sediment after centrifugation with 3500 rpm; because of the large buffer capacity of red cells this is not necessary for pH_{ery}. Electrodes in the electrolyte analyser measure concentrations in water [42]; therefore $[Cl^-]_{ery}$ is given per 1 cell water. Values for the control subjects coincide with titrimetric measurements [43]. In vitro blood buffer capacities ($-\Delta$[acid]/ΔpH) for CO_2 and lactic acid were calculated from the measurements in the corresponding equilibrated samples.

Statistics

All data are presented as means±standard errors (SE). Dependent on the number of comparisons, t-tests or analysis of variance (ANOVA) were used for significance calculations. The probability that an outlier does not belong to a sample was tested eventually [44]. Differences with $P<0.05$ were considered as significant.

Results

Anthropometry and Pathology

Table 1 shows marked reduction in both body height and body mass in the patients compared to healthy subjects. Their lung function was substantially impeded by restrictive as well as obstructive damage visible from low vital capacity and expiratory flow (FEV1, PEV); FEV1 ranged between 22 and 74%.

Blood Gases and Acid Base Status

The impaired lung function of the patients caused a reduction of ear-lobe PO_2 and SO_2 (Table 2). Generally these values were also slightly lower in males than in females. Correspondingly, PCO_2 tended to higher values in males and in patients. However, the pH was equal in all subgroups because of non-respiratory compensation visible as increased base excess in males and in patients. Venous blood pH scattered more, but there were also no systematic differences among groups (means between 7.35 and 7.38); red cell pH showed no influence of sex or illness as well (means about 7.16). In vitro buffer capacities of blood tended to higher values in all males; this was significant for acidification with CO_2 as well as lactic acid (both $P<0.05$; latter not shown in Table 2) in oxygenated blood. Concentrations of COHb (controls male 0.6±0.1%, controls female 0.4±0.1%, patients male 0.6±0.2%, patients female 0.7±0.1%) and MetHb (controls male 0.5±0.1%, controls female 0.6±0.1%, patients male 0.5±0.1%, patients female 0.5±0.1%) were low and not different among groups.

Blood Composition

[Hb] and Hct were higher in males than females, but there were no significant differences between controls and patients (Table 3). In the male patients [Hb] was negatively correlated with FEV1 ($r=-0.762$, $P<0.05$). MCHC, however, was slightly but significantly lowered in patients. They showed also slightly decreased [Cl^-] in plasma and red cells. [BPG] and [ATP] were significantly increased in the patients inspite of very low [BPG] (9.8 µmol/gHb) in the subject with the G551D mutation. Additionally there was a sex difference for [BPG] with higher concentrations in females. After equilibration [BPG] and [ATP] tended to slightly higher values (0.9 and 0.2 µmol/gHb on average, respectively, not significant) compared to native blood.

Oxygen Dissociation Curves

In the Hill plot (Fig. 1) all curves were linear (correlation coefficients better than 0.98, not corrected for the slightly decreasing pH with rising saturation) and the slopes amounted to approximately 2.6 with very little scattering in all groups (Table 4).

The standard half saturation pressures (Table 4) corresponded to known normal values in the controls. In patients P_{50}st was significantly increased by 1 mmHg (with slightly but not significantly higher values for females). When corrected to arterialized pH and PCO_2, all means were 0.8 mmHg lower. The patient with the G551D mutation presented a markedly lowered P_{50}st of 24.5 mmHg (arterialized blood 23.3 mmHg) clearly identified as

Table 2. Blood gases and acid-base status.

	n	PO_{2art}	SO_{2art}	PCO_{2art}	pH_{art}	SBE	Buffer Cap
		mmHg	%	mmHg		mmol/l	mmol/l
Controls male	6	91.4±3.0	95.9±0.3	38.0±1.6	7.430±0.006	1.3±0.7	29.9±1.2
Controlsfemale	8	99.3±1.2	96.8±0.2	34.4±1.6	7.430±0.008	−0.9±0.7	25.2±1.0
Patients male	8	64.9±3.5	91.2±1.5	41.7±1.8	7.423±0.008	3.4±0.5	28.9±0.7
Patients female	6	70.5±2.7	93.3±0.7	37.2±2.0	7.427±0.012	1.4±0.7	26.8±1.0
Anova	sex	a		a		b	a
	illness	c	d			d	

Means ± SE. art measurements in ear lobe blood. Standard base excess (SBE, 100% SO_2, standardized [Hb] of 5 g/dl, [71]) measured in venous blood. Buffer Cap: in vitro buffer capacity for CO_2 in oxygenated blood (-$\Delta[HCO_3^-]_{plasma}/\Delta$ pH). ANOVA: a $P<0.05$, b $P<0.01$ or better for differences between males and females, c $P<0.05$, d $P<0.01$ or better for differences between controls and patients.

Table 3. Substance concentrations in venous blood.

	n	[Hb]	Hct	MCHC	$[Cl^-]_{plasma}$	$[Cl^-]_{ery}$	$[BPG]_{ery}$	$[ATP]_{ery}$
		g/dl	%	g/dl	mmol/l	mmol/l H_2O	μmol/gHb	μmol/gHb
Controls male	6	15.4±0.4	45.7±0.8	33.8±0.5	103.3±0.5	73.9±1.1	13.3±1.2	4.1±0.3
Controls female	8	12.8±0.4	39.6±0.2	32.8±0.3	103.2±0.4	76.0±1.5	14.6±0.8	4.2±0.2
Patients male	8	14.7±0.4	46.5±1.5	31.9±0.4	99.6±0.5	71.9±1.9	14.1±0.8*	4.6±0.1
Patients female	6	12.9±0.4	42.0±1.3	31.8±0.6	100.3±1.2	73.0±1.3	16.7±1.5	4.3±0.3
Anova	sex	a	a				a	
	illness			c	d	c	c	d

Means ± SE. Significance levels indicated like for Table 2. MCHC and $[Cl^-]_{ery}$ corrected for 2% and 10% trapped plasma, respectively. *14.8±0.5 without the patient with the G551D mutation.

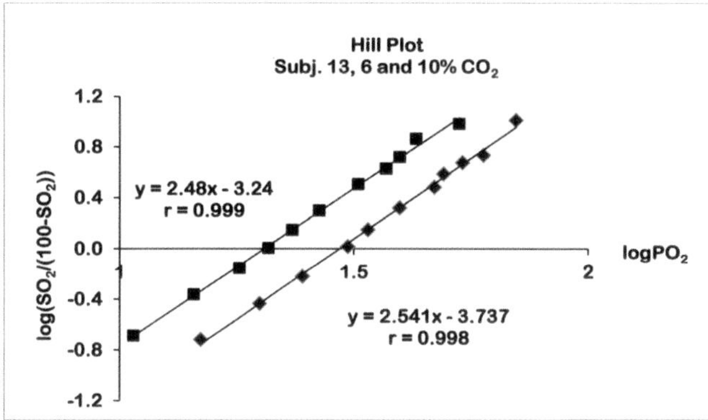

Figure 1. Two oxygen dissociation curves of one subject in the Hill plot.

an outlier ($P<0.02$). Without the latter value mean P_{50}st for the male patients rose by 0.4 mmHg.

Regression analysis including all subjects yielded a significant relation between [BPG] in the equilibrated samples and P_{50}st (Fig. 2). The male patient with the extremely low P_{50}st value fell, however, far outside of his group with a correspondingly low [BPG].

Bohr Coefficients

The Bohr coefficients (Fig. 3) for CO_2 corresponded to published data: The value was about -0.5 and decreased numerically with higher saturations ($P<0.01$ for all subjects); there was also a tendency to lower values in women. No influence of the disease was visible. The Bohr coefficients for lactic acid (Fig. 4) were generally lower numerically than for CO_2 in all groups up to 45% saturation (-0.40 to -0.45). Differences between males and females at higher SO_2 disappeared in the patients (interaction sex-illness $P<0.01$). Among the patients the subject with the G551D mutation presented the highest BC for both acids between 70 and 90% SO_2 (approx. -0.54).

Exercise Tests in Patients

At exhaustion SO_2 dropped in all patients resulting from reduced PO_2 and both respiratory and non-respiratory acidosis which caused a rise of P_{50} (Table 5). Again the subject with the G551D mutation showed the lowest P_{50} value (29.6 mmHg).

In vivo Effects

When the PO_2 values in non-equilibrated venous blood (fresh or stored in ice until measurement) were corrected with the corresponding Bohr coefficients ($BCCO_2$) to pH 7.4, they should have fallen on the individual standard ODC. However, in the range between 45 and 90% SO_2 there was a tendency for a deviation to the left (Fig. 5) in controls (-1.8 ± 0.4 mmHg, $P<0.05$) as well as in patients (-2.2 ± 0.4 mmHg, $P<0.001$). Some samples with higher values of SO_2 were not considered, because the BCs were not measured for $SO_2>90\%$. In addition there is large scattering of PO_2 in the flat part of the ODC. There was no correlation between PO_2 differences and [BPG] differences for native and equilibrated blood.

Discussion

Synopsis of Results

Our results confirm former investigations that there is a small right shift of the standard ODC in most patients with cystic fibrosis probably caused by slightly increased intraerythrocytic concentrations of organic phosphates [18,23]. This is accompanied by a constant slope of the ODC and only small changes of the Bohr coefficients. In spite of the lacking hypocapnia this reaction is similar to the typical human acclimatization to altitude but seems to be attenuated. During exercise the right shift of the ODC is enforced by hypercapnia in CF patients and a clear drawback for arterial oxygen loading. Interestingly there seems to exist an additional mechanism in controls as well as in patients: The in vivo standard ODC falls slightly left of the in vitro curve.

Blood Gases and Acid Base Status

The deterioration of lung function in the patients results in hypoxia visible in arterialized blood; a tendency to a slightly higher PCO_2 than in the controls is not significant probably because of the low number of measurements and the resting situation; when exercising the increase in PCO_2 is more marked. Measurements in 69 patients in our laboratory showed corresponding results; $PaCO_2$ increased with the severity of the illness at rest as well as during exercise [45]. This is different to healthy subjects who always show a decrease of $PaCO_2$ at high work load. The arterial oxygen saturation in patients at rest is as low as in highlanders [46,47] living 2600 m above sea level (inspiratory PO_2 approx. 120 mmHg). But in spite of a similar reduction of spirometric values the female patients show higher PO_2 and lower PCO_2 than the male patients like their healthy counterparts. Probably the long-known stimulation of respiratory brain centres by female

Table 4. Characteristics of the oxygen dissociation curves.

		P_{50}standard	Hill's n
	n	mmHg	6% CO_2
Controls male	6	26.7±0.2	2.63±0.02
Controls female	8	27.0±0.1	2.56±0.02
Patients male	8	27.7±0.5*	2.57±0.03
Patients female	6	28.0±0.3	2.61±0.03
Anova	sex		
	illness	d	

Means ± SE. Significance levels indicated as for Table 2. P_{50}standard: standard half saturation pressure calculated from the curves of blood equilibrated with 6% CO_2.*28.1±0.3 mmHg without the patient with the G551D mutation.

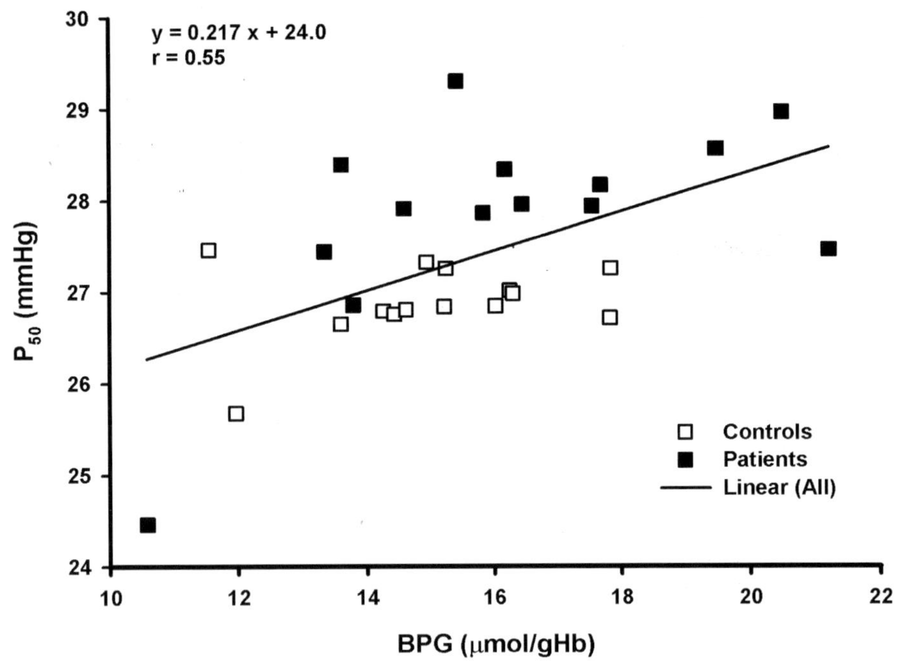

Figure 2. Dependence of P_{50}st on BPG concentration (means of equilibrated samples). Regression line for all values, correlation coefficient r different from zero ($P<0.01$).

hormones important for fetal oxygen supply is the cause (reviewed in [47]). The fact that arterialized pH is equal in all subgroups in spite of differences in PCO_2 demonstrates the importance of acid-base homeostasis for physiological functions. Non-respiratory compensation is mainly done by renal excretion/reabsorption of bicarbonate. In the patients the osmotic effect of the rise of $[HCO_3^-]$ is counteracted by a decrease of $[Cl^-]$. Also the loss of chloride via sweat glands might play a role. The slightly increased in vitro buffer capacity in both male groups is obviously caused by the higher Hb concentration. In cystic fibrosis the slight rise in bicarbonate concentration as well as the possibly increased Hb mass [21,22] help to attenuate the extracellular pH changes during exercise [48] caused by CO_2 retention.

Blood Composition

Hb concentrations showed typical sex differences but no sign of anemia in the patients. The latter might be expected in CF because of frequent problems with iron resorption. However, in

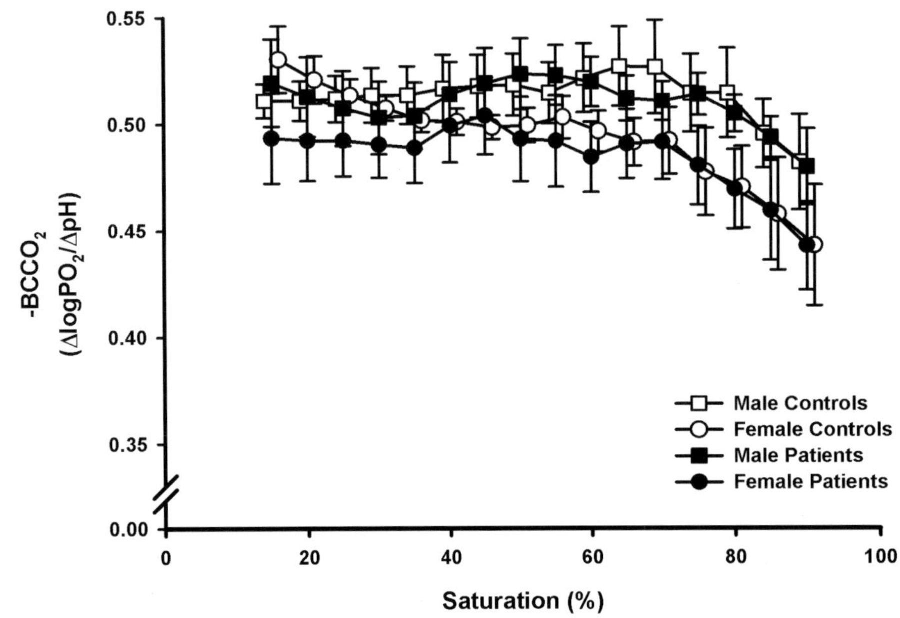

Figure 3. Saturation-dependent Bohr coefficients for acidification with CO_2 ($BCCO_2$). Means and standard errors.

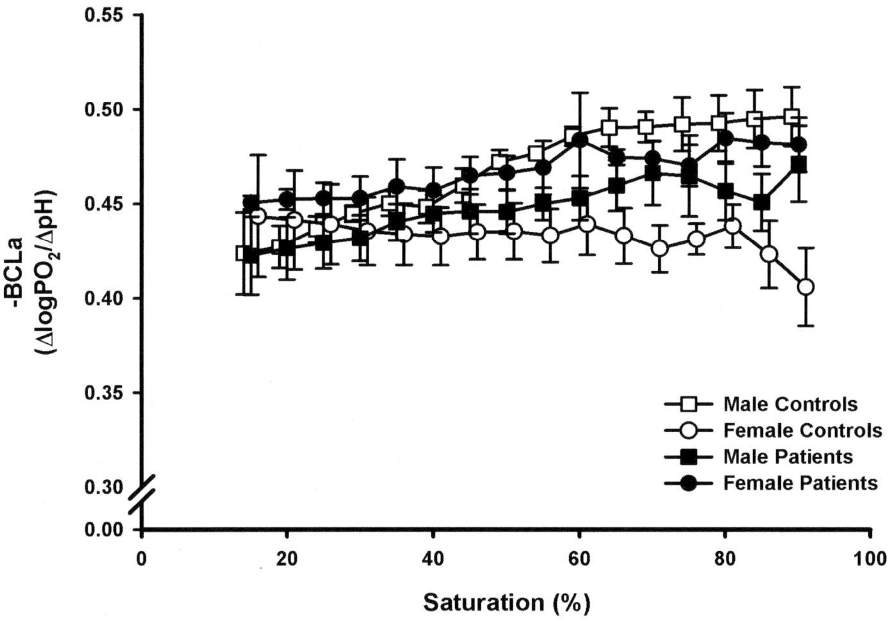

Figure 4. Saturation-dependent Bohr coefficients for acidification with lactic acid (BCLa). Means and standard errors.

our patients iron metabolism was routinely checked and deficiency was treated. One explanation for normal [Hb] in other studies might be the counteracting effects between iron deficiency and hypoxia [49]. Christoforou et al. [19] described a negative correlation of [erythropoietin] with FVC and FEV1. Such a dependency is probably the cause of the correlation between [Hb] and FEV1 in our male patients. Some authors [21,22] have even observed an increase in red cell volume in CF probably stimulated by erythropoietin which might be explained as a typical hypoxia reaction. However, only in a fraction of the corresponding studies [19,20,50,51]http://www.ncbi.nlm.nih.gov/ pubmed?term = Mc-Colley%20SA%5BAuthor%5D&cauthor = true&cauthor_-uid = 21365780 erythropoietin concentration was increased. Own unpublished measurements support the idea of chronic stimulation of erythropoesis in CF patients based on elevated erythropoietin as well as soluble transferrin receptor concentrations in a cohort of 79 CF patients. Also a low MCHC like in the patients is often related to an increased water content typical for young erythrocytes. Furthermore in patients the high level of the soluble transferrin receptor [20] might be indicative for an increased red cell production and thus a reduced erythrocytic age. However, also a link between CFTR and the function of the hypoxia inducible factor has been put forward [52] which may serve as one potential reason for a lack of increased [Hb] in CF patients.

Factors possibly increasing [BPG] and [ATP] are low SO_2 (reducing product inhibition because of BPG binding to Hb) and alkalosis (stimulating glycolysis and thus BPG synthesis). A probable explanation for the rather small increase of [BPG] and P_{50}st in CF compared to highlanders with similarly lowered arterial SO_2 and equal pH at rest (e. g. 18 µmol/g Hb in [30]) might be the different effect of physical activity: CO_2 retention causes respiratory acidosis already during moderate physical activity in the patients while highlanders effectively hyperventilate at each exercise level. In the present patient group with normal daily life and exercise therapy physical activity was obviously a factor of some importance. Additionally a low red cell age as suggested above might lead to elevated [BPG] as well as [ATP] because of high enzymatic activity [29]. The low [BPG] in the patient with the G551D mutation possibly results from changed enzyme activities because no differences in erythrocyte physiology were detectable. CFTR is incorporated into the red cell membrane (e. g. [53]), but a relation to BPG metabolism remains speculative.

[Cl^-] in red cells in part follows passively changes in plasma [Cl^-] and therefore is lowered in patients. Generally the marked concentration difference results from the high erythrocytic content of non-diffusible anions (Hb^- and organic phosphates) causing a Donnan equilibrium. Cl^- crosses the cell membrane mainly through band 3 channels. The reduction of the number of CFTR molecules in patients (e. g. [53]) does not affect this exchange [24]. Cl^- concurs with BPG for the same binding sites on Hb [54] but its affinity is lower and the small decrease of its concentration in CF is compensated for by increased [BPG].

Oxygen Dissociation Curves

The P_{50}st values of controls scatter around the normal mean value (approximately 27 mmHg) without significant sex differences. The generally higher P_{50}st in patients results from the increased [BPG] (change approx. 0.6 mmHg per µmole BPG/gHb according to [55]) while ATP plays only a minor role because of complexing with Mg^{++}. This corresponds to the typical chronic hypoxic reaction of most humans. It allows to extract more oxygen in the tissue capillaries without lowering the diffusion pressure, but it is not helpful for oxygen loading in pulmonary capillaries. In highlanders with similar reduction of arterial SO_2 P_{50}st scatters around 30 mmHg [30]. In both healthy subjects and patients the reaction (affinity change, increased ventilation and partly stimulated erythropoesis) is a sufficient compensation of moderate hypoxia at rest but maximal performance capacity is reduced. The left shift of the ODC in moles [15] living and working under comparable conditions (inspiring air with reduced O_2 and increased CO_2 content) as the patients is more reasonable but is rare in humans. Under extreme acute conditions (above 6000 m of altitude) healthy mountaineers lower their P_{50} by extreme hyperventilation [56] which is not a sustainable option for CF-

Table 5. Blood gases, acid-base status and P_{50} of patients at maximal exercise.

	n	Powermax	PO_{2art}	SO_{2art}	PCO_{2art}	pH_{art}	[Lactate]	P_{50}
		Watt/kg	mmHg	%	mmHg		mmol/l	mmHg
Patients male	7	2.2±0.3	58.9±5.4	80.1±3.1	48.3±4.0	7.240±0.018	7.9±1.1	33.1±0.9
Patients female	5	1.8±0.1	55.6±2.1	82.6±4.0	51.2±3.6	7.227±0.031	8.8±0.6	33.7±0.9

Means ± SE. Measurements in ear lobe blood. P_{50} for actual pH. All differences to rest significant for all patients as well as subgroups except SO_2 for subgroup patients female ($P<0.054$).

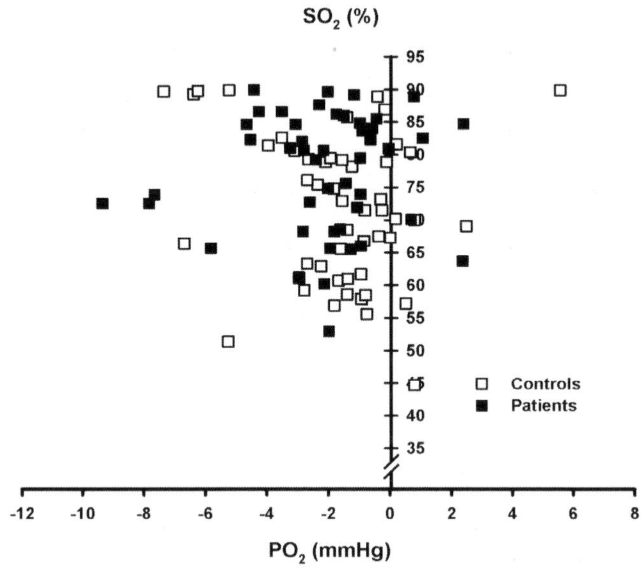

Figure 5. Deviation of in vivo PO_2 corrected to pH 7.4 from the corresponding individual standard ODC between 40 and 90% in controls and patients.

patients. For chronic acclimatization a reduction of [BPG] would be more appropriate. Surprisingly the male patient with the G551D mutation showed such an effect. One can estimate that a reduction of P_{50}st like in his blood would raise the arterial SO_2 at exhaustion in the male patients by 4%.

Interestingly in the 3 papers with P_{50}st measurements in CF patients single low P_{50}st values between 23.5 and 25.5 mmHg can be found [18,19,23]. This points to a special form of hypoxia acclimatization in some patients similar to that in moles.

The magnitude of a change in P_{50}st may reflect further compensating mechanisms. Rosenthal et al [18] showed that P_{50}st is negatively correlated with systemic oxygen delivery which depends on arterial SO_2, [Hb] and cardiac output. This means that low [Hb] or cardiac output favor a rise of P_{50}st. Indeed Arturson [57] described a P_{50}st increase with falling [Hb] in chronic pulmonary insufficiency. The present CF patients were not anemic. This might also explain why we observed a small tendency rather than a substantial change in P_{50}st.

Hill's n did not deviate much from the usually expected value of 2.7 for HbA (e.g. [55]). BPG binds to Deoxy-Hb only which may therefore increase Hill's n with rising concentration. A sligtly higher n in highlanders [30] and anemic patients [58] might be explained by this mechanism. However, the [BPG] differences between controls and patients in this study are too small to cause measurable effects.

Bohr Effect and Exercise

Similar like in altitude inhabitants [30,31] the Bohr coefficients are little changed in patients with cystic fibrosis. The coefficients for CO_2 correspond to published values [27,28,33]. They are large (numerically) at low saturation because of oxygenation dependent binding of carbamate in addition to H^+ effects during acidification with CO_2. They are lower at very high saturation; the Bohr effect disappears when all Hb molecules are in the R (relaxed) state. Anions (Cl^-, La^- and BPG) compete with CO_2 at the terminal valines (e. g. [25]). Therefore $BCCO_2$ increases at low [BPG]; this might be the cause for the rather high value in the patient with mutation G 551D. The fixed acid Bohr coefficients are small especially at low saturation compared to $BCCO_2$. The slight unexplained influence of CF on BCLa plays only a very modest role, because the peak lactic acid concentration during exercise is rather low in the patients (Table 5) compared to healthy subjects (e. g. [59]). In the lungs the Bohr effect of CO_2 is helpful for oxygen loading, when CO_2 leaves the blood, especially during hyperventilation with resulting hypocapnia during heavy exercise. In the patients with exercise hypercapnia and mostly high P_{50}st, however, an increase of $BCCO_2$ would be detrimental in this situation.

In vivo Effects

The left shift of the in vivo PO_2/SO_2 pairs relative to the in vitro standard ODCs is on an average modest (approx. 2 mmHg) but 17 differences amount to more than 4 mmHg. Differences in ODCs as well as BCs between fresh blood immediately after sampling and blood after equilibration in tonometers have occasionally been observed (e. g. [38,60]). Concentration changes of BPG, ATP, Cl^-, nitrocompounds or glutathione are possible causes. The means of [BPG] and [ATP] increase slightly but not significantly after equilibration compared to fresh venous samples explaining only 0.7 mmHg of the difference at 50% SO_2. Intraerythrocytic [Cl^-] changes are larger for a given ΔpH in vivo than in vitro resulting from exchange with the interstitial fluid [59]. Because of the opposite effects of SNO-Hb and Hb[FENO] on oxygen affinity [61] NO usually exerts no measurable influence on the ODC neither in vitro nor in vivo if no methemoglobin is formed [62–65]. In our experiments MetHb was stable. For an allosteric effect intraerythrocytic [NO] is by far too low even in Tibetans who present very high values [66]. In contrast to NO glutathione is present in millimolar concentrations in the red cells [67] and binds to oxy-Hb thus shifting the curve to the left and reducing the Bohr effect [26,68]. But a marked deficiency of extra- and intracellular glutathione possibly including erythrocytes in CF patients has been suggested [69] which might be related to the disturbed function of CFTR as glutathione transporter [52]. Very recently also an effect of glutamate on P50 was observed [70]; this substance binds to Ca^{++} channel proteins in the cell membrane and may be interchanged with muscle fibres. Thus at the moment a clear cause for the in vivo – in vitro difference of PO_2 remains unknown, but apparently it rises with SO_2. This produces a left shift of the in vivo ODC between 50 and 90% SO_2, which is an advantage for oxygen loading. Recently similar results were found at 3600 m of altitude [13,14]. Interestingly at low saturations "standardized" in vivo PO_2/SO_2 pairs tend to lie right of the in vitro curve, especially in venous blood returning from exercising muscles [36–38,55,60]. The result of this opposite changes is a markedly steepened complete in vivo oxygen dissociation curve probably in healthy subjects as well as in CF patients. Such a property is favorable for both loading and unloading of O_2 in lungs and consuming tissues.

Conclusions

The majority of the patients with cystic fibrosis in our study react to the problem of pulmonary oxygen uptake like man at altitude with a small right shift of the in vitro ODC caused by increased organic phosphate concentrations in the red cells. This improves oxygen diffusion into the consuming tissues, but is a drawback for arterialization. Healthy subjects can compensate this by hyperventilation thus reducing arterial PCO_2 with resulting left shift of the ODC during oxygenation. This is not possible for CF patients especially when CO_2 production is increased during exercise. A probably more appropriate left shift by reduction of [BPG] was observed in one patient with the G551D mutation. Also in other papers occasional left shifts can be detected. Whether this is a genetic effect, remains an intriguing question. The slope of the in vitro ODC and the Bohr coefficients were not markedly affected by the disease. Under in vivo conditions, there is a tendency for a left shift of the upper part of the ODC in both healthy controls and patients pointing to unknown affinity modifying factors which improve oxygen loading in the lungs.

Acknowledgments

The authors thank all subjects for their willing cooperation and B. Himmelsbach-Wegner for technical assistance.

Author Contributions

Conceived and designed the experiments: DB MH RB DS. Performed the experiments: AL MH RB. Analyzed the data: DB AL MH RB DS. Wrote the paper: DB AL MH RB DS. Designed the methods used for measurement and evaluation of oxygen dissociation curves: DB MH.

References

1. Cohen TS, Prince A (2012) Cystic fibrosis: a mucosal immunodeficiency syndrome. Nat Med 18: 509–519.
2. Zielenski J (2000) Genotype and phenotype in cystic fibrosis. Respiration 67: 117–133.
3. Derichs N (2013) Targeting a genetic defect: cystic fibrosis transmembrane conductance regulator modulators in cystic fibrosis. Eur Respir Rev 22: 58–65.
4. Baumann R, Bartels H, Bauer C (1987) Blood oxygen transport. In: Fishman AP, Cherniak NS, Widdicombe JG, Geiger SR, editors. Handbook of Physiology Sect. 3. Washington DC: Am. Physiol. Soc. 147–172.
5. Samaja M, Crespi T, Guazzi M, Vandegriff KD (2003) Oxygen transport in blood at high altitude: role of the hemoglobin-oxygen affinity and impact of the phenomena related to hemoglobin allosterism and red cell function. Eur J Appl Physiol 90: 351–359.
6. Weber RE (2007) High-altitude adaptations in vertebrate hemoglobins. Respir Physiol Neurobiol 158: 132–142.
7. Storz JF, Moriyama H (2008) Mechanisms of hemoglobin adaptation to high altitude hypoxia. High Alt Med Biol 9: 148–157.
8. Winslow RM (2007) The role of hemoglobin oxygen affinity in oxygen transport at high altitude. Respir Physiol Neurobiol 158: 121–127.
9. Morpurgo G, Arese P, Bosia A, Pescarmona GP, Luzzana M, et al. (1976) Sherpas living permanently at high altitude: a new pattern of adaptation. Proc Nat Acad Sci USA 73: 747–751.
10. Beall CM, Decker MJ, Brittenham GM, Kushner I, Gebremedhin A, et al. (2002) An Ethiopian pattern of human adaptation to high-altitude hypoxia. Proc Natl Acad Sci U S A 99: 17215–17218.
11. Beall CM (2007) Two routes to functional adaptation: Tibetan and Andean high-altitude natives. Proc Natl Acad Sci U S A 104 Suppl 1: 8655–8660.
12. Jürgens KD, Pietschmann M, Yamaguchi K, Kleinschmidt T (1988) Oxygen binding properties, capillary densities and heart weights in high altitude camelids. J Comp Physiol B 158: 469–477.
13. Balaban DY, Duffin J, Preiss D, Mardimae A, Vesely A, et al. (2013) The in-vivo oxyhaemoglobin dissociation curve at sea level and high altitude. Respir Physiol Neurobiol 186: 45–52.
14. Böning D, Pries AR (2013) Unknown in vivo factors influencing the oxygen dissociation curve? Respir Physiol Neurobiol 188: 79–80.
15. Campbell KL, Storz JF, Signore AV, Moriyama H, Catania KC, et al. (2010) Molecular basis of a novel adaptation to hypoxic-hypercapnia in a strictly fossorial mole. BMC Evol Biol 10: 214.
16. Huckauf H, Schäfer JH, Kollo D (1976) Oxygen affinity of haemoglobin and red cell acid-base status in patients with severe chronic obstructive lung disease. Bull Europ Physiopath Resp 12: 129–142.
17. Morgan TJ (1999) The oxyhaemoglobin dissociation curve in critical illness. Crit Care Resusc 1: 93–100.
18. Rosenthal A, Khaw KT, Shwachman H (1977) Hemoglobin-oxygen equilibrium in cystic fibrosis. Pediatrics 59: 919–926.
19. Christoforou E, Papassotiriou I, Skarmoutsou C, Doudounakis S, Stamoulakatou A, et al. (2005) Soluble transferrin receptors and tissue oxygenation in non-anaemic cystic fibrosis patients. J Cyst Fibros 4: 151–156.
20. Vichinsky EP, Pennathur-Das R, Nickerson B, Minor M, Kleman K, et al. (1984) Inadequate erythroid response to hypoxia in cystic fibrosis. J Pediatr 105: 15–21.
21. Rosenthal A, Button LN, Khaw KT (1977) Blood volume changes in patients with cystic fibrosis. Pediatrics 59: 588–594.

22. Wagener JS, McNeill GC, Taussig LM, Corrigan JJ, Lemen R (1983) Ferrokinetic and hematologic studies in cystic fibrosis patients. Am J Pediatr Hematol Oncol 5: 153–160.
23. Orzalesi MM, Motoyama EK (1973) Blood oxygen affinity in children with cystic fibrosis. Am Rev Respir Dis 107: 928–931.
24. Berghout AG, Bender SW (1984) Anion transport and 2,3-diphosphoglycerate in cystic fibrosis red blood cells. Pediatr Res 18: 1017–1020.
25. Böning D, Schünemann HJ, Maassen N, Busse MW (1993) Reduction of oxylabile CO_2 in human blood by lactate. J Appl Physiol 74: 710–714.
26. Craescu CT, Poyart C, Schaeffer C, Garel MC, Kister J, et al. (1986) Covalent binding of glutathione to hemoglobin. II. Functional consequences and structural changes reflected in NMR spectra. J Biol Chem 261 (31): 14710–14716.
27. Garby L, Robert M, Zaar B (1972) Proton- and carbamino-linked oxygen affinity of normal human blood. Acta Physiol Scand 84: 482–492.
28. Meier U, Böning D, Rubenstein HJ (1974) Oxygenation dependent variations of the Bohr coefficient related to whole blood and erythrocyte pH. Pflügers Arch 349: 203–213.
29. Schmidt W, Böning D, Braumann KM (1987) Red cell age effects on metabolism and oxygen affinity in humans. Respir Physiol 68: 215–225.
30. Schmidt W, Dahners HW, Correa R, Ramirez R, Rojas J, et al. (1990) Blood gas transport properties in endurance-trained athletes living at different altitudes. Int J Sports Medicine 11: 15–21.
31. Morpurgo G, Battaglia P, Bernini L (1970) Higher Bohr effect in Indian natives of Peruvian Highlands as compared with Europeans. Nature (Lond) 227: 387–388.
32. Humpeler E, Vogel S (1977) Oxygen affinity of hemoglobin in postmenopausal women. Pflügers Arch 372: 287–290.
33. Böning D, Draude W, Trost F, Meier U (1978) Interrelation between Bohr and temperature effects on the oxygen dissociation curve in men and women. Respir Physiol 34: 195–207.
34. Humpeler E, Amor H (1973) Sex differences in the oxygen affinity of hemoglobin. Pflügers Arch 343: 151–156.
35. Morse M, Cassels DE, Holder M, O'Connell E, Swanson A (1950) The position of the oxygen dissociation curve of the blood in normal children and adults. J Clin Invest 29: 1091–1097.
36. Rasmussen B, Klausen K, Clausen JP, Trap-Jensen J (1975) Pulmonary ventilation, blood gases and blood pH after training of the arms or the legs. J Appl Physiol 38: 250–256.
37. Sproule BJ, Mitchell JH, Miller WF (1960) Cardiopulmonary physiological responses to heavy exercise in patients with anemia. J Clin Invest 39: 378–388.
38. Böning D, Schweigart U, Tibes U, Hemmer B (1975) Influences of exercise and endurance training on the oxygen dissociation curve of blood unter in vivo and in vitro conditions. Eur J Appl Physiol 34: 1–10.
39. Barrett PM, Alagely A, Topol EJ (2012) Cystic fibrosis in an era of genomically guided therapy. Hum Mol Genet 21: R66-R71.
40. Quanjer PH, Tammeling GJ, Cotes JE, Fabbri LM, Matthys H, et al. (1993) Symbols, abbreviations and units. Working Party Standardization of Lung Function Tests, European Community for Steel and Coal. Eur Respir J Suppl 16: 85–100.
41. Hughes JM (1996) Blood gas estimations from arterialized capillary blood versus arterial puncture: are they different? Eur Respir J 9: 184–185.
42. Ben Rayana MC, Burnett RW, Covington AK, D'Orazio P, Fogh-Andersen N, et al. (2008) IFCC guideline for sampling, measuring and reporting ionized magnesium in plasma. Clin Chem Lab Med 46: 21–26.
43. Böning D, Tibes U, Schweigart U (1976) Red cell hemoglobin, hydrogen ion and electrolyte concentrations during exercise in trained and untrained subjects. Eur J Appl Physiol 35: 243–249.
44. Diem K, Lentner C (1969) Wissenschaftliche Tabellen. Geigy, AG, Basel.
45. Uhle MJ (2004) Zur Nutzbarkeit ventilatorischer Messverfahren in der Diagnostik der submaximalen Leistungsfähigkeit bei Patienten mit Zystischer Fibrose (About the usability of ventilatory measuring methods in diagnosis of submaximal exercise performance capacity in patients with cystic fibrosis) [dissertation]. Charité - Universitätsmedizin Berlin.
46. Böning D, Rojas J, Serrato M, Ulloa C, Coy L, et al. (2001) Hemoglobin mass and peak oxygen uptake in untrained and trained residents of moderate altitude. Int J Sports Med 22: 572–578.
47. Cristancho E, Reyes O, Serrato M, Mora MM, Rojas JA, et al. (2007) Arterial oxygen saturation and hemoglobin mass in postmenopausal untrained and trained altitude residents. High Alt Med Biol 8: 296–306.
48. Böning D, Rojas J, Serrato M, Reyes O, Coy L, et al. (2008) Extracellular pH defense against lactic acid in untrained and trained altitude residents. Eur J Appl Physiol 103: 127–137.
49. O'Connor TM, McGrath DS, Short C, O'Donnell MJ, Sheehy M, et al. (2002) Subclinical anaemia of chronic disease in adult patients with cystic fibrosis. J Cyst Fibros 1: 31–34.
50. Fischer R, Simmerlein R, Huber RM, Schiffl H, Lang SM (2007) Lung disease severity, chronic inflammation, iron deficiency, and erythropoietin response in adults with cystic fibrosis. Pediatr Pulmonol 42: 1193–1197.
51. Watts KD, McColley SA (2011) Elevated vascular endothelial growth factor is correlated with elevated erythropoietin in stable, young cystic fibrosis patients. Pediatr Pulmonol 46: 683–687.
52. Duranton C, Rubera I, Cougnon M, Melis N, Chargui A, et al. (2012) CFTR is involved in the fine tuning of intracellular redox status: physiological implications in cystic fibrosis. Am J Pathol 181: 1367–1377.
53. Schillers H (2008) Imaging CFTR in its native environment. Pflügers Arch 456: 163–177.
54. Rollema HS, De Bruin SA, Janssen LHM, Van Os GAJ (1975) Effect of potassium chloride on Bohr effect of human hemoglobin. J Biol Chem 250: 1333–1339.
55. Braumann KM, Böning D, Trost F (1979) Oxygen dissociation curves in trained and untrained subjects. Eur J Appl Physiol 42: 51–60.
56. West JB, Schoene RB, Milledge JS (2007) High Altitude Medicine and Physiology. London: Hodder Arnold.
57. Arturson G (1971) Changes in blood oxygen affinity during anaemia and cardiac and pulmonary insufficiency. Acta Anaesth Scand 45: 39–44.
58. Böning D, Enciso G (1987) Hemoglobin-oxygen affinity in anemia. Blut 54: 361–368.
59. Böning D, Klarholz C, Himmelsbach B, Hütler M, Maassen N (2007) Causes of differences in exercise-induced changes of base excess and blood lactate. Eur J Appl Physiol 99: 163–171.
60. Braumann KM, Böning D, Trost F (1982) Bohr effect and slope of the oxygen dissociation curve after physical training. J Appl Physiol Respir Environ Exerc Physiol 52: 1524–1529.
61. Mairbäurl H, Weber RE (2013) Oxygen transport by hemoglobin. Compr Physiol 2 : 1463–1489.
62. Head CA, Brugnara C, Martinez-Ruiz R, Kacmarek RM, Bridges KR, et al. (1997) Low concentrations of nitric oxide increase oxygen affinity of sickle erythrocytes in vitro and in vivo. J Clin Invest 100: 1193–1198.
63. Hrinczenko BW, Alayash AI, Wink DA, Gladwin MT, Rodgers GP, et al. (2000) Effect of nitric oxide and nitric oxide donors on red blood cell oxygen transport. Br J Haematol 110: 412–419.
64. von Pickardt B (2003) Wirkung NO-freisetzender Verbindungen auf die Sauerstoffbindungskurve (Effect of NO liberating substances on the oxygen dissociation curve) [dissertation]. Freie Universität Berlin.
65. Gladwin MT, Schechter AN, Shelhamer JH, Pannell LK, Conway DA, et al. (1999) Inhaled nitric oxide augments nitric oxide transport on sickle cell hemoglobin without affecting oxygen affinity. J Clin Invest 104: 937–945.
66. Erzurum SC, Ghosh S, Janocha AJ, Xu W, Bauer S, et al. (2007) Higher blood flow and circulating NO products offset high-altitude hypoxia among Tibetans. Proc Natl Acad Sci U S A 104: 17593–17598.
67. Hütler M, Pollmann C, Beneke R, Leithauser R, Böning D (2000) Measurable amount of glutathione in blood is influenced by oxygen saturation of hemoglobin. Clin Chim Acta 301: 213–217.
68. Smith JE, Lee M, Agar S, Du D (1976) Oxygen-hemoglobin equilibrium of normal and glutathione- deficient sheep. Am J Vet Res 37: 1135–1137.
69. Hudson VM (2001) Rethinking cystic fibrosis pathology: the critical role of abnormal reduced glutathione (GSH) transport caused by CFTR mutation. Free Radic Biol Med 30: 1440–1461.
70. Makhro A, Hanggi P, Goede JS, Wang J, Bruggemann A, et al. (2013) N-methyl-D-aspartate receptors in human erythroid precursor cells and in circulating red blood cells contribute to the intracellular calcium regulation. Am J Physiol Cell Physiol 305: C1123-C1138.
71. Christiansen TF (1981) An algorithm for calculating the concentration of the base excess of blood. In: Siggaard-Andersen O, editors. Proceedings of the IFCC Expert Panel on pH and blood gases held at Herved Hospital 1980. Copenhagen: Radiometer A/S. 77–81.

T Helper Cell Subsets Specific for *Pseudomonas aeruginosa* in Healthy Individuals and Patients with Cystic Fibrosis

Hannah K. Bayes[1], Stephen Bicknell[2], Gordon MacGregor[2], Tom J. Evans[1]*

1 Institute of Infection, Immunology and Inflammation, College of Medical, Veterinary and Life Sciences, University of Glasgow, Glasgow, United Kingdom, **2** West of Scotland Cystic Fibrosis Centre, Gartnavel General Hospital, Glasgow, United Kingdom

Abstract

Background: We set out to determine the magnitude of antigen-specific memory T helper cell responses to *Pseudomonas aeruginosa* in healthy humans and patients with cystic fibrosis.

Methods: Peripheral blood human memory $CD4^+$ T cells were co-cultured with dendritic cells that had been infected with different strains of *Pseudomonas aeruginosa*. The T helper response was determined by measuring proliferation, immunoassay of cytokine output, and immunostaining of intracellular cytokines.

Results: Healthy individuals and patients with cystic fibrosis had robust antigen-specific memory $CD4^+$ T cell responses to *Pseudomonas aeruginosa* that not only contained a Th1 and Th17 component but also Th22 cells. In contrast to previous descriptions of human Th22 cells, these Pseudomonal-specific Th22 cells lacked the skin homing markers CCR4 or CCR10, although were $CCR6^+$. Healthy individuals and patients with cystic fibrosis had similar levels of Th22 cells, but the patient group had significantly fewer Th17 cells in peripheral blood.

Conclusions: Th22 cells specific to *Pseudomonas aeruginosa* are induced in both healthy individuals and patients with cystic fibrosis. Along with Th17 cells, they may play an important role in the pulmonary response to this microbe in patients with cystic fibrosis and other conditions.

Editor: Dominik Hartl, University of Tübingen, Germany

Funding: The work was funded by the Wellcome Trust through the award of a Clinical Research Fellowship to HB under the Scottish Translational Medicine and Therapeutics Initiative. The funders had no role in study design, data collection and analysis, decision to publish, or preparation of the manuscript

Competing Interests: The authors have declared that no competing interests exist.

* E-mail: tom.evans@glasgow.ac.uk

Introduction

Cystic fibrosis (CF) typically results in recurrent pulmonary infections and inflammation that produces progressive respiratory failure [1,2]. The most common pathogen in these patients is *Pseudomonas aeruginosa* (PA), which produces a neutrophil dominated host response that does not, however, clear the infection [3]. Indeed, this persistent inflammatory response contributes to progressive lung injury [4,5] and thus pulmonary immune responses to *P. aeruginosa* are a potential therapeutic target.

Colonization with this bacterium results in an antibody response, which is not, however, protective [6]. In contrast, cell-mediated immunity to *P. aeruginosa* is important in host defence [7]. Recently, attention has focused on the novel T helper 17 (Th17) subset of Th cells [8]. These produce the signature cytokine IL-17 that plays a critical role in the generation and recruitment of neutrophils to sites of infection. In experimental murine models of acute pulmonary *P. aeruginosa* infection, there is evidence that Th17 cells play a key role in vaccine-induced protection [9]. Human studies have shown IL-17 is produced in CF lung, and that Th17 cells are present in the submucosa of airways from CF patients, although IL-17 is also produced from innate immune cells [10,11]. Humans typically have a very strong Th17 memory response to *Candida albicans* as well as *Staphylococcus aureus* [12,13]. However, it is not known whether there are similar memory responses to PA or whether these are altered in patients with CF.

IL-17 is commonly co-expressed with IL-22 in classic Th17 cells. IL-22 is a cytokine of the IL-10 family that has important effects on non-immune cells, promoting repair of epithelial surfaces and inducing an anti-microbial state [14]. More recently, a distinct lineage of Th cells producing IL-22 in the absence of IL-17 has been discovered, termed Th22 cells [15–18]. These cells have been found to possess a skin homing phenotype and infiltrate the skin in inflammatory disorders such as psoriasis in which IL-22 has been proposed to play a pathogenic role. In contrast, IL-22 also induces a variety of antimicrobial peptides and is important in host defence against pulmonary pathogens such as *Klebsiella pneumonia* [19]. Additionally, in a murine model of gut inflammation following infection with *Citrobacter rodentium*, IL-22 plays an important role in host defence [20,21]. In this model, IL-22 is produced both by innate lymphoid cells as well as Th22 cells [18]. IL-22 is also required to prevent dissemination of the commensal enteric bacteria from the genus *Alcaligenes* [22]. As yet, no specific pathogen or antigen has been demonstrated to elicit a human memory Th22 response.

Given that IL-22 promotes epithelial repair and induces an antimicrobial state, we hypothesised that Th22 cells could play an important role in host defence against lung infection with *P. aeruginosa* in CF and other clinical settings. Additionally, given the proposed role of Th17 cells in protection against PA infection, we hypothesized that PA-specific Th17 cells would be found in patients with CF. In order to test these hypotheses, we set out to examine the Th22, Th17 and Th1 cell responses to *P. aeruginosa* in both control and healthy individuals as well as patients with cystic fibrosis. We found that both healthy individuals as well as those with cystic fibrosis had robust antigen-specific Th17, Th1 and Th22 responses to *P. aeruginosa*. The PA-specific Th22 cells were $CCR6^+$ but lacked the skin-homing receptors CCR4 and CCR10 that have previously been found on human Th22 cells. PA-specific Th17 cells were reduced in patients with CF. These PA-specific Th cell subsets represent novel effector cells that can modulate the host anti-bacterial and inflammatory response to this pathogen and hence could be targets for novel therapeutic interventions in PA infection in CF and other conditions.

Materials and Methods

Ethics

All subjects gave informed written consent. The study was approved by West of Scotland Research Ethics Committee Number 2, a committee of the West of Scotland Research Ethics Service (WoSRES) that oversees ethical review of studies carried out on patients of the National Health Service Greater Glasgow and Clyde Health Board.

Participants and Cell Isolation

Peripheral blood samples were collected from adult CF patients attending the West of Scotland Adult CF Unit, Glasgow. Healthy individuals (controls) had no history of respiratory disease or intercurrent illness. Participant characteristics are shown in Table 1. Patients with CF attending the West of Scotland Adult CF Unit are deemed to be chronically colonized with *Pseudomonas aeruginosa* if sputum cultures remain positive for the organism after two attempts to clear the organism with combination antibiotic eradication therapy. Intermittent infection is deemed to exist when PA has been isolated and eradicated via antibiotic therapy.

PBMCs were obtained by Ficoll-Paque gradient centrifugation (GE Healthcare). $CD14^+$ monocytes were then magnetically isolated by a positive selection kit (Miltenyi Biotech). Memory $CD4^+$ T cells (purity for $CD4^+CD45RO^+$ >98%) were magnetically isolated by a negative selection kit (Miltenyi Biotech). Memory $CD4^+$ T cells were further sorted into CCR6-enriched and CCR6-depleted populations using positive selection microbeads (Stemcell Technologies). Proliferation was measured with CFSE (carboxyfluorescein diacetate succinimidyl ester; Invitrogen) or proliferation dye eFluor®450 (eBioscience) incorporated prior to cell culture.

Bacteriology

Laboratory *P. aeruginosa* (PA) strains PA103ΔpcrV and PA103-ΔUΔT [23,24] were kind gifts of Dr. Dara Frank, University of Wisconsin. Both strains have modulation of the function of the type three secretion system (T3SS), a common finding amongst CF PA strains; PA103ΔpcrV lacks the pore-forming protein of the T3SS rendering it non-functional and PA103ΔUΔT lacks the major translocation proteins (exoU and exoT) of the T3SS. Clinical non-mucoid PA strains Yorkhill 1 and Yorkhill 2, and clinical mucoid PA strain Yorkhill 5 were from CF samples (provided by Dr Craig Williams, Royal Hospital for Sick Children, Yorkhill). PA strains were grown to mid-log growth phase prior to infection.

Cell Culture

Dendritic cells (DCs) were derived from $CD14^+$ monocytes with IL-4 (500 IU/mL; Peprotech) and GM-CSF (50 ng/mL; Peprotech) for 7-days. DCs were infected with live PA strains as indicated. Ninety-minutes following infection, DCs were treated with bactericidal antibiotics (100 U/mL penicillin-streptomycin and 10 mg/mL gentamicin; both Sigma) followed by overnight incubation. Additionally, in some experiments, DCs were treated with tetanus toxoid (5 ug/mL; Calbiochem) or heat-killed preparation of Candida albicans (InvivoGen).

Infected DCs (1×10^4 cells) were cultured with autologous memory $CD4^+$ T cells (1×10^5 cells) in 96-well U-bottom plates in IMDM+Glutamax medium (Gibco Life Technologies) supplemented with 5% fetal bovine serum (Invitrogen) and 100 U/mL penicillin-streptomycin for 6-days. For polyclonal stimulation conditions, $CD4^+$ T cells were cultured with plate-bound anti-CD3 (5 ug/mL) and soluble anti-CD28 (1 ug/mL) (both eBioscience).

Measurement of $CD4^+$ T cell response

Following 6-days of co-culture, supernatants were harvested and cytokine levels measured via ELISA for IL-17A, IL-22, and IFN-γ (eBioscience).

Cell Staining and Analysis

Cells were stimulated for 5-hours with phorbol 12-myristate 13-acetate (50 ng/ml; Sigma) and ionomycin (500 ng/ml; Sigma) in

Table 1. Characteristics of participants providing peripheral blood specimens for the analysis of T helper cell responses to *Pseudomonas aeruginosa*.

	Patients with cystic fibrosis	Healthy controls
Participants (n)	8	10
Age, median (IQR), years	23 (23.5–30)	26 (24–29)
Male sex, n (%)	5 (62.5)	4 (40)
Chronic *Pseudomonas aeruginosa* colonization, n	7	na
FEV_1 median (IQR), % predicted	38.2 (35.2–44.4)	na
No. of patients with respiratory exacerbation at time of sample collection, n (%)	6 (75)	na

n, number in group; na, non-applicable; IQR, inter-quartile range; FEV_1, forced expiratory volume in 1 second.

the presence of Golgiplug (1 μl/ml; BD Pharmingen) at 37°C. Cells were fixed using 4% paraformaldehyde (VWR International) and made permeable, following extracellular staining, using Perm/Wash (BD Biosciences).

Extracellular staining was with phycoerythrin-labelled anti-CD4 (RPA-T4; eBioscience), phycoerythrin-labelled anti-αβTCR (IP26; eBioscience), phycoerythrin-Cy7-labelled anti-CCR4 (IGI; BD Pharminogen), AlexFluor®647-labelled anti-CCR9 (BL/CCR9; BioLegend), phycoerythrin-labelled anti-CCR10 (FAB 3478P; R&D), CD86 and CD40. Intracellular staining was with eFluor®660-labelled anti-IL-22 (22URTI; eBioscience), phycoerythrin-labelled anti-IL-22 (BG/IL-22; Biolegend), PerCP-Cy5.5-labelled anti-IFN-γ (4S.B3; eBioscience), and AlexFluor®488 anti-IL-17A (eBioDEC17; eBioscience). Corresponding isotype controls were used. Dead cell exclusion was achieved either by Boolean-gating based on cell scatter properties or labelling with Fixable Viability Dye eFluor®506 (eBioscience). Stained cells were analysed on either a FACSCalibur or CyAn flow cytometer (BD Biosciences). Collected data were analysed using FlowJo software (Tree Star).

Statistical analysis

Non-parametric statistical tests were used (Mann-Whitney, Kruskal-Wallis (KW), and, where appropriate, Dunn's multiple comparison test), using Prism Version 6.0 (GraphPad Software).

Results

Antigen-specific memory CD4$^+$ T cell responses exist against *P. aeruginosa* in Healthy Individuals

In order to examine antigen-dependent T cell memory responses from healthy controls and patients with CF, we isolated monocyte-derived dendritic cells (DCs) and CD4$^+$CD45RA$^-$C-D45RO$^+$ memory T cells from peripheral blood. Memory CD4$^+$ T cells were co-cultured with either uninfected DCs, DCs infected with PA, or the supernatant of such DCs, and the production of IL-17A, IL-22 and IFN-γ measured in the culture supernatant by ELISA (Figure 1).

Firstly, we examined the memory T cell responses of healthy controls. Small amounts of IL-17A were produced by T cells cultured with unstimulated DCs; this was abolished in the absence of DCs (Figure 1A). In the absence of DC infection, there was no significant production of either IL-22 (Figure 1B) or IFN-γ (Figure 1C). In contrast, co-culture of memory T cells with DCs infected with PA103 gave robust production of IL-17A, IL-22 and IFN-γ (Figure 1). This was almost completely abolished when T cells were cultured with infected DC supernatants alone (Figure 1); thus direct contact between T cells and DCs is required for cytokine production. No cytokines were produced when T cells were infected directly in the absence of DCs or when infected DCs were cultured alone in the absence of T cells (data not shown). Thus, the observed memory Th cell responses in healthy individuals were entirely dependent on physical contact between the DCs and T cells, as expected of an antigen-driven response. Cytokine production did not vary significantly following co-culture of memory T cells with DCs infected at multiplicities of infection (MOIs) between 10–60 (Figure 1D–F), suggesting even at the lowest MOI used the stimulating effect on memory T cells was already maximal.

Next, we compared this cytokine production by memory CD4$^+$ T cells in healthy individuals against different strains of PA. Similar levels of these three cytokines were produced following infection of DCs with strains of PA103 that differed in the possession of a functional type III apparatus (Figure S1). Additionally, these cytokine levels did not vary significantly between these laboratory strains and the response to PA strains isolated from patients with CF (Figure S1).

We then examined the proliferation of memory CD4$^+$ T cells of healthy individuals following co-culture with DCs alone or DCs infected with PA, using a flow cytometric method. As expected, little proliferation was seen with T cells cultured with uninfected DCs (Figure 2A). However, marked proliferation of CD4$^+$ T cell was seen in response to DCs infected with either laboratory PA103ΔUΔT (average proliferation [+/−SEM] 18.8% [+/−9.0%] for three donors) and clinical Yorkhill 5 (average proliferation [+/−SEM] 35.1% [+/−5.2%] for three donors) PA strains (Figure 2A). We also stained these cells for the presence of intracellular cytokines to determine which cells were producing the measured cytokines. IL-17 and IL-22 production in the co-cultures was predominantly by cells proliferating in response to PA (Figure 2B and C). Proliferating cells producing intracellular IL-17 and/or IL-22 were also confirmed to be αβ T cell receptor positive cells (data not shown). No intracellular cytokines were produced in DCs. Small amounts of intracellular IFN-γ were expressed by the non-proliferating CD4$^+$ memory cells following polyclonal stimulation; however, IFN-γ was only secreted from memory CD4$^+$ T cells in response to PA infected DCs (Figure 1). Collectively, these data show the existence of a classical antigen-specific memory CD4$^+$ T cell response to *P. aeruginosa* in healthy individuals with no previous history of pulmonary infection with this organism.

DC Activation following Infection with *P. aeruginosa*

To explore potential differential effects of the different PA strains on DC activation, we stained DCs for the activation markers CD86 and CD40 following infection with the different PA strains (Figure 3). Figure 3A shows representative plots of flow cytometric analysis of CD86 and CD 40 on the surface of DCs following infection with PA103ΔUΔT and Yorkhill 1 strains of PA as well as exposure to heat killed *Candida albicans*. These examples all show a marked upregulation of these activation markers on the surface of DCs. This was quantified for both CD86 and CD40 for a range of strains as shown in Figure 3B and 3C respectively. All strains tested produced an increase in expression of these markers. There was a trend towards slightly higher levels of expression in DCs infected with the PA103 strains, but this did not reach statistical significance.

Cytokine secretion by *P. aeruginosa*-specific CD4$^+$ T cells in patients with CF and controls

We then examined the cytokine responses of peripheral memory T cells in response to PA infected DCs in patients with CF compared to healthy individuals. All CF patients had a history of chronic or intermittent PA infection (Table 1). As seen in the experiments with T cells from healthy control individuals, memory CD4$^+$ T cells from patients with CF produce significant amounts of IL-17A, IL-22 and IFN-γ in response to DC infection with either laboratory or clinical PA strains compared with uninfected DCs (Figure 4A, B and C). However, the magnitude of this response between patients with CF with a history of *P. aeruginosa* infection and healthy controls was not significantly different for all three of the cytokines measured ($p>0.05$ for all strains, Kruskal Wallis).

P. aeruginosa-specific Th22, Th17 and Th1 responses in patients with CF and controls

Further to assess the Th cell subsets constituting the memory CD4$^+$ T cell response to PA, we used polyclonal re-stimulation

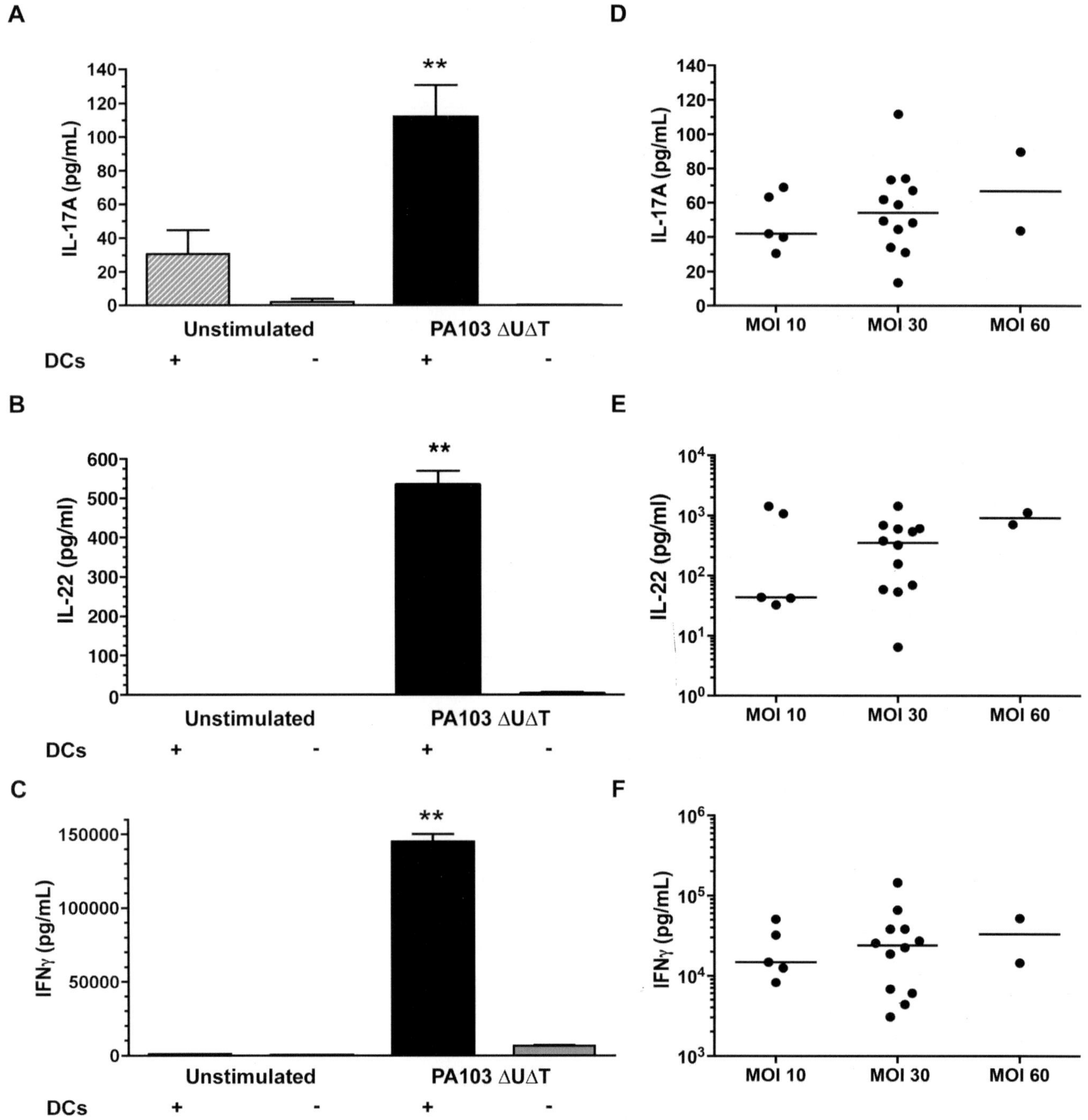

Figure 1. Cytokine production of human memory CD4$^+$ T cells in response to *P. aeruginosa*. A–C Sorted human memory CD4$^+$ T cells from healthy volunteers were co-cultured either with dendritic cells that had been infected with *P. aeruginosa* (DCs +) or with the supernatant from such infected DCs (DC −). Levels of IL-17A (**A**), IL-22 (**B**) and IFN-γ (**C**) were measured in supernatants after 6 days. DCs were infected at a MOI of 60 before culturing with T cells. Columns show the mean of triplicate determinations; error bars are ±1 standard error of mean. Results are representative of experiments in three separate individuals. **D–F**, secreted cytokine levels following DC infection at a variety of different MOIs. Each point represents a value from an individual healthy individual.

and intracellular staining of the resultant CD4$^+$ T cell populations present at the end of the co-cultures followed by flow cytometric analysis. Th1 cells are characterized by their production of IFN-γ on antigen stimulation. In humans, Th1 cells can co-produce IL-17 and IL-22, which was indeed initially classed as a Th1 cytokine [25]. To provide an unambiguous classification of the different cytokine producing cells, we adopted the following definitions. CD4$^+$ T cells expressing IFN-γ were designated as Th1 cells; Th17 cells were any IFN-γ negative cell producing IL-17A with/without IL-22; and Th22 cells were defined as those expressing IL-22 alone (Figure 5A). We used this gating strategy to quantify the proportions of memory CD4$^+$ T cells in each of these categories following stimulation with PA-infected DCs.

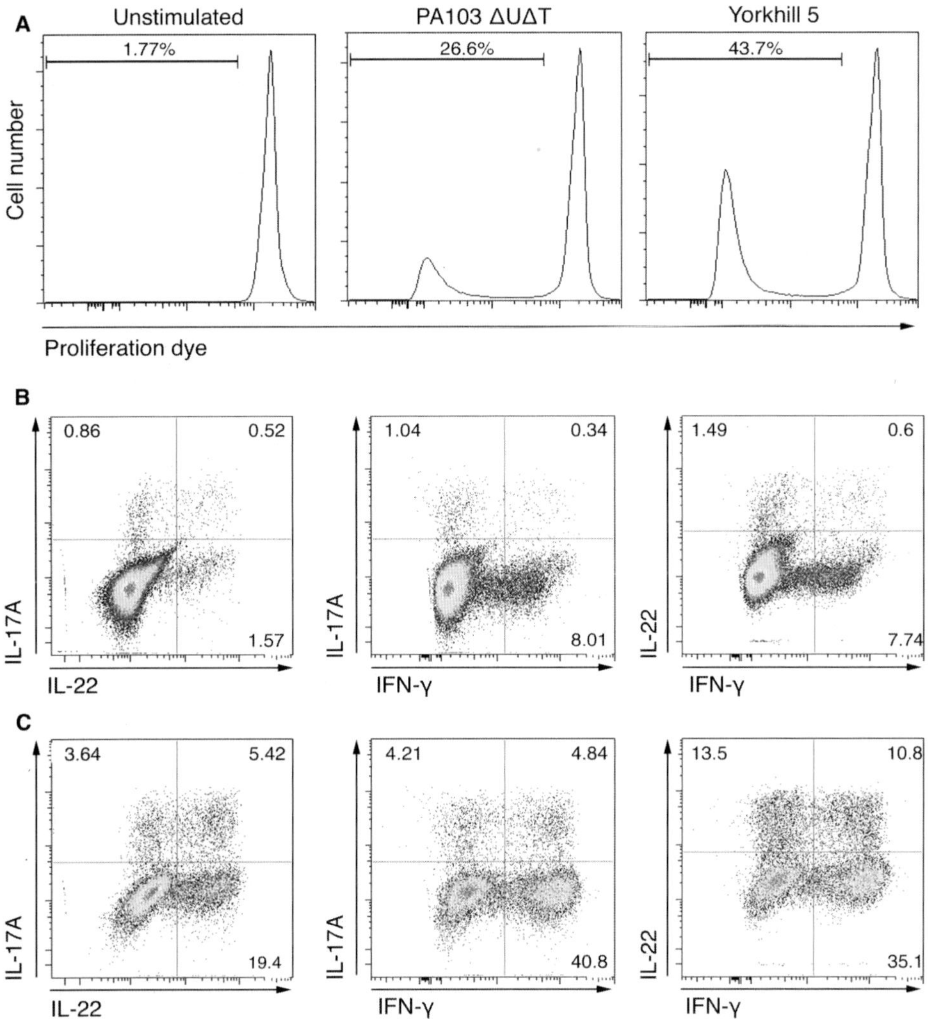

Figure 2. Cell proliferation of memory CD4$^+$ T cells following co-culture with infected dendritic cells (DCs). (**A**) Memory CD4$^+$ T cells loaded with proliferation dye were co-cultured with unstimulated DCs, DCs infected with PA103ΔUΔT MOI 30 (PA103), or DCs infected with Yorkhill 5 MOI 30 (Yorkhill 5). Panels show the distribution of the proliferation dye fluorescence in the cell population after 6-days; inset figures show the percentage of the initial population that has undergone one or more cell divisions. (**B**) Patterns of cytokine expression by non-proliferating CD4$^+$ T cells following 6-days of culture with DCs infected with Yorkhill 5. (**C**) Patterns of cytokine expression by CD4$^+$ T cells proliferating in response to culture with DCs infected with Yorkhill 5. Numbers in plot represent per cent cells in each quadrant. The experiment was repeated in 3 independent individuals with the same result.

In healthy controls (Figure 5B) and patients with CF (Figure 5C) the predominant responding population was a memory Th1 response. Within the population of IFN-γ positive cells proliferating in response to PA infected DCs, there were cells that that co-produced IL-17 and/or IL-22 (Figure 2C). Significantly, however, there were clear populations of Th22 and Th17 cells, as defined above, i.e. IFN-γ^- IL-17$^-$ IL-22$^+$ and IFN-γ^- IL-17$^+$ respectively (Figure 5). The proportion of Th1 and Th22 cells detected following co-culture with PA infected DCs was similar in healthy controls and patients with CF (see Figure S2). However, although the observed IL-17A cytokine response was of a similar magnitude (Figure 4A), there was a significantly lower proportion of Th17 cells in CF patients compared with healthy controls (Figure 5D). This was particularly evident in response to the clinical PA strains, where median percentage of Th17 cells was 5.3% in healthy controls compared with 1.04% in CF patients ($p = 0.003$).

These cytokine profiles were in distinct contrast to those obtained from memory CD4$^+$ T helper cells that were stimulated with either tetanus-toxoid treated DCs (Figure S3A, B) or heat-killed *Candida albicans* (Figure S3C, D). Tetanus-toxoid induced, as predicted, an essentially pure Th1 response. *Candida albicans*, as has been previously described [26], induced a robust Th17 response, although Th1 and Th22 cells were also evident.

Tissue-homing characteristics of-specific memory Th22 and Th17 cells

Human memory Th17 and Th22 cells characteristically express the mucosal chemokine receptor CCR6 [13,16,17]. To further verify the existence of memory Th17 and Th22 populations against PA, we sorted memory CD4$^+$ T cells on the basis of their CCR6 expression prior to culture with PA-infected DCs. This confirmed that virtually all IFN-γ negative CD4$^+$ T cell producing IL-17A and/or IL-22 (i.e. Th17 and Th22 cells) in response to PA infection were in the CCR6-enriched population (Figure 6A, B and C).

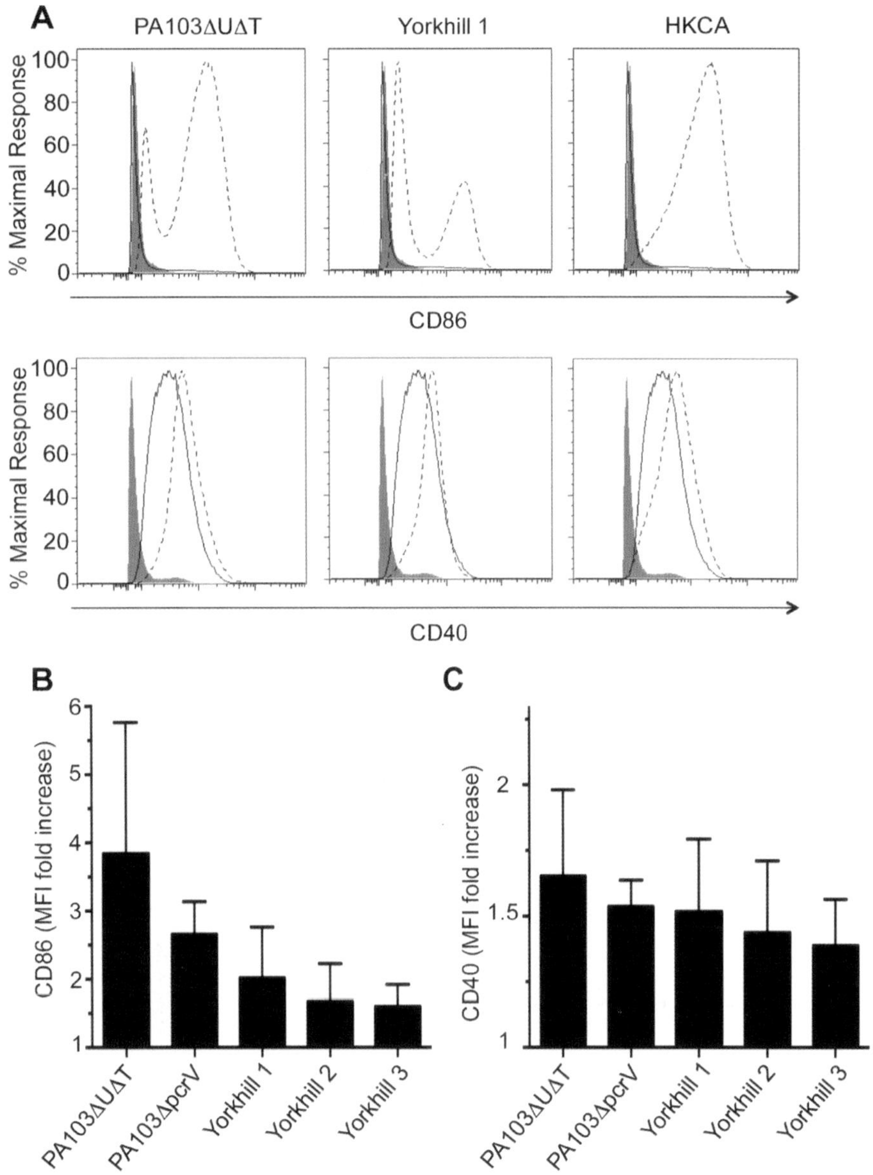

Figure 3. DC Activation following infection with different strains of *P. aeruginosa*. Levels of CD86 (**A**) and CD40 (**B**) following DC activation 24 hours following treatment with the indicated microbes. The panels show representative plots of isotype staining (solid shading), staining of unstimulated DCs (solid line) and staining following microbial treatment (dotted line). **B** and **C**, mean fold-increase in mean fluorescence intensity (MFI) of CD86 and CD40 respectively in 5 independent individuals. This was calculated as the fold-increase in MFI in infected DCs versus uninfected controls. Columns show mean and SEM.

We next addressed whether the PA-specific memory Th17 and Th22 populations demonstrated features of homing to specific tissues. Th22 cells have previously been found to demonstrate a skin-homing phenotype [13,16,17] and have been implicated in the pathogenesis of inflammatory skin conditions [15]. We thus analysed the PA-specific memory IL-22 secreting cell population for expression of the skin-homing receptors CCR4 and CCR10. In contrast to the reported properties of peripheral blood derived Th22 cells without a characterised antigen specificity [16,17], IL-22 production in response to PA infection was from memory $CD4^{+}$ T cells that did not express the skin-homing receptors CCR4 or CCR10 (Figure 6D). Additionally, we found that PA-specific IL-17A and IL-22 expressing memory T helper cells did not display the gut-homing receptor CCR9 (Figure 6D).

Discussion

The work described in this paper provides an important advance in our understanding of the human T helper response to *P. aeruginosa* and how this might influence the course of lung disease in individuals with CF who are chronically colonized with this microbe, as well as in other patients with PA infections. We found robust memory Th responses to *P. aeruginosa* in both normal individuals and in those with CF who have Pseudomonas colonization of the respiratory tract. These specific responses to *P. aeruginosa* contain Th1, Th17 and Th22 cells. This is the first time that an antigen-specific human Th22 response has been demonstrated. Moreover, these cells have a novel phenotype, lacking homing markers for skin and gut although retaining CCR6, which would allow them to respond to the ligands CCL20

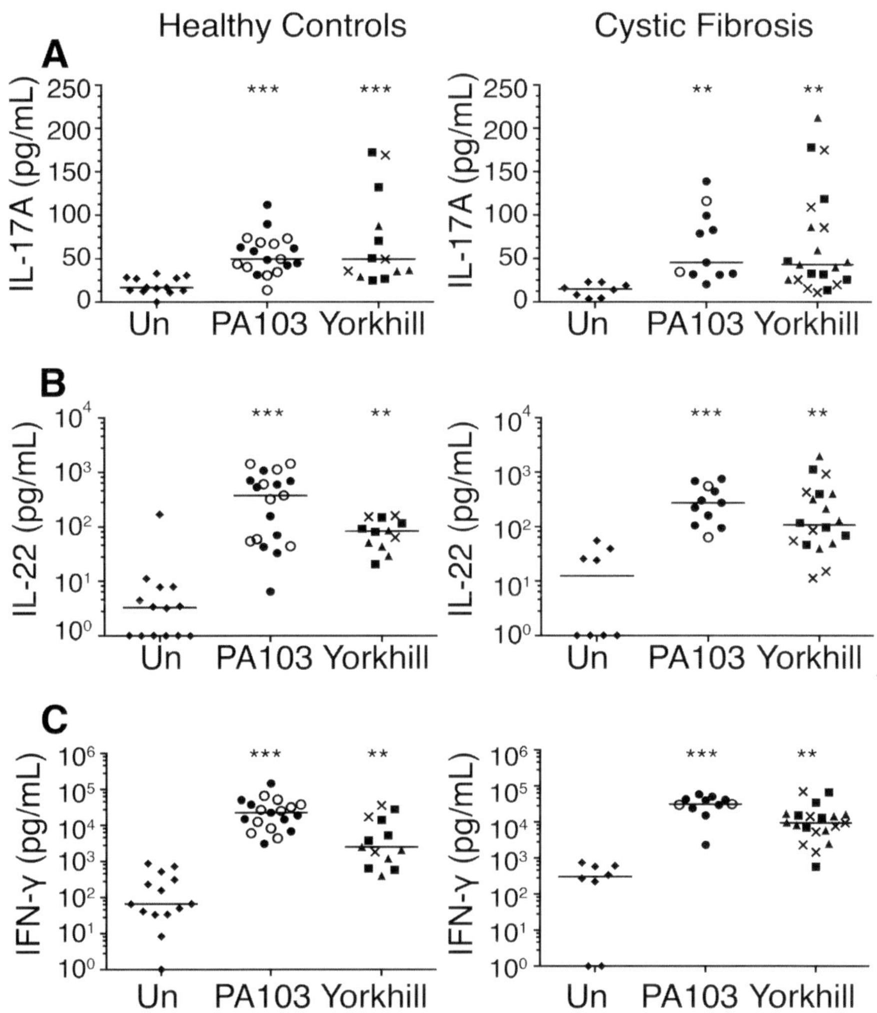

Figure 4. Cytokine production by human memory CD4⁺ T cells in healthy controls and cystic fibrosis. Human memory CD4⁺ T cells were exposed to unstimulated DCs or DCs infected with the laboratory strains (PA103) or clinical *Pseudomonas aeruginosa* strains (Yorkhill). After 6 days of co-culture levels of (**A**) IL-17, (**B**) IL-22 and (**C**) IFN-γ were measured. Each point represents the mean of triplicate wells and is the result from one individual. The different bacterial strains used are: ◆, unstimulated; ○, PA103 ΔpcrV; ●, PA103ΔUΔT; ▲, YH1; ■, YH2; ×, YH5. The line indicates the median value. Differences between infection conditions (**A–C**) were evaluated by a Kruskal-Wallis test all of which had p values <0.0009). Differences between unstimulated and infected conditions were then tested using Dunn's multiple comparison test. ** significant $p<0.01$ and *** significant $p<0.001$.

and β-defensins produced from damaged epithelia. We show that although Th22 and Th1 responses are similar in controls and patients with CF, the proportion of Th17 responding cells is significantly diminished in peripheral blood of patients with CF. Taken together, these data show that chronic airway colonization with *P. aeruginosa* could activate both Th17 and Th22 memory responses that would migrate to inflamed lung, and potentially alter the balance between inflammation, host defence and tissue repair.

The most striking finding of this study was the identification of Pseudomonal-specific Th22 cells in both healthy individuals and in those with CF. We were surprised that normal healthy controls had robust Th22 (and indeed Th1 and Th17) responses to *P. aeruginosa*, as it is generally only pathogenic in immunocompromised states. The microbe is found within the bowel flora of a minority of normal individuals, 4% in one report [27], so it would not seem likely that this is the source of bacteria to provoke a memory Th response. Indeed, the Pseudomonal-specific Th22 cells we identified did not have gut or skin homing receptors (Fig 6). Although *P. aeruginosa* is a common environmental organism, it remains unclear at what site this microbe triggers a memory T helper response. Others have also demonstrated cross-reactivity of Th17 cells against different bacterial serotypes and fungi [28,29]. We have not sought to define the antigenic component, of which there may be many, of *Pseudomonas aeruginosa* eliciting the observed Th17 and Th22 response, which might be shared with other infecting organisms and particularly with other Gram negative bacteria. The possibility of cross-reactivity of these Th cell responses remains, yet we have shown a lack of gut-homing and thus cross-reactivity with phylogenetically-related organisms in gut flora is unlikely.

In common with previous descriptions of Th22 cells in humans, the Pseudomonal-specific Th22 cells we identified were in the $CCR6^+$ population (Figure 6) [15–17]. Previous studies identified these cells as bearing skin-homing markers and a pathogenic role for these cells in psoriasis and other inflammatory skin disorders

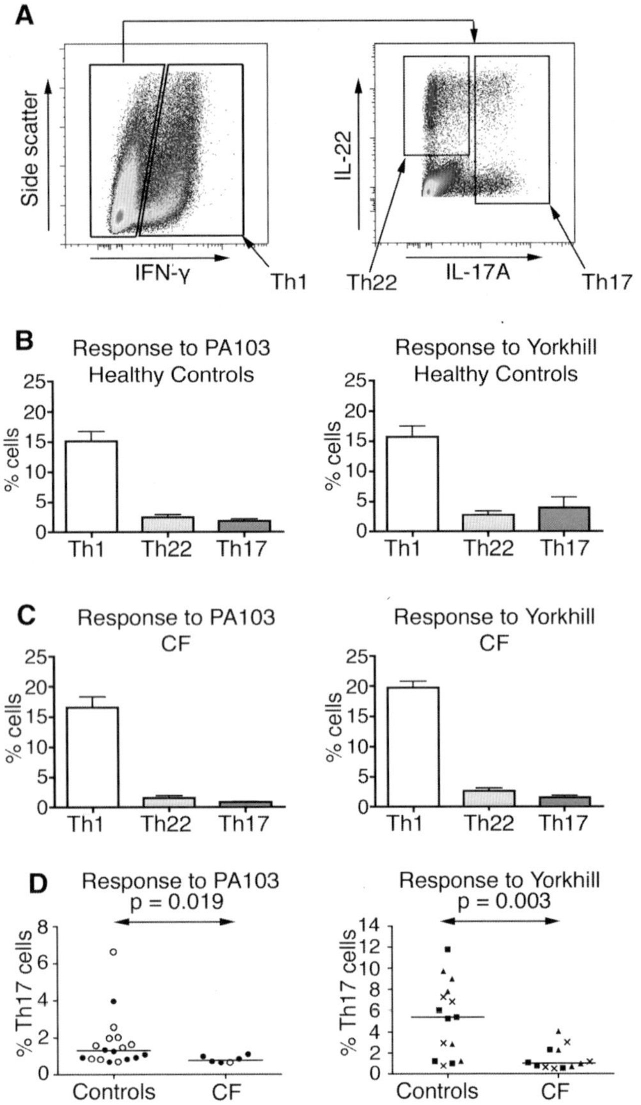

Figure 5. Memory CD4$^+$ T cells subset response to different Pseudomonas strains in CF and controls. Following co-culture with dendritic cells infected with laboratory Pseudomonas aeruginosa (PA) strains (PA103) or clinical PA strains (Yorkhill), CD4$^+$ T cells were classified into T helper cell subsets based on intracellular cytokine straining patterns, as shown for a representative patient in panel **A**. The Th1, Th17 and Th22 responses to both PA103 and Yorkhill PA strains is shown for healthy controls (**B**) and patients with CF (**C**), as a percentage of the total numbers of CD4$^+$ memory cells analysed. The columns show the mean values +/− SEM; n = 8 for CF patients and 10 for healthy controls. Panel **D** shows the proportions of PA-specific Th17 cells in CF patients compared with controls. Each point represents the result from one individual; different bacterial strains are indicated by the symbols as described in Figure 4. The line indicates the median value. Differences between controls and patients with CF (**D**) were evaluated by a Mann-Whitney test.

has been proposed. We propose that the pseudomonal-specific Th22 cells we have identified in healthy humans and patients with CF can migrate to inflamed lung, which will release the chemokines CCL20 and β-defensins, both ligands for CCR6. In relation to pulmonary recruitment, we have previously sought evidence of Th17 and Th22 recruitment within bronchoalveolar lavage (BAL) from CF patients, an approach that has significant technical limitations. We have, however, identified low level IL-22 production (IL-22 detectable in 5 of 14 CF patients, with median IL-22 levels of 12.39pg/mL) within the CF BAL and thus further implicating a potential Th22 response within the disease pathogenesis. Given its potent action in promoting epithelial repair, regulating fibrosis and mediating host defense [14,19,30], we believe that IL-22 is important in attenuating the effects of chronic pulmonary infection with *P. aeruginosa* and enhancing tissue repair. The action of IL-22 may well be modified by IL-17, as demonstrated in lung fibrosis [30]. Testing of this hypothesis will best be performed in an animal model of chronic *P. aeruginosa* lung infection. We found in general that IL-22 production in the T cell memory population was predominantly from Th22 cells more than Th17 cells (Figures 2 and 6). As outlined above, these cells would be able to migrate to inflamed tissue producing the CCR6 ligands CCL20 and β-defensins, both of which would be found in infected lung. The swift expansion of a PA-specific Th22 memory cell population would thus ensure a rapid production of an IL-22 producing cell that could migrate to the site of infection to mediate host defence and/or contribute to tissue repair.

A very recent study from Jay Kolls' group identified Pseudomonal-specific Th17 cells in the draining lymph nodes of patients with CF [31]. Intriguingly, we found a reduction in Pseudomonal-specific Th17 cells in peripheral blood of CF patients. These data suggest that this Th17 population translocates from blood to pulmonary system during the chronic pulmonary colonization with *P. aeruginosa*. Indeed, IL-17$^+$ T cells and IL-17 production has previously been observed within CF lung [10] and BAL [32], respectively. Alternatively, a recent study demonstrated that PA can induce myeloid-derived suppressor cells via flagellin stimulation [33]. These cells could act to down-regulate Th17 responses to PA, accounting for the observed reduction in PA-specific Th17 cells in CF patients.

Within the CF patient population exogenous and endogenous factors which may modulate immune function are common. For example, within our sampled CF population all patients were receiving long-term low-dose macrolide therapy and a quarter had CF-related diabetes mellitus. Nutritional status of CF patients will also be worse than age-matched controls. Controlling for such variables is problematic without a large sample size, which would be prohibitive for our described method of *ex vivo* T cell stimulation. We did however achieve adequate age matching of CF patients and controls, as well as ensuring that controls were healthy and free from conditions linked to pulmonary Th17 responses and pulmonary Pseudomonas infections, such as asthma and bronchiectasis. The data identifies and describes a previously uncharacterized Th cell response against *Pseudomonas aeruginosa* in both healthy controls and patients with CF, however generalizations to the whole heterogeneous CF population are preliminary at present.

Although this study has focussed on PA-specific Th cells in patients with cystic fibrosis, PA infections are significant in immunocompromised patients [34], in ventilator-associated pneumonia [35], following extensive burns and as a cause of infective exacerbations in patients with chronic obstructive airways disease [36]. Thus, the presence of Th22, Th17 and Th1 memory CD4$^+$ cells specific to PA may play a role in these situations as well. The balance of effects on host defence, tissue repair and systemic inflammation produced by Il-22 will likely differ between these different conditions, necessitating further experimental investigation to define the role of IL-22 and Th22 cells in each of these conditions.

In conclusion, our work has demonstrated the presence in peripheral blood of memory CD4$^+$ T cells of the Th22 lineage that are specific for *P. aeruginosa* antigens. They lack conventional skin

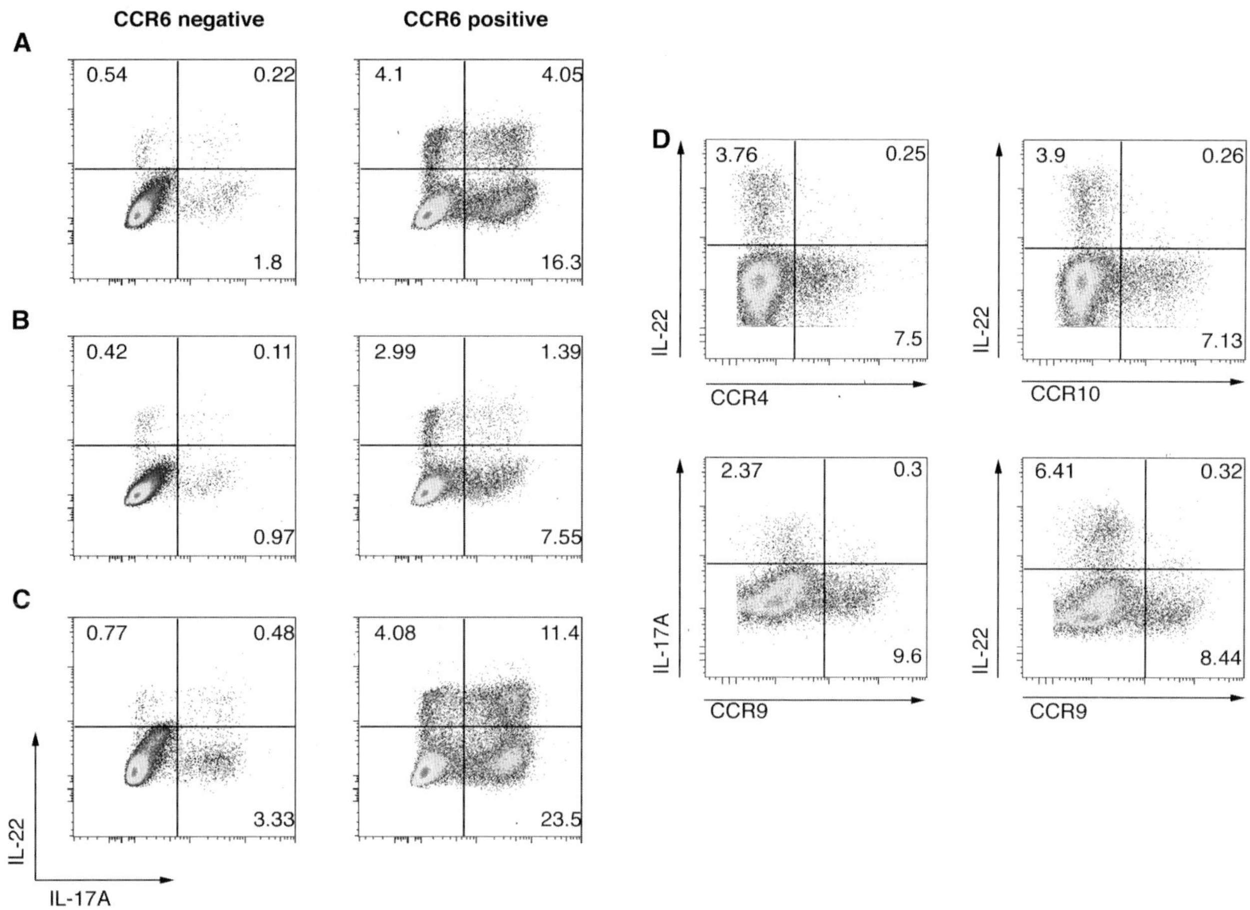

Figure 6. Tissue-homing characteristics of Pseudomonas aeruginosa-specific memory Th22 and Th17 cells. A–C Human memory CD4$^+$ T cells were sorted into CCR6-depleted (CCR6 negative) and CCR6-enriched (CCR6 positive) populations before being exposed to dendritic cells (DCs) infected with Yorkhill 5 MOI30 (**A**), DCs infected with PA103 ΔUΔT MOI30 (**B**), or stimulated with anti-CD3 and anti-CD28 which acted as a positive control by polyclonal T cell stimulation (**C**). Plots show CD4$^+$ IFN-γ negative T cells after 6-days of co-culture. **D** Memory CD4$^+$ T cells were cultured with DCs infected with PA103 ΔpcrV MOI30. Pseudomonas-specific memory CD4$^+$ T cells were analysed for expression of intracellular IL-22 or IL-17 as shown together with the skin-homing chemokine receptors CCR4, CCR10 and CCR9 as indicated. Numbers in each plot represent per cent cells in each quadrant. Results are representative of those seen in three independent individuals.

or gut homing markers but are CCR6$^+$. We propose that these cells will migrate to areas of inflamed lung under the influence of CCL20 or β-defensins. Local IL-22 within the lung could play a key role in host defence, epithelial repair and regeneration, and may be amenable to therapeutic intervention to promote healthy lung repair after damaging infection.

Supporting Information

Figure S1 Cytokine production by human memory CD4$^+$ T cells to different *Pseudomonas aeruginosa* strains. Human memory CD4$^+$ T cells from healthy volunteers (**A**, **B** and **C**) and patients with cystic fibrosis (CF) (**D**, **E** and **F**) were co-cultured with dendritic cells infected with different strains of (PA). Laboratory PA strains PA103 ΔpcrV and PA103 ΔUΔT, clinical non-mucoid strains Yorkhill 1 and 2, and the clinical mucoid strain Yorkhill 5 were used; clinical strains were derived from cystic fibrosis patients. Levels of cytokines were measured in the supernatant after 6-days of culture. Each point represents the result from one individual; an individual may be represented more than once by separate experiments. The line indicates the median value. Differences between strains were evaluated by a Kruskal-Wallis (KW) test with pairwise assessments of differences between groups made using Dunn's multiple comparison test. *, significance difference <0.05. Only minor differences were seen in the cytokine response to different strains of PA in both healthy controls and patients with CF.

Figure S2 Memory CD4$^+$ T cells subset response to different Pseudomonas strains in CF and controls. The proportion of PA specific CD4$^+$ T helper cell responses to PA103 (PA103 ΔpcrV and PA103 ΔUΔT) and Yorkhill strains (Yorkhill 1, 2 and 5) that are Th1 (**A**) or Th22 (**B**) was determined as outlined in Figure 5 in the main text. Each point represents the result from one individual; some individuals were tested against different bacterial strains as indicated by the symbols used in Figure 4. The line indicates the median value. Differences between controls and patients with CF were evaluated by a Mann-Whitney test with the p value as shown.

Figure S3 Cytokine production by human memory CD4$^+$ T cells to tetanus toxoid and heat-killed candida albicans. Human memory CD4$^+$ T cells from healthy were co-cultured with dendritic cells infected with tetanus toxoid or heat-killed candida albicans. (**A**) Patterns of cytokine expression by non-proliferating $CD4^+$ T cells following 6-days of culture with DCs infected with tetanus toxoid. (**B**) Patterns of cytokine expression by $CD4^+$ T cells proliferating in response to culture with DCs infected with tetanus toxoid. (**C**) Patterns of cytokine expression by non-proliferating $CD4^+$ T cells following 6-days of culture with DCs infected with heat-killed candida albicans (HKCA). (**D**) Patterns of cytokine expression by $CD4^+$ T cells proliferating in response to culture with DCs infected with HKCA. Numbers in plot represent percent cells in each quadrant.

Acknowledgments

We are grateful to Diane Vaughan, (Glasgow), for assistance in running the flow cytometry analyses.

Author Contributions

Conceived and designed the experiments: HKB SB GM TJE. Performed the experiments: HKB TJE. Analyzed the data: HKB TJE. Wrote the paper: HKB TJE.

References

1. Rowe SM, Miller S, Sorscher EJ (2005) Cystic fibrosis. N Engl J Med 352: 1992-2001.
2. Ratjen F, McColley SA (2012) Update in cystic fibrosis 2011. Am J Respir Crit Care Med 185: 933–936.
3. Sadikot RT, Blackwell TS, Christman JW, Prince AS (2005) Pathogen-host interactions in Pseudomonas aeruginosa pneumonia. Am J Respir Crit Care Med 171: 1209–1223.
4. Dubin PJ, Kolls JK (2007) Pseudomonas aeruginosa and the host pulmonary immune response. Expert Rev Respir Med 1: 121–137.
5. Downey DG, Bell SC, Elborn JS (2009) Neutrophils in cystic fibrosis. Thorax 64: 81–88.
6. Doring G (1989) Host response to Pseudomonas aeruginosa. Acta Paediatr Scand Suppl 363: 37–39; discussion 40.
7. Markham RB, Powderly WG (1988) Exposure of mice to live Pseudomonas aeruginosa generates protective cell-mediated immunity in the absence of an antibody response. J Immunol 140: 2039–2045.
8. Stockinger B, Veldhoen M, Martin B (2007) Th17 T cells: linking innate and adaptive immunity. Semin Immunol 19: 353–361.
9. Priebe GP, Walsh RL, Cederroth TA, Kamei A, Coutinho-Sledge YS, et al. (2008) IL-17 is a critical component of vaccine-induced protection against lung infection by lipopolysaccharide-heterologous strains of Pseudomonas aeruginosa. J Immunol 181: 4965–4975.
10. Tan HL, Regamey N, Brown S, Bush A, Lloyd CM, et al. (2011) The Th17 pathway in cystic fibrosis lung disease. Am J Respir Crit Care Med 184: 252–258.
11. Brodlie M, Corris PA, Lordan J, Ward C (2012) Interleukin-17 and cystic fibrosis lung disease. Am J Respir Crit Care Med 185: 108–109; author reply 109–110.
12. Zielinski CE, Mele F, Aschenbrenner D, Jarrossay D, Ronchi F, et al. (2012) Pathogen-induced human TH17 cells produce IFN-gamma or IL-10 and are regulated by IL-1beta. Nature 484: 514–518.
13. Acosta-Rodriguez EV, Rivino L, Geginat J, Jarrossay D, Gattorno M, et al. (2007) Surface phenotype and antigenic specificity of human interleukin 17-producing T helper memory cells. Nat Immunol 8: 639–646.
14. Wolk K, Witte E, Witte K, Warszawska K, Sabat R (2010) Biology of interleukin-22. Semin Immunopathol 32: 17–31.
15. Eyerich S, Eyerich K, Pennino D, Carbone T, Nasorri F, et al. (2009) Th22 cells represent a distinct human T cell subset involved in epidermal immunity and remodeling. J Clin Invest 119: 3573–3585.
16. Duhen T, Geiger R, Jarrossay D, Lanzavecchia A, Sallusto F (2009) Production of interleukin 22 but not interleukin 17 by a subset of human skin-homing memory T cells. Nat Immunol 10: 857–863.
17. Trifari S, Kaplan CD, Tran EH, Crellin NK, Spits H (2009) Identification of a human helper T cell population that has abundant production of interleukin 22 and is distinct from T(H)-17, T(H)1 and T(H)2 cells. Nat Immunol 10: 864–871.
18. Basu R, O'Quinn DB, Silberger DJ, Schoeb TR, Fouser L, et al. (2012) Th22 cells are an important source of IL-22 for host protection against enteropathogenic bacteria. Immunity 37: 1061–1075.
19. Aujla SJ, Chan YR, Zheng M, Fei M, Askew DJ, et al. (2008) IL-22 mediates mucosal host defense against Gram-negative bacterial pneumonia. Nat Med 14: 275–281.
20. Ota N, Wong K, Valdez PA, Zheng Y, Crellin NK, et al. (2011) IL-22 bridges the lymphotoxin pathway with the maintenance of colonic lymphoid structures during infection with Citrobacter rodentium. Nat Immunol 12: 941–948.
21. Zheng Y, Valdez PA, Danilenko DM, Hu Y, Sa SM, et al. (2008) Interleukin-22 mediates early host defense against attaching and effacing bacterial pathogens. Nat Med 14: 282–289.
22. Sonnenberg GF, Monticelli LA, Alenghat T, Fung TC, Hutnick NA, et al. (2012) Innate lymphoid cells promote anatomical containment of lymphoid-resident commensal bacteria. Science 336: 1321–1325.
23. Vallis AJ, Finck-Barbancon V, Yahr TL, Frank DW (1999) Biological effects of Pseudomonas aeruginosa type III-secreted proteins on CHO cells. Infect Immun 67: 2040–2044.
24. Sawa T, Yahr TL, Ohara M, Kurahashi K, Gropper MA, et al. (1999) Active and passive immunization with the Pseudomonas V antigen protects against type III intoxication and lung injury. Nat Med 5: 392–398.
25. Gurney AL (2004) IL-22, a Th1 cytokine that targets the pancreas and select other peripheral tissues. Int Immunopharmacol 4: 669–677.
26. Gaffen SL, Hernandez-Santos N, Peterson AC (2011) IL-17 signaling in host defense against Candida albicans. Immunol Res 50: 181–187.
27. Stoodley BJ, Thom BT (1970) Observations on the intestinal carriage of Pseudomonas aeruginosa. J Med Microbiol 3: 367–375.
28. Wuthrich M, Hung CY, Gern BH, Pick-Jacobs JC, Galles KJ, et al. (2011) A TCR transgenic mouse reactive with multiple systemic dimorphic fungi. J Immunol 187: 1421–1431.
29. Chen K, McAleer JP, Lin Y, Paterson DL, Zheng M, et al. (2011) Th17 cells mediate clade-specific, serotype-independent mucosal immunity. Immunity 35: 997–1009.
30. Sonnenberg GF, Nair MG, Kirn TJ, Zaph C, Fouser LA, et al. (2010) Pathological versus protective functions of IL-22 in airway inflammation are regulated by IL-17A. J Exp Med 207: 1293–1305.
31. Chan YR, Chen K, Duncan SR, Lathrop KL, Latoche JD, et al. (2012) Patients with cystic fibrosis have inducible IL-17(+)IL-22(+) memory cells in lung draining lymph nodes. J Allergy Clin Immunol.
32. Brodlie M, McKean MC, Johnson GE, Anderson AE, Hilkens CM, et al. (2011) Raised interleukin-17 is immunolocalised to neutrophils in cystic fibrosis lung disease. Eur Respir J 37: 1378–1385.
33. Rieber N, Brand A, Hector A, Graepler-Mainka U, Ost M, et al. (2013) Flagellin induces myeloid-derived suppressor cells: implications for Pseudomonas aeruginosa infection in cystic fibrosis lung disease. J Immunol 190: 1276–1284.
34. Pier GB, Ramphal R (2005) Pseudomonas aeruginosa. In: Mandell GL, Bennett JE, Dolin R, editors. Principles and Practice of Infectious Diseases. 6th ed. Philadelphia: Elsevier Churchill Livingstone. pp. 2587–2615.
35. Wunderink RG (2005) Nosocomial pneumonia, including ventilator-associated pneumonia. Proc Am Thorac Soc 2: 440–444.
36. Martinez-Solano L, Macia MD, Fajardo A, Oliver A, Martinez JL (2008) Chronic Pseudomonas aeruginosa infection in chronic obstructive pulmonary disease. Clin Infect Dis 47: 1526–1533.

3

Disrupted Intestinal Microbiota and Intestinal Inflammation in Children with Cystic Fibrosis and Its Restoration with Lactobacillus GG: A Randomised Clinical Trial

Eugenia Bruzzese[1], Maria Luisa Callegari[2], Valeria Raia[1], Sara Viscovo[1], Riccardo Scotto[1], Susanna Ferrari[2], Lorenzo Morelli[2], Vittoria Buccigrossi[1], Andrea Lo Vecchio[1], Eliana Ruberto[1], Alfredo Guarino[1]*

1 Department of Translational Medical Science, Section of Pediatrics, University Federico II, Naples, Italy, **2** Centro Ricerche Biotecnologiche, Università Cattolica del Sacro Cuore, Cremona, Italy

Abstract

Background & Aims: Intestinal inflammation is a hallmark of cystic fibrosis (CF). Administration of probiotics can reduce intestinal inflammation and the incidence of pulmonary exacerbations. We investigated the composition of intestinal microbiota in children with CF and analyzed its relationship with intestinal inflammation. We also investigated the microflora structure before and after *Lactobacillus* GG (LGG) administration in children with CF with and without antibiotic treatment.

Methods: The intestinal microbiota were analyzed by denaturing gradient gel electrophoresis (DGGE), real-time polymerase chain reaction (RT-PCR), and fluorescence *in situ* hybridization (FISH). Intestinal inflammation was assessed by measuring fecal calprotectin (CLP) and rectal nitric oxide (rNO) production in children with CF as compared with healthy controls. We then carried out a small double-blind randomized clinical trial with LGG.

Results: Twenty-two children with CF children were enrolled in the study (median age, 7 years; range, 2–9 years). Fecal CLP and rNO levels were higher in children with CF than in healthy controls (184 ± 146 µg/g vs. 52 ± 46 µg/g; 18 ± 15 vs. 2.6 ± 1.2 µmol/L NO_2^-, respectively; $P < 0.01$). Compared with healthy controls, children with CF had significantly different intestinal microbial core structures. The levels of *Eubacterium rectale*, *Bacteroides uniformis*, *Bacteroides vulgatus*, *Bifidobacterium adolescentis*, *Bifidobacterium catenulatum*, and *Faecalibacterium prausnitzii* were reduced in children with CF. A similar but more extreme pattern was observed in children with CF who were taking antibiotics. LGG administration reduced fecal CLP and partially restored intestinal microbiota. There was a significant correlation between reduced microbial richness and intestinal inflammation.

Conclusions: CF causes qualitative and quantitative changes in intestinal microbiota, which may represent a novel therapeutic target in the treatment of CF. Administration of probiotics restored gut microbiota, supporting the efficacy of probiotics in reducing intestinal inflammation and pulmonary exacerbations.

Editor: Stefan Bereswill, Charité-University Medicine Berlin, Germany

Funding: The study was partially supported by a grant of "Cystic Fibrosis Foundation and Therapeutics" (Account number GUARIN10A0/2009) and "Fondazione Italiana Ricerca Fibrosi Cistica" (Account number FC 23/2009). The funders had no role in study design, data collection and analysis, decision to publish, or preparation of the manuscript.

Competing Interests: The authors have declared that no competing interests exist.

* E-mail: alfguari@unina.it

Introduction

Culture-independent, molecular and metagenomic techniques have provided new insights into the complex interactions between mammalian hosts and their gut microbial species [1]. It is increasingly evident that gut microbes influence the host's metabolic and immunological activities [2,3]. Accordingly, intestinal microorganisms may influence the development of both intestinal and generalized inflammation, although the mechanism remains unclear [4,5].

In patients with cystic fibrosis (CF), the intestine is a site of inflammatory processes. Several biomarkers, including calprotectin (CLP), S100A12, IL-8, IgM, IgG, neutrophil elastase, tumor necrosis factor-α, and eosinophil cationic protein, have been used to detect intestinal inflammation in patients with CF [6]. We previously found increased concentrations of fecal CLP and rectal nitric oxide (rNO) in children with CF, suggesting that intestinal inflammation is a feature of CF [7]. This finding was confirmed by endoscopy in children with CF [8].

Recently, it was reported that patients with CF have a different pattern of intestinal microbes than do healthy controls [9–10]. The majority of bacteria present in the intestinal and respiratory tracts were represented by 8 distinct genera, and there was a microbial link between the two organ systems that was reflected in core microbiota dominated by *Veillonella* and *Streptococcus* species [11]. Further, fecal samples from CF patients consistently demonstrated reduced loads of bifidobacteria [12].

In a preliminary cross-over trial in children with CF, administration of *Lactobacillus rhamnosus* GG (LGG) was associated with a reduction in intestinal inflammation as measured by CLP and rNO concentrations [7]. Interestingly, administration of LGG was associated with a reduction in pulmonary exacerbations and hospital admissions and an improvement in the forced respiratory volume in 1 s (FEV_1) [13,14]. These data suggest that probiotics delay respiratory impairment, which is a major goal in the treatment of CF.

On the basis of these findings, we hypothesized that there exists a link between the composition of intestinal microbiota and inflammation. Although direct evidence is not available, the intestinal microenvironment in children with CF is expected to be different from that of healthy children as a consequence of Cystic fibrosis transmembrane conductance regulator (CFTR) malfunction, frequent use of antibiotics, pancreatic enzyme supplementation, and pharmacological suppression of gastric acid production. Intraluminal pH varies with the anatomical site and microbial fermentation of dietary residues; these variations may affect the composition of the bacterial community and its metabolic activity [15]. Interestingly, among children with atopy, the administration of LGG induced a global modification of intestinal microflora, suggesting that an intestinal microbiome composed of a multitude of probiotic species may protect against the development of allergic disease when compared with one dominated by a single commensal species [16].

The aims of the present study were 1) to investigate the composition of gut microbiota in children with CF as compared with healthy controls, 2) to investigate the correlation between microbial balance and intestinal inflammation, and 3) to test the hypothesis that LGG administration restores intestinal microflora and decreases inflammation in children with CF. First, we analyzed fecal microbiota by carrying out denaturing gradient gel electrophoresis (DGGE) and real-time polymerase chain reaction (RT-PCR) of fecal samples of children with CF. To investigate the effects of the administration of LGG on composition of microbiota and intestinal inflammation, 22 children with CF were enrolled in a short-term study with administration of LGG. The effect of probiotic intake on intestinal microbial structure was investigated by fluorescence *in situ* hybridization (FISH) based on the results of DGGE and RT-PCR.

Patients and Methods

Study Design

The protocol for this trial and supporting CONSORT checklist are available as supporting information; see Checklist S1 and Protocol S1.

We enrolled clinically stable children with CF who had no acute intestinal or extraintestinal diseases and had not taken antibiotics for at least two weeks. The following parameters were recorded–sex, age, body weight, CF genotype, and severity of mutations. CF genotype was classified as severe if 2 severe mutations were present, and mild if at least 1 mutation was mild, according to the mechanisms by which the mutations disrupt CFTR function [17].

Intestinal inflammation and the composition of intestinal microbiota were investigated. Stool samples were collected from healthy controls in order to investigate intestinal microbiota composition in an age-matched population. Intestinal microflora was also evaluated by FISH in an additional population of children with CF who were on antibiotic treatment. Twenty-two children with CF were enrolled in the randomized double-blind clinical trial in order to evaluate the effect of LGG on intestinal inflammation and intestinal microflora composition.

Patients were randomly assigned to the treatment or placebo arms. Patients randomized to the treatment arm received 6×10^9 CFU of LGG once daily for 1 month. Patients randomized to the placebo arm received placebo once daily for 1 month. The randomization protocol was generated by a statistician not involved in patient management. LGG and placebo formulations were masked and coded appropriately to ensure blindness. LGG formulations were composed of maltodextrin (163 mg), gelatin capsule (75 mg), LGG (60 mg), and magnesium stearate (2 mg). The placebo was composed of maltodextrin (223 mg), gelatin capsule (75 mg), and magnesium stearate (2 mg). LGG and placebo capsules were identical in appearance, taste, and color, and only a numeric code differentiated the two formulations.

Before and after administration of LGG or placebo, a microbiological investigation was carried out using FISH, and intestinal CLP concentration was measured. This study constituted a pilot study in preparation for a large trial, and it was formally registered as a clinical trial at clinicaltrials.gov (NCT 01961661). The Ethical Committee of University Federico II of Naples approved the protocol. Written informed consent was obtained for each enrolled child from the parents.

Intestinal Inflammation

Intestinal inflammation was investigated by fecal CLP and rNO production. Fecal CLP was measured by an enzyme-linked immunosorbent assay (Calprest Eurospital SpA, Trieste, Italy). Normal values for fecal CLP were 0–50 μg/g of stool; values of 50–100 μg/g were considered intermediate and required follow-up, and values >100 μg/g indicated intestinal inflammation [18].

The stable NO metabolites NO_2^- and NO_3^- were measured by the Griess reaction. rNO levels measured in healthy age-matched children were used as the normal reference [19].

Bacterial DNA Isolation

A total of 50 mg of fecal material was incubated at 37°C in lysozyme buffer (100 mM Tris-HCl, pH 8, 25% sucrose, 10 mM EDTA, and 10 mg/mL of lysozyme) for 1 h and then processed by the Maxwell® 16 System (Promega, Madison, WI, USA) using the Maxwell® 16 DNA purification kit. The extracted bacterial DNA was eluted in 400 μL of elution buffer and stored at −80°C.

DNA Amplification

The total bacterial DNA extracted from feces was used as a template in the PCR reactions. The V_2–V_3 region of the 16S rRNA gene was amplified using universal primers Hda1-GC and Hda2 [20].

Amplicons for DGGE analysis of the *Bacteroides-Prevotella* group were obtained using the primers Bac303F and Bac708R [20]. The 418-bp amplification product obtained was used as a template in nested PCR with primers Hda1-GC and Hda2 [21].

DGGE Analysis

All DGGE analyses were performed using the INGENYphorU-2x2 system (INGENY International, Amundsenweg, The Netherlands). Amplicons were analyzed on 8% polyacrylamide (40% acrylamide-bis, 37.5:1) gel with a 40% to 65% denaturing gradient of urea and formamide increasing in the direction of electrophoresis. The gel was run with a constant voltage of 80 V at 60°C for 18 h in 1× Tris-acetate buffer (pH 8.0).

The Fingerprinting II software([Bio-Rad, Hercules CA, USA) was used to compare DGGE profiles using the Pearson's similarity coefficient for comparison and the UPGMA algorithm for the dendrogram construction. The Quantity One software([version 4.6.0; Bio-Rad, Hercules CA, USA) was used for the identification and quantification of bands.

Recovery of Amplicons and Sequencing

Bands were cut from DGGE gels, eluted at 4°C for 24 h, and re-amplified according to the PCR conditions described above. The PCR products were purified using Wizard Plus® SV Minipreps-DNA Purification System (Promega) and were sequenced (BMR Genomics, Padova, Italy). Sequences obtained were analyzed using NCBI BLAST (Basic Local Alignment Search Tool) and Ribosomal Database Project (RDP).

RT-PCR

Copy numbers of the 16S rRNA gene from *Bacteroides/Prevotella* group, *Eubacterium rectale*, *Bacteroides vulgatus*, and *Bifibobacterium* were determined using previously reported primers [21–24]. Quantification was carried out in triplicate using the Light Cycler System (Roche Applied Science, Monza, Italy). Primer concentrations in the reaction mixture were 300 nM for *B. vulgatus*, *E. rectale*, and *Bifibobacterium* and 500 nM for the *Bacteroides/Prevotella* group.

Escherichia coli and *Bacteroides uniformis* were quantified using the LightCycler® TaqMan® Master mix (Roche Applied Science, Mannheim Germany). The primers and probe used to quantify *E. coli* were described by Scupham [22], and those for *B. uniformis* were published by Penders *et al.* [24].

Standard curves were obtained using reference DNA provided by the American Type Culture Collection (ATCC). Purified and quantified genomic DNA used were *Bifidobacterium infantis* ATCC 15697D, *B. vulgatus* 8482D-5, and *E. coli* ATCC 700926D-5. Genomic DNA of *E. rectale* DSM 17629, *B. uniformis* DSMZ 6597, *Bifidobacterium catenulatum* LMG 11043, *Bifidobacterium adolescentis* DSMZ 20083, and *Faecalibacterium prausnitzii* DSMZ 17677 was extracted from 5 mL of activated culture using the Genomic DNA extraction Kit [Promega] and quantified with a Qubit™ fluorometer (Invitrogen, Milan, Italy).

A standard curve was obtained by 10-fold dilutions of genomic DNA for each reference genomic DNA. The number of genomes was calculated considering the genome size; the differences in RNA copy numbers were excluded.

Sample Collection and Handling for FISH Evaluation

FISH was performed on fecal samples collected from 22 clinically stable children with CF, 20 age-matched healthy controls, and 10 children with CF on antibiotic treatment. Clinically stable children with CF were then treated with LGG([6×10^9 cfu/day) or placebo for 4 weeks, and intestinal microbiota was evaluated immediately after administration. Based on the results obtained from DGGE and RT-PCR, we used FISH to investigate the presence of *Bacteroides* and *E. rectale* since both species were consistently reduced in children with CF. *F. prausnitzii* was chosen, because it has been associated with the pathogenesis of inflammatory bowel diseases [25].

Fecal samples were fixed in Carnoy's solution and embedded in paraffin, cut longitudinally into 4-µm sections, placed on SuperFrost slides (Thermo Scientific, Italy) [26], and incubated with hybridization solution (20 mM Tris-HCl, 0.9 M NaCl, 0.1% SDS, and 1% formamide, pH 7.4) with EUB mix positive control oligonucleotide probes (100 ng of EUB I, EUBII, and EUBIII). For *Bacteroides*, *E. rectale*, and *F. prausnitzii*, the slides were incubated with hybridization buffer with 25 ng of their respective FISH probes for 45 min at 50°C and visualized using a Nikon 80i Eclipse epifluorescence microscope with a Nikon DS-U2 color camera and NIS-Elements imaging software (Nikon, Tokyo, Japan). Bacteria were quantified by count. The oligonucleotide probes used in this study were synthesized by MWG Eurofins (MWG Operon Ebersberg, Germany). All samples were analyzed with the Eub338 mix probe conjugated with fluorescein isothiocyanate (FITC, green signal) at the 5′ end (positive control that reacts with all bacteria) [27], and a species-specific probe was conjugated with a single fluorescent carbocyanine molecule (Cy3, red signal).

Statistical Analysis

Statistical analysis was performed using GraphPad Instat 3 software. A *t*-test was used to evaluate the differences in mean fecal CLP, fecal rNO, and counts of bacterial species between CF patients and age-matched healthy controls. To evaluate whether there is a possible link between intestinal inflammation and abnormalities in microbiota, patients were grouped by normal or abnormal fecal CLP concentration. The difference in the mean number of bands in the two groups was evaluated by *t*-test. The Pearson's correlation coefficient was used to investigate the correlation between intestinal inflammatory markers and the richness of intestinal microbiota, as determined by the number of bands during DGGE analysis and the specific bacterial counts (amount of bacteria by RT-PCR).

The biological diversity of microbiota in children with CF and healthy controls was estimated by the number of bands and their intensity via DGGE. The Shannon-index (H') was used to evaluate the richness of bacterial species, as it reflects the abundance of microbial species [28]. The similarity of DGGE profiles within and between groups was analyzed by the similarity coefficient. The number of bands and the Shannon index of the two groups were uniformly distributed, and the Student's *t*-test was used to evaluate the difference.

RT-PCR results are expressed as means ± SD; logarithms of the number of genomes were used if required to achieve normal distributions. Data were subjected to analysis of variance by using the GLM procedure of SAS (SAS for Windows, version 9.1). Statistical significance was set at $P \leq 0.05$.

Results

Study Population

Twenty-two children with CF were enrolled (13 males, median age of 7 years, range 2–9 years). Twelve children were homozygous, and 10 children were heterozygous for the ΔF508 mutation. Only 1 patient had a mild genotype. All enrolled patients were in stable clinical condition at the time of enrolment, as indicated by the absence of exacerbations, lack of hospitalization, and lack of treatment with steroids or antibiotics for at least two weeks before enrolment. Subjects were not receiving probiotics.

Intestinal Inflammation

The mean fecal CLP concentration was significantly higher in children with CF than in age-matched healthy controls (184±146 µg/g vs. 52±46 µg/g; $P<0.01$). Fecal CLP concentration was measured in 19 children with CF. Increased fecal CLP concentration (>100 µg/g) was measured in 63% of children with CF (12/19 subjects).

rNO concentration was measured in 12 of the 22 children with CF. The mean rNO concentration was significantly higher in children with CF than in healthy controls (18±15 vs. 2.6±1.2 µmol/L NO_2; $P<0.01$; Figure 1). The majority of children with CF (11/12) had increased concentrations of rNO, similar to our previous results [7].

DGGE Analysis

The dominant fecal bacteria among children with CF and healthy subjects were determined by DGGE analysis using Hda1-GC-Hda2 primers targeting the V2–V3 region of the 16S rRNA. The DGGE profile is shown in Figure 2. The DGGE profiles significantly differed between the two groups. Compared to controls, children with CF showed a reduced number of bands, especially in the upper part of the gel. DGGE profiles from healthy subjects appeared richer and more homogeneous than those from children with CF. The DGGE profiles from healthy controls showed a common core with similar bands detected in all samples despite slight differences in intensity. There was no such common core among children with CF whose profiles were variable, as judged by the number of samples in which common species were detected (Table 1). The analysis of DGGE gels by Fingerprint II software supported the existence of two different clusters of profiles. A dendrogram was generated from the comparison of samples of children with CF and healthy controls (Figure 3).

The differences in the number of bands and in the Shannon index (H') between children with CF and healthy controls were used to qualitatively analyze the diversity of fecal microbial communities. The analysis revealed significant differences between the two groups (Table 2). The mean number of bands in the healthy controls was 26.73±2.87 as compared with 16.00±4.54 in children with CF ($P<0.001$). The Shannon index was 2.13±0.30 in healthy controls and 1.19±0.66 in children with CF ($P<0.0001$).

The upper part of the gel was analyzed separately from the lower part, because this area contained very few bands in children with CF as compared with healthy controls (Figure 3).

A comparative analysis of the similarities among all DGGE profiles from fecal samples of children with CF and healthy controls revealed a broad range of similarity coefficients for DGGE profiles (0.00–66.31 for children with CF and 21.39–65.35 for healthy controls). The mean similarity values of total bacteria, calculated using the Hda1GC-Hda2 DGGE profiles, indicated reduced biological variability in children with CF (24.28±17.45

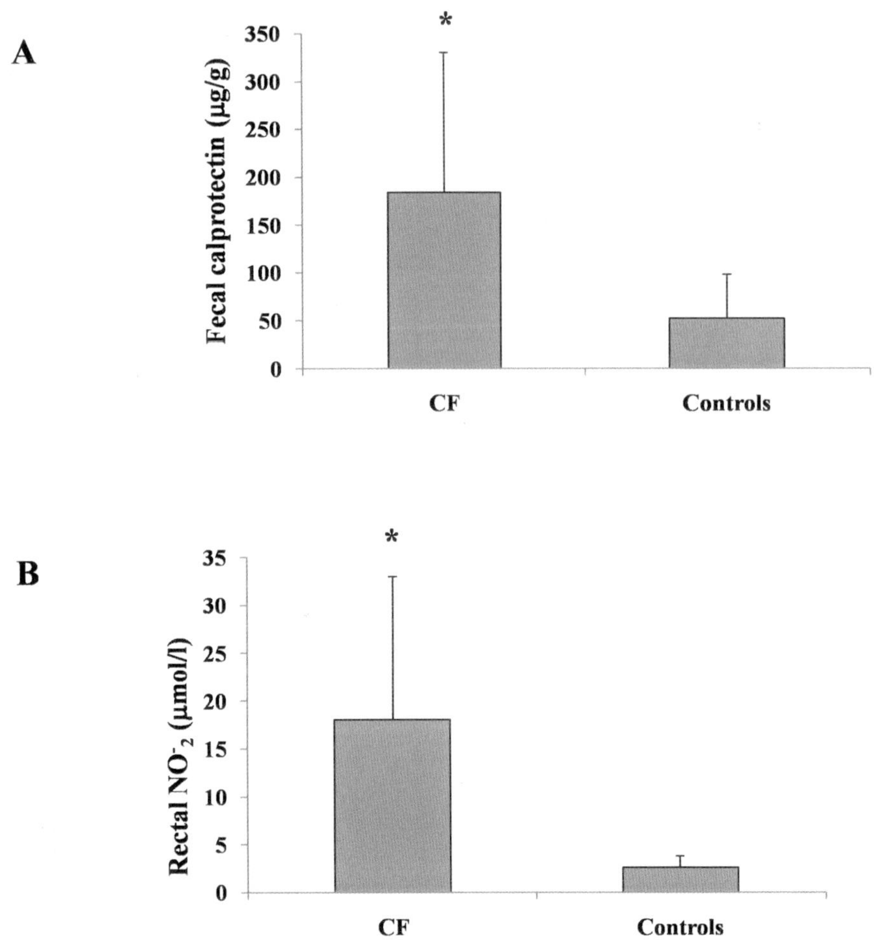

Figure 1. Intestinal inflammation markers in CF and healthy children. Fecal calprotectin (A) and rectal nitric oxide (B) concentrations in children with CF and in healthy controls ($P<0.01$).

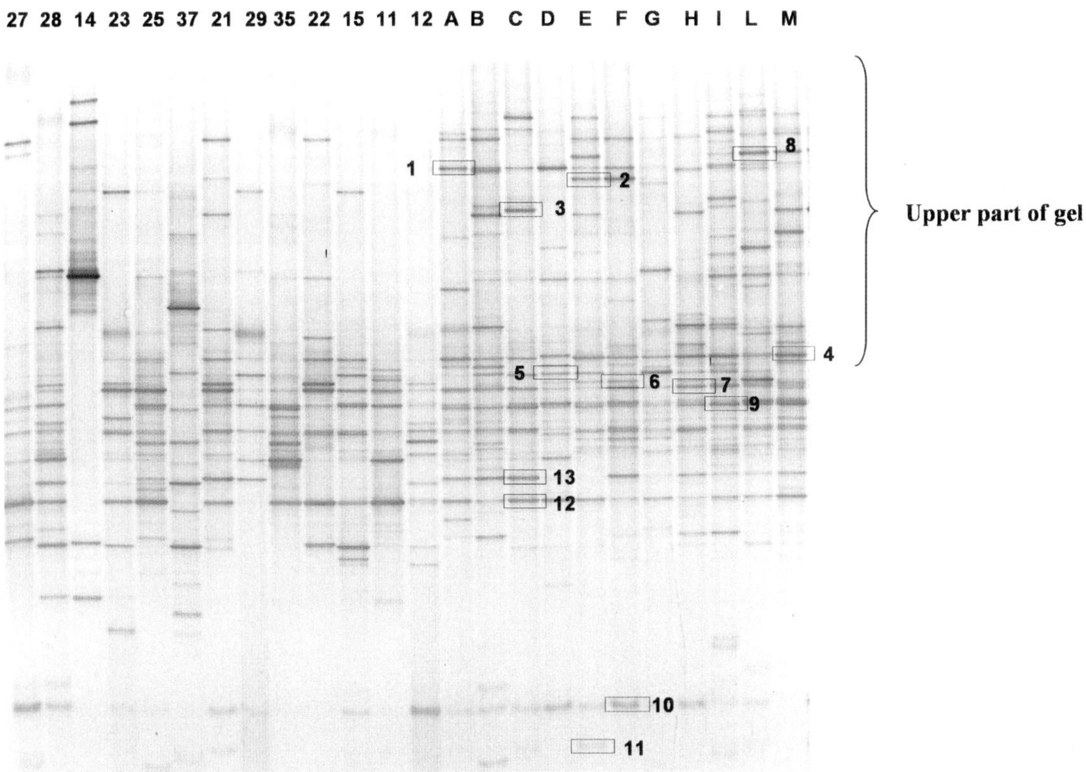

Figure 2. Microbial diversity in CF and healthy children. DGGE profiles of intestinal microbiota in children with CF (indicated by numbers) and age-matched healthy controls (indicated by letters) obtained with universal Hda1-Hda2 primers.

bands) as compared with healthy controls (43.08±9.30 bands, $P<0.0001$, Table 2).

The DGGE profile of healthy controls was characterized by two major bands with high sequence similarity to *B. vulgatus* and *B. uniformis*. These two amplicons were detected in few children with CF (Figure 4A). The dendrogram obtained by analyzing the DGGE gels of the *Bacteroides/Prevotella* group is shown in Figure 4B.

Table 1. Sequence analysis of the bands indicated in Figure 2.

Band number	% of blast similarity	Nearest species	Accession number	Presence in profiles of healthy controls (%)	Presence in profiles of children with CF (%)
1	100	*Roseburia faecis*	NR 042832	80	7.69
2	99	*Ruminococcus bromii*	L76600	27	0
3	100	*Ruminococcus gnavus*	NR036800	18	0
4	100	*Eubacterium rectale, Pseudobutyrrivibrio ruminis*	AY804151 NR026315	100	53.85
5	100	*Roseburia faecis*	AY305310	23	42.86
6	97	*Ruminococcus bromii*	NR025930	100	36.36
7	100	*Robinsoniella peoriensis Hespellia porcina Lactonifactor longoviformis*	AF445285 AF445239 NR043551	100	53.84
8	99	*Ruminococcus gauvreauii Coprococcus comes Ruminococcus torques*	NR044265 EF031542 L76604	18.18	0
9	100	*Faecalibacterium prausnitzii*	AJ413954	100	15.38
10	100	*Bifidobacterium catenulatum B. pseudocatenulatum*	NR041875 NR037117	90	53.85
11	100	*Bifidobacterium adolescentis*	GQ227713	36.36	15.38
12	100	*Faecalibacterium prausnitzii*	AJ413954	100	69.23
13	100	*Robinsoniella peoriensis Hespellia porcina Lactonifactor longoviformis*	AF445285 AF445239 NR043551	72.72	7.69

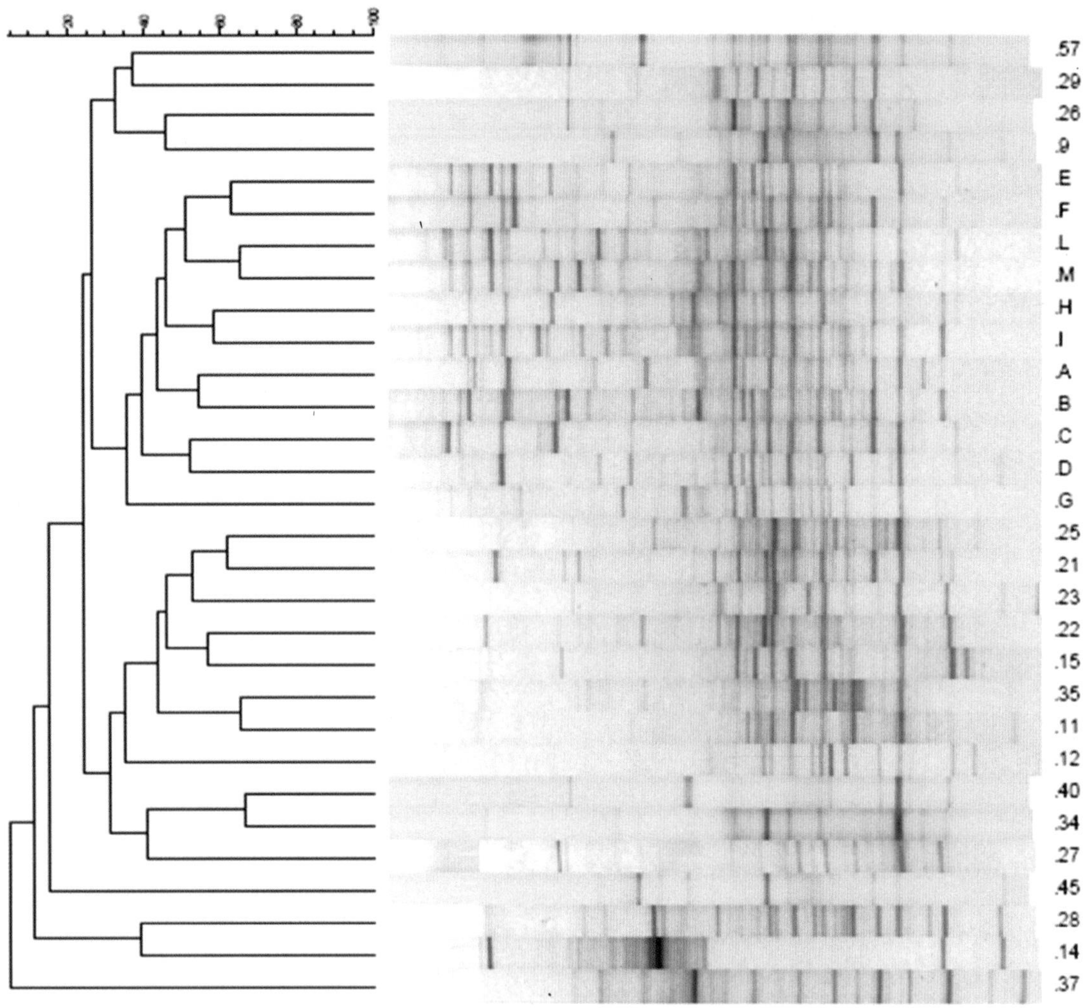

Figure 3. A hierarchical cluster analysis of the banding patterns in CF and healthy children. Dendrogram constructed using Pearson's correlation coefficients and the UPGMA algorithm of DGGE gels obtained analyzing the V2–V3 region of all fecal samples. Gels were analyzed using Fingerprinting II software (Bio-Rad). Healthy subjects are indicated with capital letters, and CF patients with numbers.

The bands isolated from the Hda1GC-Hda2 DGGE profile of healthy controls exhibited a high degree of similarity with E. rectale/Pseudobutyrivibrio ruminis, Roseburia faecis, Ruminococcus bromii, Robinsoniella peoriensis/Hespellia porcina/Lactonifactor longoviformis, F. prausnitzii, and Bifidobacterium pseudocatenulatum/B. catenulatum. Many of the species detected in

Table 2. Analysis of the V2–V3 region of DGGE profiles among children with CF and healthy controls.

Group	Diversity of microbiota by DGGE analysis		Analysis of the upper part of the DGGE gels		Microbiota similarity	
	DGGE bands (mean ± SD)	**Shannon index (mean *H'* ±SD)**	**DGGE bands (mean ± SD)**	**Shannon index (mean *H'*±SD)**	**Similarity coefficients within profiles of subjects of the same group**	**Similarity coefficients within profiles of subjects of the two groups**
Healthy controls	26,73±2,87	2,13±0,30	9,55±2,34	3,21±0,16	43.08±9.30	28.41±17.7
CF	16,00±4,54	1,19±0,66	3,95±2,93	2,55±0,27	24.28±17.45	
P-value	<0.0001	<0.0001	<0.0001	<0.0001	<0.0001	0.000

Numbers of bands (means) and Shannon index (H') obtained from DGGE profiles of the two groups. The number of bands and Shannon index were calculated for each DGGE profile and for a portion of it. The upper part of the gel corresponds to the upper part of the profile arbitrarily chosen for analysis, as shown in Fig 4. Evaluation of the similarity between microbiota of children with CF and health controls is presented as the mean of Pearson's similarity coefficients within and between groups. *P* values of <0.05 were considered statistically significant.

A

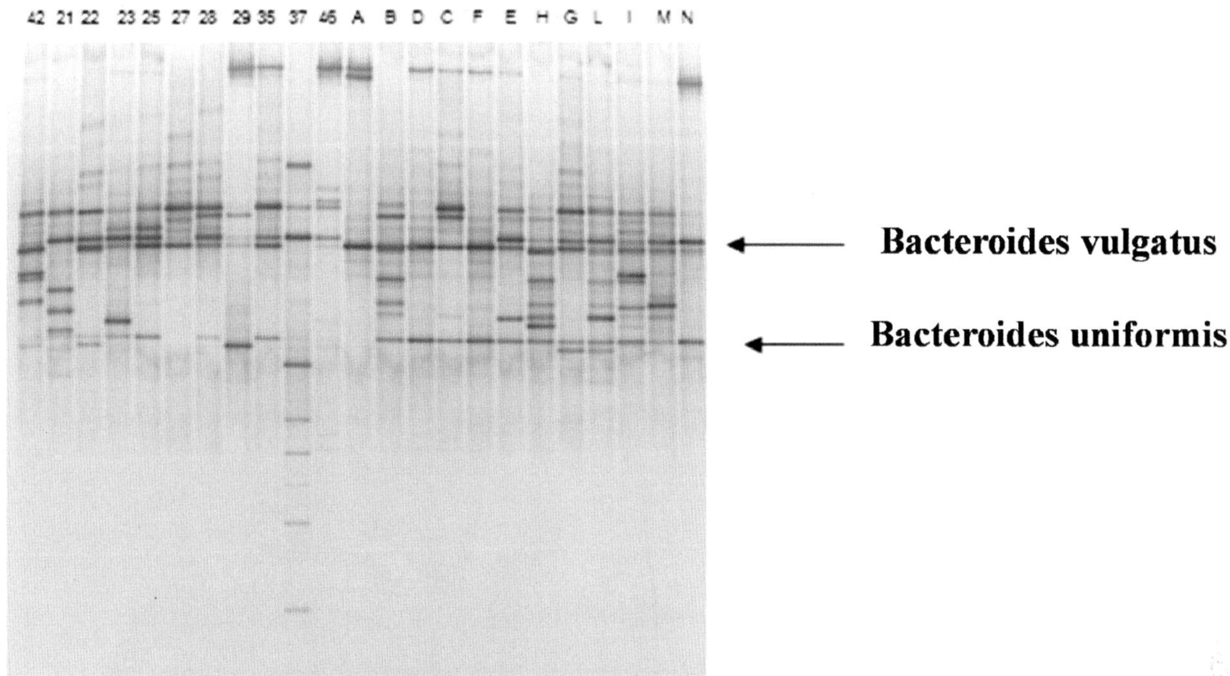
42 21 22 23 25 27 28 29 35 37 46 A B D C F E H G L I M N
Bacteroides vulgatus
Bacteroides uniformis

B

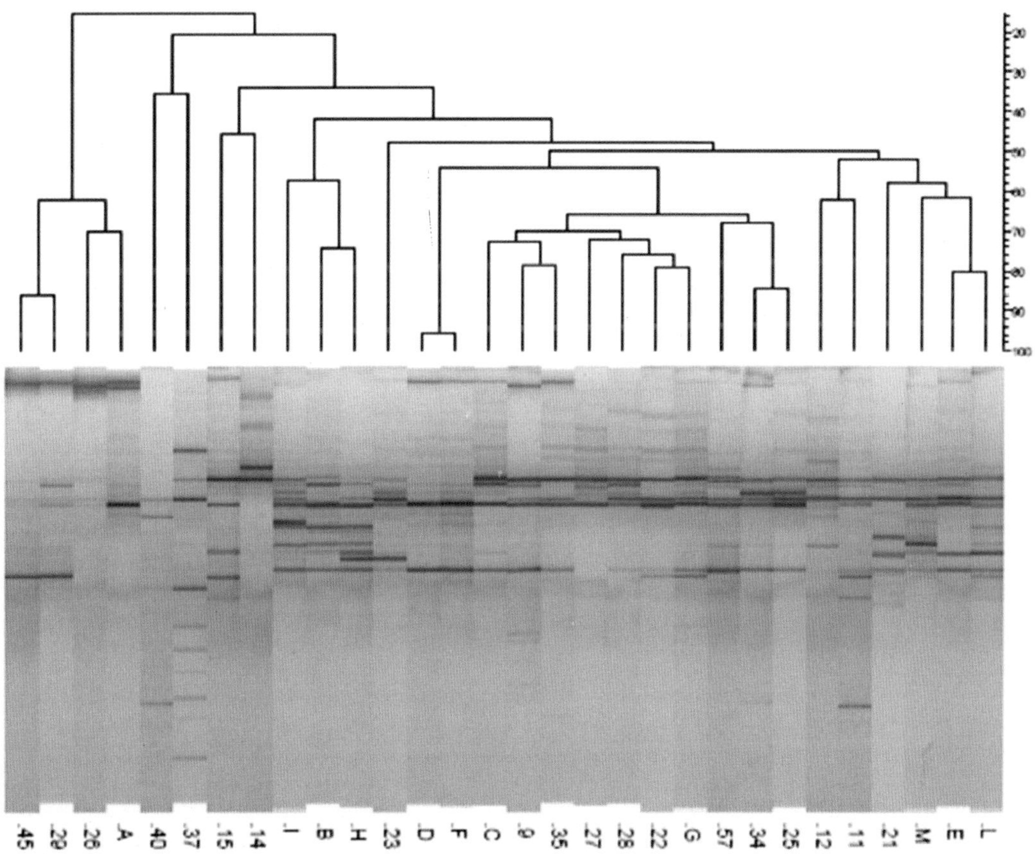
.45 .29 .26 .A .40 .37 .15 .14 .I .B .H .23 .D .F .C .9 .35 .27 .28 .22 .G .57 .34 .25 .12 .11 .21 .M .E .L

Figure 4. DGGE profiles of *Bacteroide/Prevotella* group in CF and healthy children. A, Nested DGGE of *Bacteroide/Prevotella* group profiles in children with CF (indicated by numbers) and age-matched healthy controls (indicated by letters). The bands corresponding to *Bacteroides vulgatus and Bacteroides uniformis* are reduced in children with CF as compared with healthy controls. B, Dendrogram of DGGE gel obtained using primers for analysis of *Bacteroides/Prevotella* group.

the healthy controls were not detected in the majority of children with CF; in particular, R. bromii was never detected in children with CF. Table 1 shows the identification of the bands isolated from DGGE gels and their frequency in children with CF and healthy controls.

RT-PCR Analysis

To confirm the qualitative data obtained using DGGE, a quantitative analysis was performed using RT-PCR. As shown in Figure 5, children with CF had a significant reduction in *E. rectale* and *Bacteroides* spp., mainly *B. vulgatus* and *B. uniformis*, as compared with healthy controls. Moreover, the loads of *B. catenulatum* group, *B. adolescentis*, and *F. prausnitzii* were significantly higher in the healthy controls as compared with children with CF. *E. coli* was more abundant in children with CF as compared with healthy controls, but the difference was not statistically significant.

Relationship between Intestinal Inflammation and Abnormalities in Intestinal Microbiota

We used a Pearson's correlation to evaluate the relationship between composition of intestinal microbiota and intestinal inflammation. There was no statistically significant correlation between the total number of bands and fecal CLP concentration. When subjects were grouped according to fecal CLP, the mean number of bands was higher, although not significantly, in children with fecal CLP<100 µg/g as compared with children with fecal CLP>100 µg/g (18±5 vs. 14±4; $P = 0.063$). This finding suggests a link between intestinal inflammation and reduced biodiversity of intestinal microbiota. There was a significant correlation between the number of bands in the upper part of the gel and fecal CLP concentration ($r = 0.53$; $P = 0.018$). The was no correlation between the number of individual bacterial species and fecal CLP concentration in children with CF. Furthermore, there was no correlation between rNO concentration and any specific microbial pattern.

Evaluation of Intestinal Microbiota before and after LGG Administration

We next performed a randomized, double-blind clinical trial to further investigate the composition of intestinal microflora in children with CF and to directly test the hypothesis that probiotic administration restores intestinal microflora. Therefore, we administered LGG or placebo for 4 weeks to 22 children with CF (LGG, n = 10; placebo, n = 12). We investigated the composition of intestinal microbiota before and after LGG or placebo administration by FISH. Further, we compared the results with those from age-matched healthy controls and children with CF treated with antibiotics.

The flow diagram of enrolled children is presented in Figure 6. Using DGGE, we identified *Bacteroides*, *F. prausnitzii*, and *E. rectale* as biomarkers of microbial disruption and selected specific primers for FISH analysis. The bacterial loads of *Bacteroides*, *F. prausnitzii*, and *E. rectale* were significantly reduced in children with CF as compared with healthy controls (2.5 ± 0.6 vs. $13.8 \pm 2.3 \times 10^{10}$/mL, $P<0.001$; 2.3 ± 0.7 vs. $13.4 \pm 3.1 \times 10^{10}$/mL, $P<0.001$; 4.9 ± 1.1 vs. 11.1 ± 1.3 10^{10}/mL, $P<0.001$, respectively) (Figure 7). These data confirm the results obtained by DGGE and RT-PCR. Further, a significant reduction in *Bacteroides and E. rectale* was found in children with CF who were treated with antibiotics as compared with children with CF children who were not treated with

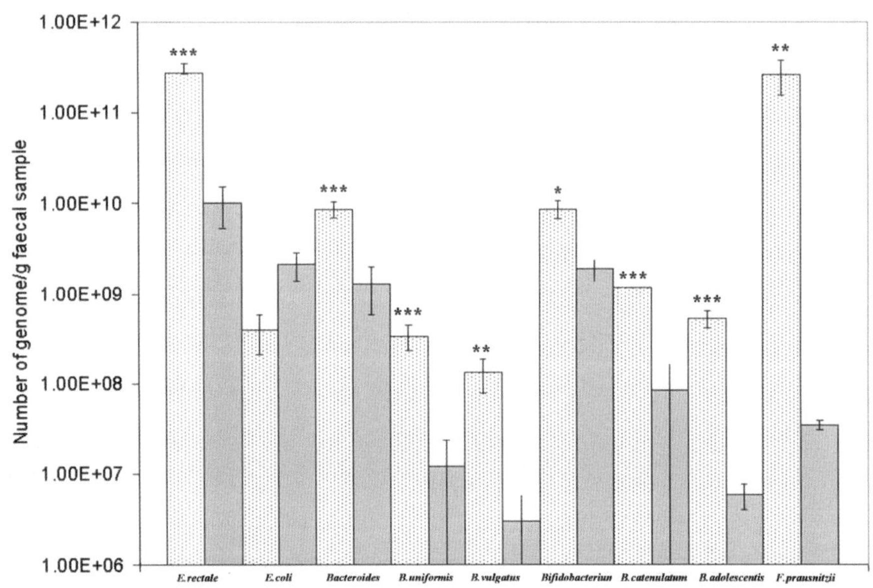

Figure 5. RT-PCR analysis of selected bacterial species in stools of CF and healthy children. Quantitative differences in *E. rectale, E. coli, Bacteroides/Prevotella group, B. uniformis, B. vulgatus, Bifidobacterium* spp., *B. catenulatum* group, *B. adolescentis*, and *F. prausnitzii* as determined by RT-PCR in children with CF and healthy individuals. Values are means ± SD. Differences indicated with *** are extremely statistically significant ($P<0.0001$); differences indicated with ** are very statistically significant ($P = 0.003$), and differences indicated with * are statistically significant ($P = 0.03$).

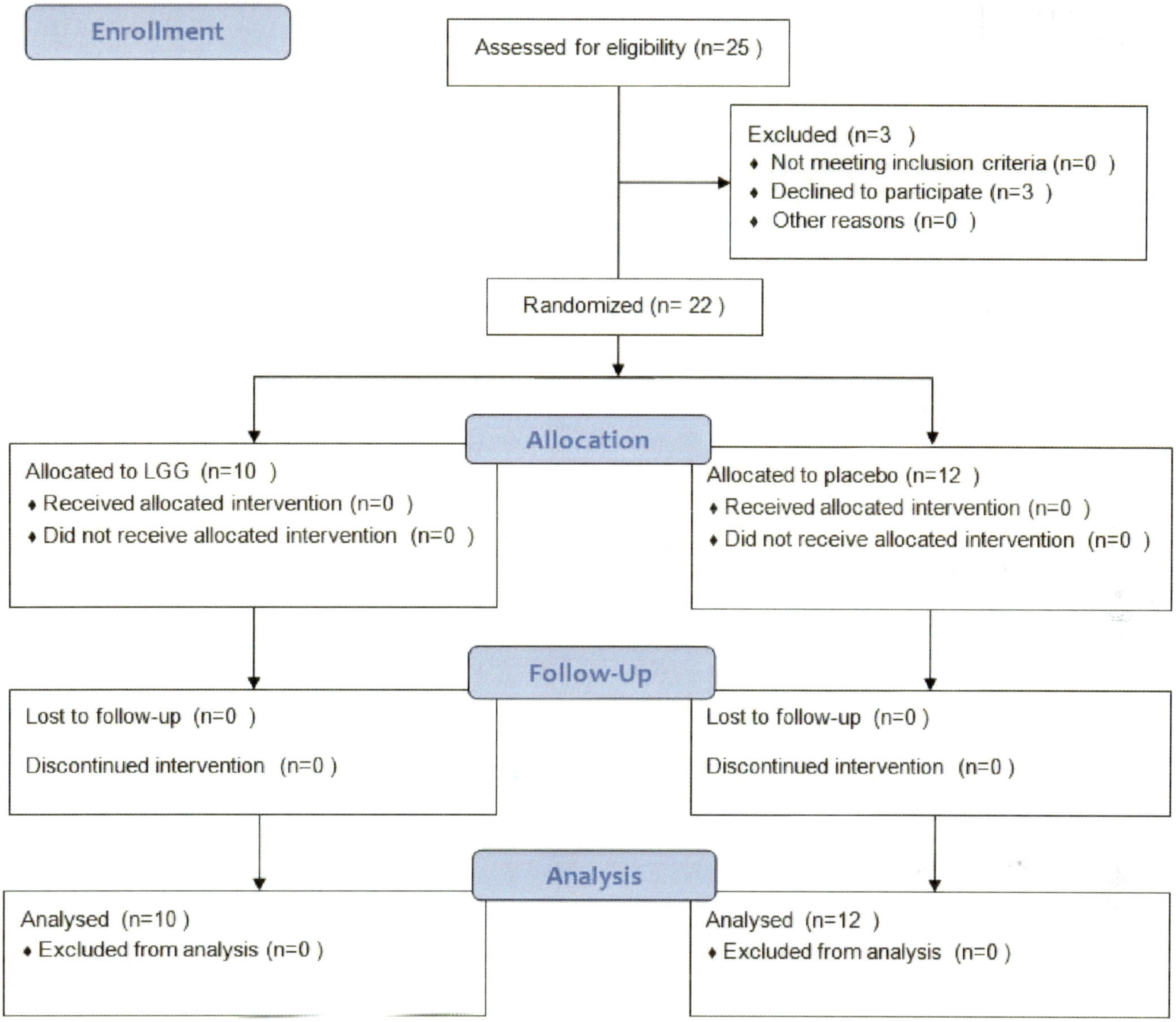

Figure 6. Flow diagram of enrolled patients.

antibiotics (2.5 ± 0.6 vs. $0.3\pm0.3\times10^{10}$/mL, $P<0.01$; 4.9 ± 1.1 vs. $0.8\pm0.5\times10^{10}$/mL, $P<0.01$, respectively). In children with CF there was also a reduction in *F. prausnitzii* counts that did not reach statistical significance (Figure 7).

Next, we investigated whether administration of LGG could restore composition of microbiota in children with CF. Children with CF treated with LGG had a significant increase in *Bacteroides* counts as compared with those treated with placebo (Table 3). There was a non-significant increase in the counts of *F. prausnitzii* in children with CF treated with LGG as compared with children with CF treated with placebo. There was no change in *E. rectale* counts after treatment with LGG (Table 3).

Intestinal inflammation was assessed by fecal CLP concentration. Children with CF who were treated with LGG showed a significant decrease in fecal CLP concentration as compared with those treated with placebo (164 ± 70 vs. 78 ± 54 µg/g, $P<0.05$; 251 ± 174 vs. 176 ± 125 µg/g, $P=0.3$, respectively; Figure 8).

Discussion

Abnormalities in intestinal microbiota have been identified in several primary intestinal diseases, often with different patterns in adults and children. However, the causal relationship between aberrations in microbiota and specific diseases remains unclear. Specific abnormalities in intestinal microbiota that are consistently associated with a pathological condition are termed "signatures." This raises the possibility that a specific pattern of intestinal microbiology maybe a "hallmark" of disease rather than contributes to pathophysiology of a disease [29].

We previously reported that intestinal inflammation is frequent in patients with CF [7]. The present study confirms that intestinal microecology is disrupted in children with CF and is significantly different from that of age-matched healthy controls. There were three specific hallmarks of the CF microbiota: 1) reduction in species richness, 2) reduction in species similarity among children with CF, and 3) a different pattern of bacterial species. A different

A

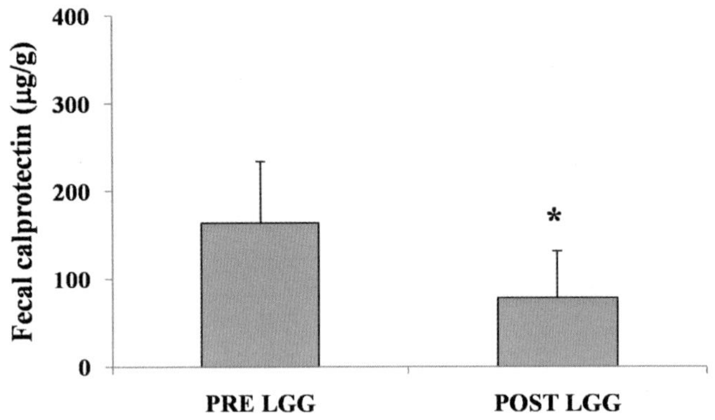

B

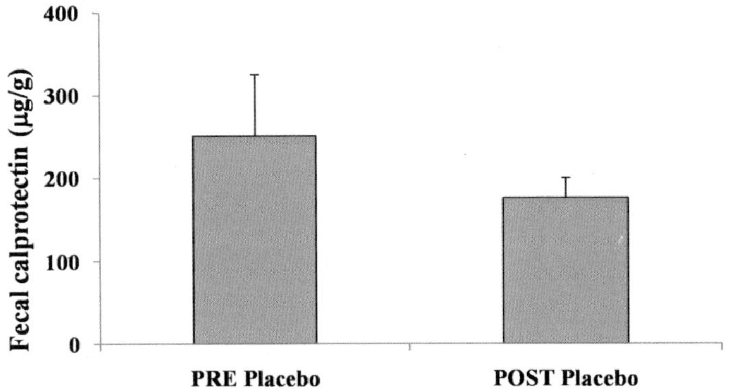

Figure 7. Quantitative analysis of different bacterial species by FISH in children with CF, healthy controls, and children with CF after antibiotic treatment. A significant reduction in the levels of *Bacteroides* spp., *Eubacterium rectale*, and *Fecalibacterium prausnitzii* spp. was observed in children with CF as compared with that in healthy controls. A further reduction in the number of *Bacteroides* spp. and *E. rectale* was observed in children with CF after antibiotic treatment as compared with that in children with CF who were not treated with antibiotics. $^{*}P<0.001$; $^{**}P<0.01$.

pattern of bacterial species in children with CF was characterized by an absence or reduction in selected species and the presence or increase in others as compared with healthy controls.

The DGGE profiles showed a reduced number of bands, indicating a reduction in biological diversity. This result was supported by the differences in Shannon index between children with CF and healthy controls. A reduction in biodiversity of microbiota is a marker of dysbiosis and is probably a consequence of selective environmental pressures [30]. However, it is also associated with intestinal inflammation, including active inflammatory bowel disease [31]. In addition to the limited biodiversity, the common "core" of bands detected in all healthy controls was absent from children with CF. Several of the profiles of children with CF did not contain the microbiologic core, and others contained only a few bands of the core. This pattern suggests that the core structure of the intestinal microbiota is disrupted in children with CF, who may have their own specific pattern. These findings apply to children with severe CF genotypes and may not hold true in milder cases of CF.

We hypothesized that the abnormal small-intestine environment of patients with CF, which is characterized by electrolyte abnormalities and an acidic pH, could select for specific bacterial genera and species. In turn, the aberrant microbiota could contribute to, rather than result from, intestinal inflammation in

Table 3. Bacterial counts before and after LGG or placebo administration in children with CF as assessed by FISH.

Bacterial species	*Bacteroides*	*F. prausnitzii*	*E. rectale*
Before LGG (n = 10)	1.7 8$\pm$0.47$\times10^{10}$/mL	2.31$\pm$0.98$\times10^{10}$/mL	4.23$\pm$1.17$\times10^{10}$/mL
After LGG	6.62$\pm$1.33$\times10^{10}$/mL*	4.77$\pm$1.3$\times10^{10}$/mL	4.82$\pm$0.85$\times10^{10}$/mL
Before placebo (n = 12)	3.07$\pm$1.05$\times10^{10}$/mL	2.25$\pm$0.96$\times10^{10}$/mL	5.54$\pm$1.77$\times10^{10}$/mL
After placebo	4.44$\pm$1.46$\times10^{10}$/mL	2.73$\pm$1.51$\times10^{10}$/mL	11.16$\pm$2.42$\times10^{10}$/mL

*$P = 0.030$.

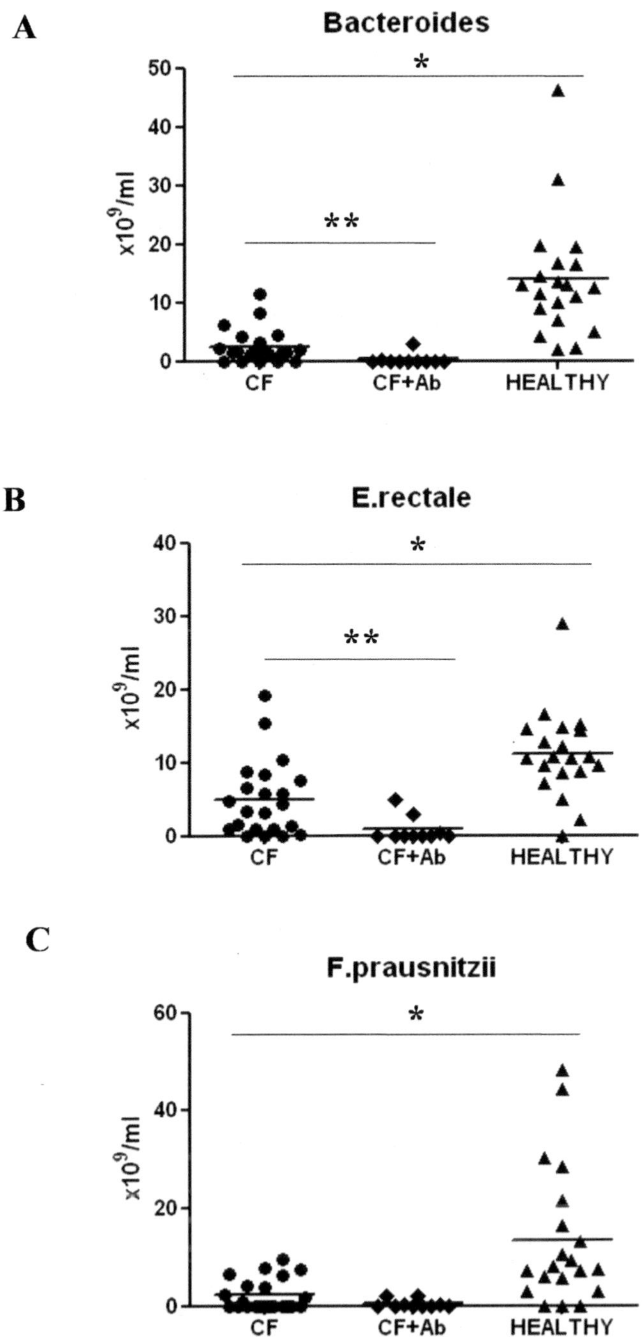

Figure 8. Modification of fecal CLP concentration before and after LGG or placebo treatment in children with CF. A significant reduction in fecal CLP was observed in children with CF after LGG treatment ($P<0.05$).

CF. The hypothesis is supported by several lines of evidence. Recently, intestinal microbiota of identical twins with Crohn's disease were molecularly analyzed; results indicated that the microbial profiles of individuals with ileal involvement significantly differed from healthy controls and from patients with colonic involvement [32]. In particular, reduced abundance of *B. uniformis* and increased abundance of *B. ovatus* and *B. vulgatus* were detected in patients with Crohn's disease with ileal involvement as compared with those with colonic involvement and in healthy controls. *B. vulgatus* was also reduced in ileal specimens from children with Crohn's disease, ulcerative colitis, and indeterminate colitis as compared with control subjects [33]. Low levels of *B. vulgatus*, *B. ovatus*, *B. uniformis*, and *Parabacteroides* spp. were also detected in patients with ulcerative colitis and irritable bowel syndrome as compared with healthy controls [34].

We found a similar reduction in the abundance of *B. uniformis* and *B. vulgatus* in children with CF as compared with healthy controls. We also identified a significant reduction in *E. rectale* in children with CF. *E. rectale* is a butyrate-producing bacteria, and butyrate is the preferred energy source for colonic mucosa, protecting it from colitis and colorectal cancer and promoting the normal development of colonic epithelial cells. Short-chain fatty acids (SCFAs) play a protective role against intestinal inflammation, and it is possible that SCFA-producing intestinal microbiota may prevent intestinal inflammation. We speculate that the reduced load of *E. rectale*, *B. vulgatus*, and *B. uniformis* found in children with CF may be involved in intestinal inflammation.

We also found a significant inverse correlation between the richness of CF microbiota and intestinal inflammation. This was most evident in children with fecal CLP concentrations >200 μg/g, who showed a significantly lower number of bands in the upper part of the gel, which corresponds to *Bacteroides* (data not shown). Administration of antibiotics further reduced the same microbial species already reduced in children with CF as compared with healthy controls.

We further investigated the role of probiotic administration on intestinal microbiota. Lynch *et al.* recently reported that LGG administration affected the overall composition of intestinal microbiota in a population of infants at high risk for asthma [16]. This finding raised the hypothesis that administration of a single probiotic strain may globally modify the microbiota, thus promoting bacterial communities that modulate host immune responses. In the present study, LGG administration restored the composition of intestinal microbiota, making it more similar to that of healthy controls. There was a concurrent reduction in intestinal inflammation, similar to previous trials [7,13]. Together with previously reported benefits for respiratory exacerbations, hospital admissions, and respiratory function, our results indicate that LGG administration modifies intestinal microbiota and ultimately contributes to its beneficial clinical effects [7,13].

In conclusion, our data provide direct evidence that intestinal microbiota are disrupted in children with CF and is associated with intestinal inflammation. Antibiotic therapy exacerbates these abnormalities. The administration of LGG may partially restore a healthy intestinal microbiota, thus promoting communities that limit intestinal inflammation and improving the disease course.

Author Contributions

Conceived and designed the clinical trial: Alfredo Guarino, Eugenia Bruzzese, Valeria Raia, Andrea Lo Vecchio. Conceived and designed the microbiological experiments: Vittoria Buccigrossi, Marialuisa Callegari, Lorenzo Morelli. Performed microbiological experiments: Vittoria Buccigrossi, Marialuisa Callegari, Susanna Ferrari. Performed clinical trial: Eugenia Bruzzese, Sara Viscovo, Riccardo Scotto, Eliana Ruberto. Contributed reagents, materials and analysis tools: Vittoria Buccigrossi, Marialuisa Callegari. Analyzed the data: Valeria Raia, Eugenia Bruzzese, Andrea Lo Vecchio. Wrote the manuscript: Eugenia Bruzzese, Marialuisa Callegari, Alfredo Guarino.

References

1. Guarino A, Giannattasio A (2011) New molecular approaches in the diagnosis of acute diarrhea: advantages for clinicians and researches.Curr Opin Gastroenterol. 27: 24–9.
2. Musso G, Gambino R, Cassader M (2011) Interactions between gut microbiota and host metabolism predisposing to obesity and diabetes. Ann Rev Med.62: 361–80.
3. Bäckhed F, Manchester JK, Semenkovich CF, Gordon JI (2007) Mechanisms underlying the resistance to diet-induced obesity in germ-free mice. Proc Natl Acad Sci U S A 104: 979–84.
4. Turnbaugh PJ, Bäckhed F, Fulton L, Gordon JI (2008) Diet-induced obesity is linked to marked but reversible alterations in the mouse distal gut microbiome. Cell Host Microbe 3: 213–223.
5. Turnbaugh PJ, Hamady M, Yatsunenko T, Cantarel BL, Duncan A, et al (2009) A core gut microbiome in obese and lean twins. Nature 457: 480–484.
6. Lee JM, Leach ST, Katz T, Day AS, Jaffe A, et al (2012) Update of faecal markers of inflammation in children with cystic fibrosis. Mediators Inflamm 948367.
7. Bruzzese E, Raia V, Gaudiello G, Polito G, Buccigrossi V, et al. (2004) Intestinal inflammation is a frequent feature of cystic fibrosis and is reduced by probiotic administration. Aliment Pharmacol Ther 20: 813–819.
8. Werlin SL, Benuri-Silbiger I, Kerem E, Adler SN, Goldin E, et al. (2010) Evidence of Intestinal Inflammation in Patients With Cystic Fibrosis. J Pediatr Gastroenterol Nutr 51: 304–308.
9. Scanlan PD, Buckling A, Kong W, Wild Y, Lynch SV, et al (2012) Gut dysbiosis in cystic fibrosis. J Cyst Fibros. 11: 454–5.
10. Duytschaever G, Huys G, Bekaert M, Boulanger L, De Boeck K, et al (2011) Cross-sectional and longitudinal comparisons of the predominant fecal microbiota compositions of a group of pediatric patients with cystic fibrosis and their healthy siblings. Appl Environ Microbiol. 77: 8015–24.
11. Madan JC, Koestler DC, Stanton BA, Davidson L, Moulton LA, et al. (2012) Serial analysis of the gut and respiratory microbiome in Cystic Fibrosis in infancy: interaction between intestinal and respiratory tracts and impact of nutritional exposures. MBio.3 pii: e00251–12.
12. Duytschaever G, Huys G, Bekaert M, Boulanger L, De Boeck K, et al (2012) Dysbiosis of bifidobacteria and Clostridium cluster XIVa in the cystic fibrosis fecal microbiota. J Cyst Fibros. pii: S1569–1993(12)00183-X.
13. Bruzzese E, Raia V, Spagnuolo MI,Volpicelli M, De Marco G, et al. (2007) Effect of Lactobacillus GG supplementation on pulmonary exacerbations in patients with cystic fibrosis: a pilot study. Clin Nutr 26: 322–328.
14. Weiss B, Bujanover Y, Yahav Y, Vilozni D, Fireman E, et al. (2010) Probiotic supplementation affects pulmonary exacerbations in patients with cystic fibrosis: a pilot study. Pediatr Pulmonol. 45: 536–540.
15. Belenguer A, Duncan SH, Holtrop G, Anderson SE, Lobley GE, et al. (2007) Impact of pH on lactate formation and utilization by human fecal microbial communities. Appl Environ Microbiol. 73: 6526–6533.
16. Cox MJ, Huang YJ, Fujimura KE, Liu JT, McKean M, et al (2010) Lactobacillus casei abundance is associated with profound shifts in the infant gut microbiome. PLoS One. 5: e8745.
17. Kerem E. (2005) Pharmacological induction of CFTR function in patients with cystic fibrosis: mutation-specific therapy. Pediatr Pulmonol 40: 183–196.
18. Fagerberg UL, Loof L, Merzoug RD, Hansson LO, Finkel Y (2003) Fecal calprotectin levels in healthy children studied with an improved assay. J Pediatr Gastroenterol Nutr 37: 468–472.
19. Canani RB, Cirillo P, Bruzzese E, Graf M, Terrin G, et al. (2002) Nitric oxide production in rectal dialysate is a marker of disease activity and location in children with inflammatory bowel disease. Am J Gastroenterol 97: 1574–1576.
20. Walter J, Tannock GW, Tilsala-Timisjarvi A, Rodtong S, Loach DM, et al. (2000) Detection and identification of gastrointestinal Lactobacillus species by using denaturing gradient gel electrophoresis and species-specific PCR primers. Appl Environ Microbiol. 66: 297–303.
21. Bartosch S, Fite A, Macfarlane GT, McMurdo ME (2004) Characterization of bacterial communities in feces from healthy elderly volunteers and hospitalized elderly patients by using real-time PCR and effects of antibiotic treatment on the fecal microbiota. Appl Environ Microbiol. 70: 3575–3581.
22. Ahmed S, Macfarlane GT, Fite A, McBain AJ, Gilbert P, et al. (2007) Mucosa-associated bacterial diversity in relation to human terminal ileum and colonic biopsy samples. Appl Environ Microbiol. 73: 7435–7442.
23. Wu X, Ma C, Han L, Nawaz M, Gao F, et al. (2010) Molecular characterisation of the faecal microbiota in patients with type II diabetes. Curr Microbiol. 61: 69–78.
24. Penders J, Vink C, Driessen C, London N, Thijs C, et al. (2005) Quantification of *Bifidobacterium* spp., *Escherichia coli* and *Clostridium difficile* in faecal samples of breast-fed and formula-fed infants by real-time PCR. FEMS Microbiol Lett. 243: 141–147.
25. Sokol H, Pigneur B, Watterlot L, Lakhdari O, Bermúdez-Humarán LG, et al. (2008) *Faecalibacterium prausnitzii* is an anti-inflammatory commensal bacterium identified by gut microbiota analysis of Crohn disease patients. Proc Natl Acad Sci U S A. 105: 16731–6.
26. Swidsinski A, Loening-Baucke V, Verstraelen H, Osowska S, Doerffel Y (2008) Biostructure of fecal microbiota in healthy subjects and patients with chronic idiopathic diarrhea. Gastroenterology. 135: 568–79.
27. Daims H, Brühl A, Amann R, Schleifer KH, Wagner M (1999) The domain-specific probe EUB338 is insufficient for the detection of all Bacteria: development and evaluation of a more comprehensive probe set. Syst Appl Microbiol. 22: 434–44.
28. Scanlan PD, Shanahan F, O'Mahony C, Marchesi JR (2006) Culture-independent analyses of temporal variation of the dominant fecal microbiota and targeted bacterial subgroups in Crohn's disease. J Clin Microbiol. 44: 3980–3988.
29. Buccigrossi V, Nicastro E, Guarino A (2013) Functions of intestinal microflora in children. Curr Opin Gastroenterol. 29(1): 31–8.
30. Marteau P (2009) Bacterial flora in inflammatory bowel disease. Dig Dis.Suppl 1: 27 99–103.
31. Takaishi H, Matsuki T, Nakazawa A, Takada T, Kado S, et al. (2008) Imbalance in intestinal microflora constitution could be involved in the pathogenesis of inflammatory bowel disease. Int J Med Microbiol 298(5–6): 463–72.
32. Dicksved J, Halfvarson J, Rosenquist M, Järnerot G, Tysk C, et al. (2008) Molecular analysis of the gut microbiota of identical twins with Crohn's disease. ISME J 2: 716–727.
33. Conte MP, Schippa S, Zamboni I, Penta M, Chiarini F, et al. (2006) Gut-associated bacterial microbiota in paediatric patients with inflammatory bowel disease. Gut 55: 1760–1767.
34. Noor SO, Ridgway K, Scovell L, Kemsley EK, Lund EK, et al. (2010) Ulcerative colitis and irritable bowel patients exhibit distinct abnormalities of the gut microbiota. BMC Gastroenterol 10: 134.

4

Cystic Fibrosis Bronchial Epithelial Cells Are Lipointoxicated by Membrane Palmitate Accumulation

Laurie-Anne Payet[1], Linette Kadri[2], Sébastien Giraud[3,4,5], Caroline Norez[1], Jean Marc Berjeaud[2], Christophe Jayle[6], Sandra Mirval[1], Frédéric Becq[1], Clarisse Vandebrouck[1], Thierry Ferreira[1]*

1 Signalisation et Transports Ioniques Membranaires, ERL CNRS 7368, Université de Poitiers, Poitiers, France, **2** Ecologie et Biologie des Interactions, UMR CNRS 7267, Université de Poitiers, Poitiers, France, **3** Service de Biochimie, CHU Poitiers, Poitiers, France, **4** Inserm U1082, Poitiers, France, **5** Faculté de Médecine et de Pharmacie Université de Poitiers, Poitiers, France, **6** Service de Chirurgie Cardiothoracique, CHU Poitiers, Poitiers, France

Abstract

The *F508del-CFTR* mutation, responsible for Cystic Fibrosis (CF), leads to the retention of the protein in the endoplasmic reticulum (ER). The mistrafficking of this mutant form can be corrected by pharmacological chaperones, but these molecules showed limitations in clinical trials. We therefore hypothesized that important factors in CF patients may have not been considered in the *in vitro* assays. CF has also been associated with an altered lipid homeostasis, *i. e.* a decrease in polyunsaturated fatty acid levels in plasma and tissues. However, the precise fatty acyl content of membrane phospholipids from human CF bronchial epithelial cells had not been studied to date. Since the saturation level of phospholipids can modulate crucial membrane properties, with potential impacts on membrane protein folding/trafficking, we analyzed this parameter for freshly isolated bronchial epithelial cells from CF patients. Interestingly, we could show that Palmitate, a saturated fatty acid, accumulates within Phosphatidylcholine (PC) in CF freshly isolated cells, in a process that could result from hypoxia. The observed PC pattern can be recapitulated in the CFBE41o$^-$ cell line by incubation with 100 μM Palmitate. At this concentration, Palmitate induces an ER stress, impacts calcium homeostasis and leads to a decrease in the activity of the corrected F508del-CFTR. Overall, these data suggest that bronchial epithelial cells are lipointoxicated by hypoxia-related Palmitate accumulation in CF patients. We propose that this phenomenon could be an important bottleneck for F508del-CFTR trafficking correction by pharmacological agents in clinical trials.

Editor: Shama Ahmad, University of Colorado, Denver, United States of America

Funding: Funding provided by Ministère de l'Enseignement supérieur et de la Recherche (http://www.enseignementsup-recherche.gouv.fr/); Vaincre La Mucoviscidose (http://www.vaincrelamuco.org/); Centre National de la Recherche Scientifique (http://www.cnrs.fr/). The funders had no role in study design, data collection and analysis, decision to publish, or preparation of the manuscript.

Competing Interests: The authors have declared that no competing interests exist.

* E-mail: thierry.ferreira@univ-poitiers.fr

Introduction

Cystic fibrosis (CF) is a genetic disease caused by mutations in the *CFTR* (CF Transmembrane conductance Regulator) gene, encoding a plasma-membrane chloride channel. Although this disease has been described for the first time in 1936 and 1938 by Franconi and Anderson, respectively, as the CF of the pancreas [1,2], the corresponding gene was identified later in 1989 [3,4]. More than 1,900 mutations of *CFTR* responsible for the disease have now been listed by the Cystic Fibrosis Genetic Analysis Consortium. The most common mutation worldwide, the deletion of phenylalanine at position 508 (*F508del-CFTR*), leads to the mistrafficking of the corresponding protein, resulting in its retention in the endoplasmic reticulum (ER) and its degradation by the ER-associated protein degradation (ERAD) pathway [5–7].

Since the *CFTR* gene discovery, many efforts have been concentrated on correcting the F508del-CFTR trafficking defect. Some molecules were found to act as pharmacological chaperones or as proteostasis modulators during the F508del-CFTR folding process in the ER, restoring its trafficking to the plasma membrane. Among these correctors, 4-PBA (sodium 4-phenylbutyrate) [8], CPX (8-cyclopentyl-1,3-dipropylxanthine) [8], VX809 [9] and miglustat [10] have been tested in clinical trials but, until now, they appeared to be less efficient *in vivo* than *in vitro* [11–14]. Our study falls within this context. We hypothesized that important factors in CF patients may have not been taken into consideration in the *in vitro* assays, therefore accounting for the clinical trial failure.

Long before the *CFTR* gene discovery, CF had already been related to an altered lipid homeostasis. Indeed, the disease had been associated since the early 60's to low concentrations of polyunsaturated fatty acids (PUFA), such as linoleic acid (C18:2, [15]) and docosahexaenoic acid (C22:6, [16–18]), in CF patient plasma and tissues. Fatty acids (FA) are the components of phospholipids (PL) and the species containing PUFA were also shown to be decreased in the plasma of CF patients, particularly phosphatidylcholine (PC) containing PUFA [19].

Nevertheless, to the best of our knowledge, there is no study that clearly determined the precise fatty acyl content of membrane phospholipids in bronchial epithelial cells from CF patients. More specifically, several studies in different cellular models demonstrated that the ratio of Unsaturated (UFA) versus Saturated Fatty Acid (SFA) phospholipid-containing species regulate crucial membrane biophysical properties and therefore control the functionality of intracellular organelles [20,21]. As an example, in previous studies using a simple eukaryotic model, the yeast *Saccharomyces cerevisiae*, we could show that SFA accumulation within PL decreases membrane fluidity [22], and induces the accumulation of misfolded proteins within the ER, which results in the induction of an ER-based response referred to as the Unfolded Protein Response (UPR). When sustained, UPR induction results in an ER-stress, which can ultimately lead to cell death by apoptosis [21]. Vesicular budding at the *Trans* Golgi network [23] and then membrane protein trafficking latter in the secretory pathway are also altered under SFA accumulation [20]. In other words, increased SFA amounts within PL impact the secretory pathway as a whole [23]. If such a process occurred in CF cells *in vivo* (*i. e.* SFA-containing PL increasing at the expense of UFA-containing species), it could alter F508del-CFTR trafficking correction by pharmacological means.

In the present study, we therefore focused on the fatty acyl content of membrane PL in bronchial epithelial cells from CF patients. We first show that Palmitate (C16:0) accumulates within PC from CF patient cells but not in the corresponding CFBE41o$^-$ cell line. Then, this CF cellular model was optimized to mimic the PL content encountered *in vivo* by adding exogenous Palmitate to the culture medium. At a concentration of 100 µM Palmitate, which results in a PC pattern very similar to the one observed in freshly isolated CF patient cells, CFBE41o$^-$ cells do not fall prey to apoptosis, but they appear to experience an ER stress. Moreover, extracellular Ca^{2+} influx and F508del-CFTR correction by pharmacological agents are significantly altered by Palmitate accumulation within PL.

Materials and Methods

Ethics Statement

The study was approved by our local institutional ethics committee (Comité de Protection des Personnes (CPP) Ouest III). All participants provided their written informed consent to participate in this study, and the ethics committee approved this consent procedure.

Freshly Isolated Bronchial Epithelial Cells

Human lung tissue was obtained from seventeen individuals: five non-CF males with a mean age of 61 yrs, two non-CF females with a mean age of 67 yrs, four *F508del/F508del-CFTR* males with a mean age of 27 yrs, and six *F508del/F508del-CFTR* females with a mean age of 28 yrs. Following lobectomy, lung samples were quickly dissected. After removal of connective tissues, cartilage and smooth muscle tissues, bronchial tubes were washed at least three times with phosphate-buffered saline (PBS, Gibco) and cut out in small segments. Epithelial cells were dissociated using enzymatic isolation for 24 h at 4°C with 0.1% protease and 0.01% deoxyribonuclease in a decontamination medium composed by Dulbecco's modified Eagle's medium-Ham's F-12 medium (DMEM/Ham's F12, Gibco) supplemented with penicillin/streptomycin 1 mg/mL (Sigma-Aldrich), amphotericin B 100 µg/mL (Sigma-Aldrich), gentamycin 0.5 mg/mL (Sigma-Aldrich) for non-CF samples and the same medium supplemented with ceftazidin 500 µg/mL (Sigma-Aldrich) and ticarcilin 500 µg/mL (Sigma-Aldrich) for CF samples. After neutralization by 10% fetal bovine serum (FBS), cells were centrifuged at 600 rpm for 6 min. Freshly isolated bronchial epithelial cells were washed three times with PBS and counted using a Malassez cell.

Cell Culture

The human CF and non-CF bronchial epithelial CFBE41o$^-$ (homozygote *F508del-CFTR*) and 16HBE14o$^-$ (wild type CFTR) cell lines were grown at 37°C in 5% CO_2 and 95% O_2 on Corning® CellBIND® surface cell culture flasks (Sigma-Aldrich), in a minimum essential medium containing L-glutamine (MEM, 31095, Gibco) and supplemented with plasmocin (5 µg/mL) and 10% serum (FBS or horse serum, HS). Frozen cells in FBS were thawed in a FBS-containing medium [24]. Two days after the thawing, cells are incubated in a medium containing 5% FBS and 5% HS during 48 h, before switching in a medium containing only HS. Culture medium was renewed at 2-day intervals. For hypoxia experiments, cells were grown into a hypoxia chamber at 37°C in 5% CO_2 and 95% N_2 during 48 h.

Fatty Acid (FA) Preparation and Cell Treatment

Palmitate preparation was described by Karaskov and colleagues [25]. Briefly, 10 mM Palmitate (Sigma-Aldrich) stocks were prepared in filtered 0.1 M NaOH and heated at 70°C. A 5% (w/v) FA-free BSA (Sigma-Aldrich) solution was prepared in double distilled H_2O and filtered. A five time more concentrated FFA/BSA solution (for example, 5 mM FFA/5% BSA) was prepared by complexing an appropriate amount of FFA to 5% BSA in a 60°C water bath. The above solution was then cooled to room temperature and diluted 1:5 in culture medium without HS to the appropriate final concentration (for example 1 mM FFA/1% BSA) for cells incubation during 16 h.

Lipid Extraction, Phospholipid Purification and Mass Spectrometry Analyses

Lipid extracts were prepared from approximately 10^5 cells, grown as indicated. Cells were harvested, washed with PBS and the cell pellets were resuspended in 1 mL of water and transferred into glass tubes with 500 µL of glass beads (diameter 0.3–0.4 mm; Sigma-Aldrich). Lipids were extracted using chloroform/methanol (2:1, v/v) and shaking on an orbital shaker (IKA® VXR basic Vibrax®, Sigma-Aldrich) at 1,500 rpm during at least 1 h. The protocol used was described by Folch et *al.* [26]. The final organic phase was evaporated and dissolved in 100 µL chloroform/methanol/H_2O (16:16:5, v/v/v) for analysis of total lipids by mass spectrometry or 100 µL dichloromethane for PL purification on a silica column (Bond ELUT-SI 100 mg 1 mL, Agilent Technologies).

Before PL purification, the silica column was washed with 3 mL methanol and 2 mL dichloromethane. Lipid samples were loaded on the top of the column. Non polar lipids were eluted by addition of 2 mL dichloromethane, and glycolipids with 3 mL acetone. PL were then eluted by 2 mL chloroform/methanol/H_2O (50:45:5, v/v/v).

To analyze PC species by ESI-MS (Electrospray Ionization Mass Spectrometry) in the positive ion mode, total lipid extracts or purified PL were evaporated and reconstituted in 1% (v/v) formic acid. The molecular profile of PC species was specifically obtained by scanning for the positive ion precursors of m/z 184, characteristic of choline phosphate. Due to material limitations, particularly with freshly isolated bronchial epithelial cells, samples were not analyzed in the negative ion mode in this study.

RT-qPCR

RNA extraction was from 10^7 cells using a commercial kit (RNeasy Mini Kit, Qiagen). Reverse transcription-PCR (RT-PCR) was done with SuperScript II (Invitrogen) using the procedure supplied by the manufacturer. Hypoxia-inducible factor 1α (*HIF1*) expression was assessed relative to Glyceraldehyde 3-phosphate dehydrogenase (*GAPDH*) expression by real-time quantitative PCR (RT-qPCR) with the GeneAmp 9500 Sequence

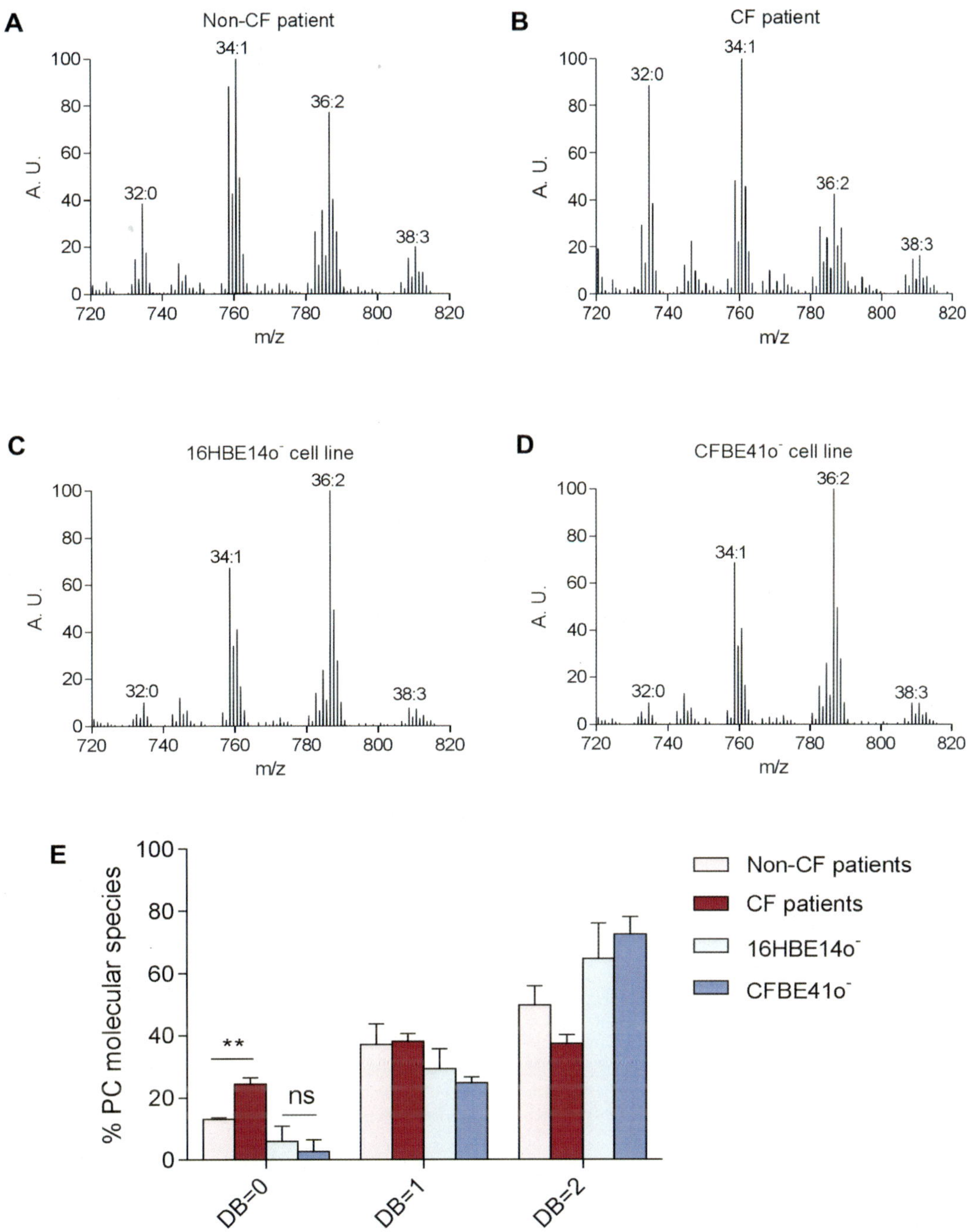

Figure 1. PC profiles of CF and non-CF cells. Characteristic PC profiles (positive ion mode) obtained from bronchial epithelial cells of A) non-CF or B) CF patient lungs, and from C) non-CF and D) CF bronchial epithelial cell lines. The total carbon chain length (x) and number of carbon-carbon double bounds (y) of the main PC molecular species are indicated (x:y). A. U., arbitrary unit. E) The relative percentage of saturated (DB = 0) versus monounsaturated (DB = 1) and diunsaturated (DB = 2) species were calculated from the mass spectra. Values are means ± SEM of at least three independent measurements. The *P*value was calculated by a two-tailed *t* test, using Graphpad Prism 6 software. **: $p<0.01$. ns: no significant difference. Schematic representations of the major PC species are included.

Detection System and SYBR Green chemistry (Applied Biosystems). The RT-qPCR primers used were: *GAPDH*, 5′-TGCACCACCAACTGCTTAGC-3′ and 5′-GGCATGGACTGTGGTCATGAG-3′; and *HIF-1α*, 5′-CATTACCCACCGCTGAAACG-3′ and 5′-TTCACTGGGACTATTAGGCTC-3′ [27].

Apoptosis Quantification

Palmitate-induced apoptosis was monitored using the cell death detection kit ELISA^{PLUS} (Roche). CFBE41o^{-} cells were seeded in 96-well plates (10,000 cells per well). 4 h later, cells were incubated with BSA-conjugated Palmitate in a serum-free medium during 16 h. After the treatment, cells were lysed and apoptosis was measured according to the manufacturer's instructions by

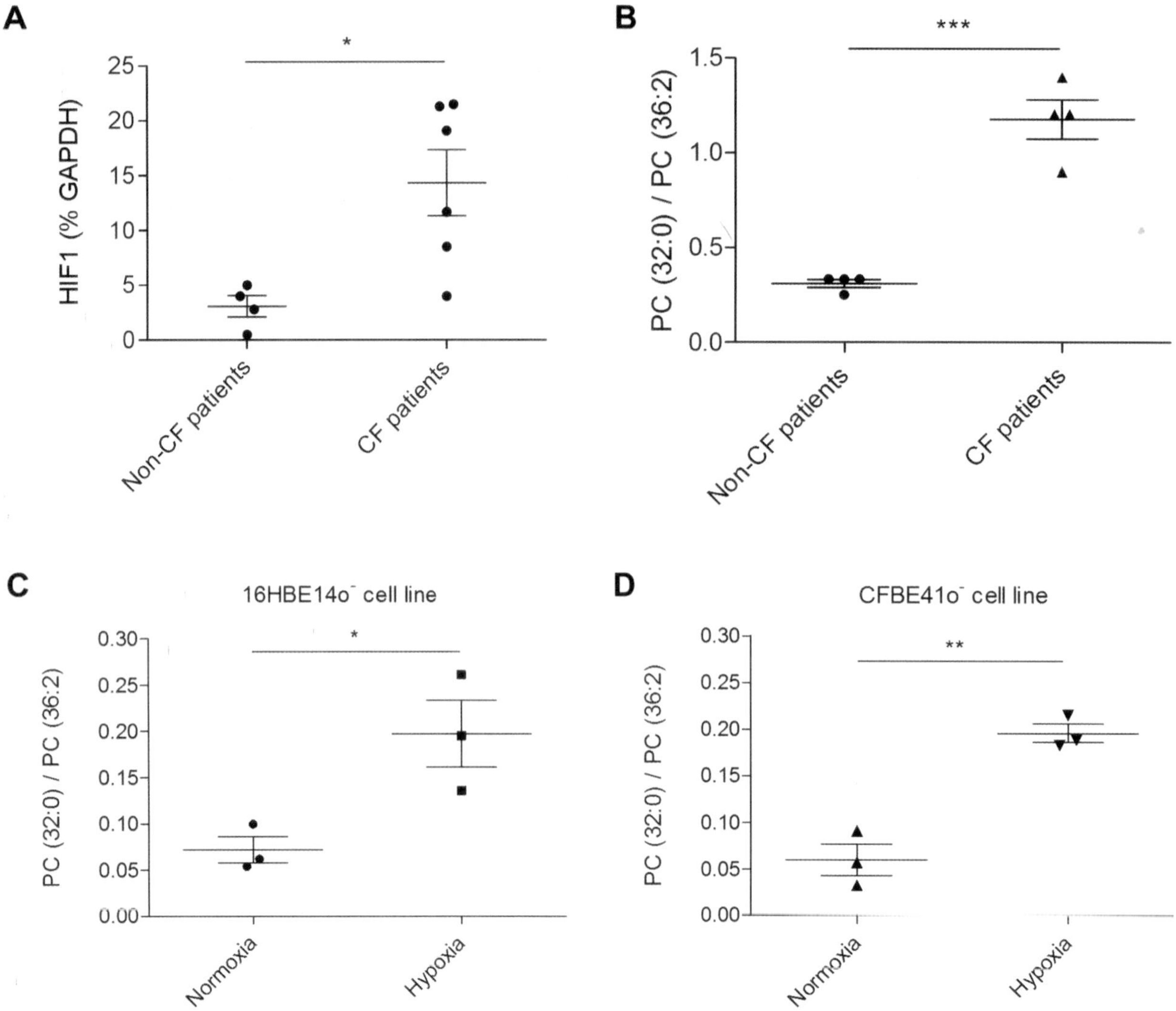

Figure 2. Relationship between PC saturation rate and hypoxia. A) *HIF1α* expression in non CF and CF patient bronchial epithelial cells, expressed as a percentage of *GAPDH*, used as a standard. Each point represents the mean of three determinations for one patient sample. Saturation rate (SR) of B) patient cells, C) non-CF and D) CF bronchial epithelial cell lines after incubation or not into a hypoxia chamber without oxygen during 48 hours. SR corresponds to the ratio PC(32:0)/PC(36:2), calculated from the mass spectra. Each point represents the mean of three determinations for one patient or one passage. Means ± SEM are indicated. The *P*value was calculated by a two-tailed *t* test, using Graphpad Prism 6 software. *: $p<0.05$. **: $p<0.01$. ***: $p<0.001$.

quantifying cytoplasmic oligonucleosomes which are indicative of apoptosis-associated DNA degradation.

Western Blot

Cells grown on a 60 mm dish were lysed by scraping after addition of 100 μL lysis buffer: Tris 10 mM pH 7.5, NP40 1% (v/v), DOC 0.5% (w/v) supplemented with a cocktail of protease inhibitors (Roche, 2%, v/v) and the phosphatase inhibitor cocktail 3 (Sigma-Aldrich, 1%, v/v). Total proteins were quantified using the bicinchoninic acid (BCA) protein assay (Sigma-Aldrich). 40 μg of total protein extract were resolved by SDS-PAGE, transferred to nitrocellulose membranes and immunoblotted with antibodies directed against the phosphorylated eukaryotic translation initiation factor 2α (P-eIF2α, Cell Signaling, 1:200), eIF2α (Cell Signaling; no. 9722, 1:500) and β tubulin (Santa Cruz Biotechnology, 1:2000). After incubation with the secondary antibody (donkey anti-rabbit IgG, or sheep anti-mouse IgG, GE Healthcare, 1:5000) conjugated to horseradish peroxidase (HRP), the bands were detected with the Immobilon Western Chemiluminescent HRP substrate (Merck Millipore, USA) or with ECL Select™ (GE Healthcare). Immunoblots were scanned and quantified by densitometry using ImageJ software.

Calcium Signal Recording

CFBE41o⁻ cells, grown till 80% of confluence on a glass slide, were incubated or not with Palmitate during 16 h. Then, they were loaded with 3 μM Fluo-4 acetoxymethyl (AM) ester (FluoProbes®) for 20 min at room temperature in a $2Ca^{2+}$ buffer solution (NaCl 118.4 mM, KCl 4.7 mM, $CaCl_2$ 2.5 mM, KH_2PO_4 1.2 mM, $MgSO_4$ 1.2 mM, $NaHCO_3$ 25 mM, Glucose 11.7 mM, pH 7.4). Global Ca^{2+} mobilization was induced by the addition of 100 μM ATP. For ER Ca^{2+} store depletion, induced by the addition of 10 μM thapsigargin, $2Ca^{2+}$ buffer solution was replaced by $0Ca^{2+}$ buffer solution (NaCl 118.4 mM, KCl 4.7 mM,

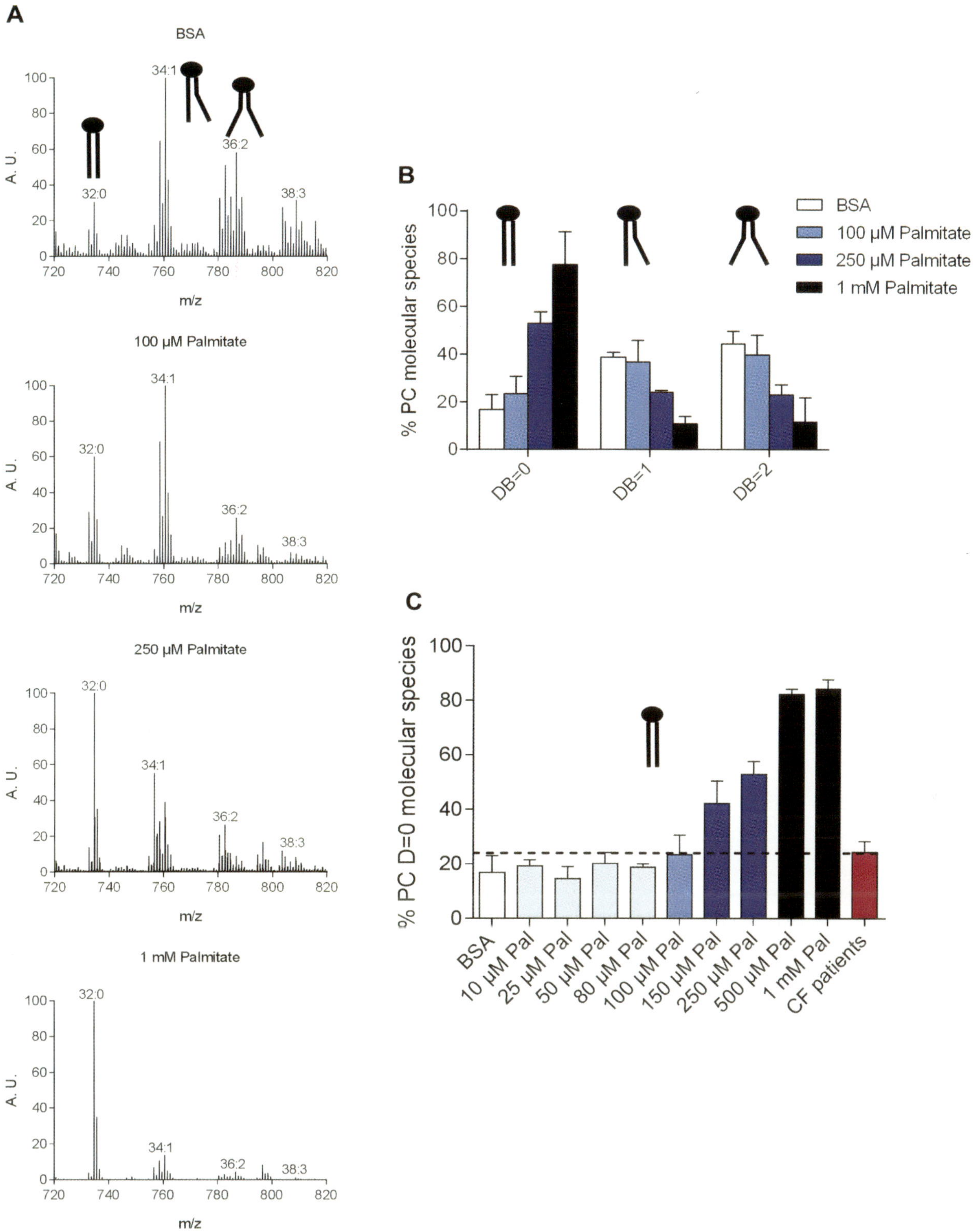

Figure 3. Effects of exogenous Palmitate intake on the fatty acyl content of PC. A) Positive ion mass spectra specific for molecular species of PC extracted from CFBE41o⁻ cells after incubation with 1% BSA, 100 μM Palmitate, 250 μM Palmitate or 1 mM Palmitate during 16 h. The total carbon chain length (x) and number of carbon-carbon double bounds (y) of the main PC molecular species (x:y) are indicated. A. U., arbitrary unit. B) Relative percentage of saturated (DB = 0) versus monounsaturated (DB = 1) and diunsaturated (DB = 2) species of CFBE41o⁻ after incubation with Palmitate at the indicated concentrations, were calculated from the mass spectra. C) Relative percentage of saturated PC species of CFBE41o⁻ cells after incubation with Palmitate concentrations ranged from 0 to 1 mM. Values are means ± SD of at least three independent measurements. Schematic representations of the major PC species are included.

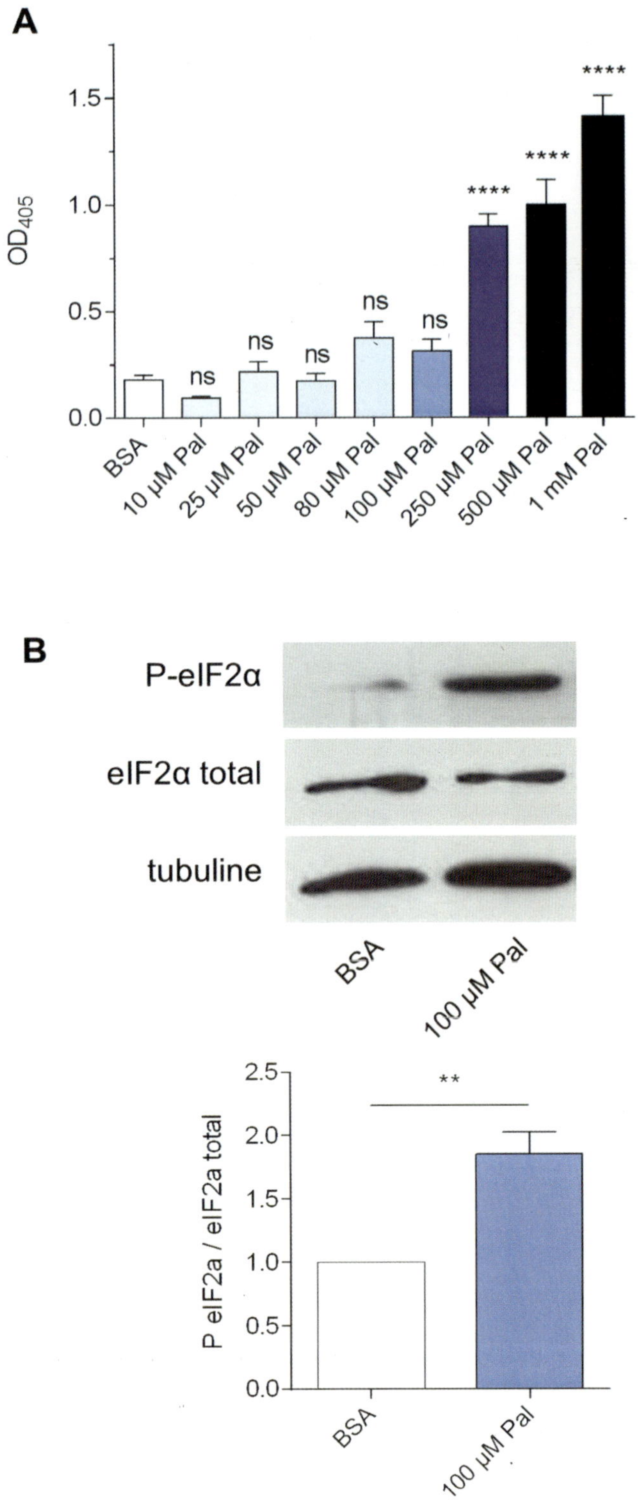

Figure 4. Effects of fatty acyl content of PC on apoptosis induction. A) Apoptosis quantification in CFBE41o$^-$ cells after incubation with Palmitate, during 16 h, using the cell death detection ELISA^{PLUS} kit (Roche). The *P*value was calculated by a One-way ANOVA test, using Graphpad Prism 6 software. ****: $P<0.0001$; ns, no significant difference compared to the control (BSA). B) Phosphorylation rate of eIF2α, an ER stress marker. Top: representative western blot of total protein extracts from CFBE41o$^-$ cells after treatment with BSA (control) or 100 µM Palmitate. Bottom: quantification of eIF2α phosphorylation as ratios of P-eIF2α versus total eIF2α, assuming a value of 1 for the ratio determined from the control. All values, obtained from five independent experiments, were normalized to a loading control (β tubulin). Means ± SEM are represented. The *P*value was calculated by a two-tailed *t* test, using Graphpad Prism 6 software. **: $p<0.01$.

KH_2PO_4 1.2 mM, $MgSO_4$ 1.2 mM, $NaHCO_3$ 25 mM, Glucose 11.7 mM, pH 7.4) just before recording. Ca^{2+} activity was assessed using a Zeiss Axio observer Z1 inverted microscope and the Carl Zeiss AxioVision Release 4.8.2 software. Fluorescence intensity of selected cells was measured every 2 sec during 5 min. Intensity profiles were normalized by dividing the fluorescence intensity of each pixel (F) by the average resting value before stimulation (F0) to generate an (F − F0/F0) image. All experiments were performed on a minimum of two different cell passages.

Iodide Efflux

The activity of swelling-dependent (Cl_{swell}), Ca^{2+}-dependent (Cl_{Ca}) and CFTR Cl^- channels was assessed on the CFBE41o$^-$ cell population by the iodide ($^{125}I^-$) efflux technique as already described [28]. Curves were constructed by plotting the rate of $^{125}I^-$ versus time. All comparisons were based on maximal values for the time-dependent rates (k = peak rates, min^{-1}), excluding the points used to establish the baseline ($k_{peak} - k_{basal}$, min^{-1}). All chemicals were from Sigma-Aldrich, except for miglustat (Toronto Research Chemicals, Canada) diluted in water, forskoline and genistein (LC Laboratories, USA) diluted in DMSO.

Results

Palmitate Accumulates within PC of Bronchial Epithelial Cells from CF Individuals, but this Accumulation is Not Directly Related to the F508del-CFTR Mutation

Lipids extracted from bronchial epithelial cells of non-CF and CF patient lung samples were analyzed by mass spectrometry. Examples of characteristic positive ion mode spectra are displayed in Figure 1A (non-CF patient) and 1B (CF patient). For peak assignment, ions were subjected to ion scan analyses as described previously [29]. In this figure, the main peaks corresponding to molecular species of PC are indicated. The detailed composition of the various PC species in each sample is displayed in Table S1 in File S1. Interestingly, the most prominent differences between non-CF and CF patients were not observed for PC species bearing PUFA chains (*e. g.* PC(38:3); compare Fig. 1A and 1B). Moreover, PC species bearing longer polyunsaturates were hardly detectable in freshly isolated bronchial epithelial cells (not-shown). Rather, the obtained PC profiles revealed that PC(32:0), a PC species bearing two saturated (*i. e.* Palmitate C16:0) side chains, was very abundant in CF patient (2-fold increase; Fig. 1B), as compared to non-CF patient cells (Fig. 1A and Table S1 in File S1). This shift towards more saturated lipids can be visualized by representing the PC Double-Bond (DB) index (Fig. 1E). As shown, in CF patients, this shift is manifested by a dramatic increase of PC with two saturated acyl chains (*i.e.* total number of double bonds in both acyl chains is zero; DB = 0) at the expense of PC with two monounsaturated acyl chains (DB = 2). As shown on Figure 1A, the most represented DB = 2 species is PC(36:2), which corresponds to a PC species bearing two Oleate chains (C18:1). To check the link between the *F508del-CFTR* mutation and Palmitate accumulation within PC, the same experiment was performed on non-CF (Fig. 1C) and CF (Fig. 1D) bronchial epithelial cell lines. Since the fatty acid composition of cells in culture is reflective of what is present in the cell culture media, the cell lines were grown in horse serum which displays a fatty acid profile that matches at best the one encountered in the human plasma [24]. Surprisingly, the two cell lines displayed the exact same PC profile, and no

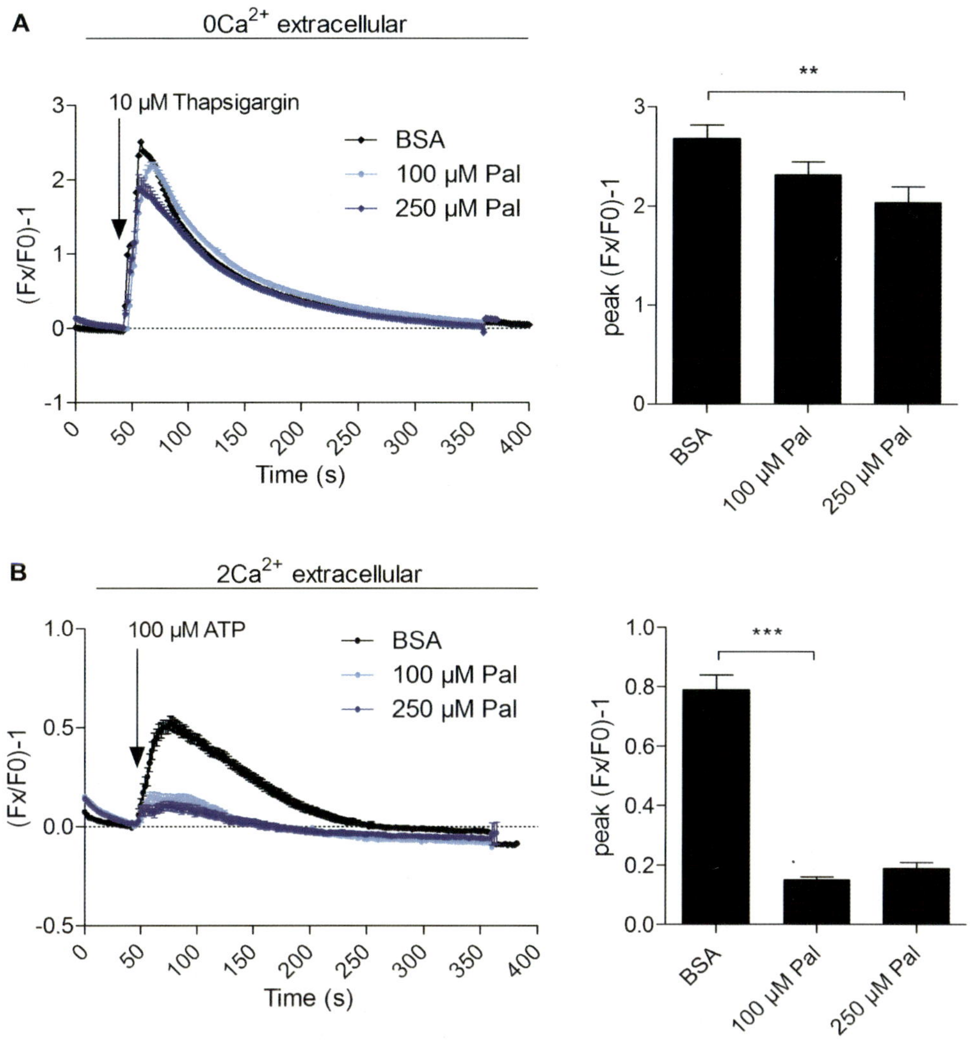

Figure 5. Effects of fatty acyl content on Ca^{2+} activity. Functional characterization of Ca^{2+} activity in CFBE41o$^-$ cells after incubation with Palmitate, using the fluorescent Ca^{2+} probe Fluo4-AM. A) Representative traces of ER Ca^{2+} store depletion induced by 10 μM thapsigargin in the absence of extracellular Ca^{2+} (left) and corresponding histograms showing peak intensity (right). B) Representative traces of global Ca^{2+} mobilization induced by 100 μM ATP in the presence of extracellular Ca^{2+} (left) and corresponding histograms showing peak intensity (right). The experiments were performed on at least 60 cells from a minimum of 2 different passages. Values are means ± SEM. The *P*value was calculated by a two-tailed *t* test, using Graphpad Prism 6 software. **: $p<0.01$. ***: $p<0.001$.

Palmitate accumulation within PC was observed in the presence of the *F508del-CFTR* mutation (compare Fig. 1C and 1D; Table S1 in File S1). Therefore, despite the fact that CFBE41o$^-$ cells are bronchial epithelial cells and that they are homozygous for the *F508del-CFTR* mutation as the cells collected from patients, they do not reflect the PC pattern observed in freshly isolated cells.

The Palmitate Accumulation within PC Could be the Result of Hypoxia

This Palmitate accumulation within PC in CF patient cells could be of physiological relevance since we have already shown that saturated PL impact the secretory pathway by altering membrane properties [22] and, as a consequence, the trafficking of plasma-membrane proteins to their final destination [20,21,23]. In order to improve the CFBE41o$^-$ model in terms of its lipid composition, we tried to figure out what could be the origin of this Palmitate accumulation within PC in the lungs of CF individuals. Based on the literature and physiological observations, we hypothesized that hypoxia could be the link between the disease and the observed Palmitate accumulation. Indeed, in CF, respiratory airways are obstructed by a thick layer of viscous mucus, which deprives the epithelial cells of oxygen [30]. Furthermore, enzymes that desaturate FA (*i. e.* which catalyze the conversion of a single bound between two carbon atoms (C-C) to a double bound (C=C) in fatty acyl chains) are oxygen-dependent [31]. In the case of a decrease in oxygen availability, they are not functional anymore and SFA tend to accumulate within the cells. Relevantly, this property was fruitfully used in yeast to provoke SFA-accumulation within PL [32]. To test this hypothesis, the expression of the hypoxia-inducible factor 1α (*HIF1α*), a transcription factor activated by the decrease in oxygen availability [33], was determined in bronchial epithelial cells from CF and non-CF patient lungs (Fig. 2A). Interestingly, *HIF1α* expression levels were significantly higher in CF patient cells compared to the non-CF ones, therefore reinforcing our original hypothesis.

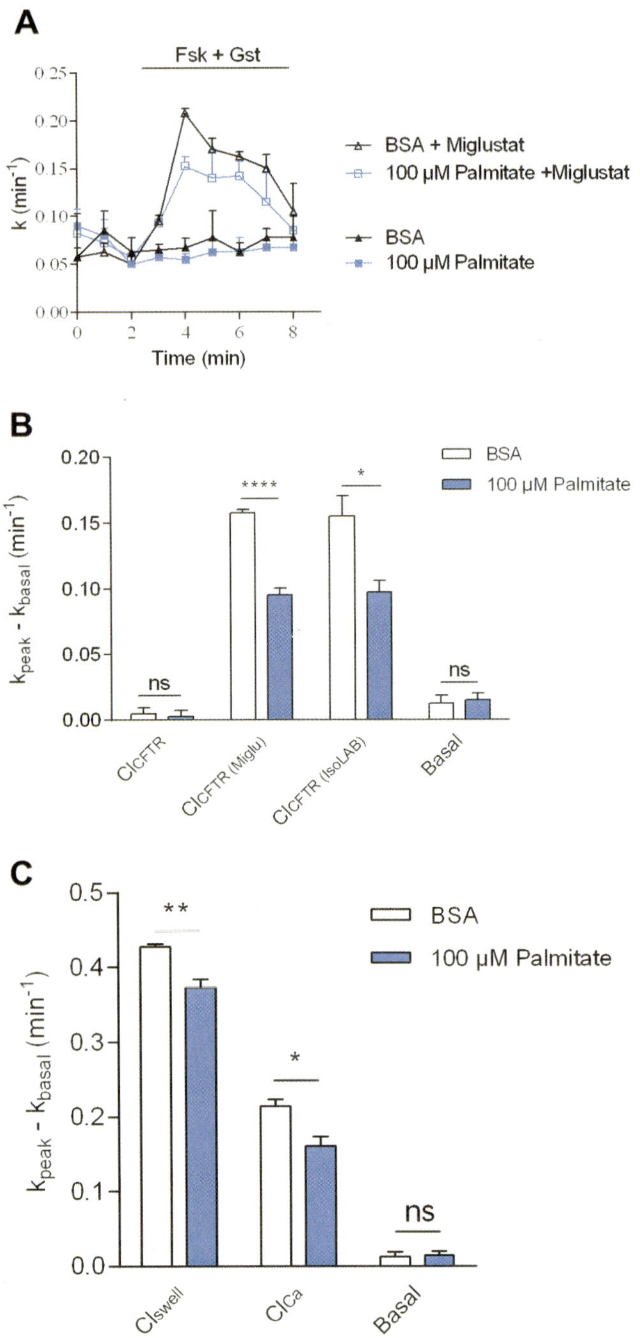

Figure 6. Effects of fatty acyl content of PC on Cl^- channels activity. A) Representative traces of iodide efflux curves obtained after stimulation of the F508del-CFTR activity by Forskoline (Fsk, 10 μM)+ Genistein (Gst, 30 μM) in CFBE41o$^-$ cells incubated or not with 100 μM Palmitate, and treated with 100 μM miglustat during 2 h. B) Histograms show the mean relative rate of F508del-CFTR activity corrected or not by miglustat (*n* = 4) or isoLAB (*n* = 4) after treatment with Palmitate. C) Histograms show the mean relative rate of Cl_{swell} after its stimulation by an osmotic shock, and Cl_{Ca} after its stimulation by the calcium ionophore A23187 (1 μM) in CFBE41o$^-$ cells treated or not with Palmitate (*n* = 4). Means ± SEM are indicated. The *P*value was calculated by a two-tailed *t* test, using Graphpad Prism 6 software. *: $p<0.05$. **: $p<0.01$. ****: $p<0.0001$. ns: no significant difference compared to the control (BSA).

In a next step, we tried to recreate the hypoxia conditions *in vitro*, by growing 16HBE14o$^-$ and CFBE41o$^-$ cells in a hypoxia chamber, where oxygen can be totally replaced by nitrogen (Fig. 2C and 2D). After 48 h under these conditions, lipids were extracted from the cells and analyzed by mass spectrometry (detailed PC compositions are given in Table S2 in File S1). To get a more quantitative vision, the saturation rate, corresponding to the ratio of the characteristic PC(32:0) over PC(36:2) species (Fig. 1) was calculated from the mass spectra obtained. The analyses revealed that the saturation rate was 4-fold higher in hypoxia than under normoxia for both cell lines. In other words, oxygen scarcity resulted in the accumulation of Palmitate within PC species. However, the saturation rates obtained under hypoxic conditions were not as spectacular as the ones observed *in vivo* (Fig. 2B). These discrepancies are likely related to the following facts/observations: *i*) the original PC(32:0) levels in both cell lines grown under normoxia were very low, even when compared to the profiles obtained from non-CF patient cells (Fig. 1E), *ii*) a 48 h incubation in the hypoxia chamber may not fully mimic the chronic hypoxia that CF patients are subjected to, and iii) complete oxygen deprivation in the hypoxia chamber reduced the cell division rate (our unpublished data), with likely impacts on PC turn-over and, as a consequence, SFA-accumulation rates within this phospholipid species.

Altogether, if these experiments clearly demonstrated that hypoxia could account for the Palmitate accumulation observed in patient lungs, the use of a hypoxia chamber to mimic the CF PC pattern in the CFBE41o$^-$ cell line showed important limitations.

Exogenous Palmitate Intake can be used to Mimic the PC Pattern Observed in Freshly Isolated CF Bronchial Epithelial Cells

In order to evaluate the impacts of Palmitate accumulation within PC in CF cells, we therefore developed an alternative strategy to improve Palmitate accumulation within the CFBE41o$^-$ cells: this consisted in supplying the culture medium with an exogenous Palmitate source. This approach proved to be efficient with different cellular models, including mammalian β-cells and hepatocytes [25,34]. BSA-conjugated Palmitate was added to the CFBE41o$^-$ cell cultures without serum at a final concentration of 1 mM, for 16 h. Lipids were extracted and purified PL were analyzed by mass spectrometry. As shown on Fig. 3A, CFBE41o$^-$ cells incubated with 1% BSA displayed a non CF-like PC profile (Fig. 1A). In contrast, when incubated with 1% BSA-1 mM Palmitate, PC(32:0) became the major, if not the only, PC species in CFBE41o$^-$ cells. These data indicate that exogenous Palmitate can be efficiently incorporated within PC, but that a concentration of 1 mM Palmitate is too high to reproduce the PC pattern observed in freshly isolated cells.

Therefore, various BSA-conjugated Palmitate concentrations, ranging from 0 to 1 mM Palmitate, were tested. The characteristic PC profiles obtained with 1% BSA, 100 μM, 250 μM and 1 mM Palmitate (Fig. 3A), showed that PC(32:0) species levels increased with Palmitate concentration in the culture medium (detailed PC compositions are given in Table S3 in File S1). More generally, increasing the exogenous Palmitate supply resulted in an increase of the saturated species (Fig. 3B, DB = 0), at the expense of the mono- and diunsaturated species (Fig. 3B; DB = 1 and DB = 2, respectively). To find the concentration which could mimic the CF PC pattern at best, we compared the DB = 0 obtained for each tested concentration with the one obtained for CF patients (Fig. 3C). 100 μM Palmitate resulted in a PC profile matching at best the CF PC pattern. Therefore, this concentration was retained for further experiments.

High PC Saturation Rates Induce Apoptosis in Bronchial Epithelial Cells

In β cells, Palmitate accumulation, obtained by the addition of 500 μM Palmitate in the culture medium, has been shown to induce apoptosis [35]. We therefore evaluated whether this could be also the case for bronchial epithelial cells under Palmitate treatment. To this aim, after incubation of CFBE41o$^-$ cells with the same range of Palmitate concentrations used for the PC profile study, induction of apoptosis was monitored using a commercial kit that measures the accumulation of cytoplasmic histone-associated DNA fragments, a characteristic trademark of apoptosis [36]. As shown on Fig. 4A, apoptosis was significantly induced in this cell type from a Palmitate concentration of 250 μM.

Interestingly, the Palmitate concentration of 100 μM, which results in a PC pattern similar to the one encountered in CF patients, was not associated with a clear-cut induction of apoptosis in CFBE41o$^-$ cells (Fig. 4A). In yeast and in β cells, apoptosis induction by SFA, and particularly Palmitate, is paralleled by the induction of an ER-based stress response, namely the UPR [21,37]. We therefore questioned if, at this Palmitate concentration, CFBE41o$^-$ cells could somehow experience such an ER-stress. In mammalian cells, UPR is composed of three independent pathways, each regulated by different proteins localized in the ER membrane: IRE1 (inositol requiring 1), ATF6 (activating transcription factor 6) and PERK (protein kinase like ER kinase). The PERK pathway is usually targeted for the study of SFA toxicity in β-cells [25,35,37,38]. PERK, after activation by an ER stress, phosphorylates the α-subunit of the eukaryotic initiation factor 2 (eIF2α). Thus, the phosphorylation rate of eIF2α can be used as a marker of the SFA-induced ER stress. As shown on Fig. 4B, incubation of CFBE41o$^-$ cells with 100 μM Palmitate resulted in a slight but significant increase of the phosphorylation rate of eIF2α, as compared to the control (BSA), suggesting that, at this Palmitate concentration, the PERK pathway is already induced.

Taken together, these data indicate that CFBE41o$^-$ cells treated with 100 μM Palmitate to mimic the PC pattern observed in freshly isolated patient cells do not fall prey to apoptosis. However, they are experiencing an ER-stress.

Effects of Exogenous Palmitate Intake on Calcium Homeostasis

SFA, and particularly Palmitate, are known to alter Ca^{2+} homeostasis in β cells and particularly ER Ca^{2+}-stores. Even if data concerning this aspect are conflicting [25,35], Cunha and collaborators showed that Palmitate-induced ER stress triggers the depletion of ER Ca^{2+} stores by the reducing ER Ca^{2+} uptake [35]. These observations were in agreement with the data from Li *et al.* who demonstrated that SFA, by increasing membrane order, inhibited the activity of the SERCA pump *in vitro*, which is responsible for the uptake of Ca^{2+} from the cytosol to the ER lumen [39].

In this context, we investigated the impacts of Palmitate accumulation within PL on Ca^{2+} homeostasis in CFBE41o$^-$ cells (Fig. 5). In agreement with previous observations, ER Ca^{2+} stores were significantly depleted after treatment with 250 μM Palmitate (Fig. 5A). However, if a decrease in the amounts of Ca^{2+} released from the ER could also be observed with 100 μM Palmitate, this result was not significant as compared to the control (Fig. 5A). The most significant effects at this Palmitate concentration could be observed on global Ca^{2+} mobilization, which results from both mobilization of ER Ca^{2+} stores and Ca^{2+} influx from the extracellular medium (Fig. 5B). These results indicate that Ca^{2+} homeostasis is affected by 100 μM Palmitate treatments of CFBE41o$^-$ cells, the main target of this alteration being the extracellular Ca^{2+} uptake by plasma membrane Ca^{2+} channels.

Effects of Exogenous Palmitate Intake on F508del-CFTR Correction by Pharmacological Agents

The fact that CFBE41o$^-$ cells experienced an ER-stress under treatment with 100 μM Palmitate suggested that, at this concentration, intracellular organelle integrity and function might be somehow affected. Indeed, SFA accumulation with PL have been shown to reduce membrane fluidity, increase lipid packing and therefore impact several biophysical processes required for protein biogenesis and trafficking, such as folding [22] and vesicular budding [23]. In CF, the F508del-CFTR is retained in the ER before its degradation by the ERAD machinery. Nevertheless, its trafficking can be corrected by pharmacological agents, such as miglustat [10], which have been shown to be less efficient in preliminary clinical trials [11–14]. We therefore hypothesized that Palmitate accumulation within the PC of CF patient cells could impact F508del-CFTR trafficking correction. To test this hypothesis, we evaluated the activity of the F508del-CFTR channel by the iodide efflux technique, after incubation of CFBE41o$^-$ cells with 100 μM Palmitate and a treatment with miglustat or isoLAB, another F508del-CFTR trafficking corrector [40], to restore F508del-CFTR trafficking. Fig. 6A shows a representative iodide efflux trace obtained for the study of the F508del-CFTR activity. Without treatment with correctors, F508del-CFTR cannot reach the plasma membrane and the relevant iodide efflux is close to zero. After treatment with miglustat, iodide efflux was restored but was 35% lower when cells were incubated with Palmitate (Fig. 6B). The same decrease in F508del-CFTR correction after Palmitate treatment was observed with isoLAB, (Fig. 6B). As plasma membrane Ca^{2+} intake was decreased under 100 μM Palmitate treatment (Fig. 5B), we wondered whether this Palmitate effect could be generalized to other membrane-embedded proteins than corrected F508del-CFTR or not. In this aim, we also tested the activity of two others chloride channels, the Cl_{Ca} channel after its stimulation by the calcium ionophore A23187, and the Cl_{swell} channel which is sensitive to cell swelling after activation by an osmotic shock (Fig. 6C). Such as corrected F508del-CFTR, iodide efflux was around 30% and 15% decreased for Cl_{Ca} and Cl_{swell} channels, respectively. These results suggest that Palmitate has global effects on plasma membrane chloride channels.

Discussion

The most common mutation responsible for CF, *F508del-CFTR*, results in a misfolded protein that cannot reach its final destination, the plasma membrane. F508del-CFTR is retained in the ER before its degradation by the ERAD machinery [5–7]. However, the trafficking to the plasma membrane of this misfolded protein can be corrected by pharmacological agents, such as miglustat [10], but their correcting properties appear to be less efficient in preliminary clinical trials. CF is also associated with an altered lipid homeostasis, with a decrease of PUFA in CF tissues and plasma [15–19]. Nevertheless, the SFA compositions of membrane PL, which have been shown to modulate crucial biophysical properties in several cellular cell types and to regulate several steps of the secretory pathway [23] and could therefore alter F508del-CFTR trafficking correction by pharmacological means, had not been studied so far.

In the present study, we show that a Palmitate accumulation occurs within CF patient bronchial epithelial cells with, as a corollary, an increase of the PC saturation rates. This accumulation is not observed in the corresponding CFBE41o$^-$ cell line under standard culture conditions (Fig. 1). We formulated the hypothesis that Palmitate accumulation could be the consequence of hypoxia, which relates to the thick layer of mucus obstructing the lungs [30], because fatty acid desaturases are oxygen-dependent [31]. Thus, we tried to culture the CFBE41o$^-$ cells in a hypoxia chamber (Fig. 2). This led to a significant increase of the PC saturation rate, but Palmitate accumulation remained too limited in these conditions to mimic the PC pattern observed in CF freshly isolated cells. Since the chronic hypoxia encountered in CF patients, and probably responsible for the Palmitate accumulation within PC, appeared to be too difficult to achieve using this method, we developed an alternative strategy consisting in feeding the cells with an exogenous Palmitate source, as already described for β cells [25]. Among the various Palmitate concentrations tested, incubation of CFBE41o$^-$ cells with 100 μM Palmitate resulted in a PC profile that appeared fairly similar to the one encountered with CF patient (Fig. 3). Interestingly, if higher Palmitate concentrations resulted in apoptosis induction (250 μM Palmitate; Fig. 4), 100 μM Palmitate did not appear obviously toxic to the cells. A closer examination revealed that incubation of CFBE41o$^-$ cells with 100 μM Palmitate resulted in an increased phosphorylation rate of eIF2α, a known marker of the SFA-induced ER stress [25,35,37,38]. Altogether, these data suggest, if extrapolated to the epithelial airway cells from CF patients, that those cells display a lipointoxication-like phenotype.

UPR induction in CF is a controversial subject. Some studies demonstrated an atypical UPR induction in CF, characterized by the lack of the PERK-eIF2α induction [41,42], while others showed the absence of ER stress in CF cells [43]. These discrepancies could result from the use of very different cellular models. We therefore propose, based on the results obtained in this study with CFBE41o$^-$ cells improved to mimic the PC pattern observed in freshly isolated CF cells (Fig. 4B), that UPR induction is not related to *F508del-CFTR* expression *per se*, but to secondary alterations in the cellular lipid composition (lipointoxication) related to hypoxia.

A very interesting point is the role of Palmitate in β-cell death and its relevance to the etiology of Type 2 diabetes. As already mentioned, such as demonstrated here for epithelial cells, β-cell exposure to long chain SFA, including Palmitate, results in ER stress [35,37], which can ultimately leads to cell death by apoptosis. This process is believed to contribute to the decrease of the β cell mass, leading to a deficient insulin secretion and therefore the development of Type 2 diabetes [44]. In CF, with the advancing patient age, the most common comorbidity is cystic fibrosis-related diabetes (CFRD) [45]. It has been shown in CF β-cells an abnormal Cl$^-$ channel function leading to thick viscous secretions obstructing the exocrine pancreas [46,47], and a significantly reduced percentage of insulin-producing cells within islets [48–51]. The data presented in this study may shed a new light on the underlying mechanisms. Indeed, one may assume that hypoxia-driven Palmitate accumulation may well be a crucial determinant for β-cell dysfunction in CFRD. Further characterization of PC composition in pancreatic cells from CF individuals will undoubtfully bring new insights in the comprehension of CFRD etiology.

In previous studies, it has been shown that Ca^{2+} homeostasis is altered in CF cells compared to non-CF cells, with a decrease of global Ca^{2+} mobilization [52,53], as a result of F508del-CFTR retention in the ER [54]. It has also been shown that ER Ca^{2+} stores are not different in both CF and non-CF cells [53]. Our data are consistent with these previous results and show that Palmitate accumulation has additive effects on calcium homeostasis disruption in CF cells.

We have also shown that increasing the saturation rate of PC has a significant impact on F508del-CFTR trafficking correction by miglustat and isoLAB. Indeed, the incubation of corrected CFBE41o$^-$ cells with 100 μM Palmitate results in the decrease of F508del-CFTR iodide efflux, reflecting the Cl$^-$ current. To account for this observation, we can formulate two hypotheses, which may be not exclusive one to the other: the decrease in Cl$^-$ current could be related to alterations in trafficking correction of the F508del-CFTR protein to the plasma membrane due to general impacts of saturated-PL on the secretory pathway, or to a loss of function of the corrected protein. High saturated-PL levels impact membrane properties in many ways. First, they tend to decrease membrane fluidity/increase membrane order, which is not compatible with most of the cellular processes that require high membrane dynamics, such as protein translocation/folding in the ER [21]. Second, they tend to increase bilayer thickness. Thickness of the hydrophobic membrane-spanning regions of an integral protein should match the thickness of the bilayer to avoid exposure of hydrophobic residues to water, a phenomenon known as hydrophobic-mismatch (for review, see [55]). As a consequence, increasing membrane thickness may have dramatic consequences on the folding, and therefore the trafficking and/or function, of membrane-embedded proteins such as the CFTR channel. Finally, PL shape itself modulates important biophysical parameters, including membrane curvature and lipid packing [23]. As shown on Fig. 1E, PC species containing two SFA display a cylindrical shape (DB = 0, Fig. 1E) while PC containing two UFA display an overall conical shape (DB = 2, Fig. 1E). Therefore, Palmitate accumulation within PC species is expected to shift the shape of the overall PC population from conical to rather cylindrical (Fig. 1E). Conical lipids are required to form areas of positive and negative curvature, and therefore SFA-related conical-PL depletion is expected to alter membrane bending. Moreover, conical lipid deprivation also results in increased lipid packing [23] which alters the recruitment of loose lipid packing-sensing proteins required for optimal budding, to nascent vesicles. Altogether, these processes could account for a global disruption of the entire secretory pathway.

Overall, SFA accumulation within membrane PL is expected to have very broad and general impacts on plasma membrane-embedded proteins in the CF cell. In fact, in this study, we measured the activity of three Cl$^-$ channels localized at the plasma membrane, namely Cl_{Ca}, Cl_{swell} and the corrected F508del-CFTR after incubation of CFBE41o$^-$ cells with 100 μM Palmitate. Even if these three Cl$^-$ channels are differently activated (Cl_{Ca} by calcium, Cl_{swell} by cell swelling, and corrected F508del-CFTR by phosphorylation and ATP hydrolysis), we could relevantly show that these Cl$^-$ channels and plasma membrane Ca^{2+} influx are impacted either in their trafficking and/or function under SFA accumulation, with, as a consequence, a significant decrease in iodide efflux (Fig. 6) and calcium intake (Fig. 5B). This strongly suggests that bronchial epithelial cells are lipointoxicated by SFA in CF patients, a process that ought to be considered for the development of future therapeutic strategies.

To conclude, if understanding the precise impacts of SFA on F508del-CFTR trafficking and/or function will require further work, such as the analysis of the delivery of the mutant form to the plasma-membrane under SFA-accumulation in overexpressing models, data presented in this study may bring some new explanations concerning the discrepancies between *in vitro* and *in vivo* effects of correctors. We propose that hypoxia-related SFA accumulation impacts on membrane properties could be an important bottleneck for F508del-CFTR trafficking correction by pharmacological means in clinical trials. Relieving lipointoxication in CF cells may well be a way to synergize corrector effects and optimize their therapeutic action.

Acknowledgments

We thank Dr. Pierre Bonnette (Hôpital Folch, Paris, France) for biopsies and human lung samples.

Author Contributions

Conceived and designed the experiments: LAP CV TF. Performed the experiments: LAP LK SG CN JMB CJ SM CV. Analyzed the data: LAP CN FB CV TF. Contributed reagents/materials/analysis tools: CJ. Wrote the paper: LAP TF.

References

1. Strandvik B (2010) Fatty acid metabolism in cystic fibrosis. Prostaglandins Leukot Essent Fatty Acids 83: 121–129.
2. Anderson D (1938) Cystic fibrosis of the pancreas and its relation to celiac disease: a clinical and pathological study. Am J Dis Child 56: 344–399.
3. Riordan JR, Rommens JM, Kerem BS, Alon N, Rozmahel R, et al. (1989) Identification of the cystic fibrosis gene: cloning and characterization of complementary DNA. Science 245: 1066–1073.
4. Rommens JM, Iannuzzi MC, Kerem B, Drumm ML, Melmer G, et al. (1989) Identification of the cystic fibrosis gene: chromosome walking and jumping. Science 245: 1059–1065.
5. Cheng SH, Gregory RJ, Marshall J, Paul S, Souza DW, et al. (1990) Defective intracellular transport and processing of CFTR is the molecular basis of most cystic fibrosis. Cell 63: 827–834.
6. Zhang F, Kartner N, Lukacs GL (1998) Limited proteolysis as a probe for arrested conformational maturation of delta F508 CFTR. Nat Struct Biol 5: 180–183.
7. Gelman MS, Kannegaard ES, Kopito RR (2002) A principal role for the proteasome in endoplasmic reticulum-associated degradation of misfolded intracellular cystic fibrosis transmembrane conductance regulator. J Biol Chem 277: 11709–11714.
8. Andersson C, Roomans GM (2000) Activation of deltaF508 CFTR in a cystic fibrosis respiratory epithelial cell line by 4-phenylbutyrate, genistein and CPX. Eur Respir J 15: 937–941.
9. Van Goor F, Hadida S, Grootenhuis PD, Burton B, Stack JH, et al. (2011) Correction of the F508del-CFTR protein processing defect in vitro by the investigational drug VX-809. Proc Natl Acad Sci U S A 108: 18843–18848.
10. Norez C, Noel S, Wilke M, Bijvelds M, Jorna H, et al. (2006) Rescue of functional delF508-CFTR channels in cystic fibrosis epithelial cells by the alpha-glucosidase inhibitor miglustat. FEBS Lett 580: 2081–2086.
11. Rubenstein RC, Zeitlin PL (1998) A pilot clinical trial of oral sodium 4-phenylbutyrate (Buphenyl) in deltaF508-homozygous cystic fibrosis patients: partial restoration of nasal epithelial CFTR function. Am J Respir Crit Care Med 157: 484–490.
12. McCarty NA, Standaert TA, Teresi M, Tuthill C, Launspach J, et al. (2002) A phase I randomized, multicenter trial of CPX in adult subjects with mild cystic fibrosis. Pediatr Pulmonol 33: 90–98.
13. Clancy JP, Rowe SM, Accurso FJ, Aitken ML, Amin RS, et al. (2012) Results of a phase IIa study of VX-809, an investigational CFTR corrector compound, in subjects with cystic fibrosis homozygous for the F508del-CFTR mutation. Thorax 67: 12–18.
14. Leonard A, Lebecque P, Dingemanse J, Leal T (2012) A randomized placebo-controlled trial of miglustat in cystic fibrosis based on nasal potential difference. J Cyst Fibros 11: 231–236.
15. Kuo PT, Huang NN, Bassett DR (1962) The fatty acid composition of the serum chylomicrons and adipose tissue of children with cystic fibrosis of the pancreas. J Pediatr 60: 394–403.
16. Underwood BA, Denning CR, Navab M (1972) Polyunsaturated fatty acids and tocopherol levels in patients with cystic fibrosis. Ann N Y Acad Sci 203: 237–247.
17. Freedman SD, Blanco PG, Shea JC, Alvarez JG (2002) Analysis of lipid abnormalities in CF mice. Methods Mol Med 70: 517–524.
18. Freedman SD, Blanco PG, Zaman MM, Shea JC, Ollero M, et al. (2004) Association of cystic fibrosis with abnormalities in fatty acid metabolism. N Engl J Med 350: 560–569.
19. Guerrera IC, Astarita G, Jais JP, Sands D, Nowakowska A, et al. (2009) A novel lipidomic strategy reveals plasma phospholipid signatures associated with respiratory disease severity in cystic fibrosis patients. PLoS One 4: e7735.
20. Pineau L, Bonifait L, Berjeaud JM, Alimardani-Theuil P, Berges T, et al. (2008) A lipid-mediated quality control process in the Golgi apparatus in yeast. Mol Biol Cell 19: 807–821.
21. Pineau L, Colas J, Dupont S, Beney L, Fleurat-Lessard P, et al. (2009) Lipid-induced ER stress: synergistic effects of sterols and saturated fatty acids. Traffic 10: 673–690.
22. Deguil J, Pineau L, Rowland Snyder EC, Dupont S, Beney L, et al. (2011) Modulation of lipid-induced ER stress by fatty acid shape. Traffic 12: 349–362.
23. Payet LA, Pineau L, Snyder EC, Colas J, Moussa A, et al. (2013) Saturated fatty acids alter the late secretory pathway by modulating membrane properties. Traffic.
24. Andersson C, Al-Turkmani MR, Savaille JE, Alturkmani R, Katrangi W, et al. (2008) Cell culture models demonstrate that CFTR dysfunction leads to defective fatty acid composition and metabolism. J Lipid Res 49: 1692–1700.
25. Karaskov E, Scott C, Zhang L, Teodoro T, Ravazzola M, et al. (2006) Chronic palmitate but not oleate exposure induces endoplasmic reticulum stress, which may contribute to INS-1 pancreatic beta-cell apoptosis. Endocrinology 147: 3398–3407.
26. Folch J, Ascoli I, Lees M, Meath JA, LeBaron FN (1951) Preparation of lipide extracts from brain tissue. J Biol Chem 191: 833–841.
27. Potiron VA, Sharma G, Nasarre P, Clarhaut JA, Augustin HG, et al. (2007) Semaphorin SEMA3F affects multiple signaling pathways in lung cancer cells. Cancer Res 67: 8708–8715.
28. Norez C, Antigny F, Becq F, Vandebrouck C (2006) Maintaining low Ca2+ level in the endoplasmic reticulum restores abnormal endogenous F508del-CFTR trafficking in airway epithelial cells. Traffic 7: 562–573.
29. Schneiter R, Brugger B, Sandhoff R, Zellnig G, Leber A, et al. (1999) Electrospray ionization tandem mass spectrometry (ESI-MS/MS) analysis of the lipid molecular species composition of yeast subcellular membranes reveals acyl chain-based sorting/remodeling of distinct molecular species en route to the plasma membrane. J Cell Biol 146: 741–754.
30. Worlitzsch D, Tarran R, Ulrich M, Schwab U, Cekici A, et al. (2002) Effects of reduced mucus oxygen concentration in airway Pseudomonas infections of cystic fibrosis patients. J Clin Invest 109: 317–325.
31. Los DA, Murata N (1998) Structure and expression of fatty acid desaturases. Biochim Biophys Acta 1394: 3–15.
32. Ferreira T, Regnacq M, Alimardani P, Moreau-Vauzelle C, Berges T (2004) Lipid dynamics in yeast under haem-induced unsaturated fatty acid and/or sterol depletion. Biochem J 378: 899–908.
33. Semenza GL (1999) Regulation of mammalian O2 homeostasis by hypoxia-inducible factor 1. Annu Rev Cell Dev Biol 15: 551–578.
34. Wei Y, Wang D, Topczewski F, Pagliassotti MJ (2006) Saturated fatty acids induce endoplasmic reticulum stress and apoptosis independently of ceramide in liver cells. Am J Physiol Endocrinol Metab 291: E275–281.
35. Cunha DA, Hekerman P, Ladriere L, Bazarra-Castro A, Ortis F, et al. (2008) Initiation and execution of lipotoxic ER stress in pancreatic beta-cells. J Cell Sci 121: 2308–2318.
36. Duke RC, Cohen JJ (1986) IL-2 addiction: withdrawal of growth factor activates a suicide program in dependent T cells. Lymphokine Res 5: 289–299.
37. Diakogiannaki E, Welters HJ, Morgan NG (2008) Differential regulation of the endoplasmic reticulum stress response in pancreatic beta-cells exposed to long-chain saturated and monounsaturated fatty acids. J Endocrinol 197: 553–563.
38. Dhayal S, Morgan NG (2011) Structure-activity relationships influencing lipid-induced changes in eIF2alpha phosphorylation and cell viability in BRIN-BD11 cells. FEBS Lett 585: 2243–2248.
39. Li Y, Ge M, Ciani L, Kuriakose G, Westover EJ, et al. (2004) Enrichment of endoplasmic reticulum with cholesterol inhibits sarcoplasmic-endoplasmic reticulum calcium ATPase-2b activity in parallel with increased order of membrane lipids: implications for depletion of endoplasmic reticulum calcium stores and apoptosis in cholesterol-loaded macrophages. J Biol Chem 279: 37030–37039.
40. da Cruz FP, Newberry S, Jenkinson SF, Wormald MR, Butters TD, et al. (2011) 4-C-Me-DAB and 4-C-Me-LAB - enantiomeric alkyl-branched pyrrolidine iminosugars - are specific and potent alpha-glucosidase inhibitors; acetone as the sole protecting group. Tetrahedron Lett 52: 219–223.
41. Nanua S, Sajjan U, Keshavjee S, Hershenson MB (2006) Absence of typical unfolded protein response in primary cultured cystic fibrosis airway epithelial cells. Biochem Biophys Res Commun 343: 135–143.
42. Blohmke CJ, Mayer ML, Tang AC, Hirschfeld AF, Fjell CD, et al. (2012) Atypical activation of the unfolded protein response in cystic fibrosis airway cells contributes to p38 MAPK-mediated innate immune responses. J Immunol 189: 5467–5475.
43. Hybiske K, Fu Z, Schwarzer C, Tseng J, Do J, et al. (2007) Effects of cystic fibrosis transmembrane conductance regulator and DeltaF508CFTR on

inflammatory response, ER stress, and Ca2+ of airway epithelia. Am J Physiol Lung Cell Mol Physiol 293: L1250–1260.
44. Butler AE, Janson J, Bonner-Weir S, Ritzel R, Rizza RA, et al. (2003) Beta-cell deficit and increased beta-cell apoptosis in humans with type 2 diabetes. Diabetes 52: 102–110.
45. Moran A, Dunitz J, Nathan B, Saeed A, Holme B, et al. (2009) Cystic fibrosis-related diabetes: current trends in prevalence, incidence, and mortality. Diabetes Care 32: 1626–1631.
46. Kopelman H, Durie P, Gaskin K, Weizman Z, Forstner G (1985) Pancreatic fluid secretion and protein hyperconcentration in cystic fibrosis. N Engl J Med 312: 329–334.
47. Kopelman H, Corey M, Gaskin K, Durie P, Weizman Z, et al. (1988) Impaired chloride secretion, as well as bicarbonate secretion, underlies the fluid secretory defect in the cystic fibrosis pancreas. Gastroenterology 95: 349–355.
48. Iannucci A, Mukai K, Johnson D, Burke B (1984) Endocrine pancreas in cystic fibrosis: an immunohistochemical study. Hum Pathol 15: 278–284.
49. Abdul-Karim FW, Dahms BB, Velasco ME, Rodman HM (1986) Islets of Langerhans in adolescents and adults with cystic fibrosis. A quantitative study. Arch Pathol Lab Med 110: 602–606.
50. Soejima K, Landing BH (1986) Pancreatic islets in older patients with cystic fibrosis with and without diabetes mellitus: morphometric and immunocytologic studies. Pediatr Pathol 6: 25–46.
51. Kelly A, Moran A (2013) Update on cystic fibrosis-related diabetes. J Cyst Fibros 12: 318–331.
52. Ribeiro CM, Paradiso AM, Schwab U, Perez-Vilar J, Jones L, et al. (2005) Chronic airway infection/inflammation induces a Ca2+i-dependent hyperinflammatory response in human cystic fibrosis airway epithelia. J Biol Chem 280: 17798–17806.
53. Antigny F, Norez C, Becq F, Vandebrouck C (2008) Calcium homeostasis is abnormal in cystic fibrosis airway epithelial cells but is normalized after rescue of F508del-CFTR. Cell Calcium 43: 175–183.
54. Antigny F, Norez C, Cantereau A, Becq F, Vandebrouck C (2008) Abnormal spatial diffusion of Ca2+ in F508del-CFTR airway epithelial cells. Respir Res 9: 70.
55. Lee AG (2003) Lipid-protein interactions in biological membranes: a structural perspective. Biochim Biophys Acta 1612: 1–40.

5

Macrolide Therapy in Adults and Children with Non-Cystic Fibrosis Bronchiectasis: A Systematic Review and Meta-Analysis

Yong-hua Gao[9], Wei-jie Guan[9], Gang Xu[9], Yan Tang, Yang Gao, Zhi-ya Lin, Zhi-min Lin, Nan-shan Zhong, Rong-chang Chen*

State Key Laboratory of Respiratory Diseases, National Clinical Research Center for Respiratory Disease, Guangzhou Institute of Respiratory Diseases, The First Affiliated Hospital of Guangzhou Medical University, Guangzhou, Guangdong, China

Abstract

Background: A systematic review and meta-analysis was conducted to evaluate the efficacy and safety of macrolide therapy in adults and children with bronchiectasis.

Methods: We searched the PUBMED, EMBASE, CENTRAL databases to identify relevant studies. Two reviewers evaluated the studies and extracted data independently. The primary outcome was the number of bronchiectasis exacerbations. Secondary outcomes included exacerbation-related admissions, quality of life (QoL), spirometry, 6-minute walk test (6MWT) and adverse events.

Results: Nine eligible trials with 559 participants were included. Six were conducted on adults, and the remaining on children. Macrolide therapy significantly reduced the number of patients experiencing one or more exacerbation in adults [risk ratio (RR) = 0.59; 95% CI, 0.40 to 0.86; P = 0.006; $I^2 = 65\%$] and children [RR = 0.86; 95% CI, 0.75–0.99; P = 0.04; $I^2 = 0\%$], but not the number of patients with admissions for exacerbation. Macrolide therapy was also associated with reduced frequency of exacerbations in adults (RR = 0.42; 95% CI, 0.29 to 0.61; $P<0.001$; $I^2 = 64\%$) and children (RR = 0.50; 95% CI, 0.35 to 0.71; $P<0.001$). Pooled analyses suggested that spirometry, including FEV_1 and FVC, were significantly improved in adults but not in children. Macrolide therapy improved the QoL (WMD, −6.56; 95% CI, −11.99 to −1.12; P = 0.02; $I^2 = 86\%$) but no significant difference in 6MWT (WMD, 4.15; 95% CI, −11.83 to 20.13; P = 0.61; $I^2 = 31\%$) and the overall adverse events (RR, 0.96; 95% CI, 0.82 to 1.13; P = 0.66; $I^2 = 0\%$) in adults. However, reports of diarrhea and abdominal discomforts were higher with macrolide therapy.

Conclusions: Macrolide maintenance therapy, both in adults and children, was effective and safe in reducing bronchiectasis exacerbations, but not the admissions for exacerbations. In addition, macrolide administration in adults was associated with improvement in QoL and spirometry, but not 6WMT. Future studies are warranted to verify the optimal populations and clarify its potential effects on antimicrobial resistance.

Editor: Michael Tunney, Queens University Belfast, Ireland

Funding: No current external funding sources for this study.

Competing Interests: The authors have declared that no competing interests exist.

* E-mail: ChenRC@vip.163.com

[9] These authors contributed equally to this work.

Introduction

Bronchiectasis is a chronic and etiologically heterogeneous airway inflammatory disease characterized by productive cough, recurrent infective exacerbations and impaired quality of life (QoL) [1]. The diagnosis and treatment of bronchiectasis has rarely been focused on, presumably due to the misperception that it is rare and can be readily managed once identified [1,2]. Although the true prevalence and burden are still unknown, recent epidemiological surveys demonstrated that the prevalence and the resultant hospitalizations are steadily increasing worldwide [3–7]. Unfortunately, current managements are mostly based on expert consensus or extrapolation from other respiratory diseases, i.e. cystic fibrosis (CF) and chronic obstructive pulmonary disease (COPD) due to a paucity of evidence-based data [1]. To date, effective long-term treatments, apart from chest clearance techniques, are lacking [1]. The development of evidence-based treatment is urgently needed to reduce the growing clinical burden of this 'orphan' disease [1,2].

Macrolides, which have considerable anti-inflammatory and immunomodulatory properties in addition to their antibacterial effects, might be effective in CF, COPD, asthma, diffuse panbronchiolitis and post-transplant bronchiolitis obliterans [8–13]. The precise mechanisms of action are unclear, but it might be associated with attenuated production of pro-inflammatory cytokines, airway mucus secretion and viscosity [14]. This provided the rationale for use in patients with non-CF bronchiectasis. Several trials have been performed to evaluate the effectiveness of macrolides for bronchiectasis maintenance treatment [15–17]. However, individual studies on the benefits of prevention from exacerbations, other clinical crucial end-points and safety of macrolides in bronchiectasis patients were of limited sample size and marked heterogeneity of results.

We conducted a systematic review and meta-analysis to evaluate the impacts of macrolides on the number of bronchiectasis exacerbations and other clinical measures, i.e. admission for exacerbations, QoL, spirometric indices and adverse events.

Materials and Methods

Literature search

We performed a literature search using PUBMED, EMBASE and CENTRAL databases for relevant studies published up to December 5th, 2013. An English language restriction was imposed. Search terms included "Macrolides", "Macrolide*", "Azithromycin", "Erythromycin", "Clarithromycin", "Roxithromycin", "Troleandomycin", "Bronchiectasis", "Bronchiect*". Searches were limited to human only and randomized controlled trials (RCTs). Additionally, we screened the reference lists of the papers identified through database search for other potentially eligible studies.

Study eligibility

Two reviewers independently (Y. G. and W.G.) performed the study selection, with differences resolved by mutual discussion and arbitration of a third reviewer (G.X.), if necessary. Studies that met the following criteria were considered potentially eligible: (1) Study design: RCTs; (2) Populations: clinically stable non-CF bronchiectasis defined by high-resolution computed tomography (HRCT); (3) Intervention: long-term macrolide treatment (≥2 months); (4) Comparison on interventions: placebo or usual care; (5) Outcomes: the primary outcome was the number of bronchiectasis exacerbations including the total number of patients experiencing one or more exacerbations as well as the frequency of exacerbation in the study period, and secondary outcomes included admissions for infective exacerbations, QoL, spirometric indices, sputum volume, 6-minute walk test (6MWT) and adverse events.

For studies reported in two or more publications, only the most complete publication was used for data extraction. Abstracts published in scientific conferences or website materials were excluded, for these studies had not been peer-reviewed and their inclusion might have biased the meta-analysis.

Data extraction

Two authors independently reviewed eligible studies and extracted the following data: first author; year of publication; study design; number of participants per treatment arm; type of macrolides, dose and duration; inclusion/exclusion criteria; length of follow-up and clinical outcomes. Any differences on data extraction were resolved by discussion and consultation of the third author (G.X.), if appropriate. Data were mainly obtained from original manuscripts when possible; when data were insufficient, we contacted the authors by e-mail, or obtained estimates from the previous meta-analyses on the topic if available [18].

Quality assessment

Two reviewers (Y. G. and W.G.) independently assessed the methodological quality of RCTs by using a validated scale (Jadad scoring system) [19] to determine how the randomization sequence was generated, how allocation was concealed and how missing outcome data were reported and analyzed, thus giving rise to a score of 0–5. Studies with a score of 3 or more were of high quality and otherwise low quality. Although concealed treatment allocation was not part of this rating scale, it was included in quality assessment. Any disagreements regarding the risk of bias assessments were harmonized by discussion and consensus.

Statistical analysis

An intervention meta-analysis was conducted using Review Manager Software 5.1.2 (Cochrane Collaboration, Oxford, UK) and STATA 12.0 software (Stata Corporation, College Station, TX, USA). Risk ratios (RR) for dichotomous variables and weighted mean difference (WMD) or standard mean differences (SMD) for continuous variables with 95% confidence intervals (95% CI) were calculated; SMD were used when studies reported different units or scales for the outcome. We measured heterogeneity by using the I^2 test [20], with suggested thresholds for low (25%-50%), moderate (50%–70%) and high (>75%) heterogeneity, respectively. Study-level data were pooled using random-effect models because of the anticipated heterogeneity with different macrolides used, different durations of therapy, different study designs and populations. For the potential sources of heterogeneity, sensitivity analyses were conducted to explore the influence of alternative statistical models (fix-effects model and random-effects model) and excluding studies with low quality on the findings. Publication bias was assessed by a funnel plot using exacerbations as an endpoint. The Egger's test was used to evaluate publication bias statistically. $P<0.05$ was considered statistically significant.

For primary outcome, subgroup analyses were also performed based on: (1) duration of treatment: ≥6 months vs. <6 months; (2) type of macrolides: azithromycin vs. erythromycin; (3) type of control group: placebo vs. usual care; (4) location of the country.

Results

Literature review

Initial literature searches retrieved 254 articles, from which 214 were screened after excluding duplicates. Following screening of the titles and abstracts, 188 citations were removed due to irrelevant publishing types or studies. Of 26 full-text citations, 9 with 559 participants fulfilled inclusion criteria [15–17,21–26]. Figure 1 describes the flow chart of our systematic review. The included studies were published between 1997 and 2013. Eight of the trials were parallel group studies [15–17,21,22,24–26] and one cross-over study [23]. Six of these studies recruited patients with adults [15–17,22,23,25] and three with children [21,24,26]. Five trials evaluated azithromycin [16,17,23,25,26], three erythromycin [15,22,24] and one roxithromycin [21]. Seven trials were placebo-controlled trials [15–17,21,22,24,26], whereas the control groups comprised usual medication care in the remaining trials [23,25]. The duration of treatment ranged from 8 weeks to 24 months. All trials reported exacerbations as either dichotomous or continuous outcomes, with six using exacerbations as primary outcomes [15–17,23,24,26]. The characteristics of the included trials are shown in Table 1.

The definition of bronchiectasis exacerbation differed among the included studies and was summarized in Table S1.

Quality Assessment

Quality assessment items are shown in Table 2. Eight trials were classified as having high quality [15–17,21–24,26] and one as low quality [25] according to Jadad scoring system. All were randomized trials, but the methods to generate the randomization

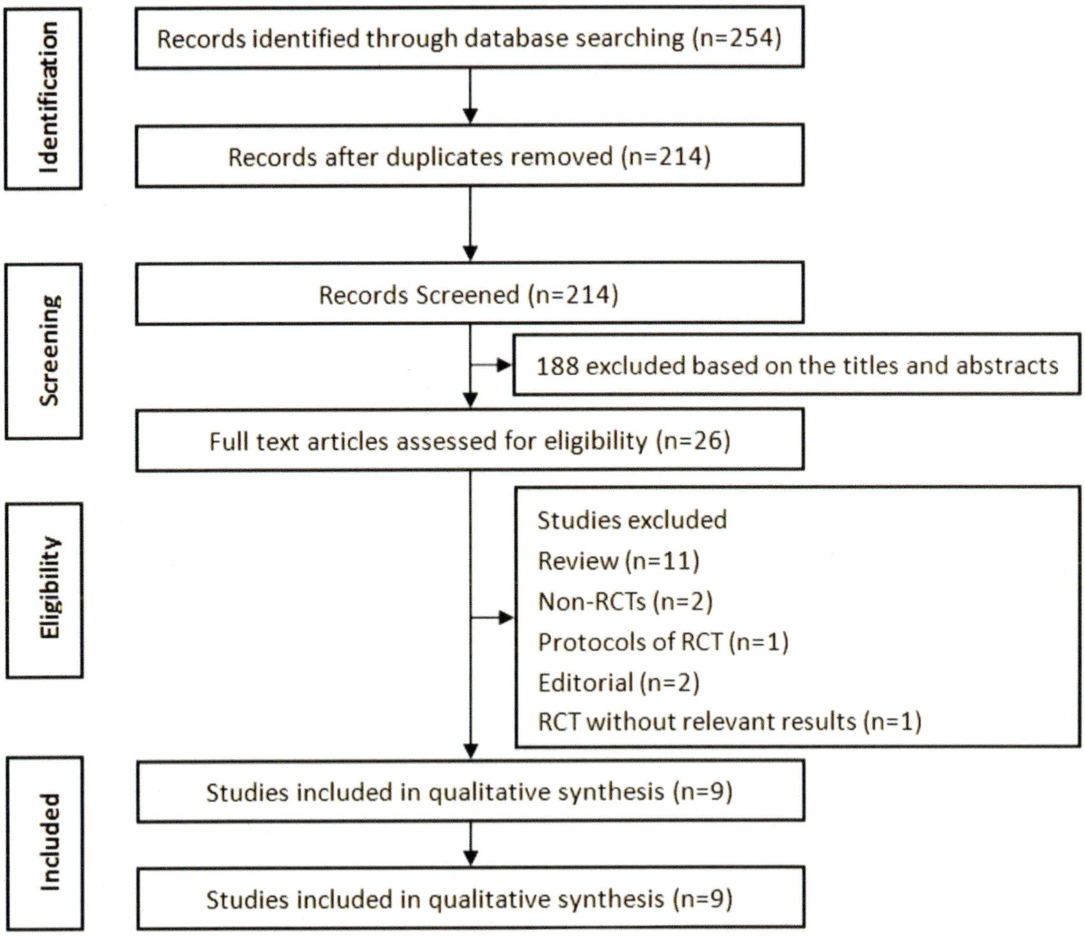

Figure 1. Flow of study selection.

sequence were accurately reported in 5 studies [15–17,23,26]. Seven studies were double-blind and placebo-controlled trials [15–17,21,22,24,26] whilst the remaining studies were open-label trials [23,25]. Seven reported concealed treatment allocation [15–17,22–24,26].

The Primary outcome: the number of patients with experiencing one or more exacerbations

The results from nine trials (n = 559) were available to examine the effects of macrolide therapy on the number of patients experiencing one or more exacerbations [15–17,21–26]. Six trials were performed in adults and the remaining one in children. When two types of exacerbation events were reported, the one as the primary outcome was included in the pooled analysis. In adults (n = 414), pooled analyses showed that the use of macrolides was associated with a significantly reduced the number of patients experiencing one or more exacerbations (RR, 0.59; 95% CI, 0.40 to 0.86; P = 0.006; Figure 2A) with a moderate among-study heterogeneity (P = 0.01; I^2 = 65%). Sensitivity analysis for alternative statistical model or excluding low quality studies did not markedly alter the overall findings. We further performed prespecified subgroup analyses to investigate the sources of heterogeneity (Table 3). There was a significantly greater benefit of macrolide therapy in reducing the number of patients experiencing one or more exacerbations in the following studies: longer treatment duration (RR = 0.59; 95% CI, 0.38 to 0.92; P = 0.02; I^2 = 77%); using placebo for control (RR = 0.63; 95% CI, 0.41 to 0.96; P = 0.03; I^2 = 74%); studies conducted in European countries (RR = 0.59; 95% CI, 0.42 to 0.82; P = 0.002; I^2 = 0%) and United States (RR = 0.25; 95% CI, 0.07 to 0.92; P = 0.04) ; and treatment with azithromycin (RR = 0.52; 95% CI, 0.41to 0.67; P<0.001; I^2 = 0%).

In children (n = 145), macrolide therapy was also associated with decreased number of patients experiencing one or more exacerbation (RR, 0.86; 95% CI, 0.75–0.99; p = 0.04, Figure 2A), with no significant among-study heterogeneity (P = 0.51; I^2 = 0%).

Primary outcome: rate of exacerbations per patient per year

The exacerbation rate was expressed as the rate ratio, which was calculated using the generic inverse variance algorithm in RevMan software. Four trials involving 430 participants reported the rate of exacerbation. Three trials were conducted in adults [15–17] and the remaining one in children [26]. In adults (n = 341), pooled analysis showed that macrolide therapy was associated with a reduction in the rate of exacerbations (RR = 0.42; 95% CI, 0.29 to 0.61; P<0.001; Figure 2B), with a moderate level of heterogeneity (P = 0.06, I^2 = 64%). A subgroup analysis according to the type of macrolides or the location of the country did not show any difference in the effect of macrolide therapy on exacerbation frequency (Table 3). Meanwhile,

Table 1. Characteristics of randomized clinical trials included in the meta-analysis.

Study/Year	Study Design	Number of subjects	Macrolides/dose/duration	Inclusion criteria/exclusion criteria	Length of follow-up
Koh YY [21]/1997	DB, RCT	25(13 treatment, 12 placebo)	Roxithromycin/(4 mg/kg) twice daily/12 weeks	**Inclusion:** Children, stable bronchiectasis, increased AR **Exclusion:** bronchopulmonary aspergillosis, CF, humoral immune deficiency, using sodium cromolyn or ICS, URTI or using antibiotics or corticosteroid in the past 1 month	12 weeks
Tsang KW [22]/1999	DB, RCT	21(11 treatment, 10 placebo)	Erythromycin/500 mg twice daily/8 weeks	**Inclusion:** 24-hr sputum>10 ml, stable idiopathic bronchiectasis. **Exclusion:** unreliable clinical attendance, adverse reactions to macrolides, lactating females.	8 weeks
Cymbala AA [23]2005	Open label, crossover, RCT	22(11 subjects, crossover)	Azithromycin/500 mg twice weekly/6 months	**Inclusion:** Age≥18 years. **Exclusion:** intolerance or allergy or sensitivity to macrolides, unable to follow instructions.	6 months
Wong C [17]2012	DB, RCT	141(71 reatment, 70 placebo)	Azithromycin/500 mg three times weekly/6 months	**Inclusion:** Age>18 years, stable bronchiectasis, 1 or more exacerbation requiring antibiotic therapy in the past year. **Exclusion:** CF, hypogammaglobulinaemia, ABPA, positive culture of NTM in the past 2 years or at screening, macrolide treatment for more than 3 months in the past 6 months, unstable arrhythmia	12 months
Altenburg J [16]/2013	DB, RCT	83(43 treatment, 40 placebo)	Azithromycin/250 mg once daily/52 weeks	**Inclusion:** Age>18 years, stable bronchiectasis, 3 or more LRTIs treated with oral or intravenous antibiotics, and 1 or more bacterial respiratory pathogens in the past year. **Exclusion:** >4 weeks macrolide therapy in the prior 3 months, using corticosteroid within 30 days screening or antimicrobial treatment for an LRTI In the last 2 weeks, allergy or intolerance to macrolides, childbearing without contraceptives or lactating females, liver disease or with elevated transaminase.	12 months
Serisier DJ [15]/2013	DB, RCT	117(59 treatment, 58 placebo)	Erythromycin/ethylsuccinate 400 mg twice daily/48 weeks	**Inclusion:** Age: 20 to 80 years, stable bronchiectasis, 2 or more exacerbations treated with intravenous antibiotics in the past year, and daily sputum production. **Exclusion:** CF, current mycobacterial disease or bronchopulmonary aspergillosis, any reversible cause for exacerbations, maintenance oral antibiotic prophylaxis, prior macrolide use except short-term, change to medications in the prior 4 weeks, smoking <6 months, positive sputum mycobacterial cultures, medications or comorbidities interactions with erythromycin	12 months
Masekela R [24]/2013	DB, RCT	31(17 treatment, 14 placebo)	Erythromycin/125 mg(≤15 Kg) or 250 mg(>15 Kg) daily/52 weeks	**Inclusion:** Age: 6 to 18 years, bronchiectasis associated with HIV, able to perform reliable PFTs. **Exclusion:** Abnormal liver function and urea/creatinine, use of carbamazepine, warfarin, cyclosporin or long-term midazolam, CF.	52 weeks

Table 1. Cont.

Study/Year	Study Design	Number of subjects	Macrolides/dose/duration	Inclusion criteria/exclusion criteria	Length of follow-up
de Diego A [25]/2013	Open label, RCT	30(16 treatment, 14 usual care)	Azithromycin/250 mg three times a week/3 months	**Inclusion:** Adults with stable bronchiectasis. **Exclusion:** CF, pulmonary surgical processes, HIV, CVID, malignancy, emphysema, ABPA, severe liver disease or diffuse interstitial pulmonary disease, intolerance to macrolides or severe liver disease.	3 months
Valery PC [26] 2013	DB, RCT	89(45 treatment, 44 placebo)	Azithromycin/30 mg/kg once a week/12–24 months	**Inclusion:** Indigenous children with age 1–8 years, HRCT confirmed bronchiectasis or chronic suppurative lung disease, 1 or more exacerbation in the past year. **Exclusion:** long-term antibiotics, receiving chemotherapy, or immunosuppressive treatment, underlying cause for bronchiectasis (i.e. CF, primary immunodeficiency), other chronic disorders (i.e. cardiac, neurological, renal or hepatic abnormality), macrolide hypersensitivity.	12–24 months

Abbreviation: DB, double-blinded; RCT, randomised controlled trials; AR, airway responsiveness; CF, cystic fibrosis; ICS, inhaled corticosteroids; URTI, upper respiratory tract infection; ABPA, allergic bronchopulmonary aspergillosis; NTM, non tuberculosis mycobacteria; LRTIs, lower respiratory tract infection; PFTs, pulmonary function test; HIV, human immunodeficiency virus; CVID, common variable immunodeficiency.

sensitivity analysis for alternative statistical model or exclusion of low quality studies did not markedly alter the overall findings.

Likewise, the use of macrolide therapy also led to reduced rate of exacerbation in children ($RR = 0.50$; 95% CI, 0.35 to 0.71; $P = 0.0001$; Figure 2B).

Secondary Outcome: bronchiectasis exacerbation-related admissions

Data on exacerbation-related admissions were available in three trials ($n = 313$) [16,17,26]. Two performed in adults [16,17], and one in children [26]. Pooled analyses in adults showed that macrolide therapy did not reduce the risk of admissions for infective exacerbations compared with control group (RR, 0.38; 95% CI, 0.08–1.94; $P = 0.25$; Figure 3). The heterogeneity was unremarkable ($P = 0.83$; $I^2 = 0\%$). A single study showed that exacerbation-related admission was also not significantly different between macrolide and placebo arms in children [26].

Secondary Outcome: health-related quality of life

Five trials conducted in adults ($n = 393$) investigated the effects of macrolide therapy on QoL [15–17,23,25]. Four assessed QoL by using St George's Respiratory Questionnaire (SGRQ) [15–17,25] and the other by using subjective report [23]. Finally, four trials ($n = 371$) were included in the pooled analyses [15–17,25]. Macrolide therapy significantly improved the SGRQ total score (WMD, −6.56 units; 95% CI, −11.99 to −1.12; $P < 0.001$; Figure 4) compared with controls. These studies were significantly heterogeneous ($I^2 = 86\%$, $P < 0.001$). Sensitivity analysis showed that removing the study with a poor quality score (Jadad score<3) [25] did not alter the results but resolved the heterogeneity (WMD, −3.75 units; 95% CI, −6.49 to −1.01; $P = 0.007$; P for heterogeneity $= 0.41$; $I^2 = 0\%$).

Table 2. Risk of bias assessment.

Study	Sequence generation	Allocation concealment	Blinding	Incomplete outcome data	Selective reporting	Other bias	Jadad score
Koh YY [21]/1997	unclear	unclear	low risk	low risk	low risk	low risk	3
Tsang KW [22]/1999	unclear	low risk	low risk	low risk	low risk	low risk	4
Cymbala AA [23]/2005	low risk	low risk	high risk	low risk	low risk	high risk	3
Wong C [17]/2012	low risk	low risk	low risk	low risk	low risk	low risk	5
Altenburg J [16]/2013	low risk	low risk	low risk	low risk	low risk	low risk	5
Serisier DJ [15]/2013	low risk	low risk	low risk	low risk	low risk	low risk	5
Masekela R [24]/2013	unclear	low risk	low risk	low risk	low risk	low risk	4
De Diego A [25]/2013	unclear	unclear	high risk	unclear	low risk	unclear	2
Valery PC [26]/2013	low risk	low risk	low risk	low risk	low risk	low risk	5

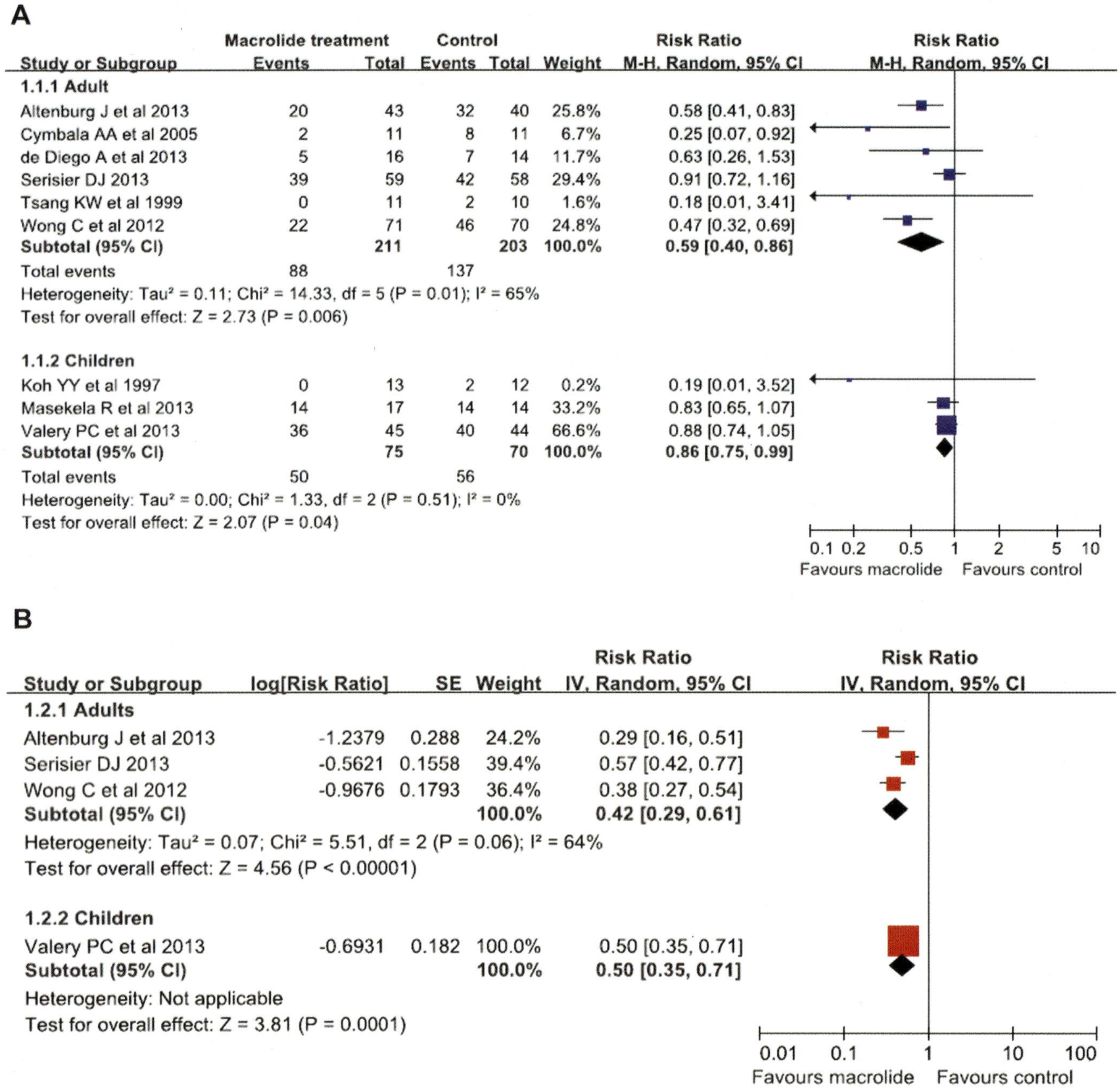

Figure 2. A. Meta-analysis of randomized controlled trials evaluating the effects of macrolide therapy on the number of patients with bronchiectasis exacerbations in adults and children. B. Meta-analysis of randomized controlled trials evaluating the effects of macrolide therapy on the rate of bronchiectasis exacerbation in adults and children.

Secondary Outcome: spirometric indices

Changes in FEV_1 from baseline. For Pre-bronchodilator FEV_1, eight trials (n = 470) were available to examine the effects of macrolide therapy on pre-bronchodilator FEV_1. Six trials (n = 414) were on adults and the remaining (n = 56) on children. In adults, pooled analyses showed that macrolide therapy yielded a significant increase in pre-bronchodilator FEV_1 (SMD 0.31; 95% CI, 0.12 to 0.51; P = 0.002, Figure 5A) without significant among-study heterogeneity ($I^2 = 0\%$, P = 0.70). In children, data from two small studies showed no between-group difference (WMD 2.19; 95% CI, −2.81 to 7.19; P = 0.39; Figure 5B). Heterogeneity was not significant ($I^2 = 0\%$, P = 0.88).

For post-bronchodilator FEV_1, data were only available from two studies conducted in adults showing a significant improvement between groups (SMD 0.33; 95% CI, 0.08 to 0.58; P = 0.008; Figure 5A) .without significant between study heterogeneity ($I^2 = 0\%$, P = 0.52).

Changes in FVC from baseline. For pre-bronchodilator FVC, six trials (n = 328) were included. Of which 5 were conducted on adults, and the other on children. Again, there were significant improvements in macrolide treatment groups compared with control groups (SMD 0.36; 95% CI, 0.13 to 0.59;

Table 3. Subgroup analysis of macrolide therapy on exacerbations in adults with bronchiectasis.

Variables	No. Patients	No. Trials	Macrolides	Controls	RR (95%CI)	P value	I^2 (%)	P value for heterogeneity
1. Number of patients with one or more exacerbation								
Total [15–17,22,23,25]	414	6	88/211	137/203	0.59(0.40–0.86)	0.006	65	0.01
Therapy duration								
≥6 months [15–17,23]	363	4	83/184	128/179	0.59(0.38–0.92)	0.02	77	0.004
<6 months [22,25]	51	2	5/27	9/24	0.56(0.24–1.32)	0.19	0	0.41
Macrolides								
Azithromycin [16,17,23,25]	276	4	49/141	93/135	0.52(0.41–0.67)	<0.001	0	0.56
Erythromycin [15,22]	138	2	39/70	44/68	0.78(0.29–2.08)	0.61	19	0.27
Controls								
Placebo [15–17,22]	362	4	81/184	122/178	0.63(0.41–0.96)	0.03	74	0.009
Non-placebo [23,25]	52	2	7/27	15/25	0.45(0.19–1.08)	0.07	25	0.25
Country location								
United States [23]	22	1	2/11	8/11	0.25(0.07–0.92)	0.04	...	...
Asia [22]	21	1	11/21	10/21	0.18(0.01–3.41)	0.26	...	...
Europe [16,25]	113	2	59/113	54/113	0.59(0.42–0.82)	0.002	0	0.88
Oceania [15,17]	258	2	130/258	128/258	0.67(0.34–1.32)	0.25	89	0.003
2. Rate of exacerbation per patients per year								
Total [15–17]	...	3			0.42(0.29–0.61)	P<0.0001	64%	0.06
Macrolides								
Azithromycin [16,17]	...	2			0.35(0.26–0.47)	P<0.0001	0	0.43
Erythromycin [15]	...	1			0.57(0.42–0.77)	p = 0.003	...	...
Country location								
Europe [16]	...	1			0.29(0.16–0.51)	P<0.01	...	...
Oceania [15,17]	...	2			0.47(0.32–0.70)	P = 0.0002	66%	0.09

P = 0.002; Figure 5A) without significant heterogeneity ($I^2 = 0\%$, P = 0.52). A single study conducted in 31 children showed no between-group differences (WMD 1.00, 95% CI, −9.48 to 11.48, P = 0.85, Figure 5B).

For post-bronchodilator FVC, data from the single study conducted in adults showed an improvement in macrolide treatment group (SMD, 0.43; 95% CI, 0.10 to 0.77; P = 0.01; Figure 5A).

Secondary Outcome: 6-minute walk test (6MWT)

Only two of the nine trials (n = 258) measured 6MWT. Pooled data showed that macrolide therapy did not increase the 6MWT compared with placebo (WMD 4.15; 95% CI, −11.83 to 20.13; P = 0.61; Figure 6). The heterogeneity was not statistically significant ($I^2 = 31\%$, P = 0.23).

Secondary Outcome: 24-hour sputum volume

Four trials [15,22,23,25] measured the effects of macrolide therapy on sputum volume presenting with various datasets including: weight or volume, mean or median etc, rendering it difficult for pooled analyses. All trials were performed in adults. There was a significant decrease in the weight of sputum with erythromycin therapy compared with placebo in the study by Serisier et al [33] [median −4.3 g; interquartile range (IQR), −7.8 to −1]. A significant improvement in mean 24-hour sputum volume was reported with erythromycin therapy by Tsang et al [22] (33.7 ml for pre-treatment vs. 23.8 for post-treatment with erythromycin, *P*<0.05; 26.2 ml for pre-treatment vs. 22.7 for post-treatment with placebo). Cymbala et al [23] reported that the mean 24-hour sputum volume was significantly decreased [15% (P = 0.005)] during the active treatment phase, and the effects of which even persisted in control phase (P = 0.028). In one study measuring the 24-hour sputum volume [25], azithromycin was associated with reduced sputum production compared with control [−8.9 (1.8) ml with azithromycin vs. 2.1 (3.4) ml with control, P<0.05)].

Adverse effects

Six trials (n = 473) presented data regarding adverse events [15–17,22,23,26]. Five trials (n = 384) were on adults and the other on children (n = 89). Available data in adults are summarized in Table 4. These studies reported comparable overall adverse events (RR, 0.96; 95% CI, 0.82 to 1.13; P = 0.66; $I^2 = 0\%$). However, patients receiving macrolides reported significantly more events of diarrhea and abdominal discomforts, but not headache, nausea, rash or sinusitis than control group. Meanwhile, the most recent three large trials also reported other various adverse events that could not be pooled for analysis. Wong et al [17] reported similar proportions of common cold, cough and chest pain in each arm. Serisier et al [15] reported a single case of suspected corrected QT

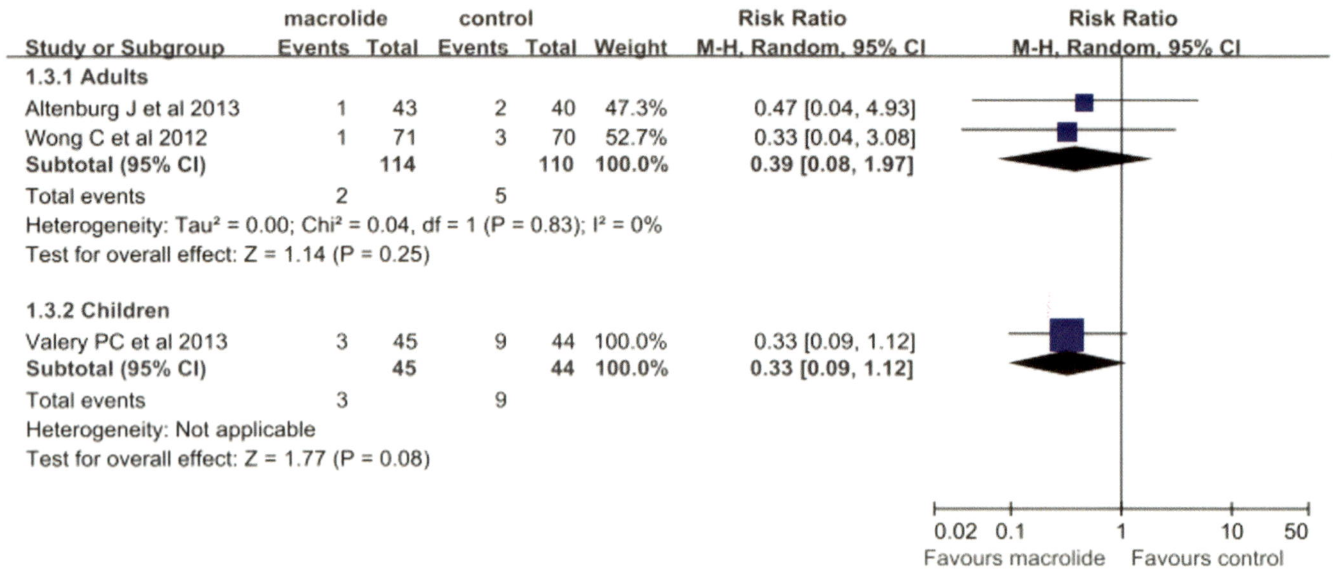

Figure 3. Meta-analysis of randomized controlled trials evaluating the effects of macrolide therapy on admission for bronchiectasis exacerbation in adults.

interval (QTc) prolongation in erythromycin group. Altenburg et al [16] reported similar proportions of auditory complaints, itching and palpitation in each arm. Three of the studies reported very small and similar numbers of adverse event in each arm to discontinue the trial medication. In children, the intervention drugs were well tolerated without serious adverse events.

Publication bias

The funnel plot for the number of patients with bronchiectasis exacerbations in adults indicated a slight asymmetry (Figure 7). However, Egger's test did not show a significant publication bias (P = 0.158). Publication bias for the rate of exacerbation in adults and the exacerbations in children was not assessed due to the limited number of studies.

Discussion

This systematic review and meta-analysis of 9 RCTs with macrolide therapy, with the duration of 2 months or more in adults and children who had stead-state bronchiectasis, indicated several meaningful findings. First, macrolide therapy significantly decreased the number of patients with exacerbations and the frequency of exacerbations, but not admissions for infective exacerbations, both in adults and children. Second, a few studies conducted in adults evidenced that macrolide therapy led to statistically significant improvement in QoL, but not 6MWT. Third, increases in FEV1 and FVC from baseline were significantly larger with macrolide therapy than with placebo or control in adults but not in children. Finally, macrolide therapy in adults might increase the risk of diarrhea and abdominal discomfort, but not overall adverse events.

We demonstrated a significantly decreased number of patients experiencing one or more exacerbations and the frequency of exacerbation with macrolide therapy in adults and children with bronchiectasis, which seemed to contradict with the 2007 Cochrane review [18]. Four recently published randomized controlled trials conducted in adults and children unanimously confirmed the beneficial effects of macrolide therapy on exacerbations. These studies contributed the majority of the weight to the pooled estimates. The subgroup analysis in adults, although not statistically significant (P = 0.44), suggested that azithromycin might have better effects on the number of patients with exacerbations than erythromycin in adults. Indeed, a recent meta-analysis [13] has demonstrated that erythromycin was associated with reduced risk of exacerbations in COPD. In addition, erythromycin was also associated with reduced rates of exacerbation. Therefore, the limited sample size, longer treatment duration and the eligible patients with a history of frequent

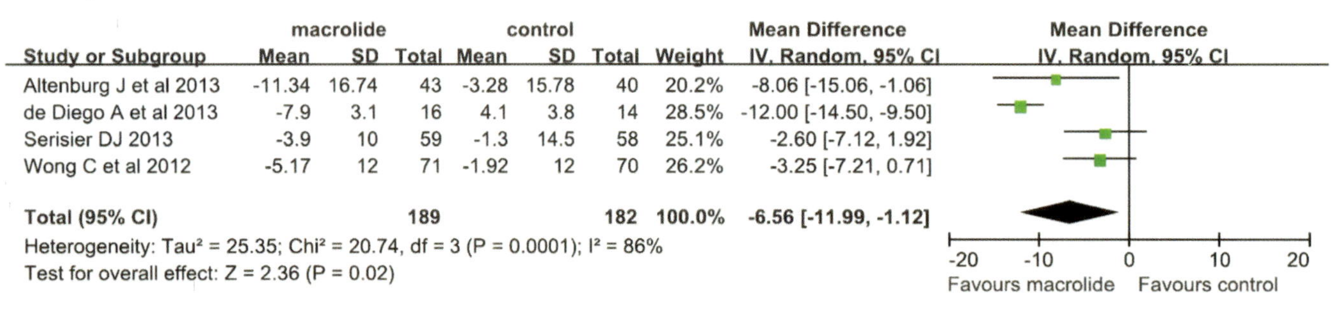

Figure 4. Meta-analysis of randomized controlled trials evaluating the effects of macrolide therapy on quality of life in adults with bronchiectasis.

A

Study or Subgroup	macrolide Mean	macrolide SD	macrolide Total	control Mean	control SD	control Total	Weight	Std. Mean Difference IV, Random, 95% CI
1.4.1 Adults-prebronchodilator FEV1								
Altenburg J et al 2013	4.39	9.06	43	-0.9	12.56	40	19.8%	0.48 [0.04, 0.92]
Cymbala AA et al 2005	-0.08	0.51	11	-0.1	0.53	11	5.4%	0.04 [-0.80, 0.87]
de Diego A et al 2013	0.06	0.03	16	0.04	0.02	14	6.8%	0.75 [0.01, 1.50]
Serisier DJ et al 2013	-0.3	5.26	59	-2.26	7.3	58	28.4%	0.31 [-0.06, 0.67]
Tsang KW et al 1999	0.14	0.6	11	-0.05	0.475	10	5.1%	0.34 [-0.53, 1.20]
Wong C et al 2012	0	0.23	71	-0.04	0.23	70	34.5%	0.17 [-0.16, 0.50]
Subtotal (95% CI)			**211**			**203**	**100.0%**	**0.31 [0.12, 0.51]**
Heterogeneity: Tau² = 0.00; Chi² = 3.02, df = 5 (P = 0.70); I² = 0%								
Test for overall effect: Z = 3.15 (P = 0.002)								
1.4.2 Adults-prebronchodilator FVC								
Altenburg J et al 2013	5.54	14.02	43	-2.6	12.59	40	27.2%	0.60 [0.16, 1.04]
Cymbala AA et al 2005	-0.03	0.67	11	-0.13	0.68	11	7.5%	0.14 [-0.69, 0.98]
de Diego A et al 2013	-0.07	0.02	16	-0.08	0.02	14	9.9%	0.49 [-0.24, 1.22]
Tsang KW et al 1999	0.12	0.98	11	0	0.57	10	7.2%	0.14 [-0.72, 1.00]
Wong C et al 2012	-0.02	0.3	71	-0.1	0.3	70	48.1%	0.27 [-0.07, 0.60]
Subtotal (95% CI)			**152**			**145**	**100.0%**	**0.36 [0.13, 0.59]**
Heterogeneity: Tau² = 0.00; Chi² = 2.11, df = 4 (P = 0.71); I² = 0%								
Test for overall effect: Z = 3.08 (P = 0.002)								
1.4.3 Adults-postbronchodilator FEV1								
Serisier DJ et al 2013	-1.6	4.6	59	-4	6.6	58	45.0%	0.42 [0.05, 0.79]
Wong C et al 2012	-0.01	0.27	71	-0.08	0.27	70	55.0%	0.26 [-0.07, 0.59]
Subtotal (95% CI)			**130**			**128**	**100.0%**	**0.33 [0.08, 0.58]**
Heterogeneity: Tau² = 0.00; Chi² = 0.41, df = 1 (P = 0.52); I² = 0%								
Test for overall effect: Z = 2.64 (P = 0.008)								
1.4.4 Adults-postbronchodilator FVC								
Wong C et al 2012	-0.01	0.3	71	-0.14	0.3	70	100.0%	0.43 [0.10, 0.77]
Subtotal (95% CI)			**71**			**70**	**100.0%**	**0.43 [0.10, 0.77]**
Heterogeneity: Not applicable								
Test for overall effect: Z = 2.53 (P = 0.01)								

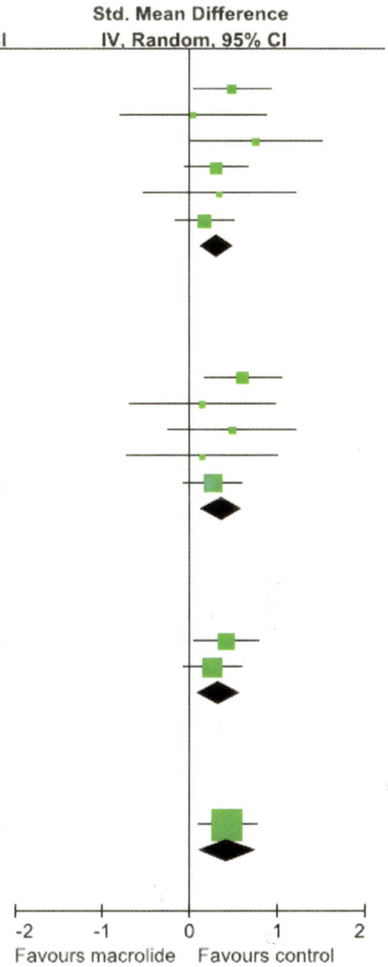

B

Study or Subgroup	macrolide Mean	macrolide SD	macrolide Total	control Mean	control SD	control Total	Weight	Mean Difference IV, Random, 95% CI
1.5.5 Children-prebronchodilator FEV1								
Koh YY et al 1997	3	6.56	13	1	7.55	12	80.8%	2.00 [-3.56, 7.56]
Masekela R et al 2013	12	18.76	17	9	13.6	14	19.2%	3.00 [-8.41, 14.41]
Subtotal (95% CI)			**30**			**26**	**100.0%**	**2.19 [-2.81, 7.19]**
Heterogeneity: Tau² = 0.00; Chi² = 0.02, df = 1 (P = 0.88); I² = 0%								
Test for overall effect: Z = 0.86 (P = 0.39)								
1.5.6 Children-prebronchodilator FVC								
Masekela R et al 2013	14	16.43	17	13	13.34	14	100.0%	1.00 [-9.48, 11.48]
Subtotal (95% CI)			**17**			**14**	**100.0%**	**1.00 [-9.48, 11.48]**
Heterogeneity: Not applicable								
Test for overall effect: Z = 0.19 (P = 0.85)								

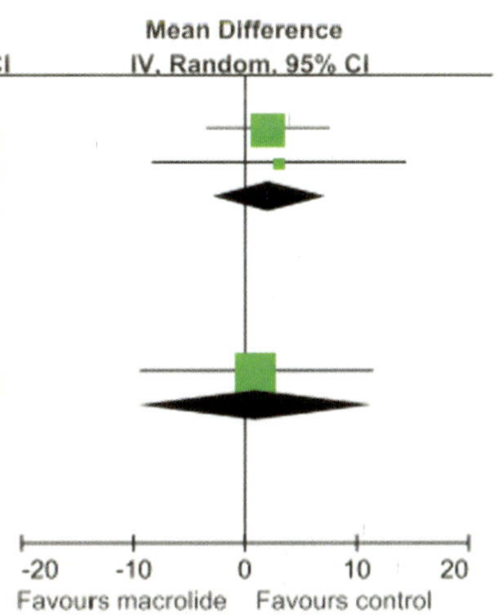

Figure 5. A. Meta-analysis of randomized controlled trials evaluating the effects of macrolide therapy on spirometric indices of FEV_1 and FVC in adults with bronchiectasis. B. Meta-analysis of randomized controlled trials evaluating the effects of macrolide therapy on spirometric indices of FEV_1 and FVC in children with bronchiectasis.

exacerbations might help explain the aforementioned outcomes. Nonetheless, further studies are still needed to explore the true effects of erythromycin on the number of patients with exacerbations in bronchiectasis. Interestingly, the results indicated that significant benefits in reducing the number of patients with exacerbations took 6 months or more to occur in adults with

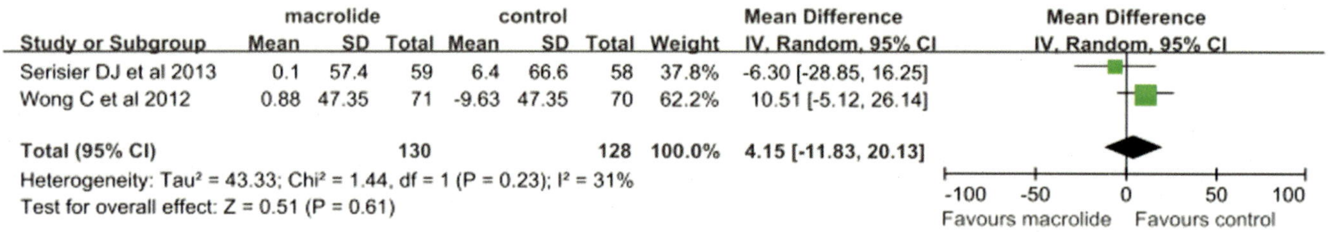

Figure 6. Meta-analysis of randomized controlled trials evaluating the effects of macrolide therapy on 6MWT in adults with bronchiectasis.

bronchiectasis, which was consistent with the findings in COPD [13]. Currently, guidelines for treatment of diffuse panbronchiolitis [27] recommended a maintenance macrolide therapy for 6 months or more, and in serious conditions, a prolonged treatment. Therefore, the optimal duration of macrolide therapy should be determined in future clinical trials. While there was a significant reduction in the number of patients with exacerbations and the rate of exacerbations, macrolide administration did not reduce the exacerbation-related admissions. However, the low rate of exacerbation-related admissions reported in two trials in adults and one in children highlighted the significance of appropriately selecting clinically relevant outcomes in future trials.

The underlying mechanisms of reduced exacerbations by macrolide therapy might be in part explained by the anti-inflammatory and immunomodulatory effects that attenuate chronic airway inflammation, inasmuch that marked airway inflammation leads to a greater risk of exacerbations [28,29]. An alternative explanation could be that macrolides alter the subtypes of P. *aeruginosa* (PA) and inhibit their adherence to respiratory epithelium as well as biofilms formation. A positive sputum culture of PA has consistently been associated with increased likelihood of infective exacerbations [29]. Macrolide therapy might have a better effect on exacerbations in patients with sputum isolation or colonization of PA than those without [15,25]. Therefore, further studies are needed to investigate the effects of macrolides on pulmonary exacerbation by stratification of PA isolation (colonization).

Changes in health related QoL and spirometric indices also appeared statistically significant in adults with bronchiectasis. Compared with placebo or control, the mean changes in the SGRQ total score among all participants outweighed the clinically significant change of 4 units [30]. Meanwhile, pooled analyses of currently available studies showed that macrolide administration also led to improvements both in FEV_1 and FVC. The beneficial effect for the QoL and spirometric indices might be explained at least in part by the decreased exacerbations in adults treated with macrolide. Previous studies showed that recurrent exacerbations not only led to progression deterioration of lung functions [31] but also one of the strong predictors of poor QoL [32]. The lack of beneficial effects of macrolide therapy for lung function in children might be related to limited studies (2 trials, 56 participants). Further research is warranted to investigate the definitive effects of macrolide therapy on spirometric indices in children with bronchiectasis.

Macrolide therapy did not significantly improve the 6MWT compared with placebo although the significant effects on spirometry were noted. Exercise capacity reflects not only respiratory but also systemic well-beings. Of note, exercise limitation might be not the crux in bronchiectasis, as evidenced by the median or mean for 500 meters or more reported in two studies [15,17].

A number of studies found significant decrease in key clinical outcomes of sputum expectoration following treatment with macrolides compared to placebo or control. One potential confounding factors is the differences in the methods of measurement, with three studies using wet volume [22,23,25] and one dry weight [15]. The optimum approach for measuring sputum volume has not been established. Despite these limitations, these studies provided preliminary supports of macrolides in reducing sputum expectoration—a crucial symptom associated with bronchiectasis.

In terms of safety, we showed that macrolides increased the risk of diarrhea and abdominal discomforts, but not overall adverse events in adults. In practice, a major concern with using macrolides for long-term therapy in respiratory diseases is the emergence of new pulmonary pathogens and increased antimicrobial resistance of airway microbiota which should be closely monitored both in individuals and the community [33]. Macro-

Table 4. Adverse events in adults with macrolides vs. control, with summary estimates across all data.

Variables	No. Patients	No. Trials	Macrolides	Controls	RR (95%CI)	P value	I^2 (%)	P value for heterogeneity
Any adverse events	384	5	97/195	98/189	0.96(0.83, 1.13)	0.66	0	0.58
Abdominal discomfort	224	2	13/114	2/110	6.20(1.43, 26.83)	0.01	0	0.78
Diarrhea	246	3	24/125	5/121	4.33(1.77, 10.58)	0.001	0	0.7
Headache	224	2	3/114	5/110	0.62(0.17, 2.29)	0.47	0	0.33
Nausea	341	3	15/173	14/168	1.03(0.52, 2.03)	0.93	30	0.24
Rash	94	2	9/54	5/50	1.67(0.60, 4.64)	0.33	0	0.62
Sinusitis	258	2	4/130	4/128	0.98(0.25, 3.86)	0.98	0	0.46

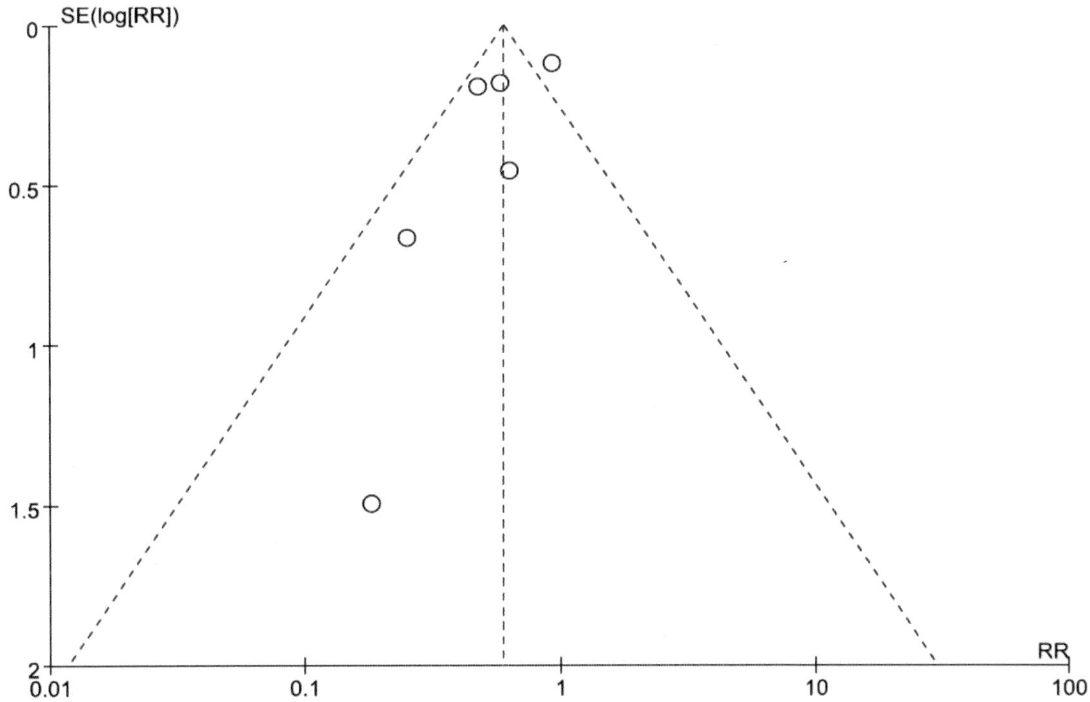

Figure 7. Funnel plot of included trials for bronchiectasis exacerbations in adults.

lides for maintenance therapy in adults has not resulted in emerging pathogens but has led to increased microbial resistance [15–17]. Studies have suggested a significant shift in the azithromycin-treated group to carriage of macrolide-resistant bacteria in children [26]. Identification of the subgroup patients who benefits more from prolonged macrolide therapy is necessary. In addition, there were no reported serious cardiovascular events in patients treated with macrolides, which resulted in significant controversies and should be closely monitored in patients with high risk of cardiovascular disorders [34,35]. Therefore, a balance between the improvement in crucial clinical endpoints, i.e. exacerbations, spirometry and QoL, and the development of antimicrobial resistance and adverse events should be well maintained.

Several limitations of this meta-analysis should be considered. First, there was significant among-study heterogeneity in: (1) subjects with different exacerbation history, age and disease severity; (2) the type, duration and dosage of macrolide treatment (Table 1); and (3) the definitions for exacerbation (Table S1). In fact, absence of a validated definition has precluded bronchiectasis exacerbation-related studies. However, it should be noted that all the included studies were RCTs comparing macrolide therapy with controls and the characteristics of patients were comparable. In addition, the random-effect model and subgroup analysis were used to account for this heterogeneity. Second, due to the limited number of studies and population, results from subgroups should be interpreted meticulously. Third, the results regarding the number of patients with one or more exacerbations in adults might be influenced by the publication bias. Although Egger's test did not show significant publication bias, the asymmetric funnel plot suggested that potential publication bias could not be ruled out. Recently published large RCTs unanimously demonstrated beneficial effects of macrolide therapy on reducing the exacerbations, rendering our conclusion unlikely to be altered by unpublished data. Nonetheless, more studies are needed to further confirm the findings. Finally, the largest study conducted in children with bronchiectasis included those who had not undergone CT scanning to confirm the presence of bronchiectasis.

In conclusion, macrolides had a benefit of preventing from exacerbations, but not admissions for exacerbation, both in adults and children with bronchiectasis compared with controls. Moreover, adults on macrolide therapy were associated with improvements in several other outcomes, including QoL, spirometric indices and reduced 24-hour sputum volume but not 6MWT and risk of overall adverse effects. Further studies are necessary to delineate the optimal agents, dose, duration of macrolide therapy, optimal population and potential antimicrobial resistance and cardiovascular risk.

Acknowledgments

We thank de Diego A for providing including the number and definition of exacerbations, Tsang KW for the definition of bronchiectasis, Serisier DJ for providing spirometric indices and Altenburg J for exacerbations,spirometric indices and quality of life from their studies.

Author Contributions

Conceived and designed the experiments: YHG WJG GX RCC. Performed the experiments: YHG WJG GX. Analyzed the data: YHG WJG GX YT YG ZYL ZML NSZ. Contributed reagents/materials/analysis tools: YHG WJG GX YT YG ZYL ZML NSZ. Wrote the paper: YHG WJG GX RCC.

References

1. Pasteur MC, Bilton D, Hill AT (2010) British Thoracic Society guideline for non-CF bronchiectasis. Thorax 65 Suppl 1: i1–58.
2. De Soyza A, Brown JS, Loebinger MR (2013) Research priorities in bronchiectasis. Thorax 68: 695–696.
3. Ringshausen FC, de Roux A, Pletz MW, Hamalainen N, Welte T, et al. (2013) Bronchiectasis-associated hospitalizations in Germany, 2005–2011: a population-based study of disease burden and trends. PLoS ONE 8: e71109.
4. Seitz AE, Olivier KN, Steiner CA, Montes de Oca R, Holland SM, et al. (2010) Trends and burden of bronchiectasis-associated hospitalizations in the United States, 1993–2006. Chest 138: 944–949.
5. Seitz AE, Olivier KN, Adjemian J, Holland SM, Prevots R (2012) Trends in bronchiectasis among medicare beneficiaries in the United States, 2000 to 2007. Chest 142: 432–439.
6. Twiss J, Metcalfe R, Edwards E, Byrnes C (2005) New Zealand national incidence of bronchiectasis "too high" for a developed country. Arch Dis Child 90: 737–740.
7. Saynajakangas O, Keistinen T, Tuuponen T, Kivela SL (1997) Bronchiectasis in Finland: trends in hospital treatment. Respir Med 91: 395–398.
8. Cai Y, Chai D, Wang R, Bai N, Liang BB, et al. (2011) Effectiveness and safety of macrolides in cystic fibrosis patients: a meta-analysis and systematic review. J Antimicrob Chemother 66: 968–978.
9. Reiter J, Demirel N, Mendy A, Gasana J, Vieira ER, et al. (2013) Macrolides for the long-term management of asthma - a meta-analysis of randomized clinical trials. Allergy 68: 1040–1049.
10. Spagnolo P, Fabbri LM, Bush A (2013) Long-term macrolide treatment for chronic respiratory disease. Eur Respir J 42: 239–251.
11. Kudoh S, Azuma A, Yamamoto M, Izumi T, Ando M (1998) Improvement of survival in patients with diffuse panbronchiolitis treated with low-dose erythromycin. Am J Respir Crit Care Med 157: 1829–1832.
12. Benden C, Boehler A (2009) Long-term clarithromycin therapy in the management of lung transplant recipients. Transplantation 87: 1538–1540.
13. Yao GY, Ma YL, Zhang MQ, Gao ZC (2013) Macrolide Therapy Decreases Chronic Obstructive Pulmonary Disease Exacerbation: A Meta-Analysis. Respiration Doi: 10.1159/000350828 (Article in press).
14. Kanoh S, Rubin BK (2010) Mechanisms of action and clinical application of macrolides as immunomodulatory medications. Clin Microbiol Rev 23: 590–615.
15. Serisier DJ, Martin ML, McGuckin MA, Lourie R, Chen AC, et al. (2013) Effect of long-term, low-dose erythromycin on pulmonary exacerbations among patients with non-cystic fibrosis bronchiectasis: the BLESS randomized controlled trial. JAMA 309 (12). 1260–1267.
16. Altenburg J, Graaff CS, Stienstra Y, Sloos JH, Haren EH, et al. (2013) Effect of azithromycin maintenance treatment on infectious exacerbations among patients with non-cystic fibrosis bronchiectasis: the BAT randomized controlled trial. JAMA 309 (12). 1251–1259.
17. Wong C, Jayaram L, Karalus N, Eaton T, Tong C, et al. (2012) Azithromycin for prevention of exacerbations in non-cystic fi brosis bronchiectasis (EMBRACE): A randomised, double-blind, placebo-controlled trial. The Lancet 380: 660–667.
18. Evans DJ, Bara AI, Greenstone M (2007) Prolonged antibiotics for purulent bronchiectasis in children and adults. Cochrane Database Syst Rev: CD001392.
19. Jadad AR, Moore RA, Carroll D, Jenkinson C, Reynolds DJ, et al. (1996) Assessing the quality of reports of randomized clinical trials: is blinding necessary? Control Clin Trials 17: 1–12.
20. Higgins JP, Thompson SG (2002) Quantifying heterogeneity in a meta-analysis. Stat Med 21: 1539–1558.
21. Koh YY, Lee MH, Sun YH, Sung KW, Chae JH (1997) Effect of roxithromycin on airway responsiveness in children with bronchiectasis: a double-blind, placebo-controlled study. Eur Respir J 10(5). 994–999.
22. Tsang KW, Ho PI, Chan KN, Ip MS, Lam WK, et al. (1999) A pilot study of low-dose erythromycin in bronchiectasis. Eur Respir J 13: 361–364.
23. Cymbala AA, Edmonds LC, Bauer MA, Jederlinic PJ, May JJ, et al. (2005) The disease-modifying effects of twice-weekly oral azithromycin in patients with bronchiectasis. Treat Respir Med 4: 117–122.
24. Masekela R, Anderson R, Gongxeka H, Steel HC, Becker PJ, et al. (2013) Lack of efficacy of an immunomodulatory macrolide in childhood HIV related bronchiectasis: A randomised, placebo-controlled trial. J Antivir Antiretrovir 5: 044–049.
25. de Diego A, Milara J, Martinez E, Palop M, Leon M, et al. (2013) Effects of Long-term Azithromycin Therapy on Airway Oxidative Stress Markers in non-Cystic Fibrosis bronchiectasis. Respirology Doi: 10.1111/resp.12130. (Article in press).
26. Valery PC, Morris PS, Byrnes CA, Grimwood K, Torzillo PJ, et al. (2013) Long-term azithromycin for Indigenous children with non-cystic-fibrosis bronchiectasis or chronic suppurative lung disease (Bronchiectasis Intervention Study): a multicentre, double-blind, randomised controlled trial. Lancet Respir Med 1: 610–620.
27. Poletti V, Casoni G, Chilosi M, Zompatori M (2006) Diffuse panbronchiolitis. Eur Respir J 28: 862–871.
28. Chalmers JD, Smith MP, McHugh BJ, Doherty C, Govan JR, et al. (2012) Short- and long-term antibiotic treatment reduces airway and systemic inflammation in non-cystic fibrosis bronchiectasis. Am J Respir Crit Care Med 186: 657–665.
29. Patel IS, Vlahos I, Wilkinson TM, Lloyd-Owen SJ, Donaldson GC, et al. (2004) Bronchiectasis, exacerbation indices, and inflammation in chronic obstructive pulmonary disease. Am J Respir Crit Care Med 170: 400–407.
30. Jones PW (2005) St. George's Respiratory Questionnaire: MCID. COPD 2: 75–79.
31. Martinez-Garcia MA, Soler-Cataluna JJ, Perpina-Tordera M, Roman-Sanchez P, Soriano J (2007) Factors associated with lung function decline in adult patients with stable non-cystic fibrosis bronchiectasis. Chest 132: 1565–1572.
32. Wilson CB, Jones PW, O'Leary CJ, Cole PJ, Wilson R (1997) Validation of the St. George's Respiratory Questionnaire in bronchiectasis. Am J Respir Crit Care Med 156: 536–541.
33. Serisier DJ (2013) Risks of population antimicrobial resistance associated with chronic macrolide use for inflammatory airway diseases. Lancet Respir Med 1: 262–274.
34. Ray WA, Murray KT, Hall K, Arbogast PG, Stein CM (2012) Azithromycin and the risk of cardiovascular death. N Engl J Med 366: 1881–1890.
35. Schembri S, Williamson PA, Short PM, Singanayagam A, Akram A, et al. (2013) Cardiovascular events after clarithromycin use in lower respiratory tract infections: analysis of two prospective cohort studies. BMJ 346: f1235.

Paracellular Transport through Healthy and Cystic Fibrosis Bronchial Epithelial Cell Lines – Do We Have a Proper Model?

Natalia Molenda[1¶], Katarina Urbanova[1¶], Nelly Weiser[1], Kristina Kusche-Vihrog[1], Dorothee Günzel[2], Hermann Schillers[1*]

1 Institute of Physiology II, University of Münster, Münster, Germany, 2 Institute of Clinical Physiology, Charité Campus Benjamin Franklin, Berlin, Germany

Abstract

It has been reported recently that the cystic fibrosis transmembrane conductance regulator (CFTR) besides transcellular chloride transport, also controls the paracellular permeability of bronchial epithelium. The aim of this study was to test whether overexpressing wtCFTR solely regulates paracellular permeability of cell monolayers. To answer this question we used a CFBE41o⁻ cell line transfected with wtCFTR or mutant F508del-CFTR and compered them with parental line and healthy 16HBE14o⁻ cells. Transepithelial electrical resistance (TER) and paracellular fluorescein flux were measured under control and CFTR-stimulating conditions. CFTR stimulation significant decreased TER in 16HBE14o⁻ and also in CFBE41o⁻ cells transfected with wtCFTR. In contrast, TER increased upon stimulation in CFBE41o⁻ cells and CFBE41o⁻ cells transfected with F508del-CFTR. Under non-stimulated conditions, all four cell lines had similar paracellular fluorescein flux. Stimulation increased only the paracellular permeability of the 16HBE14o⁻ cell monolayers. We observed that 16HBE14o⁻ cells were significantly smaller and showed a different structure of cell-cell contacts than CFBE41o⁻ and its overexpressing clones. Consequently, 16HBE14o⁻ cells have about 80% more cell-cell contacts through which electrical current and solutes can leak. Also tight junction protein composition is different in 'healthy' 16HBE14o⁻ cells compared to 'cystic fibrosis' CFBE41o⁻ cells. We found that claudin-3 expression was considerably stronger in 16HBE14o– cells than in the three CFBE41o⁻ cell clones and thus independent of the presence of functional CFTR. Together, CFBE41o⁻ cell line transfection with wtCFTR modifies transcellular conductance, but not the paracellular permeability. We conclude that CFTR overexpression is not sufficient to fully reconstitute transport in CF bronchial epithelium. Hence, it is not recommended to use those cell lines to study CFTR-dependent epithelial transport.

Editor: Shama Ahmad, University of Colorado, Denver, United States of America

Funding: Work was supported by the Deutsche Forschungsgemeinschaft SFB 629 (A6). The funders had no role in study design, data collection and analysis, decision to publish, or preparation of the manuscript.

Competing Interests: The authors have declared that no competing interests exist.

* Email: Hermann.Schillers@uni-muenster.de

¶ These authors contributed equally to this work.

Introduction

In the apical and basolateral membrane, embedded ion channels and transporters together provide for epithelial (transcellular) transport. The active transport is directly or indirectly ATP-dependent, while the passive one is driven by electrochemical gradients maintained by active transporters [1]. It is likely that the paracellular pathway is regulated in parallel with the transcellular pathway because both routes determine net transport and must work in concert as they are functionally matched to meet the transport requirements of a specific tissue [2]. On the apical membrane of epithelial cells localized cystic fibrosis transmembrane conductance regulator (CFTR) is a cyclic adenosine monophosphate (cAMP)-regulated channel, which is found in various organs like lung, pancreas, intestine, testes, and others [3,4]. CFTR is a limiting factor of the airway epithelial fluid secretion and defect of this protein results in the impaired epithelial salt and water transport, causing stasis of mucus, chronic inflammation and infection in lung. Meanwhile, over 1,900 mutations of this protein are known (http://www.genet.sickkids.on.ca) and the most common mutation causing cystic fibrosis (CF) is the deletion of phenylalanine at position 508 (F508del) [5]. The CF phenotype is the consequence of CFTR insufficiency not only in terms of its chloride conductance but also concerning its regulatory function on other ion channels and intracellular interaction partners [6–8]. In this line, CFTR is assumed to be involved in the regulation of paracellular permeability [9–12]. Paracellular transport of solutes and water is driven by the transepithelial electrochemical gradient [13] and modulated by tight junctions (TJ), a multi-protein complex, which acts as a permeability barrier [14,15]. Tight junctions allow paracellular permeation through at least two parallel pathways: i) a pore pathway - a system of charge-selective small pores (4 Å exclusion radius) and ii) a leak pathway - larger discontinuities in barrier, which lack charge and size discrimination [16]. The pore pathway has a high capacity and is responsible for the flux of specific ions and small uncharged solutes. However, through the leak pathway only a small amount of larger molecules can pass [17].

In the presented study, we compared polarized human bronchial epithelial cell line CFBE41o$^-$ transfected with wild type CFTR (wtCFTR) and mutant F508del-CFTR [18] to 16HBE14o$^-$ and CFBE41o$^-$ cell lines, to investigate the influence of CFTR and F508del-CFTR on paracellular permeability. The commonly used 16HBE14o$^-$ and CFBE41o$^-$ cell lines have the disadvantage that they do not originate from the same donor and therefore they have a different genetic background. This potential problem can be solved by the overexpression of wtCFTRwtCFTR and F508del-CFTR in the CFBE41o$^-$ cell line, which should mimic healthy and CF airway epithelia [18]. The aim of this study was to test if expression of wtCFTR in CF cells restores epithelial function, not only in terms of chloride conductance, but also regarding CFTR dependent regulation of paracellular permeability. Limiting for fluorescein flux (as a measure of paracellular solute transport) across epithelia is the protein structure and composition of TJ. Tight junction barrier function and charge selectivity are determined by claudins, a large family of integral tight junction transmembrane proteins [17]. Claudins and other TJ proteins are organized in a continuous network of parallel and interconnected strands at the lateral membranes of adjacent cells. However, permeability depends not only on microstructure regulated by molecular sieves formed by intermeshing TJ strands on the extracellular surface of opposing membranes but also on cell size [19]. Monolayers formed by small cells show more junctional length per area than large cells. Large junctional length per area means more paracellular shunts and subsequently, a higher transport capacity of these pathways. Together the transport capacity of the paracellular pathway is determined by TJ composition and cell morphology within a monolayer or a tissue. This was particularly considered in this study.

Methods

Materials

Unless specified otherwise, all chemicals were obtained from Sigma-Aldrich (Deisenhofen, Germany).

Cell Culture

The cell line 16HBE14o$^-$ was generated by the transformation of normal bronchial epithelial cells with SV40 large T-antigen [20]. The 16HBE14o$^-$ cells retain differentiated epithelial morphology by forming polarized layers with microvilli and cilia [21]; [22]. The CFBE41o$^-$ cell line was generated by transformation of cystic fibrosis (CF) tracheo-bronchial cells with SV40 and is homozygous for the F508del-CFTR mutation [23]. CFBE41o$^-$ cell line was corrected with a plasmid containing either full-length (6.2kb) wild type wtCFTR (CFBE-WT) or F508del-CFTR (4.7 kb) (CFBE-delF) cDNA [18]. All cell lines were kind gifts from Dr. Dieter C. Gruenert, California Pacific Medical Center Research Institute, San Francisco, CA, USA. Cell lines were grown in Eagle's Minimal Essential Medium (Invitrogen, Karlsruhe, Germany) and supplemented with 10% Fetal Bovine Serum (PAA Laboratories, Pasching, Austria), 2 mM L-glutamine, 50 U/ml penicillin and 50 µg/ml streptomycin. Additionally for CFBE41o$^-$ cell lines transfected with plasmids 300 µg/ml Hygromycin B (InvivoGen, San Diego, CA, USA) was added as selective agent. All cell lines were cultured in a 5% CO_2-95% air incubator at 37°C. The cell culture medium was changed three times per week. The confluent cells were trypsinized and 1.6×10^5 cells were seeded on a ThinCert cell culture inserts (12-well plate, Greiner Bio-One, Germany). The flasks and inserts were coated with a solution containing collagen type I from calf skin and human plasma fibronectin (Invitrogen, Karlsruhe, Germany). In our experiments the numbers of subcultures (P) were P4.78 for CFBE41o$^-$, P4.77.48 for CFBE-WT, P4.77.34 for CFBE-delF and P4.46 for 16HBE14o$^-$ cells. The absolute number of passages (P) as denoted by "(passages after primary isolation).(passages after immortalization).(passages after CFTR transfection).

Stimulation of Epithelial Cells

In order to activate CFTR related epithelial transport, cells were treated with 8-(4-chlorophenylthio) adenosine 3′, 5′cyclic monophosphate sodium salt (8cpt-cAMP) in final concentration of 100 µM.

Continues Transepithelial Electric Resistance (cTER) Measurements

Determination of cTER were performed as described previously [12]. Briefly, we used a cover lid for 12 well ThinCert plates equipped with 8 sets of six titanium electrodes (4 to inject current and two to measure voltage) creating a homogenous electrical field (Fig. 1). Electrical current pulses with a frequency of 125 Hz were applied at a given time interval for 1 s. The electrical resistance of cell-free ThinCert inserts (128 $\Omega \cdot cm^2$) was subtracted from TER raw data. Data acquisition and processing was performed with a 2-channel PowerLab system (26 Series, ADInstruments GmbH, Germany).

Ussing Chamber Experiments

For Ussing chamber experiments, 16HBE14o$^-$ and CFBE41o$^-$ cells were seeded on filter supports (Millicell-PCF, 0.4 µm pore size, Millipore) and grown to confluence within 7 days. Confluent cells layers on filter supports were directly mounted in conventional Ussing- chambers and both hemi-chambers were filled with 10 ml standard bath solution (in mM: 140 Na^+, 123.8 Cl^-, 5.4 K^+, 1.2 Ca^{2+}, 1.2 Mg^{2+}, 2.4 HPO_4^{2-}, 0.6 $H_2PO_4^-$, 21 HCO_3^-, 10 D(+)-glucose, pH 7.4 when equilibrated with 5% CO_2 in O_2 at 37°C). Flux measurements were carried out with and without applying voltage-clamp. After equilibration, flux tracers (fluorescein sodium salt, final concentration 100 µM) were added to the apical side and 300 µl aliquots were collected from the receiving side every 10 min and immediately replaced by fresh standard bath solution. Duplicates of fluorescein-containing samples were pipetted onto 96-well plates (140 µl/well) together with defined dilutions of fluorescein in standard bath saline for calibration and fluorescence was quantified using a plate reader (TECAN, infinite M200). Flux was calculated as increase in tracer quantity (corrected for dilution) per time unit and filter area (0.6 cm^2).

Immunostaining and Image Analysis

16HBE14o$^-$, CFBE41o$^-$ and CFBE41o$^-$ cell lines transfected with wtCFTR or F508del-CFTR were grown to confluence on ThinCert inserts, fixed in 3,7% PFA at RT for 15 min, and then permeabilized with 0.1% Triton X-100 for 5 min. After blocking with 5% goat serum in PBS for 30 min, cells were incubated for 1 h with a mouse monoclonal antibody mouse-anti-ZO-1 (zonula occludens-1) (BD Transduction Laboratories, NJ, USA), mouse-anti claudin-4 and -5 or rabbit-anti caudin-3 and -7 (1:200, Zymed/Invitrogen, San Francisco, CA) followed by labeled secondary antibody Alexa-FlourTM 488 goat anti-mouse (Molecular Probes, Inc., OR, USA) Cy2 goat anti-mouse or Cy5 goat anti-rabbit (1:1000, Jackson Immuno Research, Newmarket, UK) and DAPI 1:10000 (Invitrogen, OR, USA). Imaging was performed using a Zeiss 510 Meta laser scanning microscopy with a 63x oil objective or a Zeiss Observer Z fluorescence

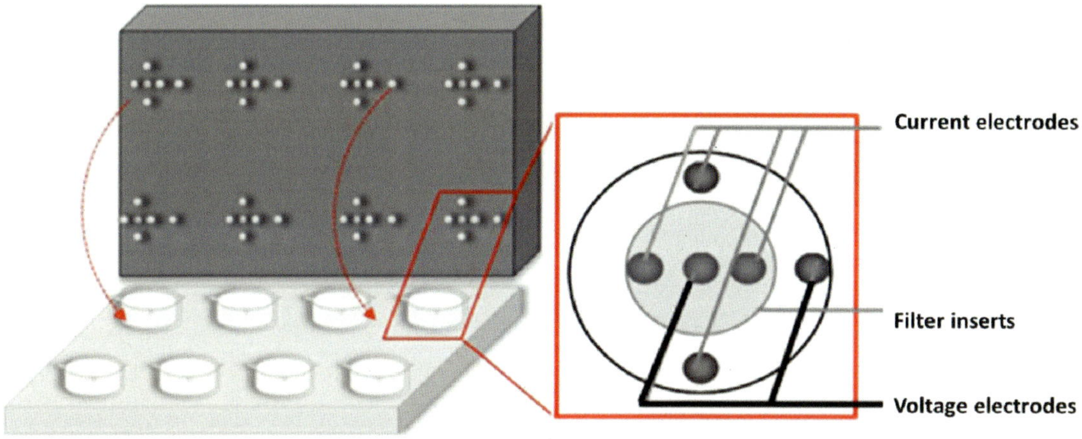

Figure 1. Scheme of the continuous transepithelial resistance measurement device (cTER). The ThinCert culture plate contains eight filter inserts with cell monolayers. The upper plate (lid) has six titanium electrodes for each insert, four electrodes to inject the current and two to measures the voltage. Electrodes are arranged in a way that resulted in a fairly homogenous electrical field.

microscope with 40x and 100x oil objectives. Fluorescence micrographs were acquired using an EMCCD camera (iXon EM+ DU-888, Andor Technology, Belfast, Ireland) and MetaMorph (Molecular Devices, Inc., CA; USA).

The length and structure of the intercellular junction of monolayers were determined after staining of cells with antibodies against ZO-1 using ImageJ image analysis software (Rasband W.S., ImageJ, National Institutes of Health, Bethesda, Maryland, USA, http://rsb.info.nih.gov/ij/, 1997–2004).

Measurement of Fluorescein Flux

The transport of the fluorescein sodium salt (fluorescein) was determined to investigate the paracellular permeability of cell monolayers grown on 12 well ThinCert inserts (all cell lines). Integrity of the monolayer was checked prior to the experiment by determination of TER. The cell monolayers were rinsed gently twice with MEM medium without phenol-red indicator and left for 1–2 hours to equilibrate in the same medium. The TER of the monolayers was measured again. A stock solution of fluorescein was mixed with fresh MEM and added to the apical compartment (end concentration 10 μM). Samples (100 μl) were withdrawn immediately and after 1 h from the apical and basolateral compartment. The flux of fluorescein across the cell layer was calculated from the net increase of the fluorescence in the basolateral compartment measured with a fluorescent microplate reader (Labsystem Fluoroskan II, GMI, Inc., USA) ($E_x = 485$ nm, $E_m = 538$ nm). Data are presented as the fluorescein flux (nmol h^{-1} cm^{-2}).

Western Blot

ProteoExtract Transmembrane Protein Extraction Kit (Calbiochem) was used for protein isolation according to the manufactures protocol 'Extraction of Membrane Proteins from Adherent Tissue Culture Cells'. Protein concentration was determined by Pierce BCA assay and 10 μg protein per lane was loaded on 12.5% polyacrylamid gels. Subsequent to SDS gel electrophoresis, proteins were blotted onto polyscreen PVDF transfer membranes (Perkin Elmer, Waltham, MA). Blots were blocked in 5% BSA before overnight incubation with primary antibodies (mouse-anti claudin-4 and -5 or rabbit-anti caudin-3, -7 and -18, all Zymed/Invitrogen, 1:1000). Peroxidase-conjugated AffiniPure $F(ab')_2$ fragment goat anti-mouse/−rabbit (1:10000, Jackson ImmunoResearch) were used as secondary antibodies and Lumi-Light^{PLUS} Western Blotting Kit (Roche, Grenzach-Wyhlen, Germany) was used for visualizationin a Fusion FX 7 image acquisition system (Vilber Lourmat, Eberhardzell, Germany).

RNA Extraction

All cell lines were grown on coated culture dishes. RNA was extracted from confluent cells using the RNeasy mini kit (Qiagen Hilden, Germany). The RNA was DNase treated (Deoxyribonuclease I, Invitrogen, Karlsruhe, Germany). The total RNA concentration and quantity were assessed by the absorbance at 260 nm using a Bio Photometer (Eppendorf, Hamburg, Germany). 1 μg of total RNA was reverse-transcribed to cDNA using SuperScript III Reverse Transcriptase (Invitrogen, Karlsruhe, Germany). For each cell line three cDNA samples from separate RNA extractions and reverse transcription reactions were employed.

Real-time PCR

Quantitative analysis of the DNA and RNA was performed in 20 μl with 1 μM each of predesigned TaqMan Gene Expression Assays (Applied Biosystems, Foster City, CA, USA) in Eppendorf Mastercycler ep realplex^4 PCR thermal cycler (Eppendorf, Hamburg, Germany). The assay ID numbers of the validated genes are as follows: Hs00357011-m1 for CFTR and Hs02758991-g1 for GAPDH (Applied Biosystems, Foster City, CA, USA). The amplification was performed as follows: an initial step at 95°C for 10 min, followed by 45 cycles of 95°C for 15 sec and 60°C for 60 sec. All samples were run in triplicate. The $2^{-\Delta\Delta CT}$ method was used to calculate the amount of gene expression [24]. CFTR mRNA expression was normalized to the parallel measured endogenous controls GADPH in each cell line. CFTR expression value of 16HBE14o$^-$ cells was defined as 1 and CFTR expression of all other cells were normalized to this value.

Statistics

Median values ± quartiles or mean ± SD are reported here. The Mann–Whitney–Wilcoxon (MWW) tests, One-way Anova analysis or Student t test were performed, respectively, to test for statistical significance. A p-value of <0.05 was accepted to indicate significant differences.

Results

Continous Transepithelial Electrical Resistance (cTER)

Epithelial cell monolayers can be characterised by cTER, which is determined primarily by the electrical resistance of the apical and basolateral cell membrane and the paracellular resistant, generated by the TJ complex [25]. A high TER value suggests a low permeability to ionic movement. TER values of 24 to 33 independent experiments showed rather large variations. Therefore, data are expressed as median [first quartile; third quartile]. Median electrical resistances of monolayers after 8–11 days in culture was 703 [854; 651] Ω*cm^2 for 16HBE14o$^-$ and 528 [616; 504] Ω*cm^2 for CFBE41o$^-$ after correction for the background contributed by the ThinCert insert and medium (Fig. 2). 16HBE14o$^-$ showed statistically significant higher TER than CFBE41o$^-$. The TER of CFBE-delF cell (470 [534; 407] Ω*cm^2) and CFBE-WT cell monolayers (431 [514; 387] Ω*cm^2) were comparable to TER of the parental CFBE41o$^-$ cell line (no statistical significance).

Stimulation of CFTR with cAMP resulted in a breakdown of resistance in all wtCFTR expressing cell monolayers. TER of 16HBE14o$^-$ cells decreased by 60% within 5 minutes (Fig. 3A) and also CFBE-WT cell monolayer shows a clear but weaker response upon CFTR stimulation (decrease of TER by 30% within 5 minutes, Fig. 3B). By contrast, TER of all F508del-CFTR expressing cells rose transiently. CFBE41o$^-$ increased by 30% and CFBE-delF by 10% respectively after stimulation with cAMP (Fig. 3A, B).

Fluorescein Flux

To distinguish between the transcellular und paracellular permeability we measured the flux of the tracer molecule fluorescein, which indicates the movement exclusively through the paracellular pathway [26]. Under control conditions fluorescein flux was comparable in all tested cell lines: 0.114 [0.191; 0.103] nmol *cm^{-2} h^{-1} for 16HB14o$^-$, 0.118 [0.167; 0.098] nmol *cm^{-2} h^{-1} for CFBE41o$^-$, 0.105 [0.185; 0.066] nmol *cm^{-2} h^{-1} for CFBE-WT and 0.125 [0.147; 0.094] nmol *cm^{-2} h^{-1} for CFBE-delF (Fig. 4A, B). Stimulation of CFTR with cAMP significantly increased fluorescein flux across the 16HBE14o$^-$ monolayers (0.317 [0.348; 0.311] nmol *cm^{-2} h^{-1}) but did not affect flux across CFBE41o$^-$ (0.125 [0.158; 0.091] nmol *cm^{-2} h^{-1}) (Fig. 4A), CFBE-WT (0.091 [0.128; 0.062] nmol *cm^{-2} h^{-1}) and CFBE-delF (0.103 [0.203; 0.081] nmol *cm^{-2} h^{-1}) monolayers (Fig. 4B). These results indicate that stimulation of CFTR affects only paracellular permeability of healthy epithelia (16HBE14o$^-$).

Because fluorescein is a negatively charged molecule, we tested if the transepithelial potential difference influenced the paracellular flux of fluorescein. First, there was no preferential direction of fluorescein transport across 16HBE14o$^-$ cell monolayers (apical to basolateral or vice-versa). Second, there was no difference in fluorescein transport in Ussing-chamber experiments when transepithelial potential difference was clamped to zero by injecting short-circuit current. The permeability to fluorescein in 16HBE14o$^-$ cell monolayers exposed to voltage clamp shows no statistically significant difference to 16HBE14o$^-$ cells without voltage clamp (n = 13). We observed the same effects for CFBE41o$^-$ cells (data not shown).

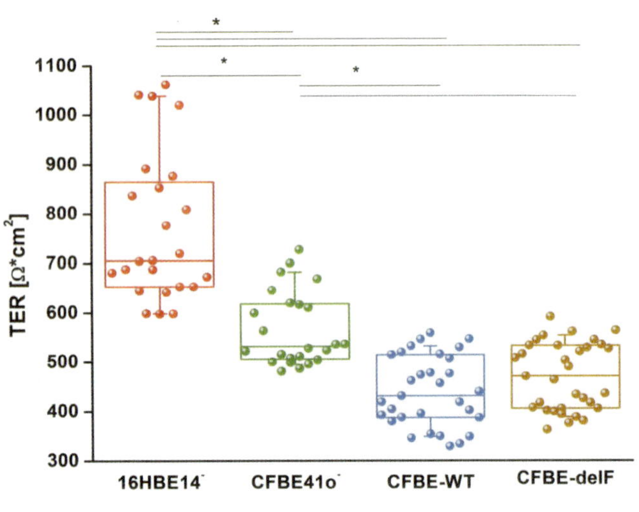

Figure 2. Continuous Transepithelial electrical resistance measurement (cTER). All cell monolayer were grown on ThinCert supports. cTER was monitored in all cell lines after they had reached confluence. 16HBE14o$^-$ cells exhibit significantly higher TER values in comparison to CFBE41o$^-$ and its transfected clones. Data are presented as a box-plots showing raw data (circles), median (horizontal line), 25 and 75 percentile (box) and SD (whiskers) (n = 24–33, $p<0.05$).

Cell Morphology

The paracellular flux depends not only on TJ structure and composition but also on junctional length (cell-cell contact length) per area. Monolayers formed by small cells show usually more junctional length per area than large cells. But junctional length depends not only on cell size but also on microstructure of cell-cell contacts (wrinkles, folds, grooves, etc.). More junctional length per area means higher transport capacity due to more paracellular shunts per area (assuming a comparable TJ protein composition). In summary the transport capacity of the paracellular pathway is determined by TJ composition and cell morphology within a monolayer or a tissue.

Morphology of TJ pathway plays an important role in paracellular permeability. TJ length per area was derived from monolayers immunolabeled for a marker of tight junctions (ZO-1) (Fig. 5A) and analysed by imaging software ImageJ. Length of 16HBE14o$^-$ TJ per µm^2 is about 30% higher compared to CFBE41o$^-$ and its transfected clones (Fig. 5C), so they have more junctional length per unit area through which electrical current and solutes can pass. 16HBE14o$^-$ cells have also more branched cell borders than the other cell lines. The ratio of persistent length to contour length is about 1.4. In contrast CFBE41o$^-$ cells show a ratio of about 1.1 (Fig. 5B). Considering these ratios allow calculating the TJ length per µm^2 for each cell line. As a result, 16HBE14o$^-$ cells show about 80% higher length of cell-cell contact per area than CFBE41o$^-$ and its transfected clones (Fig. 5C). Assuming the same TJ composition, a monolayer with smaller cells should have lower TER and higher solute flux [16]. However we observed that 16HBE14o$^-$ monolayers show significantly higher TER values than CFBE41o$^-$ and CFBE41o$^-$ clones transfected with wtCFTR or F508del-CFTR. Epithelial permeability to fluorescein, a measure of passive leakage across the epithelium was correlated to the TJ length per area (Fig. 6A, B). All cell lines show statistically indistinguishable fluorescein flux under control conditions.

Claudin Expression

Based on these results it is likely that the TJ composition differs between the investigated cell lines. Both Western blot and immuno-stainings demonstrated that 16HBE14o$^-$ and CFBE41o$^-$ cells expressed claudins-3, -4, -5 and -7 that had previously been

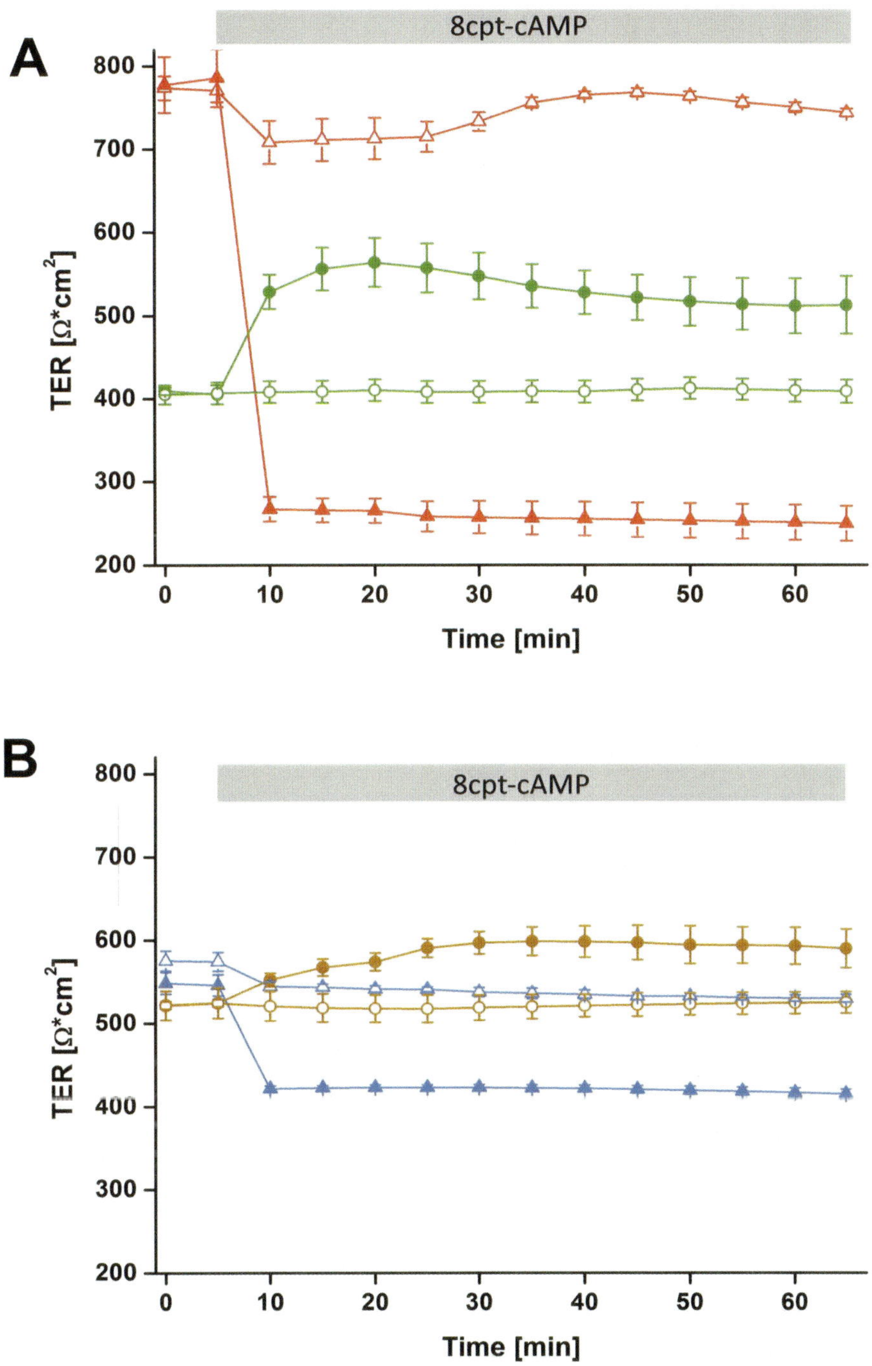

Figure 3. Changes in transepithelial electrical resistance (cTER) upon cAMP. A) 16HBE14o⁻ (triangles) and CFBE41o⁻ (circles) monolayer were grown on ThinCert supports. After 8–11 days in culture they obtained 800 and 500 Ω^*cm^2 resistance respectively. After 5 min 8cpt-cAMP was added, causing dramatic TER decrease in 16HBE14o⁻ cells (red triangles) and an increase of TER for CFBE41o⁻ (green circles). Addition of the same amount of medium to control cells (open circles and triangles) did not show any effect. **B)** CFBE-WT monolayer (blue triangles) and CFBE-delF monolayer (brown circles) were grown on ThinCert supports. After 8–11 days in culture both clones obtained 500–600 Ω^*cm^2 resistance. Stimulation with 8cpt-cAMP caused a decrease of TER in CFBE-WT cells (blue triangles) and an increase for CFBE-delF (brown circles). Addition of the same amount of medium to control cells (open circles and triangles) did not show any effect. Results are presented as mean ± SD (n = 3–6, $p < 0.05$).

described to be highly expressed in alveolar epithelial cells (Fig. 7, for rev. see [27]). No specific staining for claudin-18 could be detected (date not shown). Whereas expression for claudin-4, -5 and -7 was comparable for 16HBE14o⁻ and all CFBE41o⁻ cell clones, claudin-3 expression was considerably stronger in 16HBE14o⁻ cells than in the CFBE41o⁻ cell line and its clones, and thus independent of the presence of functional CFTR. Claudin-3 has a tightening effect on the paracellular pathway [28]. Results demonstrated that the TJ composition of 16HBE14o⁻ and CFBE41o⁻ cells is clearly different whereas CFBE41o⁻ exhibits a claudin expression, which is comparable to its clones transfected with wtCFTR or F508del-CFTR.

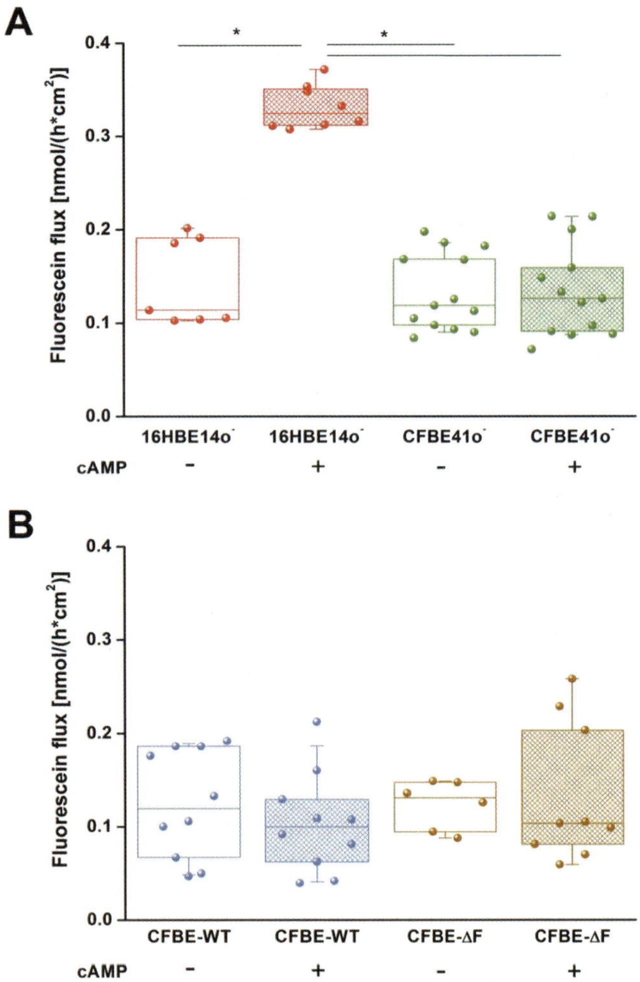

Figure 4. Paracellular permeability to fluorescein. A) Under control conditions 16HBE14o⁻ (red) and CFBE41o⁻ (green) cell lines showed a comparable fluorescein flux. Addition of cAMP significantly increased fluorescein flux of 16HB14o⁻ (red hatched box) but it did not affect CFBE41o⁻ cells (green hatched box). **B)** CFBE-WT cells (blue) and CFBE-delF (brown) do not show statistically significant differences in fluorescein flux neither under resting conditions nor upon stimulation with cAMP (hatched boxes). Data are presented as a box-plot showing raw data (circles), median (horizontal line) 25 and 75 percentile (box) and SD (whiskers) ($n = 7–13$, $p < 0.05$).

Analysis of CFTR mRNA Expression by Real-time PCR

The levels of CFTR mRNA in all cell lines were quantified by real-time PCR. CFTR expression value of 16HBE14o⁻ cells was defined as 1 and CFTR expression of all other cells were normalized to this value. CFTR mRNA levels of the other cell lines were displayed as a fold change relative to16HBE14o⁻ (Fig. 8). Vector-driven wtCFTR mRNA level in the complemented CFBE41o- clone (CFBE-WT) was 1,864 fold and not significantly higher compared to native CFTR mRNA in 16HBE14o- cells. CFBE-delF cells show an even lower mRNA expression (−0,37 fold, Fig. 8). Lowest expression of CFTR mRNA was found in CFBE41o- cells.

Discussion

We previously compared paracellular permeability of 16HBE14o⁻ and CFBE41o⁻ cell lines [12]. Both of them represent

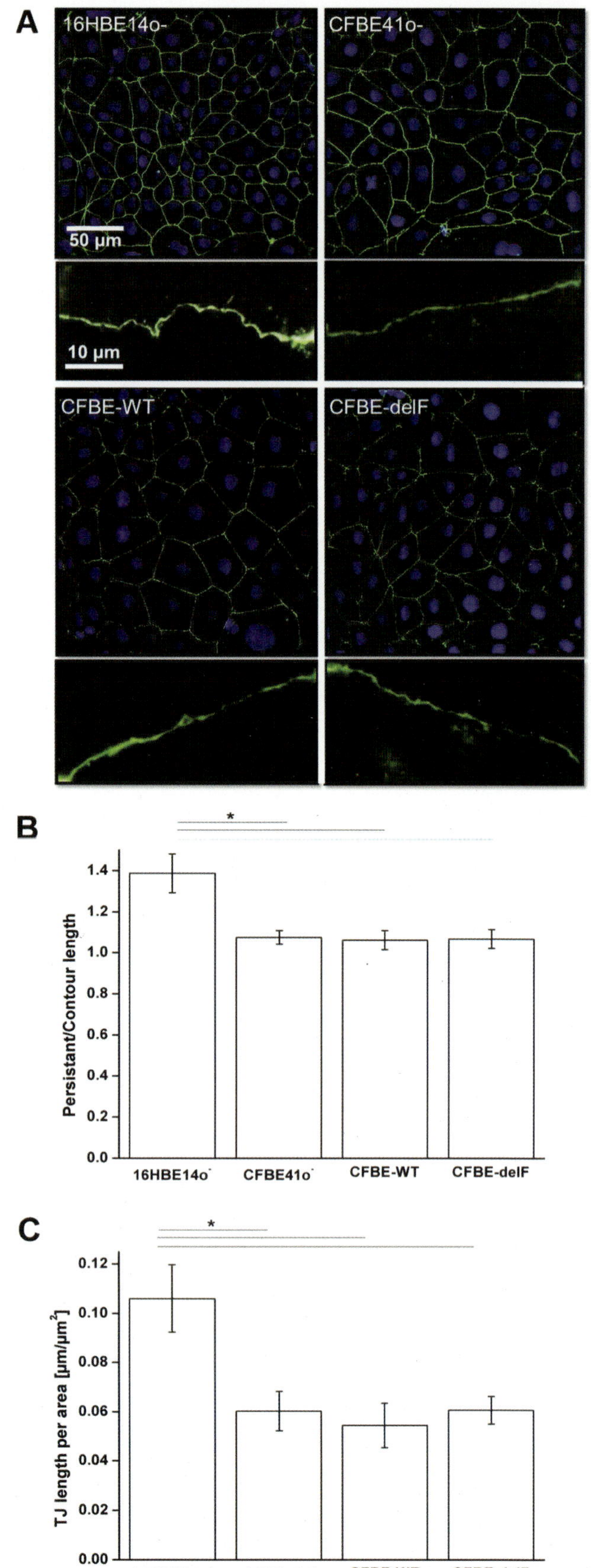

Figure 5. Differences in TJ length. A) Upper image show immunostaining of ZO-1 (green) and nuclei staining (blue). Lower

image shows magnifications of representative cell borders. **B)** Ratio of persistent length to contour length of all tested cell monolayers. 16HBE14o⁻ shows a cell-cell contact enlargement by 40% while CFBE41o⁻ cells and its transfected clones exhibit only a tiny enlargement by 10%. **C)** TJ lengths per area in μm per μm^2. 16HBE14o⁻ cells show 80% longer TJ lengths per area than CFBE41o⁻ cells. Furthermore, there is no difference in TJ lengths per area between CFBE41o⁻ cells and its transfected clones. Results are presented as mean ± SD (n = 7–8, $p<0.05$).

widely used models of the human healthy and CF bronchial epithelium. We could not completely exclude that the differences between those two cell lines originated from the fact that they came from different donors instead of different CFTR expression in cell membrane. Thus, we tested if the same relationships of TER and fluorescein flux could be observed between the CFBE-WT and CFBE-delF cells. Those clones are new models of healthy and CF epithelium, created by transfection with wtCFTR or F508del-CFTR in the parental CFBE41o⁻ cell line [18]. Under control conditions 16HBE14o⁻ showed significantly higher TER values than CFBE41o⁻ and its clones (CFBE-WT and CFBE-delF). TER of both clones is indistinguishable but significantly lower that TER of their parental cell line (CFBE41o⁻) (Fig. 2). These results are consistent with the observations of Nilsson et al., who found that CFTR overexpression in CFBE41o⁻ cells (CFBE-WT) cells reduces TER [29]. However, it was also reported that transient and stable CFTR expression in CFBE41o⁻ cells increased TER [30]. Furthermore, Illek et al. demonstrated by Ussing chambers experiments that monolayers of parental CFBE41o⁻ and both transfected clones showed similar, moderately "tight" transepithelial resistance [18]. Though, the methodology, used by these research groups was not consistent. LeSimple et al. used chop stick electrodes with an epithelial voltmeter (EVOM) [30] and Nilsson et al. an ENDOHM-6 Chamber with an EVOM [29]. Chop-stick electrodes are known for spatial constrains showing an unequal distribution of current flow through the epithelium. It is conceivable that the divergence of results is a consequence of different methods. To overcome this difficulty, we developed a six-electrode system creating a homogenous electrical field (Fig. 1) and applied electrical current pulses with a frequency of 125 Hz.

Stimulation of CFTR with cAMP resulted in the decrease of TER in both wtCFTR expressing cell lines (Fig. 3A, B). The decrease of TER by 60% and 30% in 16HBE14o⁻ and CFBE-WT cells, respectively, after CFTR stimulation was most likely caused by the increase of membrane permeability due to the activation of the CFTR chloride channel and other CFTR dependent membrane conductance [31]. In CFBE41o⁻ and CFBE-delF cells application of cAMP showed an opposite effect, TER increased by 30% and 10%, respectively (Fig. 3A, B). Also Nilsson et al. observed the same acute effect on TER by 16HBE14o⁻ and CFBE-WT cells treated with cAMP raising agents: forskolin or IBMX [29]. Obviously the second messenger cAMP induced a change in TER. Even if the mechanism is unclear, the effect on TER is linked to the presence of functional CFTR. The responses of CFBE-WT and CFBE-delF cells were clearly weaker than by 16HBE14o⁻ and CFBE41o⁻, respectively. Illek et al. suggested that CFTR expression from the transgene is not as effective at generating working channels as the CFTR endogenously expressed in 16HBE14o⁻ cells. This way they explained why cells overexpressing CFTR at mRNA level were not showing same response to CFTR stimulation as 16HBE14o⁻ cells [18]. Illek et al. generated the cell lines CFBE-WT and CFBE-delF and measured their CFTR mRNA levels shortly after stable transfection

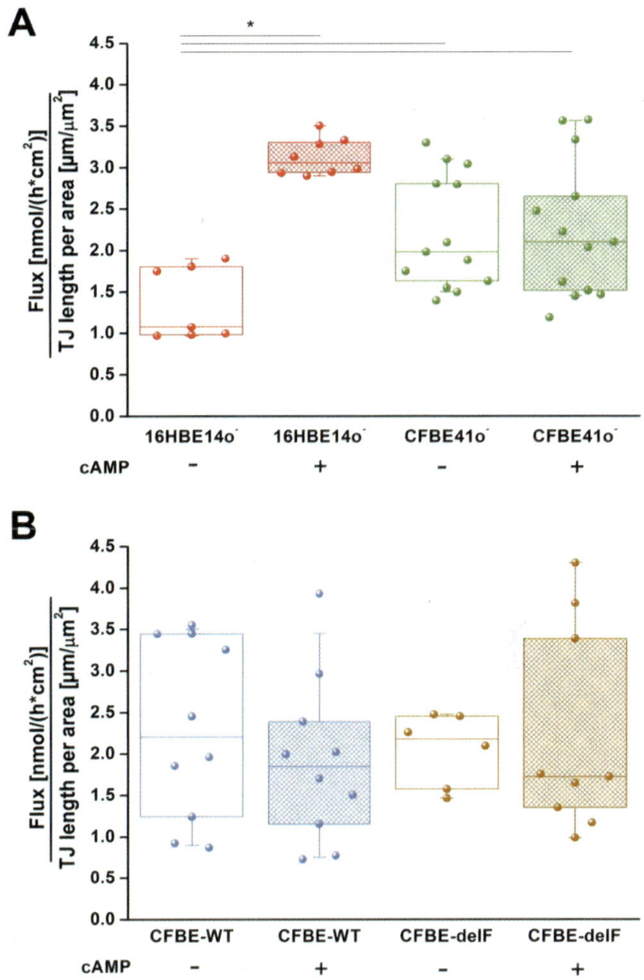

Figure 6. Fluorescein flux per TJ length. A) Calculation of flux per TJ length revealed a significant lower value for 16HBE14o⁻ cells under resting conditions (red box) compared to CFBE41o⁻ cells (green box). Stimulation with cAMP caused a 3 fold increase for 16HBE14o⁻ cells (red hatched box) while CFBE41o⁻ cells do not respond to stimulation (green hatched box). **B)** CFBE-WT cells (blue) and CFBE-delF (brown) do not show statistically significant differences in fluorescein flux per TJ length neither under resting conditions nor upon stimulation with cAMP (hatched boxes). Data are presented as a box-plot showing raw data (circles), median (horizontal line) 25 and 75 percentile (box) and SD (whiskers (n = 7–13, $p<0.05$).

(p4.77.05–p4.77.12). The expression of CFTR mRNA in the complemented cell lines was 14 to 27-fold higher (determined relative to 16HBE14o⁻). In contrast we showed that CFBE-WT do not have significantly higher CFTR expression than 16HBE14o⁻ cells (Fig. 8). Additionally in CFBE-delF mRNA expression was significantly lower than in 16HBE14o⁻ cells. One explanation could be that phenotypic stability is threatened by genetic and epigenetic changes, cell aging, and differentiation [32]. As a consequence, protein of interest expression can be reduced with time. In our experiments the numbers of subcultures (P) were P4.77.48 for CFBE-WT and P4.77.34 for CFBE-delF cells. Younger clones (lower number of P) are not available. Even Illek et al. performed measurements of transepithelial resistance and ion transport in Ussing chambers using cells p4.77.47 to p4.77.52 for CFBE-WT and p4.72.44 to p4.72.49 for CFBE-delF. Obviously the vector-driven CFTR expression in the available complemented cell lines (CFBE-WT and CFBE-delF) is not

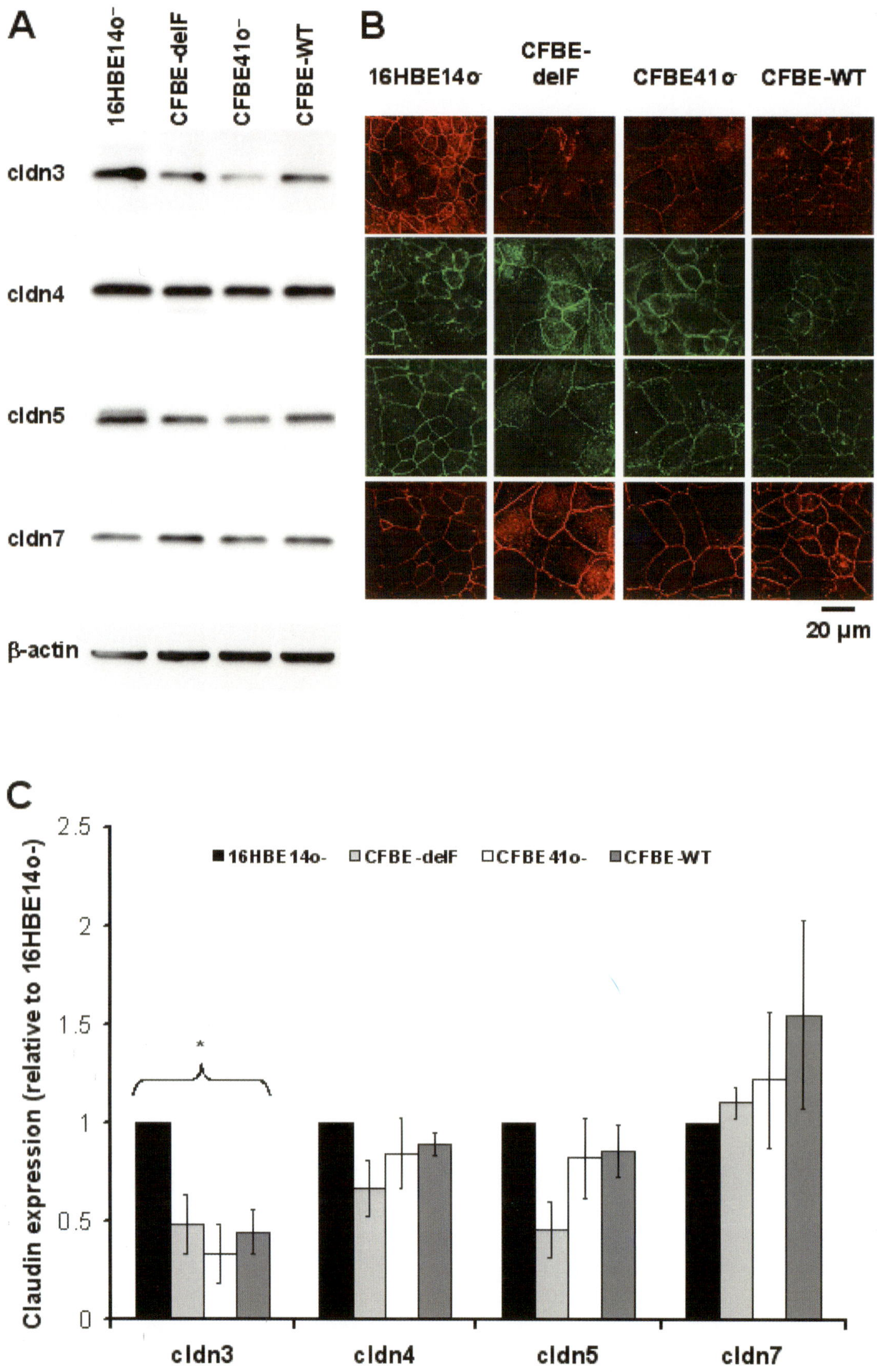

Figure 7. Detection of tight junction proteins. Presence of tight junction proteins known to be expressed in alveolar epithelial cells (claudin-3, -4, -5, -7) and their junctional localization in 16HBE14o⁻, CFBE41o⁻ cells and its transfected clones was verified by Western blot (A) and confocal laser

scanning microscopy (B). For densitometric evaluation of Western blots (C), all signals were normalized to β-actin. All values are expressed relative to the respective value detected in 16HBE14o⁻ cell layers. One-way Anova analysis revealed that claudin-3 expression differed ($p<0.05$) in 16HBE14o⁻ and CFBE41o⁻ clones, whereas claudin-4, -5 and -7 expression was not significantly different (n = 4). No claudin-18 expression was detected (not shown).

sufficient to mimic CFTR function in epithelial transport. CFTR is a key molecule for transepithelial transport which is not only determined by transcellular, but also by paracellular permeabilities and both permeabilities have to be functionally matched to comply with transport requirements of airway epithelia [2]. In a previous work, we showed with ^{14}C-mannitol flux that stimulation of 16HBE14o⁻ cells (endogenously expressing wtCFTR) with cAMP increase their paracellular permeability [12]. Here, we tested the paracellular permeability of 16HBE14o⁻, CFBE41o⁻ and its transfected clones with the marker molecule fluorescein. Fluorescein sodium salt is a fluorescent, low molecular weight compound (radius 4.5 Å) and it can be used as a marker of paracellular permeability. We performed Ussing-chamber experiments with or without applying short-circuit current to eliminate electrical potential across the epithelium. Although fluorescein has negative charge, there was no change in permeability to fluorescein from apical side to basolateral side or vice-versa. From these data, we assume that the transepithelial potential difference does not influence fluorescein flux. This is consistent with results of Koljonen et al, who used fluorescein as an alternative marker molecule for mannitol in the studies of paracellular absorption and leakage in the apical – basolateral direction in Caco-2 cell monolayers [26]. Sodium fluorescein seems to be transported actively when a pH gradient is applied between the apical and the basolateral compartment [33,34]. Therefore, we carried out all experiments under iso-pH conditions of pH 7.4 on both sides of the cell monolayer. We found that under control conditions, the fluorescein permeability of 16HBE14o⁻, CFBE41o⁻, CFBE-WT and CFBE-delF was statistically indistinguishable (Fig. 4A, B). cAMP stimulation significantly enhanced the paracellular permeability of 16HBE14o⁻ cell monolayers, but no changes in fluorescein flux were observed in CFBE41o⁻, CFBE-WT and CFBE-delF cells. These data demonstrate that expression of wtCFTR in CFBE41o⁻ is not sufficient to restore CFTR's regulatory function on paracellular transport.

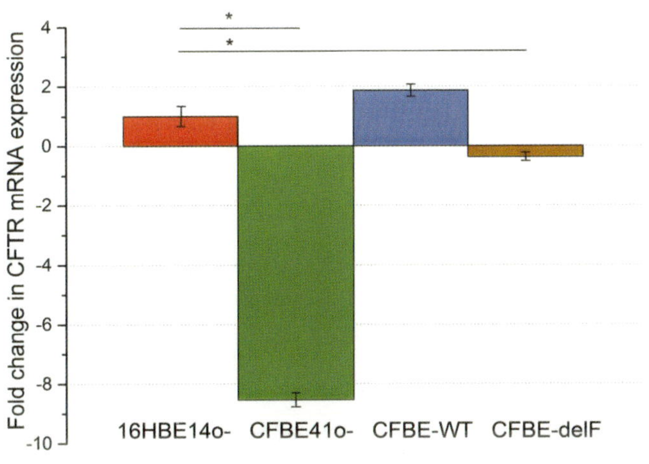

Figure 8. Expression of CFTR mRNA. The relative quantity of CFTR gene expression was calculated by the $2^{-\Delta\Delta Ct}$ method, using GAPDH as the internal reference. CFTR mRNA expression value of 16HBE14o⁻ cells was defined as 1 and expression of all other cells were normalized to this value. CFTR mRNA levels of the other cell lines were displayed as a fold change relative to16HBE14o⁻. Results are presented as mean ± SEM (n = 9–12, $p<0.001$).

To explain those discrepancies we investigated structure and morphology of cell-cell contacts. The length of cell-cell contacts per area reflects the density of paracellular pathways within a cell monolayer. Immunostaining of the TJ protein ZO-1 revealed that 16HBE14o⁻ cells are considerably smaller than CFBE41o⁻, CFBE-WT and CFBE-delF cells. Transfection with wtCFTR (CFBE-WT) or F508del-CFTR (CFBE-delF) did not influence the morphology of the cells. The smaller 16HBE14o⁻ cells show clearly longer cell-cell contacts per area than the larger CFBE41o⁻ cells and its transfected clones (Fig. 5C). Furthermore, the microstructure of 16HBE14o⁻ cell-cell contacts shows wrinkles and ruffles, while CFBE41o⁻ and its transfected clones have smooth and wrinkle-free cell borders. This structural difference could be expressed as a ratio of persistent length over contour length. Contour length is roughly the circumference of the cell while persistent length describes the real length of cell-cell contacts, enlarged by wrinkles and ruffles. A ratio of persistent length over contour length of one means that there is no enlargement of cell-cell contacts and ratio over one indicate an enlargement of cell-cell contact length by infoldings and grooves. Figure 5B shows clearly the enlargement of cell-cell contact length for 16HBE14o⁻ cell monolayers (about 40%). In contrast, the ratio for CFBE41o⁻ and its transfected clones is close to one. Together, difference of TJ length per area is further increased by the microstructure of cell-cell contacts and is two-fold larger for 16HBE14o⁻ cell monolayers than for CFBE41o⁻ and its transfected clones (Fig. 5A). If the protein composition of TJ were comparable in all four tested cell lines, 16HBE14o⁻ cells should show lowest TER and highest paracellular permeability under control conditions. Actually, the TER of 16HBE14o⁻ cells was significantly higher than those of CFBE41o⁻ and its transfected clones (Fig. 2). We could show that fluorescein flux of all cell lines was statistically indistinguishable under control conditions (Fig. 4). However, when taking into consideration the difference in TJ length, fluorescein flux per unit of 16HBE14o⁻ cells was significantly lower under control conditions and significantly higher under CFTR-stimulated conditions (Fig. 6A). The fluorescein flux of CFBE41o⁻ was not influenced by cAMP and did not show differences to those of CFBE-WT and CFBE-delF (Fig. 6A, B).

In addition to difference in size and subsequently cell-cell contact length per area, we also demonstrated differences in TJ composition between 16HBE14o⁻ cells and CFBE41o⁻ and CFBE41o⁻ clones transfected with wtCFTR or F508del-CFTR. TJ consist of many membrane and scaffolding proteins and paracellular permeability of cells depends mostly on the claudin profile. There are 27 claudins known in mammals and differences in their expression are responsible for changes in the electrolyte and solute permeability in cells layers [35]. Even subtle changes in the structure of the TJ could profoundly affect the overall permeability or the ion selectivity of an epithelium [36] [2]. We discovered significantly higher membrane expression levels of the claudin-3 in 16HBE14o⁻ in comparison with other cells (Fig.7). This could explain the observed leak tightness of this cell line. In agreement with our results, elevating claudin-3 expression of MDCK cells caused strong increased in the paracellular resistance

[28]. Recently, Lin et al. demonstrated that knockdown of the expression of either claudin 3 or 4 in ovarian carcinoma cells increased cell size and resulted in flattened morphology [37]. Cell lines investigated in this work show the same effect, since claudin 3 expression correlates with cell morphology (Fig. 5A, Fig. 7).

Nilsson et al. demonstrated that TJ integrity of $16HBE14o^-$, $CFBE41o^-$ and CFBE transfected with wtCFTR cells was reduced upon CFTR stimulation with forskolin and IBMX [29]. This suggests a possible interaction between CFTR and the TJ protein complex, probably via the cytoskeleton. Also LeSimple [30] found that CFTR trafficking but not CFTR channel function is required for proper function and organization of TJs. We observed that increasing the intracellular concentration of cAMP increases paracelluar flux of fluorescein in the $16HBE14o^-$ cells. This effect depends not solely on CFTR because even transfection with wtCFTR could not restore the ability of $CFBE41o^-$ cells to regulate paracellular permeability (Fig. 6A, B). Obviously, it is not only the missing CFTR chloride conductance which distinguishes a healthy from a CF epithelial cell.

In summary, we found that $16HBE14o^-$ cells have about 80% more junctional length per area than $CFBE41o^-$ and its transfected clones and two-fold higher claudin 3 expression. This alone is enough to explain differences in paracellular transport between $16HBE14o^-$ and $CFBE41o^-$ clones. We observed that transfection with wtCFTR in $CFBE41o^-$ cell line restores transcellular, but not the paracellular conductance. We concluded that transfection with wtCFTR in $CFBE41o^-$ cells (CFBE-WT) does not reconstitute healthy epithelium. Additionally this transfection is not as stable as originally reported [18]. Hence, cell lines investigated in this work are not suitable to study CFTR dependent epithelial transport.

Author Contributions

Conceived and designed the experiments: NM KU HS. Performed the experiments: KU NM DG NW. Analyzed the data: KU NM HS. Contributed reagents/materials/analysis tools: KK-V. Wrote the paper: KU NM HS.

References

1. Kapus A, Szaszi K (2006) Coupling between apical and paracellular transport processes. Biochem Cell Biol 84: 870–880.
2. Flynn AN, Itani OA, Moninger TO, Welsh MJ (2009) Acute regulation of tight junction ion selectivity in human airway epithelia. Proc Natl Acad Sci U S A 106: 3591–3596.
3. Sheppard DN, Welsh MJ (1999) Structure and function of the CFTR chloride channel. Physiol Rev 79: S23–S45.
4. Pilewski JM, Frizzell RA (1999) Role of CFTR in airway disease. Physiol Rev 79: S215–S255.
5. Welsh MJ, Smith AE (1993) Molecular mechanisms of CFTR chloride channel dysfunction in cystic fibrosis. Cell 73: 1251–1254. 0092-8674(93)90353-R [pii].
6. Guggino WB, Stanton BA (2006) New insights into cystic fibrosis: molecular switches that regulate CFTR. Nat Rev Mol Cell Biol 7: 426–436.
7. Kunzelmann K, Kiser GL, Schreiber R, Riordan JR (1997) Inhibition of epithelial Na+ currents by intracellular domains of the cystic fibrosis transmembrane conductance regulator. FEBS Lett 400: 341–344.
8. Treharne KJ, Xu Z, Chen JH, Best OG, Cassidy DM, et al. (2009) Inhibition of protein kinase CK2 closes the CFTR Cl channel, but has no effect on the cystic fibrosis mutant deltaF508-CFTR. Cell Physiol Biochem 24: 347–360. 000257427 [pii];10.1159/000257427 [doi].
9. Bobadilla JL, Macek M Jr, Fine JP, Farrell PM (2002) Cystic fibrosis: a worldwide analysis of CFTR mutations–correlation with incidence data and application to screening. Hum Mutat 19: 575–606.
10. Jiang C, Finkbeiner WE, Widdicombe JH, McCray PB Jr, Miller SS (1993) Altered fluid transport across airway epithelium in cystic fibrosis. Science 262: 424–427.
11. Jiang C, Finkbeiner WE, Widdicombe JH, Miller SS (1997) Fluid transport across cultures of human tracheal glands is altered in cystic fibrosis. J Physiol 501 (Pt 3): 637–647.
12. Weiser N, Molenda N, Urbanova K, Bahler M, Pieper U, et al. (2011) Paracellular Permeability of Bronchial Epithelium is Controlled by CFTR. Cell Physiol Biochem 28: 289–296. 000331742 [pii];10.1159/000331742 [doi].
13. Powell DW (1981) Barrier function of epithelia. Am J Physiol 241: G275–G288.
14. Lewis SA, Berg JR, Kleine TJ (1995) Modulation of epithelial permeability by extracellular macromolecules. Physiol Rev 75: 561–589.
15. Turner JR (2006) Molecular basis of epithelial barrier regulation: from basic mechanisms to clinical application. Am J Pathol 169: 1901–1909.
16. Anderson JM, Van Itallie CM (2009) Physiology and function of the tight junction. Cold Spring Harb Perspect Biol 1: a002584. 10.1101/cshperspect.a002584 [doi].
17. Shen L, Weber CR, Raleigh DR, Yu D, Turner JR (2011) Tight junction pore and leak pathways: a dynamic duo. Annu Rev Physiol 73: 283–309. 10.1146/annurev-physiol-012110-142150 [doi].
18. Illek B, Maurisse R, Wahler L, Kunzelmann K, Fischer H, et al. (2008) Cl transport in complemented CF bronchial epithelial cells correlates with CFTR mRNA expression levels. Cell Physiol Biochem 22: 57–68.
19. Jou TS, Schneeberger EE, Nelson WJ (1998) Structural and functional regulation of tight junctions by RhoA and Rac1 small GTPases. J Cell Biol 142: 101–115.
20. Cozens AL, Yezzi MJ, Kunzelmann K, Ohrui T, Chin L, et al. (1994) CFTR expression and chloride secretion in polarized immortal human bronchial epithelial cells. Am J Respir Cell Mol Biol 10: 38–47.
21. Ehrhardt C, Kneuer C, Fiegel J, Hanes J, Schaefer UF, et al. (2002) Influence of apical fluid volume on the development of functional intercellular junctions in the human epithelial cell line 16HBE14o-: implications for the use of this cell line as an in vitro model for bronchial drug absorption studies. Cell Tissue Res 308: 391–400.
22. Wan H, Winton HL, Soeller C, Stewart GA, Thompson PJ, et al C (2000) Tight junction properties of the immortalized human bronchial epithelial cell lines Calu-3 and 16HBE14o-. Eur Respir J 15: 1058–1068.
23. Ehrhardt C, Collnot EM, Baldes C, Becker U, Laue M, et al. (2006) Towards an in vitro model of cystic fibrosis small airway epithelium: characterisation of the human bronchial epithelial cell line CFBE41o-. Cell Tissue Res 323: 405–415.
24. Livak KJ, Schmittgen TD (2001) Analysis of relative gene expression data using real-time quantitative PCR and the 2(-Delta Delta C(T)) Method. Methods 25: 402–408. 10.1006/meth.2001.1262 [doi];S1046-2023(01)91262-9 [pii].
25. Gonzalez-Mariscal L, Chavez de RB, Lazaro A, Cereijido M (1989) Establishment of tight junctions between cells from different animal species and different scaling capacities. J Membr Biol 107: 43–56.
26. Koljonen M, Hakala KS, Ahtola-Satila T, Laitinen L, Kostiainen R, et al. (2006) Evaluation of cocktail approach to standardise Caco-2 permeability experiments. Eur J Pharm Biopharm 64: 379–387. S0939-6411(06)00157-3 [pii];10.1016/j.ejpb.2006.06.006 [doi].
27. Overgaard CE, Mitchell LA, Koval M (2012) Roles for claudins in alveolar epithelial barrier function. Ann N Y Acad Sci 1257: 167–174. 10.1111/j.1749-6632.2012.06545.x [doi].
28. Milatz S, Krug SM, Rosenthal R, Gunzel D, Muller D, et al. (2010) Claudin-3 acts as a sealing component of the tight junction for ions of either charge and uncharged solutes. Biochim Biophys Acta 1798: 2048–2057. S0005-2736(10)00248-8 [pii];10.1016/j.bbamem.2010.07.014 [doi].
29. Nilsson HE, Dragomir A, Lazorova L, Johannesson M, Roomans GM (2010) CFTR and tight junctions in cultured bronchial epithelial cells. Exp Mol Pathol 88: 118–127. S0014-4800(09)00131-2 [pii];10.1016/j.yexmp.2009.09.018 [doi].
30. Lesimple P, Liao J, Robert R, Gruenert DC, Hanrahan JW (2010) Cystic fibrosis transmembrane conductance regulator trafficking modulates the barrier function of airway epithelial cell monolayers. J Physiol 588: 1195–1209. jphysiol.2009.182246 [pii];10.1113/jphysiol.2009.182246 [doi].
31. Schwiebert EM, Benos DJ, Egan ME, Stutts MJ, Guggino WB (1999) CFTR is a conductance regulator as well as a chloride channel. Physiol Rev 79: S145–S166.
32. Barnes LM, Bentley CM, Dickson AJ (2003) Stability of protein production from recombinant mammalian cells. Biotechnol Bioeng 81: 631–639. 10.1002/bit.10517 [doi].
33. Konishi Y, Hagiwara K, Shimizu M (2002) Transepithelial transport of fluorescein in Caco-2 cell monolayers and use of such transport in in vitro evaluation of phenolic acid availability. Biosci Biotechnol Biochem 66: 2449–2457.
34. Kuwayama K, Miyauchi S, Tateoka R, Abe H, Kamo N (2002) Fluorescein uptake by a monocarboxylic acid transporter in human intestinal Caco-2 cells. Biochem Pharmacol 63: 81–88. S000629520100853X [pii].
35. Soini Y (2011) Claudins in lung diseases. Respir Res 12: 70–81.
36. Coyne CB, Gambling TM, Boucher RC, Carson JL, Johnson LG (2003) Role of claudin interactions in airway tight junctional permeability. Am J Physiol Lung Cell Mol Physiol 285: L1166–L1178.
37. Lin X, Shang X, Manorek G, Howell SB (2013) Regulation of the Epithelial-Mesenchymal Transition by Claudin-3 and Claudin-4. PLoS One 8: e67496. 10.1371/journal.pone.0067496 [doi];PONE-D-13-00995 [pii].

7

The Tumor Necrosis Factor α (-308 A/G) Polymorphism Is Associated with Cystic Fibrosis in Mexican Patients

Celia N. Sanchez-Dominguez[1], Miguel A. Reyes-Lopez[2], Adriana Bustamante[3], Ricardo M. Cerda-Flores[4], Maria del C. Villalobos-Torres[1], Hugo L. Gallardo-Blanco[5], Augusto Rojas-Martinez[1,6], Herminia G. Martinez-Rodriguez[1], Hugo A. Barrera-Saldaña[1], Rocio Ortiz-Lopez[1,6]*

1 Departamento de Bioquimica y Medicina Molecular, Facultad de Medicina, Universidad Autonoma de Nuevo Leon, Monterrey, Nuevo Leon, Mexico, **2** Laboratorio de Medicina de Conservacion, Centro de Biotecnologia Genomica, Instituto Politecnico Nacional, Reynosa, Tamaulipas, Mexico, **3** Clinica de Fibrosis Quistica, Centro de Prevencion y Rehabilitacion de Enfermedades Pulmonares Cronicas (CEPREP), Facultad de Medicina y Hospital Universitario "Dr. Jose Eleuterio Gonzalez", Universidad Autónoma de Nuevo Leon, Monterrey, Nuevo Leon, Mexico, **4** Facultad de Enfermeria, Universidad Autonoma de Nuevo Leon, Monterrey, Nuevo Leon, Mexico, **5** Departamento de Genetica, Facultad de Medicina, Universidad Autonoma de Nuevo Leon, Monterrey, Nuevo Leon, Mexico, **6** Centro de Investigacion y Desarrollo en Ciencias de la Salud, Universidad Autonoma de Nuevo Leon, Monterrey, Nuevo Leon, Mexico

Abstract

Environmental and genetic factors may modify or contribute to the phenotypic differences observed in multigenic and monogenic diseases, such as cystic fibrosis (CF). An analysis of modifier genes can be helpful for estimating patient prognosis and directing preventive care. The aim of this study is to determine the association between seven genetic variants of four modifier genes and CF by comparing their corresponding allelic and genotypic frequencies in CF patients (n = 81) and control subjects (n = 104). Genetic variants of MBL2 exon 1 (A, B, C and D), the IL-8 promoter (−251 A/T), the TNFα promoter (TNF1/TNF2), and SERPINA1 (PI*Z and PI*S) were tested in CF patients and control subjects from northeastern Mexico by PCR-RFLP.

Results: The TNF2 allele ($P = 0.012$, OR 3.43, 95% CI 1.25–9.38) was significantly associated with CF under the dominant and additive models but was not associated with CF under the recessive model. This association remained statistically significant after adjusting for multiple tests using the Bonferroni correction ($P = 0.0482$). The other tested variants and genotypes did not show any association with the disease.

Conclusion: An analysis of seven genetic variants of four modifier genes showed that one variant, the TNF2 allele, appears to be significantly associated with CF in Mexican patients.

Editor: Amit Gaggar, University of Alabama-Birmingham, United States of America

Funding: This work was supported by grants from the Consejo Nacional de Ciencia y Tecnología CONACyT (62291 and 48497) and UANL's PAICyT (1648-07) for ROL, Fondo Mixto de Fomento a la Investigación Científica y Tecnológica CONACYT – Gobierno del Estado de Tamaulipas (73578) and SIP-IPN (20080682) for MARL. The authors gratefully acknowledge scholarships from CONACyT, PIFI-IPN and Universia Santander for CNSD. The funders had no role in study design, data collection and analysis, decision to publish, or preparation of the manuscript.

Competing Interests: The authors have declared that no competing interests exist.

* E-mail: rortizlopez@gmail.com

Introduction

Gene-environment and gene-gene interactions play a role in the phenotypic expression of genetic diseases in individuals harboring the same genotype [1]. Cystic fibrosis (CF) has an estimated incidence of one in 3000 in the Caucasian population, although its frequency may vary in specific subgroups. A newborn screening study conducted in Mexico City revealed two CF-affected newborns among 7193 screened (1:3597) participants, suggesting a high frequency of CF among Mexicans [2]. Approximately 1900 mutations and variants have been reported in the CF transmembrane conductance regulator (CFTR) gene, with ΔF508 being the most prevalent mutation (50%–60%, http://www.genet.sickkids.on.ca/app). CF primarily involves epithelial cells in the respiratory tract, intestine, pancreas, bladder, and sweat glands; respiratory failure, however, is the major cause of death in CF patients [3].

Variants in genes that are involved in the inflammatory response have been studied in CF patients based on their potential effects on inflammation and host defense mechanisms. The mannose binding lectin (MBL2) gene encodes a serum acute-phase protein secreted by the liver, resembling the complement component C1q, that leads to opsonization and activation of the complement system through the classical pathway [4]. The serum concentration and complement-triggering activity of MBL depend on single-base mutations in the MBL2 gene [5–7]. These mutations may increase the susceptibility of carriers to colonization by bacterial and viral pathogens [8]. The best known genetic variants in exon 1 of the MBL2 gene are Gly54Asp (the B allele, rs1800450), Gly57Glu (the C allele, rs1800451) and Arg52Cys (the D allele, rs5030737), which are together referred to as the O allele. The interleukin 8 (IL-8) gene codes for a member of the CXC chemokine family and is mainly involved in the initiation and amplification of acute inflammatory reactions [9]. IL-8 is

Table 1. Mutations included in the kits used for the molecular diagnosis of CF patients.

Kit	Detected mutations
ASO16 Roche	DF508, G542X, G551D, R553X, W1282X, N1303K, R117H, 621+1G >T, R334W, R347P, A455E, DI507, 1717-1G >A, S549N, R560T, 3849+10Kb C >T
ASO26 Roche	DF508, G542X, G551D, R553X, W1282X, N1303K, R117H, 621+1G >T, R334W, R347P, A455E, DI507, 1717-1G >A, R560T, 3849+10KbC>T, G85E, 2307insA, G480C, A559T, R1162X, 3659delC, S1255X, R347H, 2789+5G>A, 405+3 A>C, 3120+1G>A
INNOLiPA CFTR36 Innogenetics	F508del, G542X, G551D, R553X, W1282X, N1303K, R117H, 621+1G>T, R334W, R347P, A455E, I507del, 1717-1G>A, R560T, 3849+10KbC>T, G85E, R1162X, 3659delC, 2789+5G>A, 3120+1G>A, 711+1G>T, 3905insT, S1251N, Q552X, I148T, 1898+1G>A, 394delTT, 1078delT, 2183AA>G, 2184delA, E60X, 2143delT, 711+5G>A, 3199del6, 3272-26A>G, dele2,3

produced by a wide range of cell types, such as monocytes, macrophages, and fibroblasts; it primarily mediates the activation and migration of neutrophils from peripheral blood into pathogen-infected tissue, initiating and amplifying inflammatory processes [10]. A polymorphism in position −251 of the IL-8 gene (rs4073) is associated with increased IL-8 expression [11–12]. The tumor necrosis factor alpha (TNFα) gene expresses a multifunctional pro-inflammatory cytokine secreted in response to numerous specific stimuli, such as lipopolysaccharides. This molecule induces the release of cytokines IL-6 and IL-8 and increases airway mucus production [13–14]. The −308 A TNFα promoter polymorphism (TNF2, rs1800629) has been associated with increased TNFα transcription activity relative to the normal TNF1 allele (−308 G) [15–17]. The Alpha-1-antitrypsin (AAT, SERPINA1) gene codes for an acute-phase serine protease glycoprotein that limits tissue self-damage during the inflammatory immune response. AAT deficiency, caused by the S (p.E264V, rs17580) and Z (p.E342K, rs28929474) alleles in the SERPINA1 gene, may induce liver and pulmonary disease [18]. Severe AAT deficiency is a co-dominant autosomal hereditary disorder that clinically resembles early onset pulmonary emphysema, particularly in smokers [19].

In our Cystic fibrosis clinic, we have a broad range of severity of the CF disease, even with patients carrying the same genotype. No reports on variations in modifier genes in Mexican CF patients have been previously published. Our goal was to explore polymorphisms in genes related to host defense in healthy controls and CF patients from northeastern Mexico to find differences in allelic distribution between both groups. In this study, we report the genotype and allele frequencies of seven genetic variants in four previously reported CF modifier genes: MBL, IL-8, TNFα and AAT.

Materials and Methods

Biological Samples

The study was approved by the Research and Ethics Committee of the Universidad Autonoma de Nuevo Leon University Hospital (Registry number BI09-003). After signing written informed consent, blood samples were drawn from 81 CF patients attending the Chronic Lung Disease Prevention and Rehabilitation Center (CEPREP, in Spanish) and from control subjects recruited from the University Hospital and School of Medicine (Universidad Autonoma de Nuevo Leon). Also we collected blood samples from 104 control subjects that met the following inclusion criteria: they agreed to informed consent, they were born in northeastern Mexico (the states of Nuevo Leon, Tamaulipas, Coahuila, and San Luis Potosi), and they belonged to a family with at least three ascending Mexican generations. Genomic DNA was isolated from peripheral venous blood using the phenol–chloroform method, precipitated in ethanol, and finally suspended in Tris-EDTA (pH 7.8).

Screening for the CFTR Gene Mutations

Mutation screening was performed according to the availability of resources and kits along the time. For previously screened CF patients: direct detection of ΔF508 mutation, and Roche ASO16 and 27 mutations kits, for new CF patients: direct detection of ΔF508 mutation, INNOLiPA CFTR36 probe kit and Exon

Table 2. Modifier genes analysis by PCR-RFLP adapted from previously published techniques [21–24].

Gene	Polymorphism	Primers	Enzyme	Mutant allele, bp	Normal allele, bp
MBL	Arg52Cys (D)	F: CAT CAA CGG CTT CCC AGG GCA AGA TGG G	*Mwo* I	134	109+25
	Gly54Asp (B)	R: GTC TCC TCA TAT CCC CAG GC	*Ban* I	134	95+39
	Gly57Glu (C)		*Mbo* II	78+56	134
IL-8	−251 T/A	F: GAT TCT GCT CTT ATG CCT CCA	*Mfe* I	816	520+296
		R: CCC AAG CTT GTG TGC TCT GCT GTC			
TNFα	−308 G/A	F: GGG ACA CAC AAG CAT CAA GG	*Nco* I	142	126+16
		R: AAT AGG TTT TGA GGG CCA TG			
AAT	PI*S Glu264Val	F: GAG GGG AAA CTA CAG CAC CTC G	*Taq* I$^{\alpha}$	98	78+20
		R: ACC CTC AGG TTG GGG AAT CAC C			
	PI*Z Glu342Lys	F: TAA GGC TGT GCT GAC CAT CGT C	*Taq* I$^{\alpha}$	144	123+21
		R: GGA GAC TTG GTA TTT TGT TCA ATC			

11-specific PCR and sequencing. Short descriptions of the methodologies are presented below.

PCR and electrophoresis to detect the ΔF508 mutation: PCR product was analyzed in polyachrylamide gels and the diagnosis was established comparing to molecular marker and DNAs of previously ΔF508 diagnosed patients and control subjects (98 bp band for normal allele or 95 bp band for ΔF508 mutation) [20].

Roche ASO16 and 27 kits (Roche Molecular Systems, Alameda CA, USA) or the INNOLiPA CFTR36 probe kit (Innogenetics, Ghent, Belgium). Methodology consisted of multiplex PCR reactions with biotinylated primers. After verifying the amplification in an agarose gel of 2%, the products were hybridized to membrane bound probes. A positive result was expressed as the appearance of a purple band. Both kits detected normal and mutated versions to report homozygous or heterozygous status for the CF patients. Complete list of mutations is shown in Table 1.

Exon 11- specific PCR and sequencing. Exon 11 PCR fragment was amplified and sequenced in one patient with absence of hybridization of PCR product on the normal and mutated versions of the G551D probe in the CFTR36 probe kit.

Modifier Genes Analysis

DNA from CF patients and control subjects was tested for the Gly54Asp (B allele, rs1800450), Gly57Glu (C allele, rs1800451), Arg52Cys (D allele, rs5030737), and A (wild type) alleles in exon 1 of the MBL2 gene; the −251 T/A (rs4073) allele of the IL-8 gene; the −308 G/A (TNF1/2, rs1800629) alleles of the TNFα gene; and the PI*S Glu264Val (rs17580), PI*Z Glu342Lys (rs28929474), and PI*M (wild type) alleles of the SERPINA1 gene. PCR-RFLP protocols were adapted from previously reported methods. More details are explained in Table 2 and Figure 1 [21–24].

Statistical Analysis

The SNP & Variation Suite (SVS) 7 (Golden Helix Inc., Bozeman, MA, USA) software program was used to perform all statistical analyses. The association between the tested genotypes

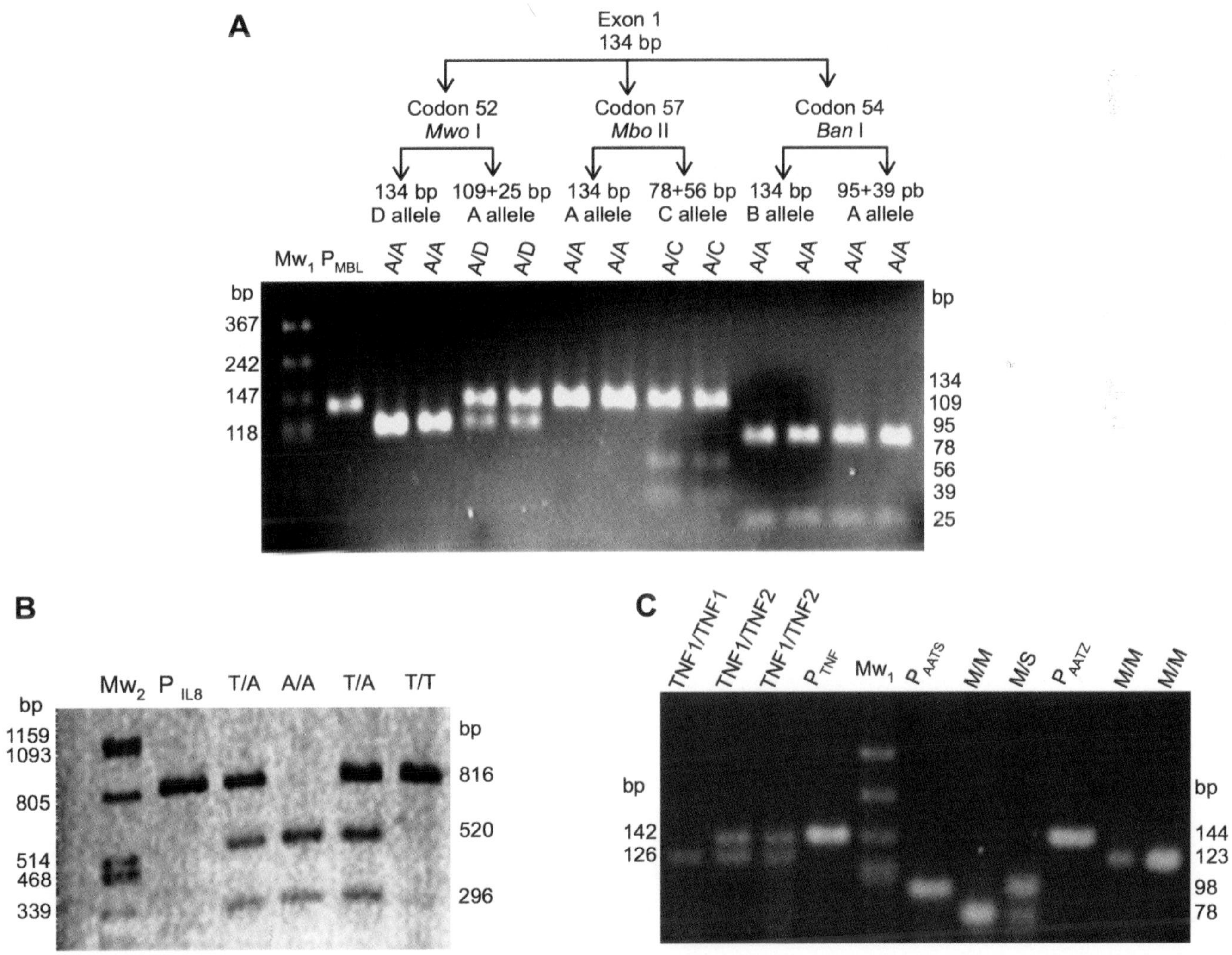

Figure 1. PCR-RFLP for the modifier genes analysis. 1A: the 134 bp PCR product from exon 1 of the MBL1 gene was digested with *Mwo* I, *Ban* I and *Mbo* II for detection of polymorphisms in the 52, 54 and 57 codons. 1B: the 816 bp PCR product from promoter region of the IL-8 gene was digested with *Mfe* I for detection of the −251 polymorphism. 1C: the 142 bp PCR product from promoter region of the TNFα gene was digested with *Nco* I for detection of the −308 polymorphism (TNF2); the 98 bp PCR product from the SERPINA1 gene was digested with *Taq* I$^{\alpha}$ for detection of the S genetic variant; the 144 bp PCR product from the SERPINA1 gene was digested with *Taq* I$^{\alpha}$ enzyme for detection of the Z genetic variant. Mw1 is the molecular marker pBs+*Msp* I, Mw2 is the molecular marker λ+*Pst* I. P_{MBL}, P_{IL8}, P_{TNF}, P_{AATS} and P_{AATZ} are undigested PCR products. The Z allele was not detected.

and CF was analyzed by correlation/trend and chi-squared (χ^2) tests under three different models (dominant, recessive, and additive) and was confirmed with the Bonferroni correction to detect the false discovery rate. Odds ratios were estimated within 95% confidence intervals. Values of $P<0.05$ were considered statistically significant. The Hardy–Weinberg Equilibrium (HWE) P-values were assessed using a chi-square test.

Results

Eighty-one CF patients and 104 control subjects were recruited for this study. Genotype frequencies for the CFTR gene are described in Table 3. A complete genotype characterization was achieved in 55.6% (n = 45) of the CF patients; in 39.5% (n = 32) of the CF patients, only one mutation was identified, and in 4.9% (n = 4) of the CF patients, both mutations remained undetected. The most prevalent genotypes were ΔF508/other (46.9%, n = 38) and ΔF508/ΔF508 (35.8%, n = 29). The overall frequency of the ΔF508 allele among CF patients was 59.3%. Ten additional mutations were detected: G542X (4.9%), S549N (3.1%), 2789+5G>A (2.5%), 3849+10 kb (1.9%), G85E, R1162X, I148T, R334W, ΔI507, and L206W (0.6% each one). Mutations in the CFTR gene were not detected in 24.7% of the total CFTR alleles.

The PCR-RFLP patterns of the seven genetic variants in the four modifier genes are shown in the Figure 1. The Z allele, and the homozygote TNF2 and AATS genotypes were not found. The genotype frequencies of modifier genes in CF patients and control subjects are shown in Table 4. The B, C, and D alleles of the MBL2 gene were grouped together and reported as the O allele. The polymorphisms were in Hardy-Weinberg equilibrium. The frequencies of the mutant alleles for CF patients and controls were: the MBL-O allele 0.231 and 0.233, the IL-8 -251T allele 0.576 and 0.569, AATS allele 0.012 and 0.014, and TNF2 allele 0.087

Table 3. CFTR genotype frequencies from 81 Mexican CF patients.

Genotype	N	%
ΔF508/ΔF508	29	35.8
ΔF508/X	26	32.1
ΔF508/G542X	5	6.2
ΔF508/3849+10 kb	3	3.7
S549N/S549N	2	2.5
G542X/X	2	2.5
ΔF508/S549N	1	1.2
ΔF508/L206W	1	1.2
ΔF508/2789+5G>A	1	1.2
ΔF508/G85E	1	1.2
2789+5G>A/2789+5G>A	1	1.2
G542X/R1162X	1	1.2
2789+5G>A/X	1	1.2
ΔI507/X	1	1.2
I148T/X	1	1.2
R334W/X	1	1.2
X/X	4	4.9
Total	81	100

X: unknown allele.

and 0.029, respectively. The TNF2 allele ($P=0.012$, Odds Ratio (OR) 3.43, 95% CI 1.25–9.38) was significantly associated with CF patients using the dominant model. This association remains statistically significant after adjusting for multiple testing using the Bonferroni correction ($P=0.0482$). The association value and the OR of the TNF2 allele were statistically significant when assessed using the additive model (Dd vs. dd) but not the recessive model (Table 5). The other genetic variants tested did not show any association.

Discussion

In the present study, the ΔF508 mutation accounted for 59.3% of the mutated CFTR alleles, a frequency that resembles the mutation frequencies of European Mediterranean countries. In this regard, this work may be comparable with modifier genes studies performed in those countries. Two previous CFTR mutation reports in the Mexican population showed ΔF508 frequencies of 40.72% [25], 45% [26] and 44.6% [27]. Differences could be explained by the clinical criteria, geographic origin and the analytical methods available at that time. The Spanish federation reported a frequency of 45%. Previous studies in the Hispanic population reported a ΔF508 allele frequency ranging from 29 to 46% [28–30]. The frequencies of the G542X, R1162X and R334W alleles reflect the Spanish heritage in the Mexican population, but the S549N and 2789+5 G>A alleles are not among the most frequent in Spain [31–32]. In this study we previously detected homozygote S549N and ΔF508/S549N genotypes with the ASO16 kit. A second patient was detected by exon 11 direct sequencing because she presented an abnormal pattern of the INNOLiPA CFTR36 kit with the normal and mutant G551D probes. This kit along with the ASO27 excluded the S549N mutation from the mutation panel, hindering the CFTR molecular diagnosis in our population. CFTR gene sequencing should be performed for new or rare CFTR mutations in Mexican population as S549N, and those mutations obtained from central Mexico patients (P750L, 846delT, 4160insGGGG and 297–1 G>A) [25], as well as for those mutations that remained undetected. It is necessary to establish an adequate diagnosis strategy based in Mexican genetic profile, considering that available commercial kits are designed mainly for Caucasian mutations profile.

In northeastern Mexico, medical care for CF patients is offered at the Cystic Fibrosis Clinic of the CEPREP (http://www.ceprep.edu.mx). Since 1987, approximately 200 patients have been diagnosed with CF based on clinical and molecular analyses. Once the diagnosis of CF is established, the rate of adherence to medical treatment and long-term medical monitoring is low, making investigations into the genetic and environmental factors that influence the outcome in CF Mexican patients difficult.

In this study, we analyzed seven variants in four modifier genes previously reported in CF patients and we found an association between CF and the TNF2 allele.

The proinflammatory role of the TNF2 allele has been demonstrated in B cell line cultures, where the TNF2 allele was more potent transcriptional activator compared to the normal TNF1 [17]. TNF2 allele has been implicated as a potent immunomediator and pro-inflammatory cytokine in the pathogenesis of several human diseases, including pulmonary diseases as CF and asthma. Patients with genotypes related to higher TNFα production had increased frequency of asthma [33]. In Mexican population TNF2 allele was found in 6.0% of asthmatic compared to 2.9% of the controls [34]. These results are similar that those we found in our study (2.9% for controls and 8.9% for CF patients).

Table 4. Modifier gene genotype frequencies (%) in CF patients and control subjects; OR, Hardy–Weinberg Equilibrium (HWE) and results of the association test with Dominant Model *P*-values.

Gene	Genotypes	Genotype Frequency in CF Patients	HWE P in CF Patients	Genotype Frequency in Controls	HWE P in Controls	OR (95% CI) Dominant Model	P-Value Dominant Model	
		N (%)		N (%)			X^2	X^2 Bonf. P
MBL2	AA	46 (57.5)	0.4210	63 (61.2)	0.1843	A 1.01 (0.62–1.65)	0.6163	1.0000
	AO	31 (38.8)		32 (31.1)		O 0.99 (0.61–1.61)		
	OO	3 (3.8)		8 (7.8)				
IL-8	AA	13 (16.5)	0.5786	19 (18.6)	0.9937	T 1.03 (0.68.1.57)	0.9194	1.0000
	AT	41 (51.9)		50 (49.0)		A 0.97 (0.64–1.48)		
	TT	25 (31.6)		33 (32.4)				
TNFα	TNF1/TNF1	66 (82.5)	0.3911	97 (94.2)	0.7608	[a]TNF1 0.30 (0.11–0.80)	0.0120	0.0482
	TNF1/TNF2	14 (17.5)		6 (5.8)		[b]TNF2 3.43 (1.25–9.38)		
	TNF2/TNF2	0 (0.0)		0 (0)				
AAT	MM	79 (97.5)	0.9104	101 (97.1)	0.8814	M 1.17 (0.19–7.01)	0.8627	1.0000
	MS	2 (2.5)		3 (2.9)		S 0.85 (0.14–5.17)		
	M/Z, S/Z, S/S, Z/Z	0 (0)		0 (0)				

CF, cystic fibrosis; OR, Odds Ratio; CI, confidence interval.
[a]TNF1 −308 G: (dd) vs. (DD, Dd),
[b]TNF2 −308 A: (DD, Dd) vs. (dd).
HW-P: *P*-value for the Hardy-Weinberg equilibrium.
X^2 Bonf. P = Chi squared test with a Bonferroni-corrected *P*-value.

By the other hand, recent studies in Mexican population reported a higher frequency of the TNF2 allele in healthy unrelated Mexican individuals (7.3%) [35]. Another report related TNF2 allele to breast cancer in Mexican patients compared to healthy women (7.5 and 24.5% respectively) [36]. Differences in TNF1 allele frequency in control subjects could be explained by sample size, methodology and characteristics of the studied group. Our study included population from Northeastern Mexico, while the other studies had different criteria as gender, living in Mexico City or been born in Mexico.

Previous studies in CF patients have shown that TNF2 is associated with a lower percentage of predicted forced expiratory volume in one second (FEV_1) and weight z scores [37]. In Mexican population, the TNF2 allele has been associated with rheumatoid arthritis [38], geriatric lipid profile [39] and spondyloarthritis [40]. This variant has also been reported to be associated with obesity and asthma [41–42]. The high frequency of the TNF2 allele in Mexican CF patients could suggest a heterozygote advantage. In Colombia, an inverse association between the TNF polymorphism and autoimmunity and TB has been reported; this association suggests the existence of a heterozygote advantage and is consistent with the hypothesis that autoimmune diseases are a consequence of natural selection for enhanced TB resistance [43–44].

MBL2, IL-8 and AAT did not show an association with the CF genotype. MBL2 had previously shown associations with different disturbances in the lung function, infection risk, and survival of CF patients [6,45–48]. In asthma, MBL has been associated with *Chlamydia pneumoniae*-specific IgG and a greater risk of developing asthma, especially in children with chronic or recurrent infection [49]. MBL levels in asthmatic children positively correlate with peripheral blood eosinophils [50]. MBL therapy may be useful in MBL-deficient patients; it may reduce the susceptibility to or enhance the recovery from bacterial infection or modify the natural history of the disease [51–53]. The IL-8 −251 polymorphism has been associated with CF lung disease severity and the differential expression of IL-8, suggesting that the IL-8 variant modifies CF lung disease severity [54]. The −251 variant has been associated with asthma, infection by respiratory syncytial virus, and chronic obstructive pulmonary disease (COPD) [10,55–56]. Finally, despite the association between AAT deficiency and COPD, studies of AAT variants and infection in CF patients have been inconclusive [57–60]. The incidence of AAT deficiency for all five phenotypic classes of the Pi*S and Pi*Z deficiency alleles is 1 in 9.8 for Canada and 1 in 11.3 for the United States. However, a previous report from our group showed very low allele frequencies of Pi*S and Pi*Z variants in a Mexican population (1.5% and 0%, respectively) [61].

In summary, the frequencies of genetic variants in the MBL2, IL-8, and AAT genes of CF patients did not show significant differences when compared to control subjects, but the TNF2

Table 5. TNF1/TNF2 association values using dominant, additive and recessive models.

Model	TNFα −308 G/−308 A OR[1] (95% CI)	*P*-value	
Dominant	TNF1 = 0.29 (0.11–0.79)	0.012[2]	0.048[3]
	TNF2 = 3.43 (1.25–9.38)		
Additive	TNF1 = NA	0.012[4]	0.049[3]
	TNF2 = 3.429 (1.25–9.38)		
Recessive	NA	NA	NA

[1]odds ratio.
[2]Chi-Squared P.
[3]Bonf. P.
[4]Correl/Trend P.

allele was significantly associated with CF patients. More studies are needed to identify the role of inflammatory mediators in the pathophysiology of CF, as emphasized in previous studies. This information is relevant because clinical trials of drugs targeting TNFα activity [62] have shown outstanding efficacy in treating chronic inflammatory diseases.

Acknowledgments

We especially acknowledge the volunteers, whose cooperation made these studies possible. The authors gratefully acknowledge Dr. Sergio Lozano for his critical reading of the manuscript and his contribution in editing the manuscript.

Author Contributions

Conceived and designed the experiments: CNSD AB ROL MARL. Performed the experiments: CNSD MCVT. Analyzed the data: HLGB RMCF. Contributed reagents/materials/analysis tools: ROL MARL HLGB. Wrote the paper: CNSD. Helped to design and revised the manuscript: HGMR HABS ARM.

References

1. Collaco JM, Cutting GR (2008) Update on gene modifiers in cystic fibrosis. Curr Opin Pulm Med 14: 559–566.
2. Velázquez A, Vela-Amieva M, Naylor EW, Chace DH (2000) Tamiz neonatal ampliado. Rev Mex Pediatr 67: 206–213.
3. Rowntree RK, Harris A (2003) The phenotypic consequences of CFTR mutations. Ann Hum Genet 67: 471–485.
4. Turner MW (1996) Mannose-binding lectin: the pluripotent molecule of the innate immune system. Immunol Today 17: 532–540.
5. Madsen HO, Satz ML, Hogh B, Svejgaard A, Garred P (1998) Different molecular events result in low protein levels of mannan-binding lectin in populations from southeast Africa and South America. J Immunol 161: 3169–3175.
6. Yarden J, Radojkovic D, De Boeck K, Macek M Jr, Zemkova D, et al. (2004) Polymorphisms in the mannose binding lectin gene affect the cystic fibrosis pulmonary phenotype. J Med Genet 41: 629–633.
7. Garred P, Larsen F, Seyfarth J, Fujita R, Madsen HO (2006) Mannose-binding lectin and its genetic variants. Genes Immun 7: 85–94.
8. Eisen DP (2010) Mannose-binding lectin deficiency and respiratory tract infection. J Innate Immun 2: 114–122.
9. Harada A, Sekido N, Akahoshi T, Wada T, Mukaida N, et al. (1994) Essential involvement of interleukin-8 (IL-8) in acute inflammation. J Leukoc Biol 56: 559–564.
10. Puthothu B, Krueger M, Heinze J, Forster J, Heinzmann A (2006) Impact of IL8 and IL8-receptor alpha polymorphisms on the genetics of bronchial asthma and severe RSV infections. Clin Mol Allergy 4: 2.
11. Hull J, Thomson A, Kwiatkowski D (2000) Association of respiratory syncytial virus bronchiolitis with the interleukin 8 gene region in UK families. Thorax 55: 1023–1027.
12. Mizunoe S, Shuto T, Suzuki S, Matsumoto C, Watanabe K, et al. (2012) Synergism between interleukin (IL)-17 and toll-like receptor 2 and 4 signals to induce IL-8 expression in cystic fibrosis airway epithelial cells. J Pharmacol Sci 118: 512–520.
13. Cowan MJ, Huang X, Yao XL, Shelhamer JH (2000) Tumor necrosis factor alpha stimulation of human Clara cell secretory protein production by human airway epithelial cells. Ann N Y Acad Sci 923: 193–201.
14. Lora JM, Zhang DM, Liao SM, Burwell T, King AM, et al. (2005) Tumor necrosis factor-alpha triggers mucus production in airway epithelium through an IkappaB kinase beta-dependent mechanism. J Biol Chem 280: 36510–36517.
15. Hajeer AH, Hutchinson IV (2000) TNF-alpha gene polymorphism: clinical and biological implications. Microsc Res Tech 50: 216–228.
16. Gambari R, Borgatti M, Lampronti I, Fabbri E, Brognara E, et al. (2012) Corilagin is a potent inhibitor of NF-kappaB activity and downregulates TNF-alpha induced expression of IL-8 gene in cystic fibrosis IB3–1 cells. Int Immunopharmacol 13: 308–315.
17. Wilson AG, Symons JA, McDowell TL, McDevitt HO, Duff GW (1997) Effects of a polymorphism in the human tumor necrosis factor alpha promoter on transcriptional activation. Proc Natl Acad Sci U S A 94: 3195–3199.
18. Kok KF, te Morsche RH, van Oijen MG, Drenth JP (2010) Prevalence of genetic polymorphisms in the promoter region of the alpha-1 antitrypsin (SERPINA1) gene in chronic liver disease: a case control study. BMC Gastroenterol 10: 22.
19. Miravitlles M, Vila S, Jardi R, de la Roza C, Rodriguez-Frias F, et al. (2003) Emphysema due to alpha-antitrypsin deficiency: familial study of the YBARCELONA variant. Chest 124: 404–406.
20. Araujo FG, Novaes FC, Santos NP, Martins VC, Souza SM, et al. (2005) Prevalence of deltaF508, G551D, G542X, and R553X mutations among cystic fibrosis patients in the North of Brazil. Braz J Med Biol Res 38: 11–15.
21. Sandford AJ, Chagani T, Spinelli JJ, Pare PD (1999) alpha1-antitrypsin genotypes and the acute-phase response to open heart surgery. Am J Respir Crit Care Med 159: 1624–1628.
22. Tin SK, Lee LY, Thumboo J, Koh DR, Fong KY (2005) PCR-RFLP genotyping for exon 1 and promoter region mutations of the human mannose binding lectin (MBL-2) gene. J Immunol Methods 303: 148–151.
23. Lee WP, Tai DI, Lan KH, Li AF, Hsu HC, et al. (2005) The −251T allele of the interleukin-8 promoter is associated with increased risk of gastric carcinoma featuring diffuse-type histopathology in Chinese population. Clin Cancer Res 11: 6431–6441.
24. Chen YP, Pfab T, Slowinski T, Richter CM, Godes M, et al. (2006) Impact of genetic variation of tumor necrosis factor-alpha on gestational hypertension. Chin Med J (Engl) 119: 719–724.
25. Orozco L, Velazquez R, Zielenski J, Tsui LC, Chavez M, et al. (2000) Spectrum of CFTR mutations in Mexican cystic fibrosis patients: identification of five novel mutations (W1098C, 846delT, P750L, 4160insGGGG and 297–1G–>A). Hum Genet 106: 360–365.
26. Villalobos-Torres C, Rojas-Martinez A, Villareal-Castellanos E, Cantu JM, Sanchez-Anzaldo FJ, et al. (1997) Analysis of 16 cystic fibrosis mutations in Mexican patients. Am J Med Genet 69: 380–382.
27. Chavez-Saldana M, Yokoyama E, Lezana JL, Carnevale A, Macias M, et al. (2010) CFTR allelic heterogeneity in Mexican patients with cystic fibrosis: implications for molecular screening. Rev Invest Clin 62: 546–552.
28. Grebe TA, Seltzer WK, DeMarchi J, Silva DK, Doane WW, et al. (1994) Genetic analysis of Hispanic individuals with cystic fibrosis. Am J Hum Genet 54: 443–446.
29. Sugarman EA, Rohlfs EM, Silverman LM, Allitto BA (2004) CFTR mutation distribution among U.S. Hispanic and African American individuals: evaluation in cystic fibrosis patient and carrier screening populations. Genet Med 6: 392–399.
30. Schrijver I, Ramalingam S, Sankaran R, Swanson S, Dunlop CL, et al. (2005) Diagnostic testing by CFTR gene mutation analysis in a large group of Hispanics: novel mutations and assessment of a population-specific mutation spectrum. J Mol Diagn 7: 289–299.
31. Aliño-Pellicer SF, Antelo-Landeira MC, Baamonde-Vidarte A, Beltrán-Bengoechea B, Berná-Torres N, et al. (2003) Federación Española contra la Fibrosis Quística. Libro Blanco de atención a la fibrosis quistica; Consumo MdSy, editor. Madrid, España.
32. Alonso MJ, Heine-Suner D, Calvo M, Rosell J, Gimenez J, et al. (2007) Spectrum of mutations in the CFTR gene in cystic fibrosis patients of Spanish ancestry. Ann Hum Genet 71: 194–201.
33. Shmarina G, Pukhalsky A, Petrova N, Zakharova E, Avakian L, et al. (2013) TNF gene polymorphisms in cystic fibrosis patients: contribution to the disease progression. J Transl Med 11: 19.
34. Jimenez-Morales S, Velazquez-Cruz R, Ramirez-Bello J, Bonilla-Gonzalez E, Romero-Hidalgo S, et al. (2009) Tumor necrosis factor-alpha is a common genetic risk factor for asthma, juvenile rheumatoid arthritis, and systemic lupus erythematosus in a Mexican pediatric population. Hum Immunol 70: 251–256.
35. Vargas-Alarcon G, Ramirez-Bello J, Juarez-Cedillo T, Ramirez-Fuentes S, Carrillo-Sanchez S, et al. (2012) Distribution of the IL-1RN, IL-6, IL-10, INF-gamma, and TNF-alpha Gene Polymorphisms in the Mexican Population. Genet Test Mol Biomarkers 16: 1246–1253.
36. Gomez Flores-Ramos L, Escoto-De Dios A, Puebla-Perez AM, Figuera-Villanueva LE, Ramos-Silva A, et al. (2013) Association of the tumor necrosis factor-alpha −308 G>A polymorphism with breast cancer in Mexican women. Genet Mol Res 12: 5680–5693.
37. Hull J, Thomson AH (1998) Contribution of genetic factors other than CFTR to disease severity in cystic fibrosis. Thorax 53: 1018–1021.
38. Rodriguez-Carreon AA, Zuniga J, Hernandez-Pacheco G, Rodriguez-Perez JM, Perez-Hernandez N, et al. (2005) Tumor necrosis factor-alpha −308 promoter polymorphism contributes independently to HLA alleles in the severity of rheumatoid arthritis in Mexicans. J Autoimmun 24: 63–68.
39. Parra-Rojas I, Ruiz-Madrigal B, Martinez-Lopez E, Panduro A (2006) Influence of the −308 TNF-alpha and −174 IL-6 polymorphisms on lipid profile in Mexican subjects. Hereditas 143: 167–172.
40. Vargas-Alarcon G, Casasola-Vargas J, Rodriguez-Perez JM, Huerta-Sil G, Perez-Hernandez N, et al. (2006) Tumor necrosis factor-alpha promoter polymorphisms in Mexican patients with spondyloarthritis. Hum Immunol 67: 826–832.
41. Castro-Giner F, Kogevinas M, Imboden M, de Cid R, Jarvis D, et al. (2009) Joint effect of obesity and TNFA variability on asthma: two international cohort studies. Eur Respir J 33: 1003–1009.
42. Wu H, Romieu I, Sienra-Monge JJ, del Rio-Navarro BE, Anderson DM, et al. (2007) Parental smoking modifies the relation between genetic variation in tumor necrosis factor-alpha (TNF) and childhood asthma. Environ Health Perspect 115: 616–622.

43. Correa PA, Gomez LM, Anaya JM (2004) [Polymorphism of TNF-alpha in autoimmunity and tuberculosis]. Biomedica 24 Supp 1: 43–51.
44. Correa PA, Gomez LM, Cadena J, Anaya JM (2005) Autoimmunity and tuberculosis. Opposite association with TNF polymorphism. J Rheumatol 32: 219–224.
45. Buranawuti K, Boyle MP, Cheng S, Steiner LL, McDougal K, et al. (2007) Variants in mannose-binding lectin and tumour necrosis factor alpha affect survival in cystic fibrosis. J Med Genet 44: 209–214.
46. Muhlebach MS, MacDonald SL, Button B, Hubbard JJ, Turner ML, et al. (2006) Association between mannan-binding lectin and impaired lung function in cystic fibrosis may be age-dependent. Clin Exp Immunol 145: 302–307.
47. Davies JC, Turner MW, Klein N (2004) Impaired pulmonary status in cystic fibrosis adults with two mutated MBL-2 alleles. Eur Respir J 24: 798–804.
48. Haerynck F, Van Steen K, Cattaert T, Loeys B, Van Daele S, et al. (2012) Polymorphisms in the lectin pathway genes as a possible cause of early chronic Pseudomonas aeruginosa colonization in cystic fibrosis patients. Hum Immunol 73: 1175–1183.
49. Nagy A, Kozma GT, Keszei M, Treszl A, Falus A, et al. (2003) The development of asthma in children infected with Chlamydia pneumoniae is dependent on the modifying effect of mannose-binding lectin. J Allergy Clin Immunol 112: 729–734.
50. Uguz A, Berber Z, Coskun M, Halide Akbas S, Yegin O (2005) Mannose-binding lectin levels in children with asthma. Pediatr Allergy Immunol 16: 231–235.
51. Garred P, Pressler T, Lanng S, Madsen HO, Moser C, et al. (2002) Mannose-binding lectin (MBL) therapy in an MBL-deficient patient with severe cystic fibrosis lung disease. Pediatr Pulmonol 33: 201–207.
52. Summerfield JA (2003) Clinical potential of mannose-binding lectin-replacement therapy. Biochem Soc Trans 31: 770–773.
53. Kilpatrick DC (2003) Introduction to mannan-binding lectin. Biochem Soc Trans 31: 745–747.
54. Hillian AD, Londono D, Dunn JM, Goddard KA, Pace RG, et al. (2008) Modulation of cystic fibrosis lung disease by variants in interleukin-8. Genes Immun 9: 501–508.
55. Heinzmann A, Ahlert I, Kurz T, Berner R, Deichmann KA (2004) Association study suggests opposite effects of polymorphisms within IL8 on bronchial asthma and respiratory syncytial virus bronchiolitis. J Allergy Clin Immunol 114: 671–676.
56. Arinir U, Klein W, Rohde G, Stemmler S, Epplen JT, et al. (2005) Polymorphisms in the interleukin-8 gene in patients with chronic obstructive pulmonary disease. Electrophoresis 26: 2888–2891.
57. Mahadeva R, Stewart S, Bilton D, Lomas DA (1998) Alpha-1 antitrypsin deficiency alleles and severe cystic fibrosis lung disease. Thorax 53: 1022–1024.
58. Mahadeva R, Westerbeek RC, Perry DJ, Lovegrove JU, Whitehouse DB, et al. (1998) Alpha1-antitrypsin deficiency alleles and the Taq-I G–>A allele in cystic fibrosis lung disease. Eur Respir J 11: 873–879.
59. Meyer P, Braun A, Roscher AA (2002) Analysis of the two common alpha-1-antitrypsin deficiency alleles PiMS and PiMZ as modifiers of Pseudomonas aeruginosa susceptibility in cystic fibrosis. Clin Genet 62: 325–327.
60. Frangolias DD, Ruan J, Wilcox PJ, Davidson AG, Wong LT, et al. (2003) Alpha 1-antitrypsin deficiency alleles in cystic fibrosis lung disease. Am J Respir Cell Mol Biol 29: 390–396.
61. Sanchez-Dominguez CN, Buenfil-Lozano JA, Molina-Guajardo CA, Borjas-Almaguer OD, Castillo-Lartigue A, et al. (2008) Frequency of S and Z alleles for alpha-1-antitrypsin and tumor necrosis factor alpha −308 promoter polymorphism in northeastern Mexico. Allergy Asthma Proc 29: 406–410.
62. Kim J, Remick DG (2007) Tumor necrosis factor inhibitors for the treatment of asthma. Curr Allergy Asthma Rep 7: 151–156.

CFTR Mutations Spectrum and the Efficiency of Molecular Diagnostics in Polish Cystic Fibrosis Patients

Ewa Zietkiewicz[1]*, Ewa Rutkiewicz[1], Andrzej Pogorzelski[2], Barbara Klimek[1], Katarzyna Voelkel[1], Michał Witt[1,3]

1 Department of Molecular and Clinical Genetics, Institute of Human Genetics, Polish Academy of Sciences, Poznan, Poland, **2** Department of Pneumology and Cystic Fibrosis, Institute of Tuberculosis and Lung Diseases, Rabka, Poland, **3** International Institute of Molecular and Cell Biology, Warsaw, Poland

Abstract

Cystic fibrosis (CF) is caused by mutations in the cystic fibrosis transmembrane regulator gene (*CFTR*). In light of the strong allelic heterogeneity and regional specificity of the mutation spectrum, the strategy of molecular diagnostics and counseling in CF requires genetic tests to reflect the frequency profile characteristic for a given population. The goal of the study was to provide an updated comprehensive estimation of the distribution of *CFTR* mutations in Polish CF patients and to assess the effectiveness of INNOLiPA_*CFTR* tests in Polish population. The analyzed cohort consisted of 738 patients with the clinically confirmed CF diagnosis, prescreened for molecular defects using INNOLiPA_*CFTR* panels from Innogenetics. A combined efficiency of INNOLiPA *CFTR_19* and *CFTR_17_TnUpdate* tests was 75.5%; both mutations were detected in 68.2%, and one mutation in 14.8% of the affected individuals. The group composed of all the patients with only one or with no mutation detected (109 and 126 individuals, respectively) was analyzed further using a mutation screening approach, i.e. SSCP/HD (single strand conformational polymorphism/heteroduplex) analysis of PCR products followed by sequencing of the coding sequence. As a result, 53 more mutations were found in 97 patients. The overall efficiency of the CF allele detection was 82.5% (7.0% increase compared to INNOLiPA tests alone). The distribution of the most frequent mutations in Poland was assessed. Most of the mutations repetitively found in Polish patients had been previously described in other European populations. The most frequent mutated allele, F508del, represented 54.5% of Polish CF chromosomes. Another eight mutations had frequencies over 1%, 24 had frequencies between 1 and 0.1%; c.2052-2053insA and c.3468+2_3468+3insT were the most frequent non-INNOLiPA mutations. Mutation distribution described herein is also relevant to the Polish diaspora. Our study also demonstrates that the reported efficiency of mutation detection strongly depends on the diagnostic experience of referring health centers.

Editor: Klaus Brusgaard, Odense University Hospital, Denmark

Funding: This work was supported by the grant from Polish Scientific Committee KBN-NN401-020-435 to EZ. The funders had no role in study design, data collection and analysis, decision to publish, or preparation of the manuscript.

Competing Interests: The authors have declared that no competing interests exist.

* E-mail: zietkiee@man.poznan.pl

Introduction

Cystic fibrosis (CF; MIM 219700) is the most frequent autosomal recessive disease among Caucasians; its median incidence in Europe is 1 in 3,500 [1] and ranges from 1 in 1,350 to 1 in 25,000, depending on the population under study [2]. The disease is caused by mutations in the cystic fibrosis transmembrane regulator (*CFTR*) gene (Ensembl ENSG00000001626) [3]. The comprehensive list of the *CFTR* mutations, maintained at the Cystic Fibrosis Mutation Database (CFMDB) (www.genet.sickkids.on.ca/cftr), was approximately 1950 as of November 2013.

The most frequent *CFTR* mutation, F508del, accounts for ~66% CF chromosomes in the general Caucasian population [4–5]. Few other widely spread mutations reach worldwide frequencies >1%, less than twenty have frequencies between 0.1 and 1.0%, and the majority are found only in certain geographical regions, populations or "private" (reported in singular families). Local frequencies of the most common mutations vary among populations [4–5], with founder effect(s) shown to be responsible for a number of them. The strong allelic heterogeneity has a direct bearing on the strategy of molecular diagnostics and counseling in CF. In order to increase the rate of *CFTR* mutation detection and to correctly evaluate the residual risk of being a CF carrier after molecular analysis, it is essential that genetic tests are designed based on the frequency profile characteristic for a given population and that the sensitivity to detect mutations is as high as possible [4–6].

The most recent publication regarding the prevalence of *CFTR* mutations in Poland is now more than 12 years old [7]; the other three papers investigated only a limited number of mutations [8–9] or a specific subpopulation of adult CF patients [10].

The goal of the present study was to provide an updated comprehensive estimation of the distribution of *CFTR* mutations in Poland, based on the analysis of a representative cohort of CF patients. At the same time, we aimed to assess the effectiveness of INNOLiPA (IL) *CFTR* tests (Innogenetics) in PL (Polish) population.

Results

Two IL tests, *CFTR_19* and *CFTR_17 TnUpdate*, used to examine a cohort of 738 PL CF patients, revealed mutations in

66.8% and 8.7% of the CF alleles, respectively (a combined efficiency of 75.5%). Two mutations were found in 68.2%, and of one mutation in 14.8% of the patients, and no mutation was identified in 17.1% of PL CF patients (Table 1). Of the 36 most frequent European-wide *CFTR* mutations targeted by both IL tests, 22 were found in at least one individual (Table 2).

All the CF patients without two IL mutations were analyzed further using PCR - SSCP/HD - sequencing approach. Among fifty-six non- IL mutations revealed in 99 patients, forty-five were already reported in the CFMDB, and eleven were novel, never described before (Table 2). All migration variants detected by SSCP/HD were confirmed /explained by dideoxy sequencing.

Two of the non-IL CFMDB mutations were relatively frequent. The c.2052_2053insA (legacy name, l.n.2184insA) was found in 15 (1.0%) analyzed chromosomes, and the c.3468+2_3468+3insT (l.n.3600+2insT) – in 11 (0.7%). Both mutations were in a compound heterozygosity, in most cases with F508del, and in singular patients with another CF mutation (Table 2); in two patients, no mutations in trans were found. In the Clinical and Functional Translation of CFTR database (CFTR2; www.cftr2.org), c.2052_2053insA has been reported as causing pancreatic insufficiency (PI); here, most of the patients were PI but some were pancreatic sufficient (PS); the same was observed for patients carrying c.3468+2_3468+3insT.

Two other CFMDB mutations affected the c.1210-12T_n_1210-34_35TG_m site in intron 9 (l.n.IVS8-T_n/TG_m). Specific SSCP/HD patterns (confirmed by sequencing) allowed unambiguous differentiation of the T_n alleles associated with variable size of the adjacent TG repeat. Among nineteen T_5 alleles found in the whole analyzed cohort, eight (42%) were in cis with TG_{12-13}; these compound alleles were not found in 300 analyzed control chromosomes. The T_5_TG_{12} combination was found in six patients (in three with F508del in trans, in three as the only mutation identified). The T_5_TG_{13} was found in two patients (in one as the only mutation, in one with c.2012delT in trans). The IVS9 T_5_TG_{12-13} compound alleles have been described in the CFTR2 database as having "varying consequences". Here, the CF manifestation in the majority of patients carrying these alleles was relatively mild.

Of the remaining non-IL CFMDB mutations, 13 were found on 2 5 chromosomes each, and 28 were found on a single chromosome each. Eleven were amino acid substitutions whose deleterious consequence was not supported by strong negative SVM (Support Vector Machine) values. Three of them (R352Q, Q359R and D1152H) were in a compound heterozygosity with F508del, six (E217G, I506, V562L, G723V, D924N and L967S) had no accompanying mutation in trans. These nine substitutions were tentatively considered causative, but their pathogenic character requires further studies. Another substitution, G576A (SVM +1.73), was found in three patients, in cis with a deleterious R668C allele (SVM -1.61); the latter was also present without G576A, in two patients (in one with c.1585-1G>A in trans). In the UMD-CFTR database (www.umd.be/CFTR), G576A and R668C have been reported in cis; in the CFTR2 database both mutations are described as having "varying consequences". Three of our patients carrying R668C were PI, and two appeared PS; PS/PI status was independent on the presence of G576A. We considered R668C a pathogenic mutation, and G576A – an associated element of a compound allele. Finally, S912L (SVM +2.12), found in a single chromosome with F508del in trans, has been reported in the CFMDB as pathogenic only if in cis with c.3067–3072del6; since the latter was not found in the analyzed patient, we considered S912L a neutral polymorphism.

Of the eleven novel changes, seven affected the length of the CFTR protein by: (i) introducing a premature STOP codon (two); (ii) introducing a frameshift or changing the protein length (three); (iii) changing the conserved splicing site positions (two); all were considered pathogenic mutations. They were present in a single patient each (major manifestation indicated in parentheses), and most were in trans with F508del: L165X (PI; chloride values: 88 and 90 mmol/L); V1327X (meconium ileus, MI; no chloride data available); c.341_353del13bp (PI; chloride values: 131, 143 and 147 mmol/L); c.3376_3379delGAAG (PI; chloride values: 97 and 90); c.2908+3A>C (PS; chloride values: 117, 119 and 182 mmol/L). The c.1116+2T>A (no chloride data available) was in trans with Q1412X; for the c.2817_2820delTACTC (PS; normal chloride values: 33 and 52 mmol/L), no second mutation was identified.

In case of three novel amino acid substitutions (G27V, R153I and I752V), the possibility that a change represented a non-pathological polymorphism was examined. None of these alleles was found in 300 healthy chromosomes from Polish general population, neither reported in the NCBI database for human single nucleotide polymorphisms, which encompassed data from the 1000Genome project (www.ncbi.nlm.nih.gov/SNP; build 137). The SVM values indicated strongly deleterious effect of both R153I and G27V on the protein stability (−2.61 and −1.92, respectively), and both positions were conserved in the comparative analysis with orthologues from several Eutherian species (www.ensembl.org); R153I and G27V were therefore assumed to be pathogenic mutations. R153I was found in two unrelated patients with pulmonary manifestation and a known CF mutation on another allele (F508del or c.3528delC); the first patient had elevated chloride values (94 and 98 mmol/L), and no chloride data were available for the second patient. G27V was found in a single patient with PI and pulmonary symptoms (chloride values >100 mmol/L), and was accompanied by F508del on another allele. The deleterious consequence of I752V (found in a single

Table 1. Mutation detection efficiency using INNOLiPA tests: *CFTR19* and *CFTR17TnUpdate.*

Mutations detected in a patient	Number of CF patients	Alleles with no mutation identified	Alleles with CF mutations detected using INNOLiPA tests		Further molecular analysis
			CFTR_19	*CFTR_17 TnUpdate*[a]	
both	503 (68.1%)	0	888 (60.2%)	118 (8.0%)	Not necessary
one	109 (14.8%)	109	98 (6.6%)	11 (0.7%)	Yes
none	126 (17.1%)	252	0	0	Yes

Legend: [a] I148T included in CFTR-17TnUpdate was not counted as a mutation if not in cis with c.3067-72del6 (l.n. 3199del6); c.1210(-12)T_n site in intron 9 (l.n.IVS8-T_n) without data on the associated TG repeat was not counted as a mutation.

Table 2. Mutations found in the analyzed cohort of 738 Polish CF patients, sorted according to the position in the gene.

Exon / intron (legacy)	Exon / intron (Ensembl)	Protein change	SVM value	cDNA (HGVS nomenclature)	gDNA (cDNA +132 bp)	Number of PL CF chromosomes	Reference [a]	Mutations in trans
Pathogenic mutations								
1	1	L15Ffs10X		c.43delC	175delC	1	CFMDB	1717-1G>A
2	2	G27V	−1.92	c.80G>T	212G>T	1	Novel	F508del
2	2	S18RfsX16		c.54-5940_273 +10250del21kb	exon2,3del21kb	66	IL19	various CF mutations
i2	i2	IVS2_Donor		c.164+1G>A	296+1G>A	3	CFMDB	various CF mutations
3	3	G85E	−2.61	c.254G>A	386G>A	1	IL17	unknown
3	3	E60X		c.178G>T	310G>T	0	IL17	x
3	3	L88IfsX22		c.262_263delTT	394delTT	0	IL17	x
4	4	E92K	−1.92	c.274G>A	406G>A	2	CFMDB	c.164+1G>A; c.2051-2AA>G
4	4	L101X		c.302T>G	434T>G	1	CFMDB	c.3717+12191C>T
4	4	K114IfsX5		c.341_353del13bp	473del13bp	1	Novel	F508del
4	4	R117H	−0.35	c.350G>A	482G>A	5	IL17	F508del; 2x unknown
4	4	R117C	−2.07	c.349C>T	481C>T	2	CFMDB	S1206X;1x unknown
4	4	L137_L138insT		c.412_413insACT	L138ins	1	CFMDB	F508del
4	4	R153I	−2.61	c.458G>T	590G>T	2	Novel	F508del; c.3527delC
i4	i4	IVS4_Donor		c.489+1G>T	621+1G>T	5	IL17	F508del; c.489+1G>T
5	5	L165X		c.494T>A	626T>A	1	Novel	F508del
i5	i5	IVS5_Donor		c.579+1G>T	711+1G>T	0	IL19	x
i5	i5	IVS5_Donor		c.579+3A>G	711+3A>G	2	CFMDB	2,3del21kb; c.2052-3insA
i5	i5	IVS5_Donor		c.579+5G>A	711+5G>A	0	IL17	x
7	8	F311L	−0.90	c.933C>G	965C>G	2	CFMDB	2x F508
7	8	G314R	−0.58	c.940G>A	1072G>A	4	CFMDB	various CF mutations
7	8	F316LfsX12		c.948delT	1078delT	1	IL17	unkown
7	8	R334W	−2.41	c.1000C>T	1132C>T	6	IL17	various CF mutations
7	8	I336K	−2.07	c.1007T>A	1139T>A	2	CFMDB	2,3de21kb; F508del
7	8	R347P	−2.27	c.1040G>C	1172G>C	11	IL17	various CF mutations
i7	i8	IVS8_Donor		c.1116+2T>A	1248+2T>A	1	Novel	Q1412X
9	10	A455E	−2.61	c.1364C>A	1496C>A	0	IL17	x
i9	i10	IVS10_Donor		c.1392+1G>A	1524+1G>A	1	CFMDB	c.3816-7delGT
10	11	S466X		c.1397C>G	1529C>G	1	CFMDB	G542X
10	11	I507del		c.1519_1521delATC	1651delATC	2	IL19	F508del
10	11	F508del		c.1521_1523delCTT	1654delCTT	805	IL19	various CF mutations
i10	i11	IVS11_Acceptor		c.1585-1G>A	1717-1G>A	27	IL19	various CF mutations
11	12	G542X		c.1624G>T	1756G>T	25	IL19	various CF mutations
11	12	G551D	−1.24	c.1624G>T	1756G>T	5	IL19	various CF mutations
11	12	Q552X		c.1654C>T	1786C>T	0	IL19	x
11	12	R553X		c.1657C>T	1789C>T	14	IL19	various CF mutations
11	12	R560T	−1.92	c.1679G>C	1811G>C	0	IL19	x
i12	i13	IVS13_Donor		c.1766+1G>A	1898+1G>A	6	IL19	various CF mutations
i12	i13	IVS13_Donor		c.1766+1G>C	1898+1G>C	1	CFMDB	F508del
13	14	H620P	−1.73	c.1859A>C	1991A>C	1	CFMDB	F508del
13	14	R668C//G576A	−1.61//1.73	c.2002C>T//c.1727G>C	2134C>T// 1859G>C	5 [b]	CFMDB// rs1800098	c.1585-1G>A; 4 unknown
13	14	L671X		c.2012delT	2143delT	27	IL17	various CF mutations
13	14	K684SfsX38		c.2051_2052delAAinsG	2183AA>G	10	IL17	various CF mutations
13	14	K684NfsX38		c.2052delA	2184delA	0	IL17	x
13	14	Q685TfsX4		c.2052_2053insA	2184insA	15	CFMDB	various CF mutations[c], 1 unknown

Table 2. Cont.

Exon / intron (legacy)	Exon / intron (Ensembl)	Protein change	SVM value	cDNA (HGVS nomenclature)	gDNA (cDNA +132 bp)	Number of PL CF chromosomes	Reference [a]	Mutations in trans
13	**14**	L732X		c.2195T>G	2327T>G	1	CFMDB	F508del
14A	**15**	R851X		c.2551C>T	2683C>T	3	CFMDB	various CF mutations
14A	**15**	I864SfsX28		c.2589_2599del11bp	2721del11bp	2	CFMDB	F508del; 2,3del21kb
i14B	**i16**	IVS16_Donor		c.2657+2_2657+3insA	2789+2insA	1	CFMDB	F508del
i14B	**i16**	IVS16_Donor		c.2657+5G>A	2789+5G>A	0	IL17	unkown
15	**17**	Y919C	−1.02	c.2756A>G	2888A>G	1	CFMDB	unknown
15	**17**	H939HfsX27		c.2817_2820delTACTC	2949delTACTC	1	Novel	unkown
i15	**i17**	IVS17_Donor		c.2908+3A>C	3040+3A>C	1	Novel	F508del
i16	**i18**	IVS18_Donor		c.2988+1G>A	3120+1G>A	0	IL19	x
17A	**19**	I1023_V1024del		c.3067_3072delATAGTG	3199del6	0	IL19	x
i17A	**i19**	IVS19		c.3140-26A>G	3272-26A>G	9	IL19	various CF mutations
17B	**20**	L1065R	−1.90	c.3194T>G	3326T>G	1	CFMDB	F508del
17B	**20**	Y1092X		c.3276C>A	3408C>A	1	CFMDB	R334W
i18	**i21**	IVS21_Donor		c.3468+2_3468+3insT	3600+2insT	11	CFMDB	various CF mutations[d], 1 unknown
18	**21**	E1126EfsX7		c.3376_3379delGAAG	3508delGAAG	1	Novel	F508del
19	**22**	R1158X		c.3472C>T	3604C>T	2	CFMDB	F508del; R553X
19	**22**	R1162X		c.3484C>T	3616C>T	1	IL17	F508del
19	**22**	L1177SfsX15		c.3528delC	3659delC	4	IL17	various CF mutations
19	**22**	S1206X		c.3617C>A	3749C>A	1	CFMDB	R117C
i19	**i22**	IVS22		c.3717+12191C>T	3849+10kbC>T	58	IL17	various CF mutations
20	**23**	G1244R	−2.62	c.3730G>C	3862G>C	1	CFMDB	F508del
20	**23**	S1251N	−2.28	c.3752G>A	3884G>A	0	IL19	x
20	**23**	L1258FfsX7		c.3773_3774insT	3905insT	0	IL19	x
20	**23**	V1272VfsX28		c.3816_3817delGT	3944delGT	1	CFMDB	c.1392+1G>A
20	**23**	W1282X		c.3846G>A	3978G>A	9	IL19	various CF mutations
21	**24**	N1303K	−2.62	c.3909C>G	4041C>G	18	IL19	various CF mutations
22	**25**	V1327X		c.3979delG	4111delG	1	Novel	F508del
22	**25**	S1347PfsX13		c.4035_4038dupCCTA	c.4167dupCCTA	1	CFMDB	2,3del21kb
23	**26**	Q1382X		c.4144C>T	4276C>T	1	CFMDB	F508del
23	**26**	Q1412X		c.4234C>T	4366C>T	2	CFMDB	F508del; c.1116+2T>A
i23	**i26**	IVS26_Donor		c.4242+1G>T	4374+1G>T	1	CFMDB	F508del
Sequence changes of uncertain pathogenic effect, tentatively counted as mutations								
6A	**6**	E217G	0.30	c.650A>G	782A>G	1	CFMDB; rs1219109046	unknown
7	**8**	R352Q	−0.01	c.1055G>A	1187G>A	1	CFMDB; rs121908753	F508del
7	**8**	Q359R	0.33	c.1076A>G	1208A>G	1	CFMDB	F508del
i8	**i9**	IVS9		c.1210-12T_5_1210-34_35 $(TG)_{12}$	1332-12T_n_-34TG_m	6	CFMDB	F508del; 3x unknown
i8	**i9**	IVS9		c.1210-12T_5_1210-34_35 $(TG)_{13}$	1332-12T_n_-34TG_m	2	CFMDB	2143delT; 1x unknown
i8	**i9**	IVS9		c.1210-12T_8	1332-12T_n	1	Novel	unknown
10	**11**	I506V	−0.21	c.1516A>G	1648A>G	1	CFMDB; rs1800091	unknown
12	**13**	V562L	0.79	c.1684G>C	1816G>C	1	CFMDB; rs1800097	unknown
13	**14**	G723V	0.44	c.2168G>T	2300G>T	1	CFMDB; rs200531709	unknown
15	**17**	D924N	0.03	c.2770G>A	2902G>A	1	CFMDB; rs201759207	unknown

Table 2. Cont.

Exon / intron (legacy)	Exon / intron (Ensembl)	Protein change	SVM value	cDNA (HGVS nomenclature)	gDNA (cDNA +132 bp)	Number of PL CF chromosomes	Reference [a]	Mutations in trans
15	**17**	L967S	0.27	c.2900T>C	3032T>C	1	CFMDB; rs1800110	unknown
18	**21**	D1152H	0.50	c.3454G>C	3586G>C	1	CFMDB; rs75541969	F508del
Sequence changes considered as lacking pathogenic effect								
4	**4**	I148T	2.04	c.443T>U	575T>U	4	IL19[e]	unknown
13	**14**	I752V	0.35	c.2254A>G	2386A>G	1\	Novel[f]	F508
15	**17**	S912L	2.12	c.2735C>T	2867C>T	1	CFMDB[g] ; rs121909034	F508

Legend: [a] IL19 i 17 – mutations included in the INNOLiPA tests (see below); CFMDB – non-INNOLiPA mutations present in the CTFR mutation database; novel – mutations first reported in this study; [b] in three chromosomes R668C with G576A in trans; [c] F508del, c.1585-1G>A, G542X, N1303K or c.579+3A>G; [d] F508del, G542X, R553X or N1303K; [e] not pathogenic if not in cis with c.3067-72del6 (l.n.3199del6); [f] not pathogenic – see explanation the text; [g] not pathogenic if not in cis with G1244V.
[a]Mutations detected by two INNOLiPA_CFTR tests (legacy names): IL19 (INNOLiPA_*CFTR*19): F508del; G542X; N1303K; W1282X; G551D; 1717-1G>A; R553X; *CFTR*dele2,3(21kb); I507del; 711+1G>T; 3272-26A>G; 3905insT; R560T; 1898+1G>A; S1251N; I148T; 3199del6; 3120+1G>A; Q552X.
IL17 (INNOLiPA_*CFTR*17_TnUpdate): 621+1G>T; 3849+10kbC>T; 2183AA>G; 394delTT; 2789+5G>A; R1162X; 3659delC; R117H; R334W; R347P; G85E; 1078delT; A455E; 2143delT; E60X; 2184delA; 711+5G>A; polymorphism 5T/7T/9T.

patient with F508del on another allele) was not supported by the SVM value (+0.35); the patient was PS and had ambiguous chloride values (45, 64 and 83 mmol/L). In addition, I752 (although present in Primates) was not conserved in other Mammalian species. I752V was therefore considered to represent a rare neutral polymorphism rather than a pathogenic mutation.

An atypical allele of the length polymorphism in intron 9, with an even number of T-s associated in cis with the TG_{12}, IVS9 T_8_TG_{12}, was identified in one patient with MI and failure to thrive. No mutation in trans was found and no RNA was available from the patient to experimentally confirm the effect of this mutation on *CFTR* expression. However, given that a similar change (T_6 allele) was reported in the UMD-CFTR database as pathogenic, we tentatively considered the T_8 allele to be a CF mutation.

MLPA (multiplex ligation-dependent probe amplification) analysis was performed to detect the potential presence of large exonic deletions in 58 patients with only one mutation and in 46 of 100 patients with no pathogenic mutations identified in the IL tests combined with the SSCP/HD screening. No changes indicative of the presence of unknown large exonic deletions were identified.

Discussion

Using both *CFTR_19* and *CFTR_17TnUpdate* tests allowed identification of *CFTR* mutations in 75.5% of the CF chromosomes. SSCP/HD-based screening detected 53 more sequence changes assumed to be pathogenic mutations. After the extended screening of the CFTR coding sequence, the second mutation was found in 71 of the 109 patients with one IL mutation (Table 3). Among the 126 patients without IL mutations, one mutation was found in 20 and two in 6 individuals. The residual proportion of CF patients with none of the mutations detected was 13.6% (100/738), i.e. 3.5% less than after using only IL tests. The combined efficiency of *CFTR* mutations detection (82.5%) represented 7.0% increase compared to the IL tests alone. These results indicate that IL panels, which are among the most popular CF-diagnostic tests used in Europe, may not optimal for the mutation detection in PL population. The most frequent non-IL alleles identified in this study (i.e. c.2052_2053insA; c.3468+2_3468+3insT; IVS9 T_5_TG_{12-13}; R668C; G314R) should be included in the PL population screening panel. Mutation distribution described herein is also relevant to the Polish; according to the Polish Press Agency, the rapport of the Polish Ministry of Foreign Affairs issued in July 2013 estimated the size of Polish diaspora at over 18 million people, with the major centers in US, Canada, Germany, UK and other countries (see also www.wikipedia.org/wiki/Polish_diaspora). The aforementioned mutations could be considered when testing these populations.

On the other hand, even the extended screening procedure left over 17% of *CFTR* mutations unidentified. It has to be kept in mind that, for budgetary reasons, sequencing was performed when an altered migration pattern of an amplicon was detected in the SSCP/HD analysis. Our long experience with the SSCP/HD technique indicates that using appropriate conditions allows detecting ~85–90% of the existing sequence changes. Applying this estimate to the 158 chromosomes with no identified mutation, one may assume that 10–15% of them (~16–24 chromosomes) could harbor sequence change undetected due to technical reasons. Nevertheless, this would still leave over 130 chromosomes with no identified mutation. The presence of large novel exonic deletions, not detectable using SSCP/HD-based approach, was excluded by MLPA analysis performed in ~60% of the chromosomes with no identified mutation. Undetected mutations could therefore be located in the gene regions, which were not targeted in the screening procedure, such as deep intronic sequences or regulatory regions [12]. Also, when estimating mutation detection efficiency, the accuracy of the clinical diagnosis is an important issue, as discussed below.

Heterogeneity of the clinical manifestation may render clinical diagnosis of some cases difficult. This problem had already been noted in one of the previous studies on *CFTR* mutations, where patients had been divided into groups of "CF classical, atypical and doubtful" [7]. In this context it is also worth mentioning that the estimates of CF incidence in PL population differ, very likely reflecting differences in diagnostic schemes [2]. The most-cited source, indicating the incidence of 1:2300, is now 40 years old [13]. The more recent estimates provide much lower values, ranging from 1:5000 [14], 1:6000 cited in WHO 2002 report [15] to 1:7500 for Southeastern Poland estimated for a 1-year period of

Table 3. Comparison of the efficiency of mutation detection efficiency using INNOLiPA tests and teh follow-up screening (SSCP/HD and sequencing).

Overall mutations detected in a patient	Proportion of patients	CF mutations per patient detected in INNOLiPA tests	Additional CF alleles detected in the follow-up phase	Number of CF patients
both	**78.6%**	both	n.a.	503
"	"	one	1	71[a]
"	"	none	2	6
one	**7.8%**	none	1	20[b,c]
"	"	one	0	38[c]
none	**13.6%**	none	0	38[c]+62

Legend: [a] including six alleles with $T_5\_TG_{12-13}$ in intron 9; [b] including four alleles with $T_{5or8}\_TG_{12-13}$ in intron 9; [c] also analyzed by MLPA

2009–2010 [16]. Some of the discrepancies in the mutation detection efficiency across populations and studies may reflect this type of inaccuracies.

To illustrate potential impact of the care center on the correct clinical diagnosis and thus on the efficiency of mutation detection, we compared the results obtained for two subgroups of our cohort (Fig. 1): patients from the national CF reference center (Institute of Tuberculosis and Lung Diseases in Rabka; N = 368) and from other health centers (general pediatric hospitals in Poznan and other cities, excluding Warsaw (see below); N = 370). The success of the IL tests (detection of both mutations) was 79% in Rabka and 58% in other centers ($p<0.0001$; Pearson's chi square test). After the extended gene screening, the number of patients with no mutations detected remained significantly ($p<0.0001$) higher in patients from the general pediatric centers (~23%) than in patients from the specialized CF center in Rabka (~5%). The observed discrepancy can be interpreted as indicating the lower rate of a successful clinical CF diagnosis outside the reference center. Of note, among the patients from Rabka with only one or with no mutation found, ~80% had high sweat chloride values; in the corresponding group from the peripheral centers, high chloride values were reported only in ~50% of the patients, while the other half had ambiguous chloride values or no test results had been reported.

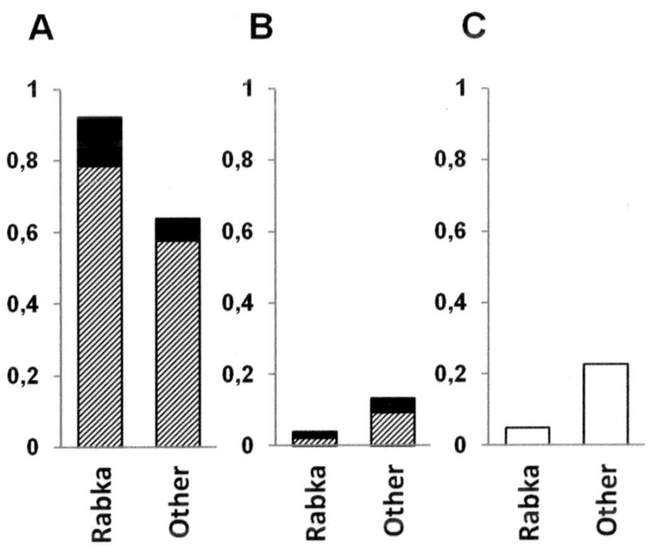

Figure 1. *CFTR* mutation detection efficiency in PL CF patients from different health centers. A. Both mutations identified. B. One mutation identified. C. No mutation identified. Diagonal stripes – INNOLiPA mutations; solid black – non-INNOLiPA mutations. Rabka – Institute of Tuberculosis and Lung Diseases in Rabka; Other – other health care centers in Poland.

The efficiency of non-IL mutations detection was almost 5 times higher in the patients with one IL mutation than in those with no IL mutation (non-IL mutation found in ~65% and ~13% of the chromosomes, respectively, see Table 3). This discrepancy appears consistent with the scenario that some individuals of the former group (composed mostly of patients from outside of Rabka) were in fact misdiagnosed as CF. In addition, in over 20% of the patients with no mutation found, the clinical diagnosis was based on the presence of MI. While MI occurs in 10–20% of all CF patients at birth [17], a considerable proportion (20–50%) of newborns with MI may not in fact have CF [18–19].

In conclusion, taking into account that up to ~10% of the whole analyzed cohort could have been incorrectly diagnosed as CF, it is possible that the real efficiency of mutation detection would be higher than the estimated 85%; similar correction would apply to the estimated mutation frequencies.

Our study group consisted mostly of CF patients from the Western and Southern PL. In order to assess the mutation spectrum in the whole country, we compared our data with those obtained in the Institute of Mother and Child in Warsaw, where most of the patients were from the Central and Northeastern Poland (Prof. Jerzy Bal, personal communication). The data (based on direct sequencing of the coding region) were only available for patients (N = 480) with both mutations detected (the total number of analyzed CF patients and of patients with only one mutation detected were not provided). To compare data from both laboratories, we calculated allele frequencies in a subset of our patients, with both mutations identified. F508del frequency in this subset was significantly higher than in the full cohort (67.2% vs 54.5%, $p = 0.000$; Pearsons's chi square), which most probably results from the possible presence of misdiagnosed patients, as discussed above; the adjusted frequencies for other mutations did not differ between both subsets of our cohort. Three mutations in our reduced data set were significantly ($p<0.03$) less frequent than in Warsaw (F508del: 67.2% vs 71.8%; G542X: 1.98% vs 2.92%; N1303K: 1.47% vs 2.92%), while two mutations were significantly more frequent (c.3468+2_3468+3insT: 0.86% vs 0.10%; c.489+1G>T: 0.43% vs 0%; G314R: 0.34% vs 0%). The discrepancies between data from our laboratory and from Warsaw may reflect regional differences in samples origin.

The most frequent *CFTR* mutations found in PL patients (>0.1%, as suggested in the recommendations regarding selection

Table 4. Distribution of the most frequent CFTR mutations detected in CF patients from Poland, compared with Central and Southeastern European populations.

Mutations[a]	*Poland*	*Czechs*	*Slovakia*[c]	*Germany*	*Lithuania*	*W. Ukraine*	*E. Hungary*	*Romania*[c]	*Bulgaria*	*Serbia*	*Greece*
Number of chromosomes	*1476*	*1200*	*856*	*700*	*98*	*264*	*80*	*256*	*208*	*352*	*874*
F508del	**54.54**[b]	67.42[d]	66.80[d]	72.00[d]	52.0	54.17	70.00	56.3	65.38[d]	72.28[d]	53.40
exon2,3del21kb (l.n.CFTRdele2,3_21kb)	**4.47**	5.75	2.26	1.2[f]	2.0	4.17	5.00	1.6	NA	0[e]	0.34[e]
c.3717+12191C>T (l.n.3849+10kbC>T)	**3.93**	1.67[e]	4.28	1.00[e]	NA	0.76	0	0.4[e]	1.44	0[e]	0.11[e]
c.2012delT (l.n.2143delT)	**1.83**	0.92	1.10	0.71	0	1.14	0	0[e]	0	0[e]	0[e]
c.1585-1G>A (l.n.1717-1G>A)	**1.83**	0.33[e]	NA	0.86	0	0.38	1.25	0.4	0	0[e]	0[e]
G542X	**1.69**	2.00	4.06[d]	1.43	0	2.65	3.75	3.9	3.37	2.57	3.90[d]
R347P	**1.57**	0.92	1.10	1.57	0	0	1.25	NA	1.44	0[e]	0.11[e]
N1303K	**1.22**	2.42	2.03	2.29	2.0	4.92[d]	5.00	0.8	6.73[d]	0	2.63
c.2052-2053insA (l.n.2184insA)	**1.02**	0.42	1.58	0.57	0	7.20[d]	5.00[d]	0	0.48	0.28	0[e]
R553X	**0.95**	0.50	0.90	2.29	4.2[d]	0.38	0	NA	0	0	0
c.3468+2−3insT (l.n.3600+2insT)	**0.75**	0.25	NA	0[e]	0	NA	0	NA	0	0	0[e]
c.2051–2052AA>G (l.n.2183AA>G)	**0.68**	0.08	NA	0.57	0	0.38	0	0.8	0	0	1.38
W1282X	**0.61**	0.58	0.50	0.71	1.0	2.27	0	2.3[d]	0.96	0	0.67
c.3140-26A>G (l.n.3272-26A>G)	**0.61**	0.67	0.50	0.86	0	0.76	0	0.4	0	0	0.81
l.n.IVS8 T_5_TG_{12-13}	**0.54**	NA	NA	NA	0	NA	NA	NA	NA	0	NA
R334W	**0.41**	0.25	NA	0.29	0	0.76	0	0.4	0	0.28	0.81
c.1766+1G>A (l.n.1898+1G>A)	**0.41**	1.42[d]	0.50	0	0	1.14	0	NA	0	0	0.11
c.489+1G>T (l.n.621+1G>T)	**0.34**	0.42	NA	0.14	0	0.76	0	0.8	0	2.86[d]	5.72[d]
R117H	**0.34**	NA	NA	0.29	0	0	0	0.4	0	0	0.23
G551D	**0.34**	2.91[d]	0.50	1.00	0	0	0	0	0	0	0.34
G314R	**0.37**	0	NA	0	0	0	0	NA	0	0	0
R668C	**0.34**	0	NA	0	0	0	0	NA	0	0	0
c.3528delC (l.n.3659delC)	**0.27**	0.17	NA	0.57	0	0	0	NA	0	0	0
c.164+1G>A (l.n.296+1G>A)	**0.20**	0.08	NA	0	0	0	0	NA	0	0	0
R851X	**0.20**	0.08	NA	0	0	0	0	NA	0	0	0
I336K	**0.14**	0.58	NA	0.45	0	0	0	NA	0	0	0
R1158X	**0.14**	0.08	NA	0	0	0	0	NA	0	0	1.03
E92K	**0.14**	0.08	NA	0	0	0.38	0	NA	0	0	0
R153I	**0.14**	0	NA	0	0	0	0	NA	0	0	0
c.579+3A>G (l.n.711+3A>G)	**0.14**	0.17	NA	0	0	0	0	NA	0	0	0.69
c.2589–2599del11bp (l.n.2721-31del11bp)	**0.14**	0.08	NA	0	0	0.38	0	NA	0	0	0
I507del	**0.14**	0.08	NA	0.15	0	0	0	0	0	0.28	0.69
R117C	**0.14**	0.08	NA	0.15	0	0	0	NA	0	0	0.23

Table 4. Cont.

Mutations[a]	*Poland*	*Czechs*	*Slovakia*[c]	*Germany*	*Lithuania*	*W. Ukraine*	*E. Hungary*	*Romania*[c]	*Bulgaria*	*Serbia*	*Greece*
Number of chromosomes	*1476*	*1200*	*856*	*700*	*98*	*264*	*80*	*256*	*208*	*352*	*874*
F311L	**0.14**	0	NA	0	0	0	0	NA	0	0	0
Q1412X	**0.14**	0	NA	0	0	0	0	NA	0	0	0
Other reported	**1.52**	8.51	NA	7.10	2.0	1.14	7.50	3.8	12,03	4.28	17.83
Not detected	**17.5**	0.50	13.89	4.57	35.8	16.29	6.25	27.7	8.17	17.43	9.15
Estimated efficiency of INNOLiPA tests	**75.5**	**89.9**	**84.0**	**88.7**	**61.2**	**74.6**	**87.5**	**69.1**	**80.3**	**78.7**	**73.3**

Legend: Data are given in %. [a] non-INNOLiPA mutations are in bold, and a novel mutation is underlined; [b] very close to the earlier estimate of 54% based on a much smaller study group of PL patients [7]; [c] only selected segments of the gene have been screened; [d] frequency significantly higher or [e] lower than in Polish cohort (p<0.005, Pearsons's chi square); [f] [5]; NA– not analyzed/not available; Poland (mostly Southern and Western Poland; this study); Czech Republic [21]; Slovakia (based on [21]); Germany [22]; Lithuania [23]; Western Ukraine [24]; East Hungary [25]; Romania [26]; Bulgaria [27]; Serbia [28]; Greece [29].

of mutation panels [20]), listed in Table 4, were compared to those reported for several Central and Southeastern European countries [21–29]. The overall efficiency of the IL tests in Polish patients (75.5%; 87% in Rabka and 65% in Polish peripheral centers) was within the range reported for other populations (61–90%; see Table 4). Please note, that the highest efficiencies of testing for INNOLiPA mutations have been reported in the countries with a long-standing tradition of genetic CF testing. These data lend even further support to the observation that the reported efficiency of genetic tests in a given population strongly depends on the quality of clinical diagnostics performed in referring care centers from a given country or region.

The frequency of F508del (~54.5%), was similar to the estimates for Western Ukrainians, Lithuanians, Romanians and Greeks but significantly ($p<0.006$; Pearsons's chi square) lower than for Germans, Czechs, Slovaks, Bulgarians, and Serbs; this shows that the decreasing North-South gradient of F508del frequency across Europe [4] does not hold in Eastern Slav populations. The relatively high frequency of exon2.3del21kb alias *CFTR*dele2,3(21 kb) (~4.5%) was consistent with its Slavic origin [30]. The frequency of Israeli c.3717+12191C>T (l.n.3849+10kbC>T) [4] was significantly elevated in Poland (3.9%) and Slovakia compared to most of the examined populations (Czechs, Germany, Romania, Serbia, Greece, $p<0.005$), possibly indicating the Ashkenazi-Jewish contribution; in contrast, the frequency of another Israeli mutation, W1282X [4,12], was significantly lower in Poland (0.61%) than in Romania ($p<0.006$). The Eastern European c.2012delT (l.n.2143delT) [12] was found in Poles at the relatively high frequency (1.83%) compared to Czechs, Slovaks, Western Ukrainians and Germans, and was absent elsewhere, including Romania, Serbia and Bulgaria; its increased frequency may suggest PL origin of the c.2012delT. The frequency of Mediterranean c.1585-1G>A (l.n.1717-1G>A) [4–5] was 1.83%, significantly ($p<0.005$) higher than in several other Slavic populations, while that of another Mediterranean mutation, N1303K [4], was 1.22%, significantly ($p<0.005$) lower than in Western Ukraine, Bulgaria, Serbia and Hungary.

Among non-IL mutations, the frequency of c.2052–2053insA (l.n.2184insA, ~1.0%) was significantly ($p<0.005$) lower than 7.2% or 5.0% reported for Western Ukraine or Eastern Hungary, respectively [24,25]. This confirms the proposed "Galician" origin of this mutation and indicates that Poland is at the decreasing side of its distribution. The c.3468+2_3468+3insT (originally reported in a single PL individual [7]), accounted for ~0.75% PL CF chromosomes; so far, it has been reported only in Poles and in Czechs [21]. The regional origin of Polish patients carrying this insertion (Southeastern part of PL) and the homogeneous SNP-based background haplotype (not shown) indicate that this is probably a founder mutation. G314R, a novel missense change found in 0.37% of the studied CF chromosomes, might be another PL founder mutation. These observations would have to be confirmed by screening for c.3468+2_3468+3insT and G314R in a larger numbers of CF patients from other neighboring European populations.

The relatively high frequency (0.54%) of IVS9 $T_5\_TG_{12-13}$ (without R117H in cis) in PL patients could not be compared with other populations. While TG_{12-13} in cis with T_5 are known to contribute to less efficient splicing of exon 10 and to abnormal phenotype [31–32], most of the CF tests do not determine the length of the TG repeat, and reporting the T_5 in intron 9 (l.n.IVS8-T_5) as a pathogenic mutation has been recommended only if in cis with R117H [12].

Materials and Methods

Ethics Statement

The research protocol was approved by the Ethics Committee of the Medical University in Poznan. Genetic data referred to in the manuscript were collected over many years as a component of a routine hospital diagnostic procedure. As such, they are covered by an implied consent, which – according to the local Institutional Review Board – does not require signing additional informed consent form and is documented by the fact of a patient subjecting to the diagnostic procedure. All further analyses were based on the archival data that were stored in the database with no current connection to the patients' identifiers.

Patients

The samples, referred for molecular diagnosis during the period of 1995–2011, originated from different care centers (predominantly Institute of Tuberculosis and Lung Diseases in Rabka, ~50%; and pediatric clinical hospitals from Poznan, ~25%); patients represented mostly Western and Southern PL. The initial diagnosis of CF was based on standard criteria [6,33], which included one or more of the characteristic clinical features (most often: chronic obstruction/ infection of the respiratory tract; gastrointestinal abnormalities; failure to thrive; meconium ileus, MI; exocrine pancreatic insufficiency) and/or at least two positive sweat chloride tests in pilocarpine iontophoresis (>60 mmol/L). Chloride measurements were not collected for newborns and very young children, consistent with the well-known observation that no sweat tests are reliable during the first years of age (e.g. [34]); in particular, for most of the patients with MI no chloride data were available.

Mutation screening

The group of unrelated CF patients (N = 738) had been sequentially examined using IL tests: *CFTR_19* and – if two mutations were not detected – *CFTR_17TnUpdate*. IL reverse dot blot kits rely on the DNA amplification and hybridization with a membrane-immobilized set of probes (Line Probe Assay). The probes correspond to the normal and mutated alleles, covering 36 most frequent European *CFTR* mutations. The procedure was performed as indicated by the manufacturer (InnoGenetics, Ghent, Belgium; see also [35]).

To comprehensively determine the population frequency profile of *CFTR* mutations, a follow-up molecular screening was performed. All the patients with only one IL mutation (N = 109) and with no mutation found (N = 126) were analyzed using SSCP/HD (single strand conformational polymorphism and heteroduplex) technique as described in [11]. Briefly, specific primer pairs were designed for each of the 27 *CFTR* exons, and the 5' and 3' UTR regions; to achieve the length of each amplicon <340 bp some exons were analyzed as overlapping fragments. For the SSCP/HD analysis, PCR-amplified segments were denatured and separated in 7 or 8% polyacrylamide (29:1) in 0.5x or 1xTBE gels (optionally with ~2 M urea and 10% glycerol) were run at 8–10 W for 20–40 h at RT or 4°C. Primer sequences, PCR conditions and detailed conditions used to separate each of the analyzed fragments are available from the authors upon request.

Nucleotide changes underlying all the detected SSCP/HD migration variants were resolved by direct sequencing of the PCR products (BigDyeTerminator v3.1 on an ABI Prism 3130XL Analyzer, Applied Biosystems); trace files were checked and edited using FinchTV1.3.1. (Geospiza Inc.). Sequences were evaluated manually using Chromas 1.45 software and FASTA sequence comparison algorithm (http://fasta.bioch.virginia.edu/fasta_www2).

Finally, 2/3 of the samples, in which one or both mutations remained unidentified, were examined for possible intragenic rearrangements using MLPA technique with SALSA MLPA Kit P091-B1 CFTR (MRC-Holland). This P091-B1 CFTR probemix contains probes for each of the 24 *CFTR* exons and a second probe for exons 6, 14, 17 and 24. In addition, the probemix P091-B1 contains a mutation specific that detects the wildtype allele of the F508del mutation.

The effect of amino acid changes on the protein stability was examined using SNPs3D online software (www.snps3d.org); the negative SVM value (<−0.5) was assumed to indicate a deleterious effect.

Nomenclature of mutations

The currently recommended numbering of the gene exons (www.ensembl.org) and the protein or cDNA-based HGVS nomenclature of mutations were used throughout the text; the commonly used legacy name (l.n.), if mentioned, was given in parentheses.

Acknowledgments

We thank Prof. Jerzy Bal for sharing unpublished data on CFTR screening performed in the Institute of Mother and Child, Warsaw, and Ms Lidia Pawlik for help in retrieving clinical data from the database in Rabka.

Author Contributions

Conceived and designed the experiments: EZ MW. Performed the experiments: ER BK KV. Analyzed the data: EZ ER AP. Contributed reagents/materials/analysis tools: AP. Wrote the paper: EZ. Revised manuscript critically for important intellectual content: ER AP BK KV MW. Final approval of the version to be published: EZ ER AP BK KV MW.

References

1. Southern KW, Munck A, Pollitt R, Travert G, Zanolla R, et al. (2007) ECFS CF Neonatal Screening Working Group. A survey of newborn screening for cystic fibrosis in Europe. *J Cyst Fibros* 6: 57–65.
2. Farrell PM (2008) The prevalence of cystic fibrosis in the European Union. *J Cyst Fibros* 7: 450–453.
3. Kerem B-S, Rommens JM, Buchanan JA, Markiewicz D, Cox TK, et al. (1989) Identification of the cystic fibrosis gene: genetic analysis. *Science* 245: 1073–80.
4. Estivill X, Bancells C, Ramos C (1997) Geographic distribution and regional origin of 272 cystic fibrosis mutations in European populations. The Biomed CF Mutation Analysis Consortium. *Hum Mutat* 10: 135–54.
5. Bobadilla JL, Macek M Jr, Fine JP, Farrel PM (2002) Cystic Fibrosis: A worldwide analysis of CFTR mutations-correlation with incidence data and application to screening. *Hum Mutat* 19: 575–606.
6. Dequeker E, Stuhrmann M, Morris MA, Casals T, Castellani C, et al. (2009) Best practice guidelines for molecular genetic diagnosis of cystic fibrosis and CFTR-related disorders—updated European recommendations. *Eur J Hum Genet* 17: 51–65.
7. Aznarez I, Bal J, Casals T, Estivill X, Moral N, et al. (2000) Analysis of mutations in the CFTR gene in patients diagnosed with cystic fibrosis in Poland (in Polish). *Med Wieku Rozwoj* 4: 149–59.
8. Bal J, Maciejko D, Mazurczak T, Potocka A, Krawczak M, et al. (1991) Frequency of the cystic fibrosis mutation delta F508 in Poland. *Hum Genet* 86: 329.
9. Bal J, Maciejko D, Mazurczak T (1995) The type and frequency of mutations in CFTR gene occurrence in patients with cystic fibrosis in Poland - implication of results obtained from genetic counseling and diagnostic screening (in Polish). *Pediatr Pol* 70: 627–32.
10. Witt M, Pogorzelski A, Bal J, Rutkiewicz E, Majka L, et al. (1999) Frequency of mutations and genotypes of the CFTR gene in cystic fibrosis adults in Poland (in Polish). *Pneumonol Alergol Pol* 67:137–41.

11. Zietkiewicz E, Nitka B, Voelkel K, Skrzypczak U, Bukowy Z, et al. (2010) Population specificity of the *DNAI1* gene mutation spectrum in primary ciliary dyskinesia (PCD). *Respir Res* 11: 174.
12. Castellani C, Cuppens H, Macek Jr M, Cassiman JJ, Kerem E, et al. (2008) Consensus on the use and interpretation of cystic fibrosis mutation analysis in clinical practice. *J Cyst Fibros* 7: 179–96.
13. Bożkowa E, Golebiowska H, Rutkowski J, Nowakowska A, Holzer J (1971) Epidemiologia mukowiscydozy u dzieci w Polsce (in Polish). *Ped Pol* 46: 677–684.
14. Colombo C, Littlewood J (2011) The implementation of standards of care in Europe: state of the art. *J Cyst Fibros* 10S2: S7–15.
15. WHO Report (2004) The molecular genetic epidemiology of cystic fibrosis; www.who.int/ genomics/publications/en/HGN_WB_04.02_report.pdf.
16. Słuszniak A, Kurtyka Z, Lemańska D (2011) Neonatal mass screening for cystic fibrosis in south-east Poland (in Polish). *Przegl Lek* 68: 59–62.
17. Kerem E, Corey M, Kerem B, Durie P, Tsui LC, et al. (1989) Clinical and genetic comparisons of patients with cystic fibrosis, with or without meconium ileus. *J Pediatr* 114: 767–73
18. Fakhoury K, Durie PR, Levison H, Canny GJ (1992) Meconium ileus in the absence of cystic fibrosis. *Arch Dis Child* 67s: 1204–6.
19. Gorter RR, Karimi A, Sleeboom C, Kneepkens CM, Heij HA (2010) Clinical and genetic characteristics of meconium ileus in newborns with and without cystic fibrosis. *J Pediatr Gastroenterol Nutr* 50: 569–72.
20. Grody W, Cutting G, Klinger K, Richards CS, Watson MS, et al. (2001) Laboratory standards and guidelines for population-based cystic fibrosis carrier screening. *Genet Med* 3: 149–54.
21. Krenkova P, Piskackova T, Holubova A, Balascakova M, Krulisova V, et al. (2012) Distribution of CFTR mutations in the Czech population: Positive impact of integrated clinical and laboratory expertise, detection of novel/de novo alleles and relevance for related/derived populations. *J Cyst Fibros* S1: 1569–1993.
22. Dork T, Mekus F, Schmidt K, Bosshammer J, Fislage R, et al. (1994) Detection of more than 50 different CFTR mutations in a large group of German cystic fibrosis patients. *Hum Genet* 94: 533–42.
23. Giannattasio S, Bobba A, Jurgelevicius V, Vacca RA, Lattanzio P, et al. (2006) Molecular basis of cystic fibrosis in Lithuania: incomplete CFTR mutation detection by PCR-based screening protocols. *Genet Test* 10: 169–73.
24. Makukh H, Krenkova P, Tyrkus M, Bober L, Hancarova M, et al. (2010) A high frequency of the cystic fibrosis 2184insA mutation in Western Ukraine: genotype–phenotype correlations, relevance for newborn screening and genetic testing. *J Cyst Fibros* 9: 371–5.
25. Ivady G, Madar L, Nagy B, Gonczi F, Ajzner E, et al. (2011) Distribution of CFTR mutations in Eastern Hungarians: relevance to genetic testing and to the introduction of newborn screening for cystic fibrosis. *J Cyst Fibros* 10:217–20.
26. Frentescu L, Brownsell E, Hinks J, Malone G, Shaw H, et al. (2008) The study of cystic fibrosis transmembrane conductance regulator gene mutations in a group of patients from Romania. *J Cyst Fibros* 7: 423–8.
27. Angelicheva D, Calafell F, Savov A, Jordanova A, Kufardjieva A, et al. (1997) Cystic fibrosis mutations and associated haplotypes in Bulgaria – a comparative population genetic study. *Hum Genet* 99: 513–520.
28. Radivojevic D, Djurisic M, Lalic T, Guc-Scekic M, Savic J, et al. (2004) Spectrum of cystic fibrosis mutations in Serbia and Montenegro and strategy for prenatal diagnosis. *Genet Test* 8: 276–280.
29. Kanavakis E, Efthymiadou A, Strofalis S, Doudounakis S, Traeger-Synodinos J, et al. (2003) Cystic fibrosis in Greece: molecular diagnosis, haplotypes, prenatal diagnosis and carrier identyfication amongst high-risk individuals. *Clin Genet* 63: 400–409.
30. Dork T, Macek Jr M, Mekus F, Tummler B, Tzountzouris J, et al. (2000) Characterization of a novel 21-kb deletion, CFTRdele2,3(21kb), in the CFTR gene: a cystic fibrosis mutation of Slavic origin common in Central and East Europe. *Hum Genet* 106: 259–68.
31. Cuppens H, Lin W, Jaspers M, Costes B, Teng H, et al. (1998) Polyvariant mutant cystic fibrosis transmembrane conductance regulator genes – the polymorphic (TG)m locus explains the partial penetrance of the T5 polymorphism as a disease mutation. *J Clin Invest* 101: 487–496.
32. Groman JD, Hefferon TW, Casals T, Bassas L, Estivill X, et al. (2004) Variation in a repeat sequence determines whether a common variant of the cystic fibrosis transmembrane conductance regulator gene is pathogenic or benign. *Am J Hum Genet* 74: 176–9.
33. Rosenstein BJ, Cutting GR (1998) The diagnosis of cystic fibrosis: a consensus statement. *J Pediatr* 132: 589–595.
34. Traeger N, Shi Q, Dozor AJ (2013) Relationship between sweat chloride, sodium, and age in clinically obtained samples. *J Cyst Fibros* S1: 569–1933.
35. Heaney DL, Flume P, Hamilton L, Lyon E, Wolff DJ (2006) Detection of an apparent homozygous 3120G>A cystic fibrosis mutation on a routine carrier screen. *J Molec Diagn* 8: 137–140.

9

Characterization of Defects in Ion Transport and Tissue Development in Cystic Fibrosis Transmembrane Conductance Regulator (CFTR)-Knockout Rats

Katherine L. Tuggle[1,2], Susan E. Birket[1,3], Xiaoxia Cui[4], Jeong Hong[1,5], Joe Warren[4], Lara Reid[4], Andre Chambers[4], Diana Ji[4], Kevin Gamber[4], Kengyeh K. Chu[6,7], Guillermo Tearney[6,8], Li Ping Tang[1], James A. Fortenberry[1], Ming Du[1,9], Joan M. Cadillac[9], David M. Bedwell[1,10], Steven M. Rowe[1,3], Eric J. Sorscher[1,3], Michelle V. Fanucchi[1,2]*

1 Gregory Fleming James Cystic Fibrosis Research Center, University of Alabama at Birmingham, Birmingham, Alabama, United States of America, **2** Department of Environmental Health Sciences, School of Public Health, University of Alabama at Birmingham, Birmingham, Alabama, United States of America, **3** Department of Medicine, University of Alabama at Birmingham, Birmingham, Alabama, United States of America, **4** SAGE Labs, Inc., St. Louis, Missouri, United States of America, **5** Department of Cell, Developmental, and Integrative Biology, University of Alabama at Birmingham, Birmingham, Alabama, United States of America, **6** Wellman Center for Photomedicine, Harvard Medical School, Massachusetts General Hospital, Boston, Massachusetts, United States of America, **7** Department of Dermatology, Massachusetts General Hospital, Boston, Massachusetts, United States of America, **8** Department of Pathology, Massachusetts General Hospital, Boston, Massachusetts, United States of America, **9** Animal Resources Program, Office of the Vice President for Research, University of Alabama at Birmingham, Birmingham, Alabama, United States of America, **10** Department of Microbiology, University of Alabama at Birmingham, Birmingham, Alabama, United States of America

Abstract

Animal models for cystic fibrosis (CF) have contributed significantly to our understanding of disease pathogenesis. Here we describe development and characterization of the first cystic fibrosis rat, in which the cystic fibrosis transmembrane conductance regulator gene (CFTR) was knocked out using a pair of zinc finger endonucleases (ZFN). The disrupted *Cftr* gene carries a 16 base pair deletion in exon 3, resulting in loss of CFTR protein expression. Breeding of heterozygous ($CFTR^{+/-}$) rats resulted in Mendelian distribution of wild-type, heterozygous, and homozygous ($CFTR^{-/-}$) pups. Nasal potential difference and transepithelial short circuit current measurements established a robust CF bioelectric phenotype, similar in many respects to that seen in CF patients. Young $CFTR^{-/-}$ rats exhibited histological abnormalities in the ileum and increased intracellular mucus in the proximal nasal septa. By six weeks of age, $CFTR^{-/-}$ males lacked the vas deferens bilaterally. Airway surface liquid and periciliary liquid depth were reduced, and submucosal gland size was abnormal in $CFTR^{-/}$ animals. Use of ZFN based gene disruption successfully generated a CF animal model that recapitulates many aspects of human disease, and may be useful for modeling other CF genotypes, including CFTR processing defects, premature truncation alleles, and channel gating abnormalities.

Editor: Prosper N. Boyaka, The Ohio State University, United States of America

Funding: This work was supported by CF Foundation Grant R464-CR07 (www.cff.org) and NIH P30 DK072482 (www.nih.gov) to EJS and R01 HL116213 to SMR. The funders had no role in study design, data collection and analysis, decision to publish, or preparation of the manuscript.

Competing Interests: The authors have read the journal's policy and have the following conflicts: XC, JW, LR, AC, DJ and KG are full-time employees of SAGE Labs, Inc., which sells genetically engineered rats and provides custom model creation services. KKC, EJS, SMR, and GT have filed a patent application related to use of µOCT technology in airways. The application serial number is PCT/US12/52553, entitled "Method for functional investigation of respiratory airways a nd other ciliated tissues using µOCT," filed August 27, 2012. No financial benefit has yet been derived from this application by any author. SMR receives research support from the NIH, the Cystic Fibrosis Foundation (CFF), the American Lung Association, Synedgen Inc., and Forest Research Institute for basic and translational research. SMR also receives support from CFF Therapeutics (CFFT), Vertex Pharmaceuticals, PTC Therapeutics, N30 Therapeutics, and Novartis to conduct clinical trials related to the treatment and control of cystic fibrosis. SMR receives unrestricted research support for consulting services to Novartis, Kala Pharmaceuticals, Celtaxys Inc., and Bayer Healthcare. SMR receives no personal income from any of the sponsors noted above. GT receives research support from iLumen, Ninepoint Medical, Merck Research Laboratories, Canon, Samsung, and Air Liquide Medical Gases. GT. receives personal income from Ninepoint Medical, Terumo Corporation, and MIT through patent licensing arrangements. GT also receives consulting income from Samsung Advanced Institute of Technology and Ninepoint Medical. EJS receives research support from NIH, CFF, and CFFT. EJS serves as a scientific consultant to Genzyme, Pfizer, and Gilead. He receives consulting income from Gilead. KLT, SEB, JSH, LPT, JAF, MD, JMC, DMB, and MVF have no conflicts of interest to disclose.

* E-mail: fanucchi@uab.edu

Introduction

Cystic fibrosis (CF) is the most common lethal recessive genetic disorder among individuals of European descent, affecting 1 in every 2,500–3,500 newborns each year [1]. The disease is characterized by multi-system pathology, including respiratory complications, intestinal obstruction, exocrine pancreatic disease, hepatoductal blockage, and absence of the vas deferens [2]. The predominant cause of morbidity and mortality in CF results from chronic pulmonary infection and inflammation. CF is caused by mutations in the cystic fibrosis transmembrane conductance regulator (CFTR) gene, encoding an anion channel expressed in epithelial and other tissues.

A variety of CF mice have been generated since the discovery of *Cftr* in 1989 [3,4]. The mouse models, while presenting with CF-related intestinal disease, fail to recapitulate many other manifestations observed in patients. Nonetheless, CF mice have provided a valuable tool for testing pharmaceutical and other interventions, and investigating contributors to pathogenesis, including CF modifier genes [5]. Porcine [6] and ferret [7] CF models exhibit a respiratory phenotype closely resembling that observed in humans, although prolonged gestational period, time to sexual maturation, expense, and specialized care requirements have significantly limited their widespread use.

The development of a CF rat (*Rattus norvegicus*) would provide a number of advantages in comparison with available animal models of CF. First, the rat has a very short gestational period (21–23 days) and time to sexual maturity (8 weeks), allowing rapid colony propagation, breeding studies, and characterization of animals as they mature shortly after birth. Second, there is considerable interest regarding airway glandular function as a mediator of CF respiratory failure [8]. Airway submucosal glands are believed to underlie considerable pathology observed in human CF lungs. Rats are an attractive model in this context because, unlike mice but similar to humans, rats develop extensive submucosal glands throughout the trachea to the level of bronchi [9]. Third, relative to mice, rats are considerably larger in size, even during the early postnatal period, allowing for larger tissue samples to be collected from animals and ease performing surgical procedures [10]. Rats are also a traditional species for pharmacology and toxicology research due to their well-defined pharmacokinetic and biodistribution profiles [11,12]. Previous CF studies have sometimes required transgenic mice for efficacy, with safety studies conducted in rat; however, a CF rat model would facilitate pharmaceutical efficacy and safety studies of potential therapeutic molecules in the same species. Finally, because rats have been well studied in the laboratory for years, there is a large body of literature regarding normal physiology and a vast array of laboratory tools and reagents (i.e. antibodies, siRNA, other genomic probes) readily available for the study of chaperone, binding partner, and other protein based analyses relevant to disease mechanism that would be very difficult to obtain for ferret or pig.

Recent advances in gene manipulation techniques have provided a number of opportunities for developing genetically modified animals other than mouse. Zinc-finger endonuclease (ZFN) technology, for example, allows targeting of user-defined site-specific mutations that generate knockout animals with high efficiency and over a shorter time line than embryonic stem-cell targeting used in many species other than mouse [13,14]. Here, we describe the generation of a $CFTR^{-/-}$ rat by pronuclear microinjection of ZFNs and its characterization. The disease phenotypes observed in young (21–44 days postnatal) $CFTR^{-/-}$ animals, which closely resemble human manifestations, suggest the rat model will be useful for studies of CF pulmonary pathogenesis and drug development.

Materials and Methods

Ethics Statement

This study was carried out in compliance with the Guide for the Care and Use of Laboratory Animals of the National Institutes of Health. Protocols were approved by the SAGE Labs, Inc. or University of Alabama at Birmingham (UAB) Institutional Animal Care and Use Committee (IACUC; SAGE Approval Number 001.02, UAB Approval Number 09479). All surgeries were performed under sodium pentobarbital or ketamine/xylazine/acepromazine anesthesia with all efforts made to minimize animal suffering.

Generation of the Model

ZFN mRNA preparation. *Cftr* specific ZFNs were obtained from the CompoZr product line (Sigma, St. Louis, MO). mRNA was prepared from each construct, linearized with XhoI and modified using MessageMax and Poly(A) polymerase tailing kits (Epicentre Biotechnology). Samples were purified, quantified, and transfected at a 1:1 ratio into rat C6 cells for activity validation.

Animal husbandry. Derivation and breeding of animals was conducted at SAGE Labs (microinjection and founder identification/breeding) operated under approved animal protocols overseen by the SAGE IACUC. Sprague Dawley rats (Ntac:SD) from Taconic Farms (Hudson, New York) were used for microinjection. Animals were bred with housing in standard cages maintained on a 12 h light/dark cycle with *ad libitum* access to food and water. Routine health monitoring of the colony was performed at IDEXX (Columbia, MO) and indicated no evidence of infection with known serious pathogens.

Microinjection. Four to five week-old female donors were injected with 20 units of pregnant mare serum gonadotropin (PMS) followed by injection of 50 units hCG after an additional 48 h, and immediately mated with stud males. Fertilized eggs were harvested a day later. *Cftr* ZFN mRNA was microinjected at 10 ng/ml into the pronucleus of fertilized eggs. Following microinjection, 25–30 eggs were transferred into each pseudo-pregnant female, leading to birth of the founder generation.

Founder identification and breeding. Tail or toe biopsies were used for genomic DNA extraction and analysis as described previously [15]. Primers flanking the target site were forward 5′- AATATCTGGGTGGGCAGTTG and reverse 5′-TTGTTTGCAAGATTGCCCTT. Primers used to detect larger deletions were LD forward 5′-TACGCAATGCCAAGAAGTCA; LD reverse 5′-GAGGATGTTGGGAAGCTTTG. A founder was selected and bred with wild-type to obtain heterozygous animals, and sibling mating of heterozygotes resulted in homozygous SD-$CFTR^{tm1sage}$ rats (termed $CFTR^{-/-}$).

Characterization of the Model

Animals. All animal experiments at UAB were conducted in accordance with UAB IACUC approved protocols. Male and female Sprague-Dawley $CFTR^{+/-}$ rats were paired and housed in HEPA filtered ventilated cages with a 12 hour light/dark cycle and provided sterilized food and water *ad libitum*. Litters remained with lactating dams until weaning. Heterozygous rats were separated from wild-type and $CFTR^{-/-}$ littermates. Heterozygous animals exhibited growth and survival rates similar to wild-type, did not develop intestinal obstruction, and presented with normal dentition and complete male reproductive organs. In preliminary studies, CFTR heterozygotes also exhibited similar bioelectric and other characteristics to wild-type. In order to preclude any subtle confounding variables, CFTR+/− carriers were excluded from data analysis shown in this manuscript. Wild-type and $CFTR^{-/-}$ animals were provided water and standard rodent chow (pellet and ground) with a supplemental diet of DietGel 76A (Clear H_2O). A subset of wild-type and $CFTR^{-/-}$ pups were also provided 1× GoLytely (Braintree Laboratories, Inc) at weaning as a means to reduce gastrointestinal complications.

PCR genotyping. DNA analysis of litters was performed by extracting tail snip genomic DNA prepared in 500 μL lysis buffer (200 mM NaCl, 100 mM Tris-HCl, 5 mM EDTA, 0.25% Tween-20) with 1 mg Proteinase K (Sigma P6556) overnight at room temperature, followed by 60°C incubation to complete tissue lysis. DNA was obtained by standard techniques with 2-propanol, 70% ethanol, and DNA stored TE buffer (10 mM Tris-HCl, 1 mM EDTA) at −20°C. For PCR, 1 µL of DNA was mixed with 8 µL H_2O, 10 µL JumpStart Taq ReadyMix (Sigma P2893), and 0.5 µL each primer (forward 5′-GCAGCTCACTGGTC-GATCTT, reverse 5′-GACACTATATTCACAAGGGAGAG). PCR conditions were 95°C for 5 minutes, followed by 35 cycles of 95°C for 30 seconds, 60°C for 30 seconds, and 68°C for 40 seconds, with a fixed cycle at 68°C for 5 minutes. This PCR resulted in amplification of a 172-bp DNA fragment for the wild-type *Cftr* allele and a 156-bp DNA fragment (16-bp deleted) for mutant *Cftr*. PCR products were resolved on a 3.5% agarose gel.

Western blotting. Lung tissue was homogenized in TBS on ice followed by lysis in RIPA buffer (ThermoScientific, Rockford, Il) with Halt protease inhibitor cocktail (ThermoScientific). Protein was quantitated using the BCA assay (ThermoScientific), samples mixed with 4× sample buffer, and incubated at 37°C for 10 minutes. Equal amounts of protein (20 µg) were loaded into each lane, resolved by SDS-PAGE, and blotted onto PVDF membranes. Wild-type Sprague-Dawley rat lung extract (Sc-2396, Santa Cruz Biotechnology, Inc, Dallas, Tx) was used as an additional positive control for CFTR detection. Blocking was with 1% rabbit serum followed by incubation with goat anti-CFTR primary antibody (1:200 Sc-8909) overnight at 4°C, and subsequent rabbit anti-goat HRP conjugated secondary antibody (1:5000 Sc-2768) for 1 hour at room temperature. Labeled proteins were detected using SuperSignal West Femto ECL kit (ThermoScientific).

Histology. Left lung lobes were cannulated and inflation fixed with 1% paraformaldehyde at 30 cm pressure for 30–60 minutes, followed by storage in 10% buffered formalin. Nasal tissue was collected, mandible removed, and nasal passages flushed retrograde with 10% buffered formalin followed by immersion in formalin until processed [16]. Nasal samples were decalcified for 4–5 days in Immunocal (Decal Chemical Corporation, Tallman, NY) solution, and rinsed thoroughly. The nasal cavity was sectioned into four regions at specific anatomic sites as described previously [17,18]. All other tissues were harvested, immersion fixed in 10% buffered formalin or 70% ethanol/formalin and stored at 4°C until processed. Tissues were embedded in paraffin, sectioned, and stained with hematoxylin and eosin (H&E) for evaluation by a board certified veterinary pathologist. Nasal, tracheal, lung, and intestinal tissues were stained with alcian blue periodic acid Schiff (AB-PAS) for identification of mucosubstances. Sections were imaged on an Olympus BX-41 microscope with a digital Q-color 5 camera (Olympus) using Q Capture imaging software (Q Imaging, Surrey, Canada) [19].

Quantitation of intracellular mucus in the nasal septa. The amount of stored mucosubstance in upper respiratory epithelium was estimated by quantifying the area of AB-PAS positive tissue per unit basement membrane. Septa from proximal nasal samples were evaluated at 20×, providing 4–6 fields (entire length of septa) per animal. Images were imported into ImageJ (NIH) and colors separated using the RGB stack feature. Using a green channel, areas of interest were outlined using the polygon tool and maximum threshold set for each image to include all stained intracellular mucus.

Morphometric analysis of tracheal tissue. Tracheas were imaged at 4× and 20× magnification followed by analysis with ImageJ (NIH) using protocols modified from Meyerholz *et al.* [20]. For each animal, three tracheal sections were studied (with a minimum distance of 15 µm between sections) using the following parameters. Lumenal circumference was determined by measuring the apical surface of the epithelium. Cartilage area was quantified by outlining cartilaginous tissue in the tracheal ring, measuring the area, and summing area for all cartilage in each image. Maximal cartilage thickness was evaluated by determining the perpendicular distance between outer boundaries of cartilage rings, with epithelial thickness represented by the distance between the basement membrane (on the serosal surface) and the apical membrane lumenally. Submucosal gland area was determined by circling and measuring both serous and mucus components of the gland structures. Submucosal gland intracellular mucus was assessed by outlining the entire submucosal gland area (same protocol as for quantitation of intracellular mucus in the nasal septa), in order to define the extent of intracellular mucosubstance. The percent of intracellular mucus was determined as the ratio of intracellular mucus/total submucosal gland area.

Bioelectric Measurements

Nasal potential difference. Rats were anesthetized with ketamine (200 mg/kg), acepromazine (0.6 mg/kg), and xylazine (30 mg/kg) by intraperitoneal injection. Potential difference was measured using AgCl electrode and electronic data capture (AD Instruments) as previously described for mouse and human [21,22]. Nasal cavities were perfused sequentially with 1) Ringer solution containing 140 mM NaCl, 5 mM KCl, 1 mM $MgCl_2$, 2 mM $CaCl_2$, 10 mM HEPES, and 100 µM amiloride (pH 7.3); 2) Cl^-free Ringer solution (6 mM Cl^-, pH 7.3) with amiloride; and 3) Cl^-free Ringer solution, amiloride, and forskolin (20 µM). Each condition was studied for 5 to 10 minutes until a stable signal was achieved. Traces were interpreted in a blinded fashion.

Tracheal short-circuit current (I_{SC}). Tracheas were excised, sectioned into 3–4 segments, and opened longitudinally along the dorsal surface. Segments were mounted as flat sheets in modified Ussing chambers (area ~0.031 cm^2) maintained at 37°C and bubbled vigorously with 95% O_2:5% CO_2.

I_{SC} measurements were performed under voltage clamp conductions using MC8 equipment and P2300 Ussing chambers (Physiologic Instruments, San Diego, CA). Tissue segments were equilibrated for 10 minutes in regular Ringer solution that contained (in mM) 120 NaCl, 25 $NaHCO_3$, 3.33 KH_2PO_4, 0.83 K_2HPO_4, 1.2 $CaCl_2$, 1.2 $MgCl_2$, and 10 mannitol to establish a baseline and then tested by one of the following experimental protocols:

1. Administration of amiloride (100 µM) to inhibit the epithelial sodium channel (ENaC), followed by sequential addition of forskolin (10 µM) to activate cAMP-dependent CFTR current, ATP (10 µM) to activate Ca^{2+}- activated chloride channel (CaCC) transport, and bumetanide (100 µM) to block transepithelial Cl^- transport.
2. Administration of $CFTR_{Inh}$-172 (10 µM) to block constitutively active CFTR dependent chloride current, followed by sequential addition of amiloride, ATP, and bumetanide as above.

Changes in I_{SC} attributable to ion transport agonists and inhibitors were calculated following achievement of a stable plateau for several minutes. ATP-sensitive I_{SC} was measured as the highest current value for each sample [21].

Ileal I_{SC} measurements. Tissue segments approximately 8 mm in length sectioned 5 cm above the cecum were stripped of the serosa (visceral peritoneum) and longitudinal/circular muscle layers of the intestinal wall, opened longitudinally along the mesenteric border, and incubated in TTX (Tetrodotoxin, 3.3×10^{-4} µM in PBS) for 10 min to block action potential dependent sodium channels. Segments were mounted as flat sheets onto sliders (area ~0.09 cm^2) and I_{SC} measured under voltage clamp conditions using MC8 equipment and P2300 Ussing chambers (Physiologic Instruments, San Diego, CA) as previously described [23]. Bath solutions were gently stirred and gassed with 95% O_2:5% CO_2.

Regular Ringer solution was utilized for monitoring I_{SC} as above. Low Cl^- Ringer contained (in mM) 1.2 NaCl, 25 $NaHCO_3$, 3.33 KH_2PO_4, 0.83 K_2HPO_4, 1.2 $CaCl_2$, 1.2 $MgCl_2$, 141 Na gluconate, and 10.8 mannitol. Sliders with mounted ileum were equilibrated for 10 minutes in Ringer solution followed by 10 minutes of recording; mucosal side chambers were changed to 1:1 regular Ringer:low Cl^- Ringer. Indomethacin (10 µm) was added to both chambers to block ion transport associated with phospholipase C or A2 activity induced by seromuscular stripping. After 30 minutes of incubation, forskolin (10 µm) and IBMX (3-Isobutyl-1-methylxanthine, 100 µm) were added to both chambers, followed by glybenclamide (200 µM) to block forskolin-activated CFTR short-circuit current.

In all experiments, fully stimulated current was obtained within 3 minutes of forskolin addition. Pulse during voltage clamp measurements was imposed every second after forskolin/IBMX stimulation, and every 20 seconds following other drug treatments.

Micro Optical Coherence Tomography (µOCT)

Tissue preparation. Tracheal tissue was excised, immediately placed on Gelfoam soaked in DMEM/F12 1: 1 media, and incubated under physiologic conditions (37°C, 5% CO_2, and 100% humidity) using an environmentally controlled chamber (Pathology Devices, Westminster, MD). Tracheas were equilibrated for 30 minutes before analysis.

Image acquisition. Measurements of functional microanatomic parameters in tracheal tissue, including measurement of (i) airway surface liquid (ASL) depth, the aqueous layer lining the airway epithelium, (ii) periciliary liquid (PCL) depth, the thin aqueous gel surrounding the cilia, (iii) ciliary beat frequency (CBF), and (iv) velocity of mucociliary transport (MCT) were performed using Micro-Optical Coherence Tomography (µOCT), a high-speed, high-resolution microscopic reflectance imaging modality [24]. µOCT methods for investigation of airway epithelia and quantitative image analysis have been previously described [24,25]. In brief, the µOCT instrument provides cross sectional images of epithelium with a transverse and axial resolutions of approximately 2 µm and 1 µm, respectively. This resolution is sufficient to directly visualize and quantify parameters including ASL depth, PCL depth, CBF, and MCT rate without using exogenous dyes or particles. Acquisition speed is 20,480 Hz line rate, resulting in 40 frames per second at 512 lines per frame.

Image analysis. Quantitative analysis of ASL and PCL depths were characterized directly by geometric measurement of the respective layers, and images over several frames captured the length of fully extended cilia. CBF was investigated by Fourier analysis of the reflectance due to beating cilia. MCT rate was determined using time elapsed and distance traveled of native particulates in the mucus over multiple frames. Images were acquired at randomly chosen locations on the mucosal surface with the optical beam scanned along the longitudinal axis of the trachea.

Bronchoalveolar lavage fluid cell differentials. Tracheas were cannulated and lungs lavaged with 2.0 mL PBS (7.4 pH). Cells were collected by instilling 2.0 mL phosphate buffered saline (pH 7.2) and the lavage centrifuged onto slides (Cytospin). Slides were stained using Hema 3 stain kit (Fisher Scientific, Kalamazoo, MI) [26]. A minimum of 300 cells were counted per animal.

Complete Blood Counts (CBC) and serum chemistry. Blood (200–500 µL) was collected from the brachial artery into EDTA tubes and processed for CBC by ANATECH Diagnostics (Smyrna, GA). For serum chemistry, whole blood (300–500 µL) was processed in serum separator tubes and allowed to clot at room temperature for 1 hour. Supernatant was obtained by centrifugation at 10,000×*g* for 10 minutes, with serum placed in a fresh tube and frozen at −80°C. Samples were thawed and analyzed on an Abaxis VetScan using a Comprehensive Diagnostic Profile rotor (500–1038, Union City, CA).

Statistical analysis. Data are expressed as mean ± SEM or as individual data points. Statistical significance was determined using unpaired, two-tailed Student's t-test or one-way ANOVA using Prism (GraphPad, LaJolla, CA). For survival analysis, Kaplan-Meier survival curves were plotted and statistical significance determined using the logrank test for trend. P values ≤0.05 were considered significant.

Results

Microinjection and Founder Identification

A pair of ZFNs was confirmed to cleave the target site within exon 3 of *Cftr*, shown in Figure 1A. Following microinjection and embryo transfer, 44 pups were born to six recipients, 18 of which carried at least one mutant allele. The mutations ranged from 9 bp to hundreds of base pairs in length. Seven founders carried the same 9 bp deletion (Figure 1B), presumably due to microhomology within the target site, as discussed previously [15]. One founder was mosaic, harboring wild type *Cftr* allele, an allele with a 16 bp deletion and an allele with a 479 bp deletion. Larger deletions were observed to span the junction of exon 3/intron 3. Heterozygous rats with the 16 bp deletion (a frameshift in the reading frame leading to premature termination in exon 4) (Figure 1C), were used to establish a breeding colony.

Litter Demographics

Four breeding pairs of $CFTR^{+/-}$ rats gave rise to 332 pups from 30 litters with an average litter size of 11 pups. Litters were analyzed by PCR (Figure 2B) and found to have a genotype distribution of 27.1% wild-type, 49.4% heterozygous, and 23.5% $CFTR^{-/-}$, a result similar to the expected 1:2: 1 inheritance pattern. Western blot of whole lung homogenates from wild-type and $CFTR^{-/-}$ animals confirmed that the 16 bp deletion resulted

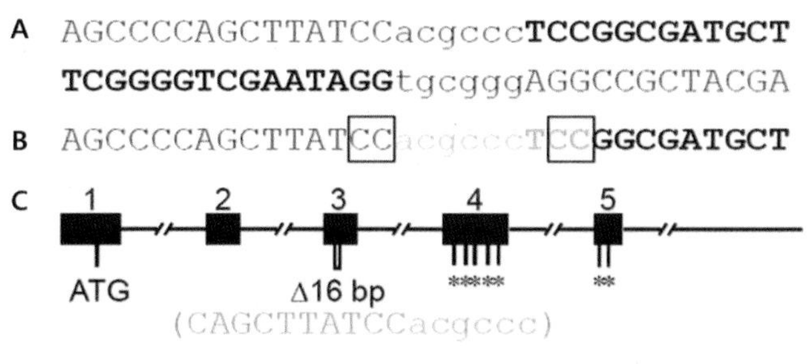

Figure 1. Targeting in exon 3 of *Cftr*. (A) ZFN recognition site sequence. The two ZFN binding sites are in bold uppercase. Cleavage site is in lower case. (B) Nine base pair deletion recovered in multiple founders. The deleted sequence is shown in gray. Microhomology that may have favored this deletion is marked in boxes. (C)Schematic of the gene structure of the first 5 exons of rat *Cftr*. Exons are shown by filled rectangles with exon number above. ATG, position of the translational start codon; Δ16 bp marks the position of 16 bp deletion, with nucleotide sequence below). *indicates premature stop mutations introduced by the 16 bp deletion in exon 3.

in loss of CFTR protein expression (Figure 2C and Figure S3). At birth, body weight and overall body size were similar between wild-type and CFTR$^{-/-}$ animals; however, begining in the second week following birth, CFTR$^{-/-}$ rats gained weight more slowly than wild-type littermates (Figure 2A, 2D). Survival of CFTR$^{-/-}$ rats was similar to wild-type until weaning, but was greatly reduced by 6 weeks (30% vs 99%, $p \leq 0.05$; Figure 2E). Mortality was associated with weight loss secondary to gastrointestinal complications (including obstruction, see also below). Addition of GoLytely to water resulted in significantly improved survival rates of CFTR$^{-/-}$ animals at 6 weeks of age (30% vs 64%, $p \leq 0.05$; Figure 2E).

Ileal Tissue

CFTR$^{-/-}$ rats developed intestinal obstruction after weaning and exhibited significant weight loss and decreased survival. Histological evaluation of small intestine demonstrated epithelial cell sloughing and crypts dilated with mucus, as well as a qualitative increase in bacterial load (Figure 3A). Ileal tissue was evaluated for CFTR short-circuit current phenotype by Ussing chamber measurements. Wild-type ileal tissue exhibited a strong forskolin-stimulated current (150±49 μA/cm^2), which was absent in CF rats (8±6 μA/cm^2, $p<0.0001$; Figures 3B, C).

Stored Mucosubstances in Airway Epithelium of the Proximal Septa

The respiratory epithelium of the nasal septum, immediately posterior to the upper incisors, was evaluated and labeled for intracellularly stored mucosubstance. Both wild-type and CFTR$^{-/-}$ animals had normally developed epithelium consisting of a pseudostratified columnar epithelium comprised of both goblet and ciliated epithelial cells. CFTR$^{-/-}$ animals had elevated levels of intracellular mucus that encompassed a significant portion of the airway epithelial cytosol (Figure 4A, Table 1), resulting in cells from CF animals appearing thicker and swollen ("stuffed") compared to wild-type.

Nasal Potential Difference Measurements

To characterize electrophysiology of the upper airway, transepithelial potential difference was monitored in response to a series of pharmacologic ion channel regulators. CFTR$^{-/-}$ rats had no evidence of Cl^- dependent secretion upon stimulation of CFTR mediated Cl^- transport by Cl^- free Ringer with forskolin (3.8±0.6 mV), whereas changes were robust in wild-type littermates (−9.3±2.7 mV, $p \leq 0.01$; Figure 4B, C). There were no differences between CF and non-CF following perfusion with amiloride. These measurements indicate a bioelectric phenotype consistent with absence of CFTR in the nasal airways, but without concomitant increase in amiloride sensitive voltage, the conventional ion transport pathway associated with sodium reabsorption.

Morphometric Analysis of Tracheal Rings

Tracheal morphology in young CF animals appeared grossly similar between wild-type and CFTR$^{-/-}$ genotypes (Figure 5); however, morphometric analysis revealed important differences attributable to absent CFTR (Table 1). While lumenal circumference was not significantly different between wild-type and CFTR$^{-/-}$ rats at 3–6 weeks after birth, cartilage area was significantly diminished in CF animals. CF rats also exhibited reduced tracheal gland area (~50% compared to wild-type) even after normalization for tracheal lumen circumference. Additionally, at all time points during the 3–6 week growth period, alcian blue positive (AB+) staining of submucosal glandular cells was decreased in CF versus wild-type rats, suggesting that glandular maturation in the CF animals was delayed in comparison to age-matched controls.

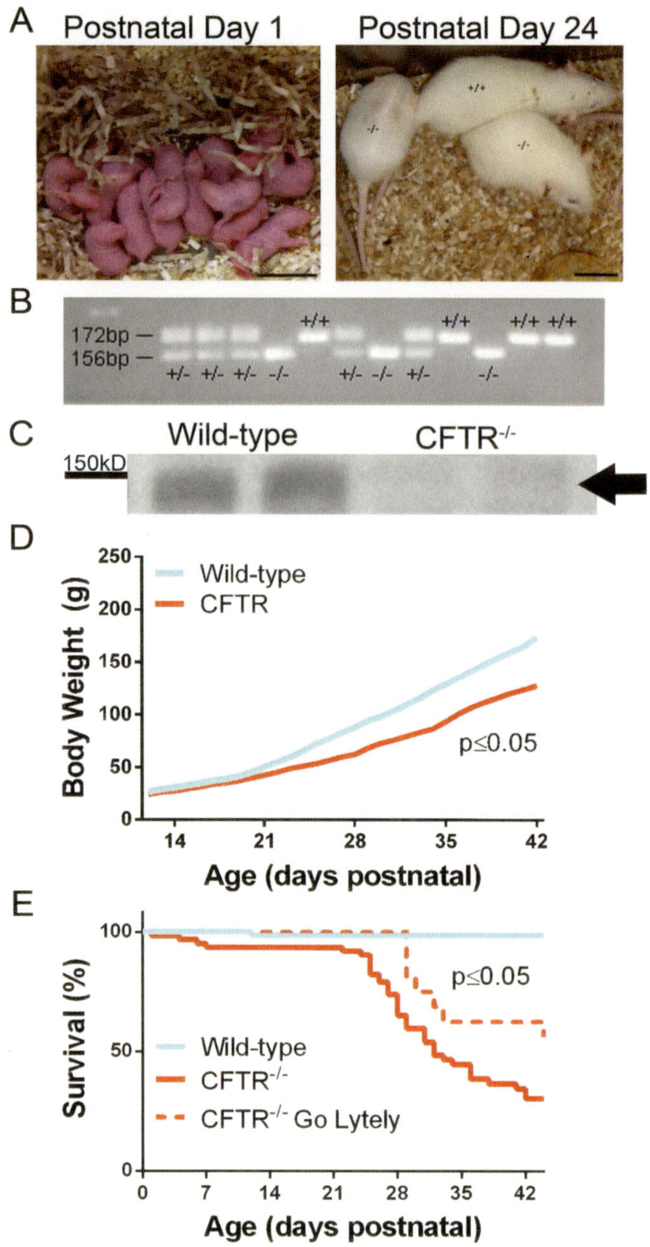

Figure 2. Generation of CFTR$^{-/-}$ rats. (A) Animals at days 1 and 24 postnatal. (B) Results of PCR genotyping from a representative litter. (C) Western blot indicating expression of CFTR in wild-type rats and absence of CFTR protein from lungs of CFTR$^{-/-}$ animals. Arrow - CFTR. (D) Body weight values (mean ± SD) from wild-type and CFTR$^{-/-}$ rats from 12 to 44 days postnatal. (E) Survival curve for CFTR$^{-/-}$ rats from postnatal day 1 to 44 ($p<0.05$ for all groups, n = 12–67 animals/group).

Tracheal I_{SC} Measurements

Baseline I_{SC} of freshly excised trachea was significantly lower in CFTR$^{-/-}$ animals compared to wild-type (Figure 5B), a finding predominantly attributable to $CFTR_{Inh}$-172 sensitive current. To determine the contribution of Na^+ transport to basal currents,

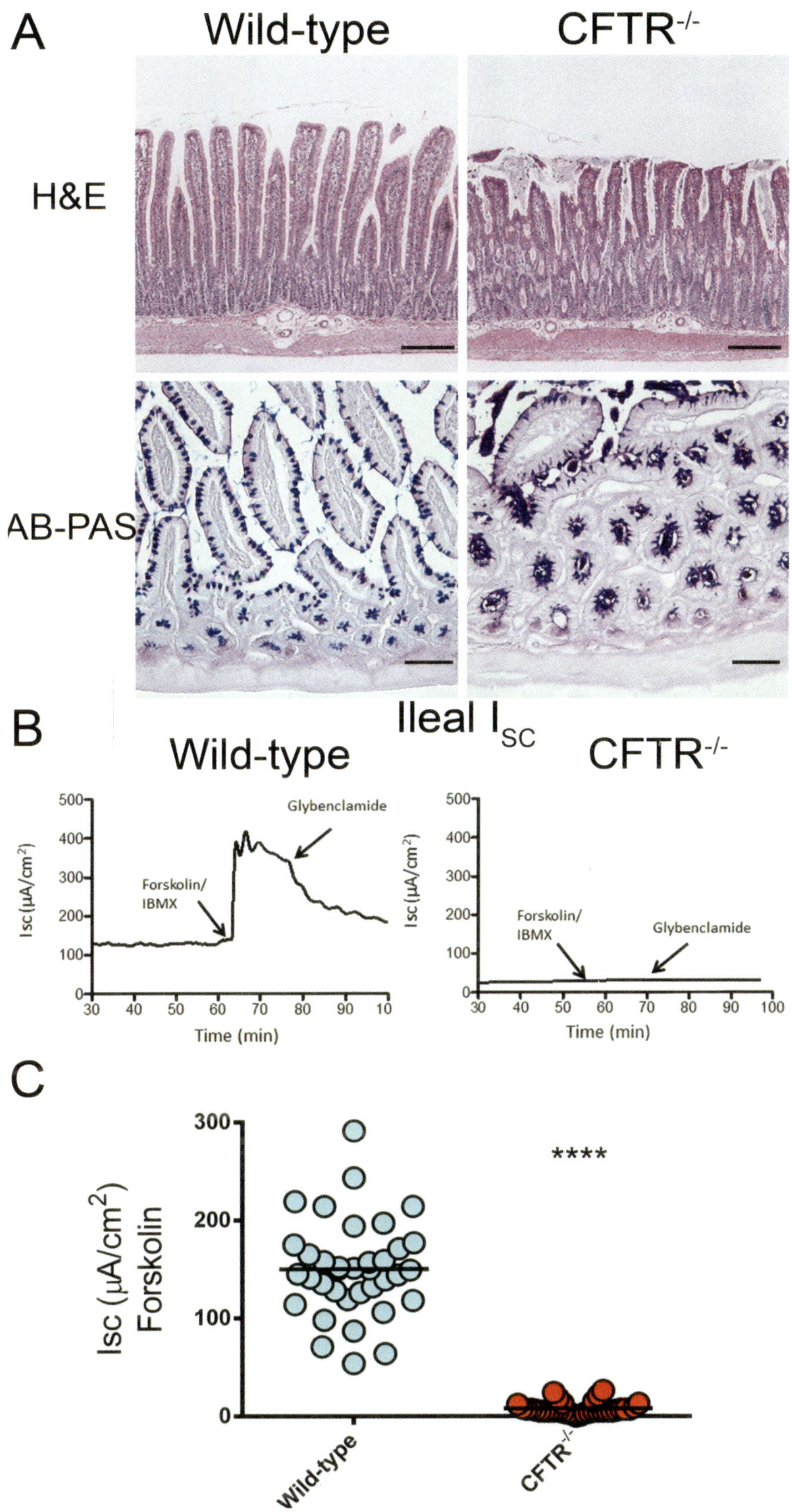

Figure 3. Histology and short-circuit current measurements from small intestines of wild-type and CFTR$^{-/-}$ rats. H&E (bar = 200 µm) and AB-PAS (bar = 100 µm) stained sections of the small intestines from wild-type and CFTR$^{-/-}$ rats. (n = 3–5 animals/group) (B) I_{SC} tracings from wild-type and CFTR$^{-/-}$ rat ileum. (C) Summary of forskolin stimulated current measurements from ileal sections. (n = 5 animals/group) ****$p \leq 0.0001$.

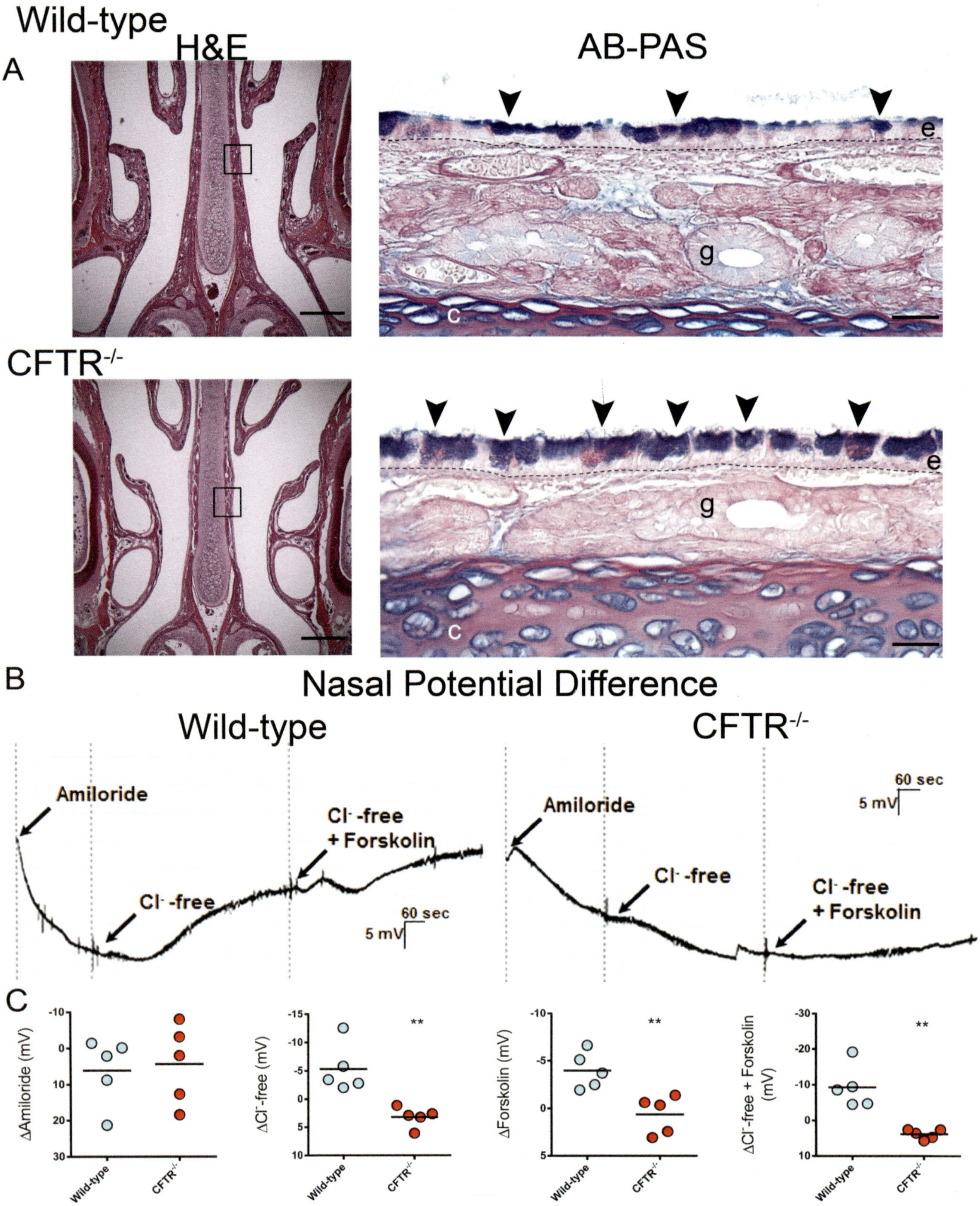

Figure 4. Proximal nasal histology and nasal potential difference measurements. (A) Low power magnification (4×) H&E stained sections from the proximal nasal passages bar = 500 μm. 20× images of ABPAS stained nasal septa from boxed areas bar = 25 μm. Arrowheads, cells swollen with intracellular mucus; e, respiratory epithelium; g, submucosal gland; dashed line (–), basement membrane (n = 4 animals/group) (B) NPD tracings from wild-type and CFTR$^{-/-}$ rats. (C) Summary data from NPD measurements for Δamiloride, ΔCl$^-$-free Ringers, Δforksolin, and ΔCl$^{-/-}$free Ringers+ forskolin. (n = 5 animals/group) **p≤0.01.

Table 1. Morphometric analysis of respiratory tissue from 3–6 week old wild-type and CFTR$^{-/-}$ rats.

	Wild-type	CFTR$^{-/-}$
Nasal Septa		
Intracellular mucus/basement membrane (μm^2/μm)	3.5±0.9	7.5±0.9*
Trachea		
Lumen circumference (mm)	5.5±0.3	5.1±0.2
Cartilage area (mm^2)	0.63±0.06	0.42±0.03**
Cartilage area/lumenal circumference (mm^2/mm)	0.11±0.01	0.08±0.01*
Maximum cartilage thickness (mm)	0.20±0.01	0.17±0.01
Epithelial thickness (μm)	11.5±0.7	9.9±1.09
Submucosal gland area (mm^2)	0.057±0.005	0.032±0.006*
Submucosal gland area/lumenal circumference (mm^2/mm)	0.016±0.001	0.006±0.001*
Submucosal gland intracellular mucus (μm^2)	7409±1481	2877±752*
% intracellular mucus	12±2	8.4±2

Values shown as mean ± SEM (n = 4–6 animals/group).
*p≤0.05, **p≤0.001 (Student's t-test).

amiloride was added apically (Figure 5B, left panel). The reduction in I_{SC} was similar for both wild-type and CFTR$^{-/-}$ rats (49±11 μA/cm^2 and 64±21 μA/cm^2, respectively; Figure 5C) indicating comparable levels of sodium transport irrespective of CFTR expression (Figure 5B, left panel; a finding similar to the nasal ion transport phenotype, Figure 4). Subsequent addition of forskolin did not confer substantial I_{SC} activation in either group, suggesting CFTR may be constitutively active in wild-type sections, diminishing the additional activation otherwise expected from forskolin. In contrast, ATP stimulated current was much greater for CFTR$^{-/-}$ animals (although maximal Cl^- currents for both genotypes were comparable and inhibited by addition of bumetanide), suggesting a compensatory increase of ATP-dependent Cl^- transport in the absence of functional CFTR, as also seen in humans [27]. To confirm that CFTR was constitutively active in wild-type animals, an alternative protocol was developed to test this interpretation (Figure 5B, right panel). Using the modified assay, wild-type rats demonstrated a baseline current of 547±102 μA, while current was far less (61±17 μA) in CFTR$^{-/-}$ animals. Addition of CFTR$_{Inh}$-172 reduced the current in wild-type by 304±63 μA, demonstrating high level basal CFTR activity, whereas CFTR$_{Inh}$-172 had minimal effect on constitutive current in CFTR$^{-/-}$ rats (9±7 μA, p≤0.001). ATP sensitive currents were strongly inhibited by the addition of bumetanide.

Measurement of Functional Airway Microanatomy

We used μOCT to visualize and quantify the functional microanatomy of the airway surface (Figure 6). Excised tracheas from wild-type animals had significantly greater ASL depth compared to CFTR$^{-/-}$ rats (p≤0.05; Figure 6). In addition, PCL thickness was reduced in CFTR$^{-/-}$ animals (p≤0.05). Ciliary beat frequency and mucociliary transport were not different between wild-type and CFTR$^{-/-}$ groups.

CFTR$^{-/-}$ Male Rats Exhibit Bilateral Absence of the Vas Deferens

Evaluation of gross genitourinary anatomy revealed absence of the vas deferens in 6 week old CFTR$^{-/-}$ male rats (Figure 7). When sections from 6 month old males were evaluated histologically, only connective tissue and vasculature were observed with no evidence of the vas identified (data not shown).

CF rats have Abnormal Dentition

Incisors of wild-type rats presented with yellow-brown enamel while CFTR$^{-/-}$ rats exhibited white incisors (Figure 8A). Wild-type rats maintained normally filed teeth while CF animals exhibited grossly malformed dentition, possibly due to defective physiological trimming. Without intervention, incisors of CF rats developed dental malformations, including curvature of the incisors and penetration of the hard palate (Figure 8B).

Lung and Major Exocrine Tissues from CFTR$^{-/-}$ Rats are without Pathology or Inflammatory Cell Infiltrates During Early Life

Pulmonary sections from wild-type and CFTR$^{-/-}$ rats appear to develop normally from days 22 to 42 (Figure S1). In addition, BAL profiles were not different between genotypic groups, indicating the absence of overt pulmonary inflammation. Pancreas and liver from young animals were also histologically normal (Figure S2).

Hematology and Serum Chemistry

Hypoalbuminemia, decreased total protein, and increased blood urea nitrogen (Table S1) were observed in CFTR$^{-/-}$ rats. Because many animals experienced substantial weight loss prior to euthanasia, these findings may be attributable in part to malnourishment and poor hydration. Serum electrolytes (Ca^{2+}, Na^+, K^+) were not different between wild-type and CFTR$^{-/-}$ groups (Table S1). A trend towards increased blood glucose levels was observed in CF animals with very high values in a subset (data not shown) which is currently under investigation.

Red blood cells, hemoglobin, and hematocrit were all within normal range for young animals. Total white blood cell counts were not different between groups, although the differential was influenced by genotype (Wild-type: 21±4% neutrophils and 76±4% circulating lymphocytes, CFTR$^{-/-}$ animals: 52±5% neutrophils and 44±6% circulating lymphocytes), likely attributable to gastrointestinal or other stress-related complications observed in CFTR$^{-/-}$ animals.

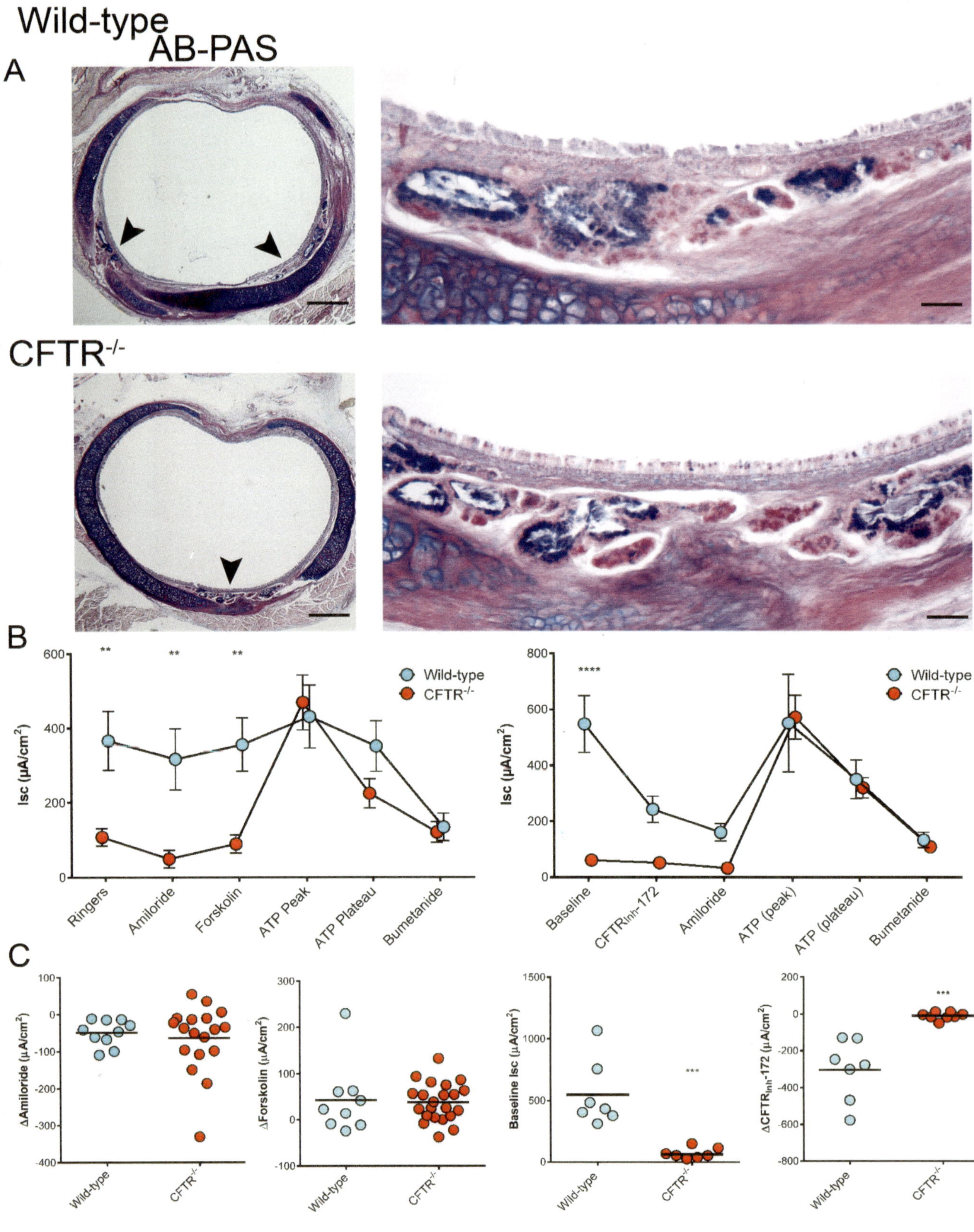

Figure 5. Tracheal histology and short circuit current measurements. (A) AB-PAS stained tracheal sections from 6 week old rats. Submucosal glandular tissue indicated by arrowheads. Low magnification bar = 500 μm, high magnification bar = 50 μm (B & C) Summary data from Ussing chamber short circuit current measurements. Panels on right depict a modified protocol designed to specifically detect baseline (constitutive) CFTR function. (n = 3–6 animals/group) $^{**}p \leq 0.01$, $^{***}p \leq 0.001$, $^{****}p \leq 0.0001$.

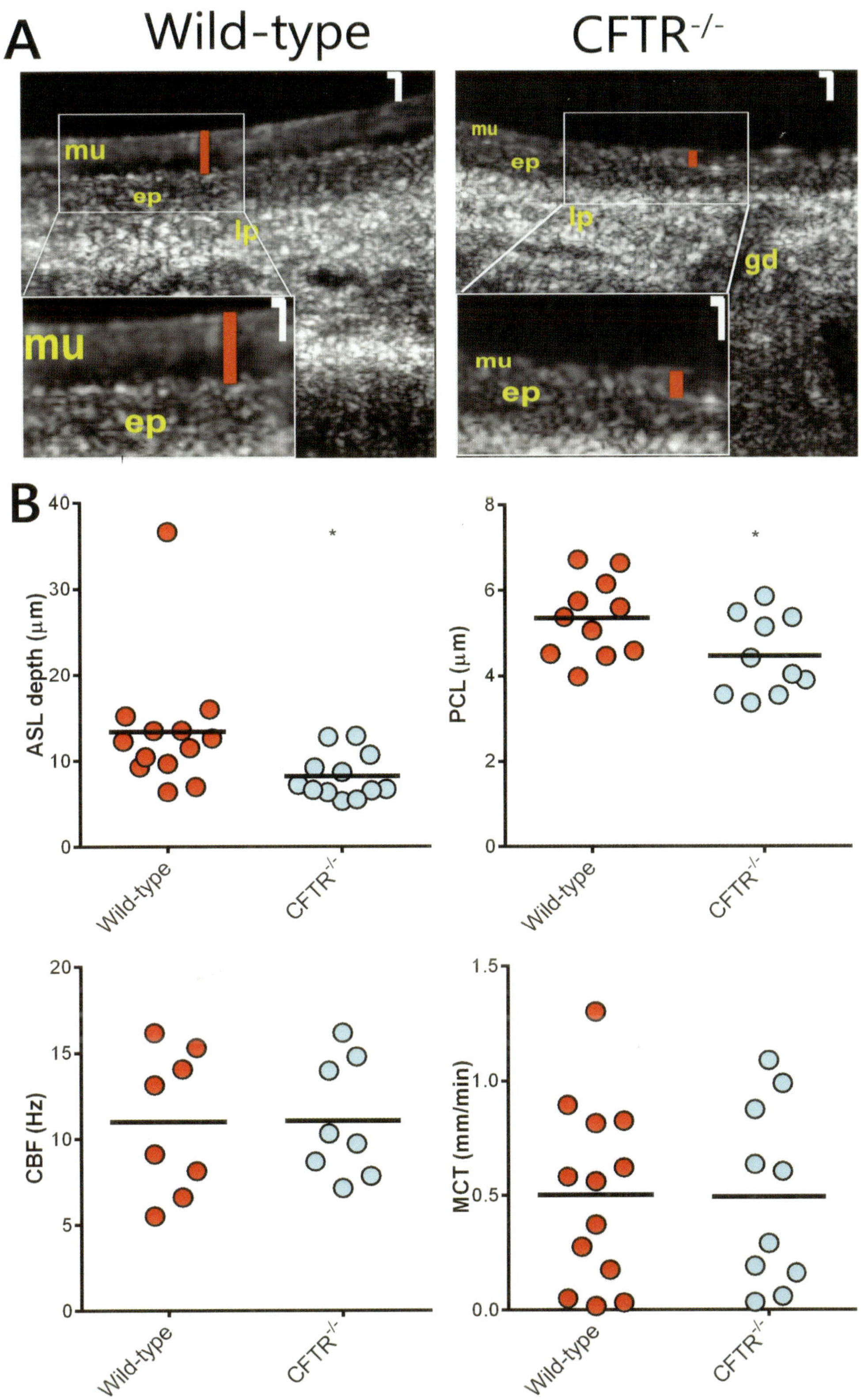

Figure 6. Functional anatomy of rat trachea. (A) Representative time-averaged μOCT images of wild-type and CFTR$^{-/-}$ tracheas. Higher magnification insets (bottom left corner) show differences in ASL height between wild-type and CFTR$^{-/-}$ animals. White magnification bar = 10 μm. Red bars indicate ASL height. Mucus layer (mu), epithelium (ep), lamina propria (lp), and gland duct (gd) are also visualized. (B) Summary data for airway surface liquid depth (ASL), periciliary liquid depth (PCL), ciliary beat frequency (CBF), and mucociliary transport (MCT). (n = 8–13 animals/group) *$p \leq 0.05$.

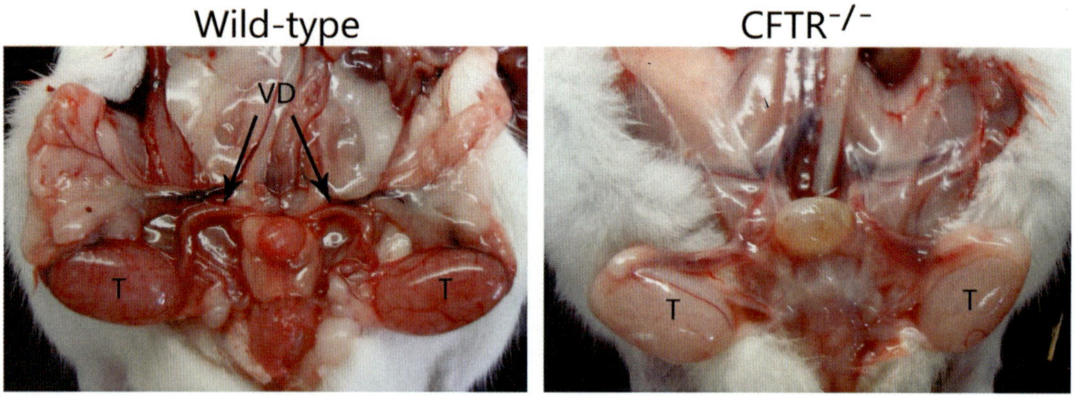

Figure 7. Male CFTR$^{-/-}$ rats have bilateral absence of the vas deferens by 6 weeks of age. Wild-type males (left) have an intact reproductive tract. CFTR$^{-/-}$ males (right) develop other reproductive organs, but exhibit absent vas at 6 weeks. T, testis; VD, vas deferens. (n = 3 animals/group).

Discussion

We present here a novel cystic fibrosis rat with a number of phenotypic characteristics that resemble the human disease. The CF rat furnishes a new opportunity to investigate (i) developmental processes that affect disease progression and severity, (ii) the impact of CFTR and other ion channels with regard to ASL depth in CF airways, (iii) contributions of ASL and PCL abnormalities to manifestations of CF respiratory pathology, and (iv) the role of CFTR in mucus synthesis and release.

Developmental defects attributable to absent CFTR have received considerable recent attention, including abnormal airway remodeling and tracheal formation [20], deficient levels of growth hormone [28], absent vas deferens [7,29], and problems with enamel deposition in teeth [30–33]. Similar to CF pig [20] and human subjects [20,34], we observed reduced tracheal circumference and a loss of submucosal gland area in the CF rat model (Figure 2), supporting the notion that CFTR may play a critical role during normal lung development [20]. The CF rat offers an ideal opportunity to monitor phenotypes such as these more longitudinally than has been practical in the past (e.g. from intrauterine tissue formation to adulthood).

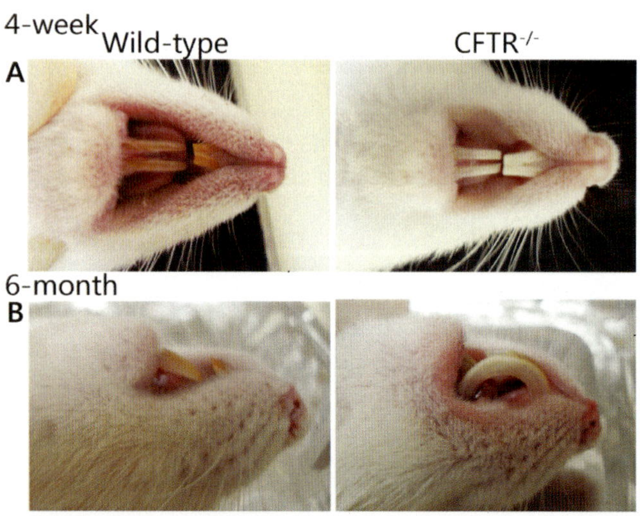

Figure 8. CF rats have abnormal dentition. (A) Wild-type rats (left) have yellowish-brown enamel while CFTR$^{-/-}$ rats (right) exhibit bright white incisors. (B) Incisors from CF rats exhibit uncontrolled growth and penetrate the hard palate. (n = 3 animals/group).

The rat model will also serve as a valuable resource for investigating developmental events that lead to abnormalities of the male reproductive tract. The majority (~99%) of men with CF are sterile due to degeneration or complete absence of the vas deferens [35]. In both the CF pig and ferret, the vas deferens is poorly formed or absent at birth [7,29]. The most commonly utilized CF animal model, the mouse, does not exhibit this feature. CF rats have lost the vas deferens by 6 weeks of age. The role of chloride secretion versus intracellular or other CFTR functions with regard to vas deferens involution are not well understood, but can be more readily characterized *in vitro* and *in vivo* using this new animal model. The rat may also facilitate experiments intended to determine the extent to which vas tissue destruction can be ameliorated by early (e.g. prenatal) therapeutic intervention.

Another area of increasing interest is the development of dental complications in CF subjects. Similar to observations in mice [33], CFTR$^{-/-}$ rats exhibit white incisors compared to yellow dentition of wild-type littermates (Figure 8A). Moreover, by three months of age CF rats demonstrate grossly malformed upper and lower incisors, characterized by curved dentition and penetration of the hard palate (Figure 8B). Additional studies are in progress to determine whether this phenotype is the result of (i) dysregulated growth and/or (ii) reduced wearing of the teeth, and the extent to which hypomineralization or other defects in enamel contribute to the findings [30,31,33,36]. Human data indicate that many CF patients have diminished mineralization of enamel [37–40] which may predispose to development of caries. The rat represents an ideal means of further investigating this feature of clinical CF.

The relationship of ASL depth to pathogenesis of cystic fibrosis lung disease has engendered considerable controversy. Previous studies have concluded that depleted ASL is primarily responsible for cystic fibrosis pulmonary damage, and associated with defects in ciliary extension [41]. The present results in CFTR$^{-/-}$ animals indicate ASL depletion in lower airways (Figure 6) that is qualitatively and quantitatively very similar to that noted in human subjects [42], but without evidence of overt respiratory pathology (Figure S1). Our findings establish that defective ASL hydration can occur for several weeks without resulting in manifestations of a CF pulmonary phenotype. While spontaneous lung disease is absent in very young CF rats, it is important to note that the animals described here have been housed in HEPA

Table 2. Summary of phenotypes across numerous CF species.

	Human	Mouse	Pig	Ferret	Rat
Increased Stored Nasal Mucus	NR	Yes [52]	Yes [51]	NR	Yes
Airway Surface Hydration	NR	Depleted [55]	Not Depleted [47]	NR	Depleted
Sodium Hyperabsorption	Yes [41,56], No [57]	Yes [58], No [59]	No [47]	No [48]	No
Hypoplastic Tracheal Submucosal Glands	Inconclusive [20,34]	NR	Hypoplastic at birth [20]	NR	Hypoplastic 21–42 DPN
Intestinal Obstruction	13–17% MI, 7–8% DIOS in childhood [60]	0–95% OB at weaning [4][a]	100% MI [61]	50–100% MI [7]	~70% OB between weaning and 42 DPN
Vas deferens	~99% CBAVD [35]	Normal	Degenerate or absent vas at birth [29]	Degenerate or absent vas at birth [7]	Vas absent before 42 DPN
Dentition	Abnormal [37–39]	Abnormal [33]	Abnormal [31]	NR	Abnormal

CBAVD – congenital bilateral absence of the vas deferens, DIOS – distal intestinal obstruction syndrome, DPN – Days postnatal, NR – Not reported, MI – meconium ileus, OB – Obstruction.
[a]Background strain and/or CFTR genotype dependent.

filtered ventilated cages. Future studies will determine whether older animals maintained under more natural housing conditions develop evidence of lower respiratory involvement. If such experiments fail to elicit a CF phenotype, the findings would indicate that defects in ASL and PCL hydration by themselves do not represent a proximate cause of CF pathology. The rat model will therefore furnish a valuable means to address unanswered questions regarding airway surface hydration and cystic fibrosis pathogenesis.

Decreased ASL depth has classically been attributed to Na^+ hyperabsorption as a consequence of absent CFTR [43–46]. Similar to what has recently been reported in CF pig [47] and ferret [48], the cystic fibrosis rat does not exhibit sodium hyperabsorption in either nasal or lower airways. Although amiloride-sensitive sodium transport is not significantly different between wild-type and $CFTR^{-/-}$ rats, ASL depth is markedly diminished (Figures 4 and 5). The abrogation of constitutively active CFTR fluid secretion may provide part of the explanation for ASL depletion in CF animals (as opposed normal levels of ASL observed in the CF porcine model) [47]. Our findings therefore suggest that CFTR (rather than ENaC) serves as the dominant regulator of ASL depth in the rat airway *in vivo*.

It has recently been argued that mucus in cystic fibrosis lungs is excessively viscous due to loss of CFTR dependent bicarbonate secretion, and that the newly formed mucus gel fails to properly expand [49]. We observed markedly increased mucus stores (i.e. cells appear 'stuffed' with mucins; Figure 4) in epithelial cells from the proximal nasal septa of CF compared to non-CF rats. Histological findings such as these are compatible with an intrinsic defect in mucus secretion/release [50]. CF pigs develop mucous cell hyperplasia [51] qualitatively similar to that observed in our young $CFTR^{-/-}$ animals, and CF mice have also been reported to exhibit a phenotype characterized by measurably increased numbers of mucous cells [52]. Based on findings shown in Figure 4 and Table 1, the rat model should be useful for investigating CFTR-dependent airway mucin synthesis, expansion, and release.

The generation of the first $CFTR^{-/-}$ rat using zinc finger nuclease technology suggests a clear path to other CF animal models with specific mutations relevant to therapeutic development, including animals that express F508del or CFTR premature truncations alleles. The advantages of a rat model for CF drug development include robust and multi-organ bioelectric and histological findings, ease of breeding, short gestation, manageable expense, availability of antibodies and other reagents for mechanistic studies, and standard use for pharmacokinetic and drug toxicity analysis.

In summary, the $CFTR^{-/-}$ rat exhibits many features of the CF phenotype found in human subjects and CF animal models (summarized in Table 2), including defects in airway mucus production (Figure 4), tracheal development (Table 1), airway surface and periciliary fluid depth (Figure 6), nasal mucus (Figure 4), dentition (Figure 8), and involution of the vas deferens (Figure 7). Bioelectric findings in rat are also informative and demonstrate significantly diminished periciliary fluid without evidence of ENaC hyperactivity. Moreover, unlike the CF ferret or pig, the $CFTR^{-/-}$ rat does not present with meconium ileus at birth. Only after weaning do large numbers of animals develop intestinal blockage, which appears similar to the distal intestinal obstruction syndrome observed in children and adults with cystic fibrosis [53]. Complications due to intestinal obstruction can be managed by use of dietary modification (Figure 2). The new CF rat model will provide a very useful resource for longitudinal studies of tissue development, electrophysiology, and other end-points relevant to disease mechanism in the future.

Supporting Information

Figure S1 Analysis of lung tissue from CF rats. (A) Lung histology of wild-type and $CFTR^{-/-}$ animals. Magnification bar = 200 μm (n = 7–11 animals/group) (B) Total cell counts and cell differential of BAL in wild-type and CF rats (n = 4 animals/group).

Figure S2 Histology of pancreas and liver from CF rats. H&E stained paraffin sections of (A) pancreas and (B) liver from 22–44 day old wild-type and $CFTR^{-/-}$ rats. Magnification bar = 100 μm (n = 3–5 animals/group).

Figure S3 Expanded western blot (see Figure 2). Western indicating absence of CFTR protein from lungs of $CFTR^{-/-}$ animals and expression of CFTR in wild-type samples. Arrow - rat CFTR (~150 kD as previously reported [54]); *indicates likely CFTR degradation product commonly observed in CFTR preparations. This experiment has been repeated three times in separate animals with similar results.

Table S1 CBC and serum chemistry for wild-type and CFTR−/− rats.

Acknowledgments

We thank the UAB Comparative Pathology and CMBD Core Laboratories for processing samples. We also thank the UAB Animal Resource Program staff, who have assisted with breeding and rat husbandry. The authors also thank Dr. Trenton Schoeb for his review and analysis of tissue sections.

Author Contributions

Conceived and designed the experiments: KLT SEB XC DMB SMR EJS MVF. Performed the experiments: KLT SEB JH JW LR AC DJ LPT JF MD MVF. Analyzed the data: KLT SEB KKC GT MD DMB SMR EJS MVF. Contributed reagents/materials/analysis tools: KKC GT. Wrote the paper: KLT SEB XC MD EJS MVF. Coordinated Collaboration: KG. Provided veterinary care and assisted with animal husbandry: JMC.

References

1. Grosse SD, Boyle CA, Botkin JR, Comeau AM, Kharrazi M, et al. (2004) Newborn screening for cystic fibrosis: evaluation of benefits and risks and recommendations for state newborn screening programs. MMWR Recomm Rep 53: 1–36.
2. Derichs N (2013) Targeting a genetic defect: cystic fibrosis transmembrane conductance regulator modulators in cystic fibrosis. Eur Respir Rev 22: 58–65.
3. Riordan JR, Rommens JM, Kerem B, Alon N, Rozmahel R, et al. (1989) Identification of the cystic fibrosis gene: cloning and characterization of complementary DNA. Science 245: 1066–1073.
4. Guilbault C, Saeed Z, Downey GP, Radzioch D (2007) Cystic fibrosis mouse models. Am J Respir Cell Mol Biol 36: 1–7.
5. Carvalho-Oliveira I, Scholte BJ, Penque D (2007) What have we learned from mouse models for cystic fibrosis? Expert Rev Mol Diagn 7: 407–417.
6. Rogers CS, Hao Y, Rokhlina T, Samuel M, Stoltz DA, et al. (2008) Production of CFTR-null and CFTR-DeltaF508 heterozygous pigs by adeno-associated virus-mediated gene targeting and somatic cell nuclear transfer. J Clin Invest 118: 1571–1577.
7. Sun X, Sui H, Fisher JT, Yan Z, Liu X, et al. (2010) Disease phenotype of a ferret CFTR-knockout model of cystic fibrosis. J Clin Invest 120: 3149–3160.
8. Pilewski JM, Frizzell RA (1999) Role of CFTR in airway disease. Physiol Rev 79: S215–255.
9. Smolich JJ, Stratford BF, Maloney JE, Ritchie BC (1978) New features in the development of the submucosal gland of the respiratory tract. J Anat 127: 223–238.
10. Mashimo T, Serikawa T (2009) Rat resources in biomedical research. Curr Pharm Biotechnol 10: 214–220.
11. Aitman TJ, Critser JK, Cuppen E, Dominiczak A, Fernandez-Suarez XM, et al. (2008) Progress and prospects in rat genetics: a community view. Nat Genet 40: 516–522.
12. Jacob HJ (1999) Functional genomics and rat models. Genome Res 9: 1013–1016.
13. Urnov FD, Rebar EJ, Holmes MC, Zhang HS, Gregory PD (2010) Genome editing with engineered zinc finger nucleases. Nat Rev Genet 11: 636–646.
14. Cui X, Ji D, Fisher DA, Wu Y, Briner DM, et al. (2011) Targeted integration in rat and mouse embryos with zinc-finger nucleases. Nat Biotechnol 29: 64–67.
15. Carbery ID, Ji D, Harrington A, Brown V, Weinstein EJ, et al. (2010) Targeted genome modification in mice using zinc-finger nucleases. Genetics 186: 451–459.
16. Fanucchi MV, Hotchkiss JA, Harkema JR (1998) Endotoxin potentiates ozone-induced mucous cell metaplasia in rat nasal epithelium. Toxicology and Applied Pharmacology 152: 1–9.
17. Young JT (1981) Histopathologic examination of the rat nasal cavity. Fundam Appl Toxicol 1: 309–312.
18. Harkema JR, Hotchkiss JA, Harmsen AG, Henderson RF (1988) In vivo effects of transient neutrophil influx on nasal respiratory epithelial mucosubstances. Quantitative histochemistry. Am J Pathol 130: 605–615.
19. Fanucchi MV, Bracher A, Doran SF, Squadrito GL, Fernandez S, et al. (2012) Post-exposure antioxidant treatment in rats decreases airway hyperplasia and hyperreactivity due to chlorine inhalation. Am J Respir Cell Mol Biol 46: 599–606.
20. Meyerholz DK, Stoltz DA, Namati E, Ramachandran S, Pezzulo AA, et al. (2010) Loss of cystic fibrosis transmembrane conductance regulator function produces abnormalities in tracheal development in neonatal pigs and young children. Am J Respir Crit Care Med 182: 1251–1261.
21. Solomon GM, Konstan MW, Wilschanski M, Billings J, Sermet-Gaudelus I, et al. (2010) An international randomized multicenter comparison of nasal potential difference techniques. Chest 138: 919–928.
22. Pyle LC, Fulton JC, Sloane PA, Backer K, Mazur M, et al. (2010) Activation of the cystic fibrosis transmembrane conductance regulator by the flavonoid quercetin: potential use as a biomarker of ΔF508 cystic fibrosis transmembrane conductance regulator rescue. Am J Respir Cell Mol Biol 43: 607–616.
23. Dawson DC (1977) Na and Cl transport across the isolated turtle colon: parallel pathways for transmural ion movement. J Membr Biol 37: 213–233.
24. Liu L, Chu KK, Houser GH, Diephuis BJ, Li Y, et al. (2013) Method for quantitative study of airway functional microanatomy using micro-optical coherence tomography. PLoS One 8: e54473.
25. Rutland J, Cole PJ (1981) Nasal mucociliary clearance and ciliary beat frequency in cystic fibrosis compared with sinusitis and bronchiectasis. Thorax 36: 654–658.
26. Brand JD, Ballinger CA, Tuggle KL, Fanucchi MV, Schwiebert LM, et al. (2012) Site-specific dynamics of CD11b+ and CD103+ dendritic cell accumulations following ozone exposure. Am J Physiol Lung Cell Mol Physiol 303: L1079–1086.
27. Clarke LL, Boucher RC (1992) Chloride secretory response to extracellular ATP in human normal and cystic fibrosis nasal epithelia. Am J Physiol 263: C348–356.
28. Rosenberg LA, Schluchter MD, Parlow AF, Drumm ML (2006) Mouse as a model of growth retardation in cystic fibrosis. Pediatr Res 59: 191–195.
29. Pierucci-Alves F, Akoyev V, Stewart JC, Wang LH, Janardhan KS, et al. (2011) Swine models of cystic fibrosis reveal male reproductive tract phenotype at birth. Biol Reprod 85: 442–451.
30. Arquitt CK, Boyd C, Wright JT (2002) Cystic fibrosis transmembrane regulator gene (CFTR) is associated with abnormal enamel formation. J Dent Res 81: 492–496.
31. Chang EH, Lacruz RS, Bromage TG, Bringas P, Welsh MJ, et al. (2011) Enamel pathology resulting from loss of function in the cystic fibrosis transmembrane conductance regulator in a porcine animal model. Cells Tissues Organs 194: 249–254.
32. Dabrowska E, Błahuszewska K, Minarowska A, Kaczmarski M, Niedźwiecka-Andrzejewicz I, et al. (2006) Assessment of dental status and oral hygiene in the study population of cystic fibrosis patients in the Podlasie province. Adv Med Sci 51 Suppl 1: 100–103.
33. Wright JT, Kiefer CL, Hall KI, Grubb BR (1996) Abnormal enamel development in a cystic fibrosis transgenic mouse model. J Dent Res 75: 966–973.
34. Sturgess J, Imrie J (1982) Quantitative evaluation of the development of tracheal submucosal glands in infants with cystic fibrosis and control infants. Am J Pathol 106: 303–311.
35. Jarzabek K, Zbucka M, Pepiński W, Szamatowicz J, Domitrz J, et al. (2004) Cystic fibrosis as a cause of infertility. Reprod Biol 4: 119–129.
36. Wright JT, Hall KI, Grubb BR (1996) Enamel mineral composition of normal and cystic fibrosis transgenic mice. Adv Dent Res 10: 270–274; discussion 275.
37. Azevedo TD, Feijó GC, Bezerra AC (2006) Presence of developmental defects of enamel in cystic fibrosis patients. J Dent Child (Chic) 73: 159–163.
38. Ferrazzano GF, Sangianantoni G, Cantile T, Amato I, Orlando S, et al. (2012) Dental enamel defects in Italian children with cystic fibrosis: an observational study. Community Dent Health 29: 106–109.
39. Primosch RE (1980) Tetracycline discoloration, enamel defects, and dental caries in patients with cystic fibrosis. Oral Surg Oral Med Oral Pathol 50: 301–308.
40. Jagels AE, Sweeney EA (1976) Oral health of patients with cystic fibrosis and their siblings. J Dent Res 55: 991–996.
41. Boucher RC (2007) Evidence for airway surface dehydration as the initiating event in CF airway disease. J Intern Med 261: 5–16.
42. Song Y, Namkung W, Nielson DW, Lee JW, Finkbeiner WE, et al. (2009) Airway surface liquid depth measured in ex vivo fragments of pig and human trachea: dependence on Na+ and Cl- channel function. Am J Physiol Lung Cell Mol Physiol 297: L1131–1140.
43. Chinet TC, Fullton JM, Yankaskas JR, Boucher RC, Stutts MJ (1994) Mechanism of sodium hyperabsorption in cultured cystic fibrosis nasal epithelium: a patch-clamp study. Am J Physiol 266: C1061–1068.
44. Boucher RC, Stutts MJ, Knowles MR, Cantley L, Gatzy JT (1986) Na+ transport in cystic fibrosis respiratory epithelia. Abnormal basal rate and response to adenylate cyclase activation. J Clin Invest 78: 1245–1252.
45. Boucher RC, Cotton CU, Gatzy JT, Knowles MR, Yankaskas JR (1988) Evidence for reduced Cl- and increased Na+ permeability in cystic fibrosis human primary cell cultures. J Physiol 405: 77–103.
46. Cotton CU, Stutts MJ, Knowles MR, Gatzy JT, Boucher RC (1987) Abnormal apical cell membrane in cystic fibrosis respiratory epithelium. An in vitro electrophysiologic analysis. J Clin Invest 79: 80–85.
47. Chen JH, Stoltz DA, Karp PH, Ernst SE, Pezzulo AA, et al. (2010) Loss of anion transport without increased sodium absorption characterizes newborn porcine cystic fibrosis airway epithelia. Cell 143: 911–923.

48. Fisher JT, Tyler SR, Zhang Y, Lee BJ, Liu X, et al. (2013) Bioelectric Characterization of Epithelia from Neonatal CFTR Knockout Ferrets. Am J Respir Cell Mol Biol 49: 837–844.
49. Chen EY, Yang N, Quinton PM, Chin WC (2010) A new role for bicarbonate in mucus formation. Am J Physiol Lung Cell Mol Physiol 299: L542–549.
50. Garcia MA, Yang N, Quinton PM (2009) Normal mouse intestinal mucus release requires cystic fibrosis transmembrane regulator-dependent bicarbonate secretion. J Clin Invest 119: 2613–2622.
51. Chang EH, Pezzulo AA, Meyerholz DK, Potash AE, Wallen TJ, et al. (2012) Sinus hypoplasia precedes sinus infection in a porcine model of cystic fibrosis. Laryngoscope 122: 1898–1905.
52. Tarran R, Grubb BR, Parsons D, Picher M, Hirsh AJ, et al. (2001) The CF salt controversy: in vivo observations and therapeutic approaches. Mol Cell 8: 149–158.
53. Houwen RH, van der Doef HP, Sermet I, Munck A, Hauser B, et al. (2010) Defining DIOS and constipation in cystic fibrosis with a multicentre study on the incidence, characteristics, and treatment of DIOS. J Pediatr Gastroenterol Nutr 50: 38–42.
54. Collaco A, Marathe J, Kohnke H, Kravstov D, Ameen N (2010) Syntaxin 3 is necessary for cAMP- and cGMP-regulated exocytosis of CFTR: implications for enterotoxigenic diarrhea. Am J Physiol Cell Physiol 299: C1450–1460.
55. Jayaraman S, Song Y, Vetrivel L, Shankar L, Verkman AS (2001) Noninvasive in vivo fluorescence measurement of airway-surface liquid depth, salt concentration, and pH. J Clin Invest 107: 317–324.
56. Boucher RC (2004) New concepts of the pathogenesis of cystic fibrosis lung disease. Eur Respir J 23: 146–158.
57. Itani OA, Chen JH, Karp PH, Ernst S, Keshavjee S, et al. (2011) Human cystic fibrosis airway epithelia have reduced Cl- conductance but not increased Na+ conductance. Proc Natl Acad Sci U S A 108: 10260–10265.
58. Grubb BR, Vick RN, Boucher RC (1994) Hyperabsorption of Na+ and raised Ca(2+)-mediated Cl- secretion in nasal epithelia of CF mice. Am J Physiol 266: C1478–1483.
59. Livraghi-Butrico A, Kelly EJ, Wilkinson KJ, Rogers TD, Gilmore RC, et al. (2013) Loss of Cftr function exacerbates the phenotype of Na(+) hyperabsorption in murine airways. Am J Physiol Lung Cell Mol Physiol 304: L469–480.
60. van der Doef HP, Kokke FT, van der Ent CK, Houwen RH (2011) Intestinal obstruction syndromes in cystic fibrosis: meconium ileus, distal intestinal obstruction syndrome, and constipation. Curr Gastroenterol Rep 13: 265–270.
61. Rogers CS, Stoltz DA, Meyerholz DK, Ostedgaard LS, Rokhlina T, et al. (2008) Disruption of the CFTR gene produces a model of cystic fibrosis in newborn pigs. Science 321: 1837–1841.

A Little CFTR Goes a Long Way: CFTR-Dependent Sweat Secretion from G551D and R117H-5T Cystic Fibrosis Subjects Taking Ivacaftor

Jessica E. Char[1], Marlene H. Wolfe[1], Hyung-ju Cho[1], Il-Ho Park[1], Jin Hyeok Jeong[1], Eric Frisbee[1], Colleen Dunn[2], Zoe Davies[2], Carlos Milla[2], Richard B. Moss[2], Ewart A. C. Thomas[3], Jeffrey J. Wine[1,2,3]*

1 Cystic Fibrosis Research Laboratory, Stanford University, Stanford, California, United States of America, **2** Department of Pediatrics, Stanford University School of Medicine, Stanford, California, United States of America, **3** Department of Psychology, Stanford University, Stanford, California, United States of America

Abstract

To determine if oral dosing with the CFTR-potentiator ivacaftor (VX-770, Kalydeco) improves CFTR-dependent sweating in CF subjects carrying G551D or R117H-5T mutations, we optically measured sweat secretion from 32–143 individually identified glands in each of 8 CF subjects; 6 F508del/G551D, one G551D/R117H-5T, and one I507del/R117H-5T. Two subjects were tested only (−) ivacaftor, 3 only (+) ivacaftor and 3 (+/−) ivacaftor (1–5 tests per condition). The total number of gland measurements was 852 (−) ivacaftor and 906 (+) ivacaftor. A healthy control was tested 4 times (51 glands). For each gland we measured both CFTR-independent (M-sweat) and CFTR-dependent (C-sweat); C-sweat was stimulated with a β-adrenergic cocktail that elevated $[cAMP]_i$ while blocking muscarinic receptors. Absent ivacaftor, almost all CF glands produced M-sweat on all tests, but only 1/593 glands produced C-sweat (10 tests, 5 subjects). By contrast, 6/6 subjects (113/342 glands) produced C-sweat in the (+) ivacaftor condition, but with large inter-subject differences; 3–74% of glands responded with C/M sweat ratios 0.04%–2.57% of the average WT ratio of 0.265. Sweat volume losses cause proportionally larger underestimates of CFTR function at lower sweat rates. The losses were reduced by measuring C/M ratios in 12 glands from each subject that had the highest M-sweat rates. Remaining losses were estimated from single channel data and used to correct the C/M ratios, giving estimates of CFTR function (+) ivacaftor = 1.6%–7.7% of the WT average. These estimates are in accord with single channel data and transcript analysis, and suggest that significant clinical benefit can be produced by low levels of CFTR function.

Editor: Giuseppe Novelli, Tor Vergata University of Rome, Italy

Funding: This work was supported by Cystic Fibrosis Foundation Therapeutics, Grant WINE08A0 to JJW. http://www.cff.org/research/cfft/. The funders had no role in study design, data collection and analysis, decision to publish, or preparation of the manuscript.

Competing Interests: The authors have declared that no competing interests exist.

* E-mail: wine@stanford.edu

Introduction

Genetic mutations that reduce CFTR-mediated anion conductance ($G_{anion} = nP_O\gamma$) cause cystic fibrosis (CF). Over 1,000 mutations are known or predicted to reduce CFTR channel number (n), open probability (P_O), and/or conductance (γ), and 127 of these have been identified as disease-causing mutations [1]. A complex set of interacting pathophysiological consequences follows large reductions in CFTR function, most resulting from defective ion and fluid transport. The most efficient way to stop this cascade is to correct the defective gene or protein. Ivacaftor (VX-770, Kalydeco) increases P_O in a wide variety of CFTR mutations as well as WT CFTR [2]. VX-770 was shown to improve the function of G551D in cultured cells [3], and patients having at least one G551D mutation treated with oral ivacaftor showed marked clinical improvement [4,5], leading to FDA approval of ivacaftor for use in G551D patients. Recently, ivacaftor was shown to improve CFTR-dependent ion transport in human airway epithelial cells carrying an R117H mutation [6], and trials are now underway to determine if ivacaftor will be clinically beneficial for patients with R117H-5T mutations.

Most CFTR mutations are rare, and marked phenotypic differences can occur in patients having the same mutations [7,8,9]. Therefore, n-of-1 studies are informative. With that in mind, a bioassay was developed that compares the volume of CFTR-independent and CFTR-dependent sweat secretion gland-by-gland for ~50 individually identified glands within each subject [10]. On the premise that the therapeutics of interest will act directly on CFTR, we treated individual glands as the units of analysis, providing sufficient statistical power to determine efficacy for individual subjects in n-of-1 studies.

The assay takes advantage of two parallel pathways for sweat secretion: a CFTR-independent, cholinergic pathway stimulated with methacholine ('M-sweat') and a β-adrenergic pathway that is CFTR-dependent ('C-sweat') [10]. When C-sweating is expressed as a function of M-sweating, the assay gives a near-linear readout of CFTR function over a wide range: i.e. the C-sweat/M-sweat ratio for carriers of one CFTR mutation is 50% that of non-CF controls, while the ratio for CF subjects is zero. However, at very low levels of CFTR function the C-sweat assay departs from linearity and becomes less sensitive: at present it doesn't detect C-sweating in most pancreatic sufficient (PS) CF subjects, who are

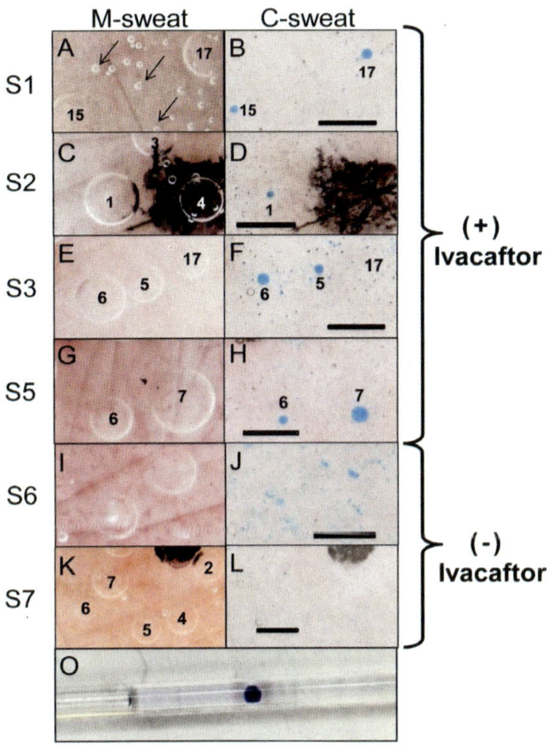

Figure 1. CFTR independent (M-sweat) and CFTR dependent (C-sweat) secretion in G551D CF subjects. Each image shows a small region (~1.5 mm^2) of the stimulated field of sweat glands (full imaged field is 0.63 cm^2) for each subject. Images for S1-3 and S5 were (+) ivacaftor and S6, 7 (−) ivacaftor. A portion of each field was selected to show glands that responded (or not) to the β-adrenergic cocktail (right column). (A-B). S1, male. Arrows in (A) point to air bubbles in the oil. (C-D) S2, female. (D) Shows the single sweat gland that responded to the β-adrenergic stimulus in this experiment. The dark stain is an ink spot on the freckle used for image registration. (E-F) S3, female. This subject had high background staining. (G-H) S5, male. (I-J) S6, female, (-) ivacaftor. This subject showed the most background staining of any subject in this series. (K-L) S7, female, (−) ivacaftor. (O) C-sweat collected in 2 µl constant bore capillary from S1 (+) ivacaftor. Calibration bars =0.5 mm.

known to have some residual CFTR function [10]. The sweat volume bioassay is thus complementary to the sweat chloride test, which does discriminate between CF patients based on their pancreatic status, but which can't discriminate CF heterozygotes from WT subjects [10]. Both tests benefit by using an organ that is unaffected by the progressive, destructive changes that occur in many other CFTR-expressing organs [11].

Given the assay's present inability to discriminate between PI and PS subjects, it was important to determine if it could detect functional efficacy of ivacaftor in CF subjects carrying the G551D mutation, where its clinical efficacy has already been demonstrated [4,5]. Therefore, in the present study we measured the efficacy of ivacaftor in 4 individuals of G551D/F508del genotype. In addition, we wanted to use the assay with patients having mutations for which clinical efficacy of ivacaftor is presently unknown. Therefore, we also used the assay to measure the efficacy of ivacaftor in two CF subjects with R117H-5T mutations.

Materials and Methods

Subjects

The study was approved by the Institutional Review Board of Stanford University. After written informed consent, six adults with genotypes G551D/F508del, one with G551D/R117H-5T and one with I507del/R117H-5T were enrolled, along with a healthy control. All CF subjects were classified as having cystic fibrosis by the Stanford Cystic Fibrosis Center on the basis of elevated sweat chloride levels, CFTR mutations, and clinical indications. The healthy control subject was genotyped by the Molecular Pathology Laboratory, Stanford University Medical Center and was free of any CFTR mutations and had (TG)12-7T and (TG)10-9T.

Two subjects were tested only off drug, three only on drug, and two were tested both off and on. There were no adverse events. Seven subjects had been enrolled in multi-center studies of ivacaftor and were studied either during the open label period, during the month prior to the start of open label, or both. One G551D subject who was not enrolled in an ivacaftor trial was studied off drug prior to FDA approval and then on-drug after starting ivacaftor as prescribed by his physician.

Ratiometric measurement of sweat secretion from identified individual glands

We used the single gland, ratiometric, optical assay for CFTR secretory function as described by Wine *et al.* [10]. In brief, a specific region of skin on the volar forearm was sequentially injected intradermally with methacholine to stimulate CFTR-independent sweating (M-sweat) and then with a cocktail of agents that blocked M-sweating and produced CFTR-dependent sweating (C-sweat). Bubbles of sweat from single glands were captured in an oil layer, visualized by oblique lighting or dye-partioning, and digitally imaged at 30 sec intervals. The individual glands were identified by location as follows: a region of interest (ROI) was defined by counting bubbles of M-sweat starting at the center of the field and spiraling outward until ~50 individual glands were numbered. For each identified gland the increases in M- and C-sweat volumes over time were measured. Plots of volume vs. time were made at 5-6 min intervals for selected glands to latencies and rates of volume increase. Plots correlating M- and C-sweat volumes were based on M-sweat volumes at the end of 15 min, and C-sweat volumes/2 at the end of 30 min. In the plots of M- and C-sweat correlations, each point represents the average volume for a single identified gland based on all trials where the gland was measured.

To provide a common, meaningful basis of comparison among the CF subjects, we obtained a mean C/M ratio of 0.2651 from testing six healthy controls subjects [10], set that value =100%, and expressed the responses of the CF subjects with reference to it. Proportionality between CFTR-dependent and CFTR-independent secretory function, i.e., the constancy of the C/M ratio across glands, is compromised by sweat volume losses via ductal absorption and physical capacitance [10], as well as by finite losses into the oil from very small bubbles in spite of extensive water saturation of the oil (P.M. Quinton, personal communication). Indeed, the C/M values showed a positive relation to M-sweat rates, consistent with proportionally less sweat volume loss in the faster secreting glands. To take advantage of this relationship for each subject, we plotted the C/M ratio for the 12 highest M-sweat secreting glands, in which sweat loss is much reduced and the C/M ratio is expected to be relatively constant. A further correction factor was obtained by using single channel

Table 1. G551D/F508del subjects.

			Gland numbers			Gland volumes/rates				Ratios			
ID	**G**	**TestDate**	**MCh glands (n)**	**Cktl glands (n)**	**C/M n glands (%)**	**MCh Avg. Final Vol. (nl/gland)**	**MCh Rate Estimate nl/gl/min**	**Cktl Avg Final Vol (pl/gl)**	**Cktl Rate (pl/gl/min)**	**C mean/ M mean**	**% WT**	**% WT (Highest 12 M-sweat)**	**% WT (Hi-12, Loss-Corrected)**
S1 G551D/F508del (−) ivacaftor													
S1	M	10/20/2011	71	0	0%	75.83	5.06	0	0	0.00%	0.00%	-	—
S1	M	1/13/2012	85	0	0%	64.58	4.31	0	0	0.00%	0.00%	-	—
S1	M	2/4/2012	75	0	0%	71.34	4.76	0	0	0.00%	0.00%	-	—
S1 (−) Averages			**77**	**0**	**0%**	**70.58**	**4.71**	**0**	**0**	**0.00%**	**0.00%**	**0.00%**	**0.00%**
S1 G551D/F508del (+) ivacaftor													
S1	M	3/23/2012	82	13	16%	70.99	4.73	152	5.06	0.11%	0.42%	-	—
S1	M	4/10/2012	71	15	21%	91.91	6.13	105	3.52	0.06%	0.22%	-	—
S1	M	4/17/2012	66	11	17%	97.02	6.47	110	3.66	0.06%	0.22%	-	—
S1 (+) A xverages			**73**	**13**	**18%**	**86.64**	**5.78**	**122**	**4.08**	**0.07%**	**0.29%**	**0.64%**	**1.59%**
S2 G551D/F508del (−) ivacaftor													
S2	F	2/2/2012	99	0	0%	28.61	1.91	0	0	0.00%	0.00%	-	—
S2	F	3/20/2012	100	0	0%	29.16	1.94	0	0	0.00%	0.00%	-	—
S2 (−) Averages			**99.5**	**0**	**0%**	**28.88**	**1.93**	**0**	**0**	**0.00%**	**0.00%**	**0.00%**	**0.00%**
S2 G551D/F508del (+) ivacaftor													
S2	F	5/8/2012	82	4	5%	35.55	2.37	11	0.37	0.02%	0.06%	-	—
S2	F	5/15/2012	90	1	1%	29.16	1.94	2	0.07	0.00%	0.01%	-	—
S2 (+) Averages			**86**	**2.5**	**3%**	**32.36**	**2.16**	**7**	0.22	**0.01%**	**0.04%**	**0.13%**	**2.75%**
S3 G551D/F508del (+) ivacaftor													
S3	**F**	**7/24/2012**	**90**	**21**	**23%**	**45.03**	**3.00**	**95**	**3.18**	**0.11%**	**0.41%**	**0.58%**	**2.27%**
S5 G551D/F508del (+) ivacaftor data													
S5	**M**	**11/2/2012**	**58**	**29**	**50%**	**78.94**	**5.26**	**703**	**23.42**	**0.45%**	**1.74%**	**3.07%**	**4.11%**
S6 G551D/F508del (−) ivacaftor data													
S6	**F**	**2/2/2012**	**143**	**0**	**0%**	**14.37**	**0.96**	**0**	**0**	**0.00%**	**0.00%**	**0.00%**	**0.00%**
S7 G551D/F508del (−) ivacaftor data													
S7	**F**	**2/13/2012**	**123**	**0**	**0%**	**32.16**	**2.14**	**0**	**0**	**0.00%**	**0.00%**	**0.00%**	**0.00%**
Summary (−) ivacaftor: 4 G551D subjects													
Sums or Averages			**852**	**0**	**0%**	**36.50**	**2.43**	**0**	**0**	**0.00%**	**0.00%**	**0.00%**	**0.00%**
Summary (+) ivacaftor 4 G551D subjects													
Sums or Averages			**906**	**317**	**29%**	**42.93**	**2.84**	**267**	**6.80**	**0.29%**	**1.15%**	**1.84%**	**4.07%**

Summary of results for CF subjects with G551D mutations. Six adult G551D CF subjects were tested. Table is arranged by subject and condition, each row shows the results for a single test or means/sums when multiple tests were performed. Subjects had been taking ivacaftor for at least 3 weeks prior to (+) ivacaftor testing. Columns labeled 'gland numbers' show the number of glands that secreted to an intradermal injection of MCh, then to the β-adrenergic cocktail at the same site (C-sweat), and the ratio of the two expressed as a percentage. Columns labeled 'gland volumes/rates' show the average final M-sweat or C-sweat volumes per gland expressed as nanoliters for a 15 min period (M-sweat) or 30 min period (C-sweat) followed by average rates (per min, per gland). The 4 columns labeled 'ratios' show: 1) the mean C-sweat rate as a percent of the mean M-sweat rate; 2) the C/M ratios as a percentage of the average C/M ratio of 0.2651 obtained for 6 control subjects [10]; 3) that value for the 12 glands having the highest M-sweat rates; and 4) the value for the 12 highest glands after correcting for sweat volume loss.

measures of P_O and γ for R117H [12] and mRNA transcript measurements of n [13] to provide an independent estimate of unpotentiated R117H-5T channel function. We then subtracted the C/M measure from the predicted single channel value to obtain an estimate of the amount of fluid loss, and added this back for a final, best estimate of CFTR function (see discussion). For G551D, our corrected C/M values were compared with single channel measures made (±) ivacaftor [14,15].

The small volumes of C-sweat observed for the CF subjects made us alert to possible artifacts. In addition to other criteria [10], we also used pipets to collect C-sweat from three CF subjects after optically recording secretion in the presence of ivacaftor. The small amounts collected were in accord with the optical measurements. We tried but failed to collect any C-sweat from CF subjects (−) ivacaftor. Skin staining seen in some experiments (−) ivacaftor (e.g. **Fig. 1L**) had no detectable volume and could not be dislodged by the collecting pipet. Such staining was seen variably in 6 experiments done prior to 2/13/2012 when it was eliminated by a rinse procedure between the M-sweat and C-sweat trials. All (+) ivacaftor trials were done with minimized background

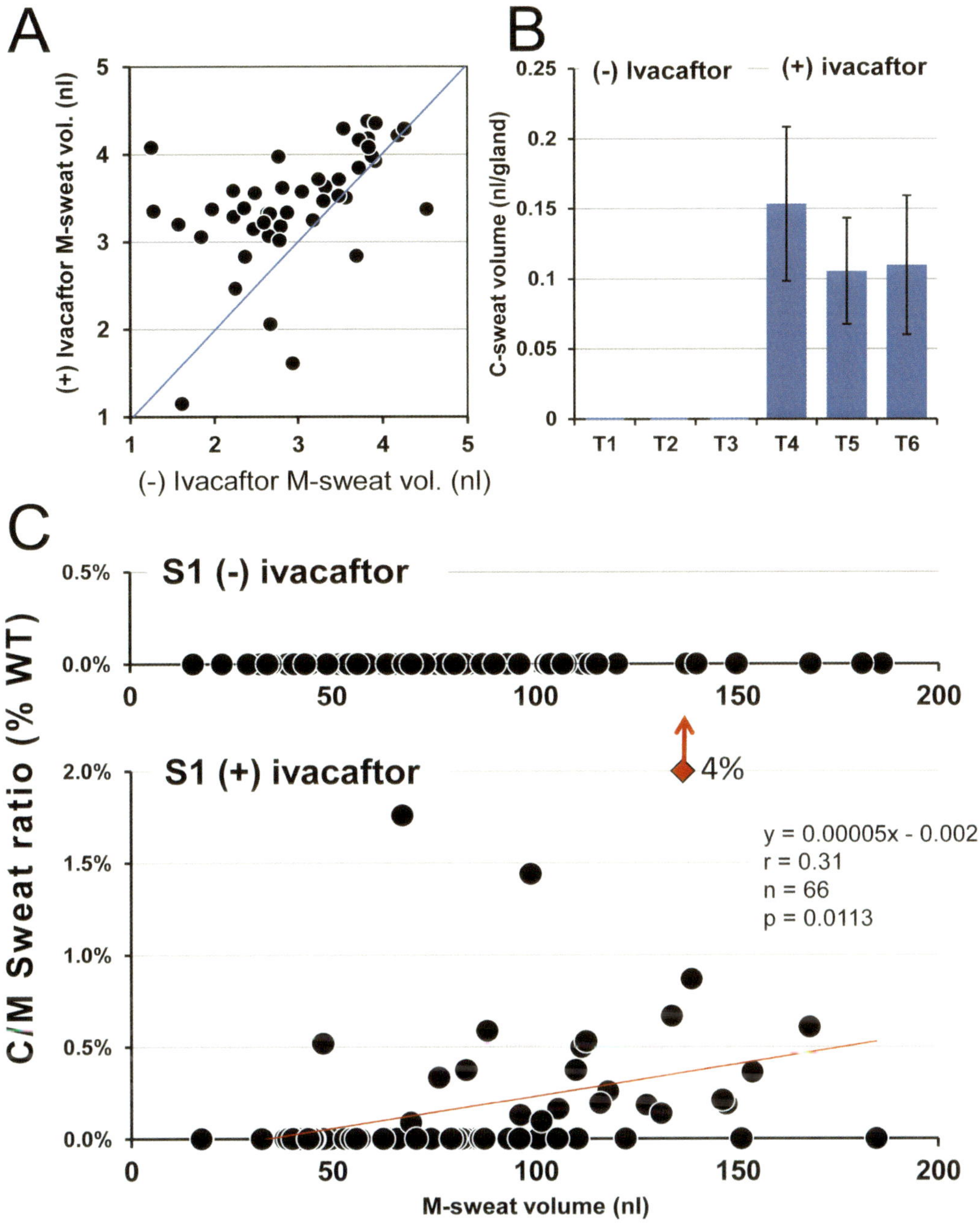

Figure 2. M- and C-sweat secretion (±) ivacaftor for CF subject 1: male, F508del/G551D. (A) Larger M-sweat responses (+) ivacaftor were seen (uniquely) in this subject. Scatter plot shows gland-by-gland volumes measured 7.5 min post MCh injection before any appreciable mergers for 46 glands. Each point is the average of 2–3 measures (2.93 measures per gland per condition), log transformed. Value (−) ivacaftor are on the x-axis and (+) ivacaftor on the y axis. Mean volume at the 7.5 min time point was 28.7±20 vs. 38.35±20 nl^{-gland}, $p = 0.004$, paired t-test on log transformed data. Diagonal line shows equivalence. (B) Bar graphs showing mean C-sweat volumes ± ivacaftor; 3 tests in each condition; zero C-sweat seen (−) ivacaftor. (C) Gland-by-gland sweat secretion (±) ivacaftor. Each point in these graphs is jointly determined by the mean of M-sweat responses (x axis) and C-sweat/M-sweat ratios expressed as a% of the mean WT C/M ratio (y axis). Top graph with truncated y axis shows measurements (−) ivacaftor. Each point is mean ratio measured in 1–3 tests (mean 2.1 tests) for each of 94 identified glands. C-sweating and hence ratio was zero for all glands. Bottom graph, (+) ivacaftor. 25/66 glands produced C-sweat on 1–3 trials (average 1.56 trials). The dark outlined red diamond and arrow show an outlier gland (G19) which secreted ~10 times more than the mean of all responding glands on each of 3 (+) ivacaftor trials. Red line is linear fit.

and hence had reduced chances of false positives, but extremely low levels of secretion might have been missed in 3 (−) ivacaftor tests done before the rinse procedure.

Statistical Analysis

Single, identified sweat glands were the units of analysis for the within-subject comparisons in our "n-of-1" analyses [10]. Paired t-tests on log transformed data, Pearson r, ANOVA, and mixed

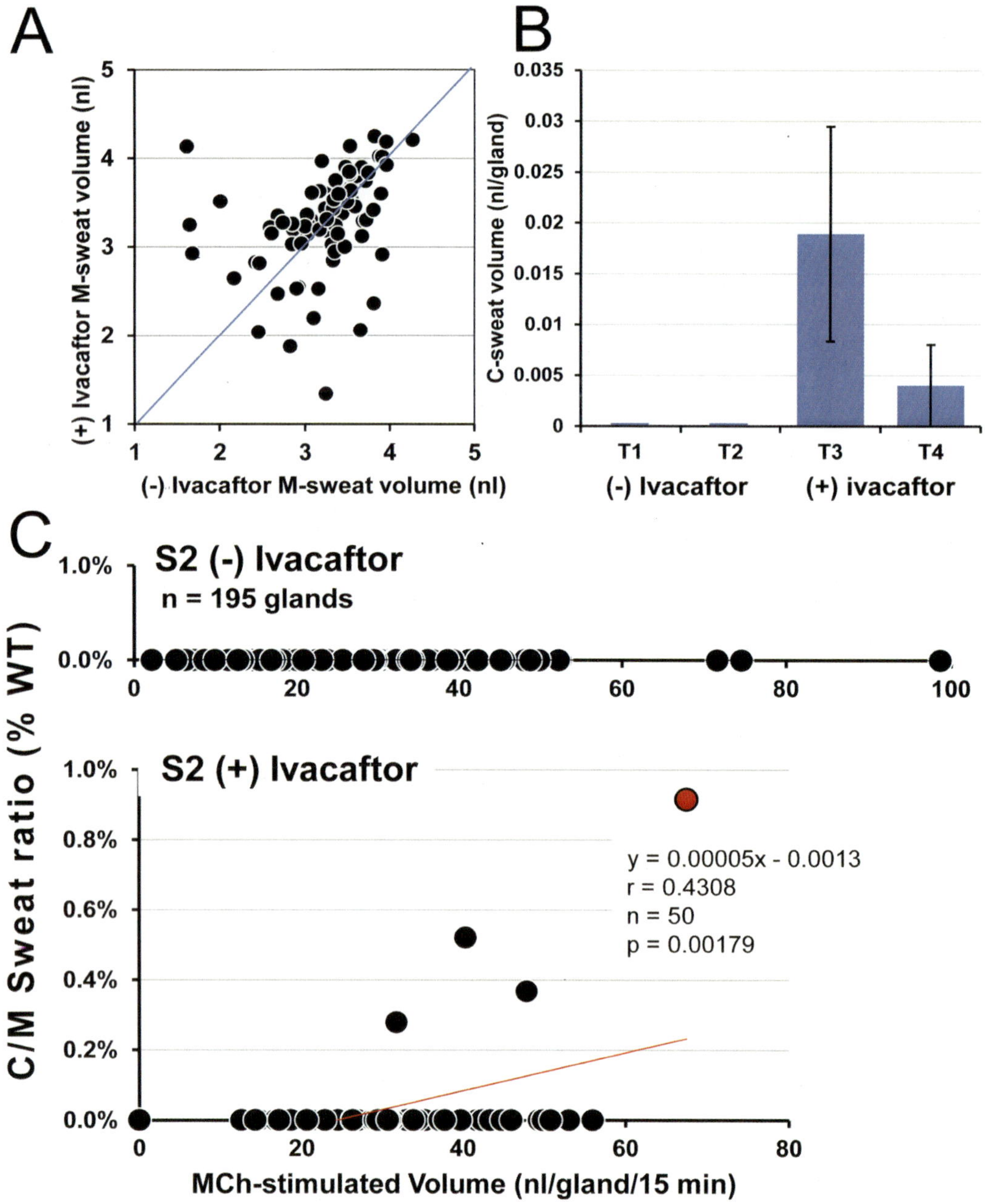

Figure 3. M- and C-sweat secretion (±) ivacaftor for CF subject 2: female, F508del/G551D. (A) M-sweat responses were unchanged by ivacaftor in this subject. Each point is log transformed values for a single pre-test and mean of 2 post-test measures for each of 87 glands. Mean volumes were 28.2±12.5 vs. 31.9±14.6 nl^{-gland}, pre and post, n = 87 glands $p = 0.12$, paired t-test on log transformed data, plotted as in Fig. 2A. (B) Bar graphs show C-sweat volumes (mean ± SEM) for (±) ivacaftor conditions; 2 tests in each condition. One (−) ivacaftor test was at a different site. (The means are based on glands 1–50). (C) Gland-by-gland C-sweat secretion ± ivacaftor. Each symbol shows correlations for each gland between mean M-sweat volumes (x axis) vs. C-sweat/M-sweat ratio expressed as a% of mean WT value (y axis). (Top graph, truncated y axis) shows measurements (−) ivacaftor. Each point is M-sweat volume for a single test for 195 identified glands at two sites; C-sweat was zero. (Bottom graph) shows measurements (+) ivacaftor (mean of 2 tests). Four of 87 glands produced C-sweat, only one gland secreted on both tests (red symbol). Red line is linear fit. This was the smallest response observed for any subject (+) ivacaftor.

models regression with lmer() from the lme4 package in R (see methods, ref [10]) were used as appropriate.

The ratio of the average rates of M- and C-sweat produced per gland (averaged over 15 min for M-sweat and 30 min for C-sweat) is the main index of sweat production, and we use it here to estimate the proportion of CFTR function in various conditions relative to a sample of healthy controls. However, for CF subjects, virtually no glands produced C-sweat in the (-) ivacaftor condition, and the majority still failed to produce measurable C-sweat (+) ivacaftor. We assume that glands sometimes secrete amounts of sweat that fail to exceed the threshold resulting from subtractive processes [10]. To assess this assumption, we dichotomized the C-sweat response as 0, if there is no observed secretion, and 1, otherwise. With this recoding, the average recoded C-sweat response is simply the *probability* that a gland produces C-sweat on

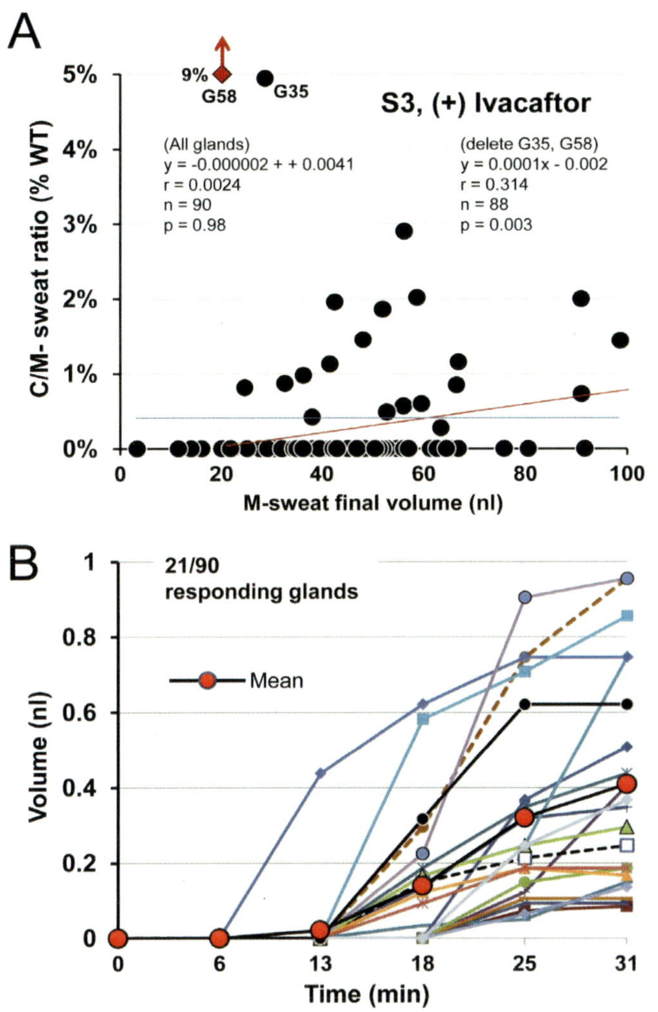

Figure 4. C-sweat secretion (+) ivacaftor in CF subject 3: female, F508del/G551D. S4 was tested only once, (+) ivacaftor. (A) Gland-by-gland correlations of M- and C-sweating using the same conventions as above. M-sweat was measured for 90 glands of which 21 also produced C-sweat with C/M ratios of 0.3% to 5% of the mean WT ratio. (B) Volume vs. time plots for C-sweating of each responding gland. β-adrenergic cocktail injected at time 0, and no observations were made during the first 3 min when atropine was taking effect and when the site was rinsed and dried before reapplying oil. Note slow time course of response.

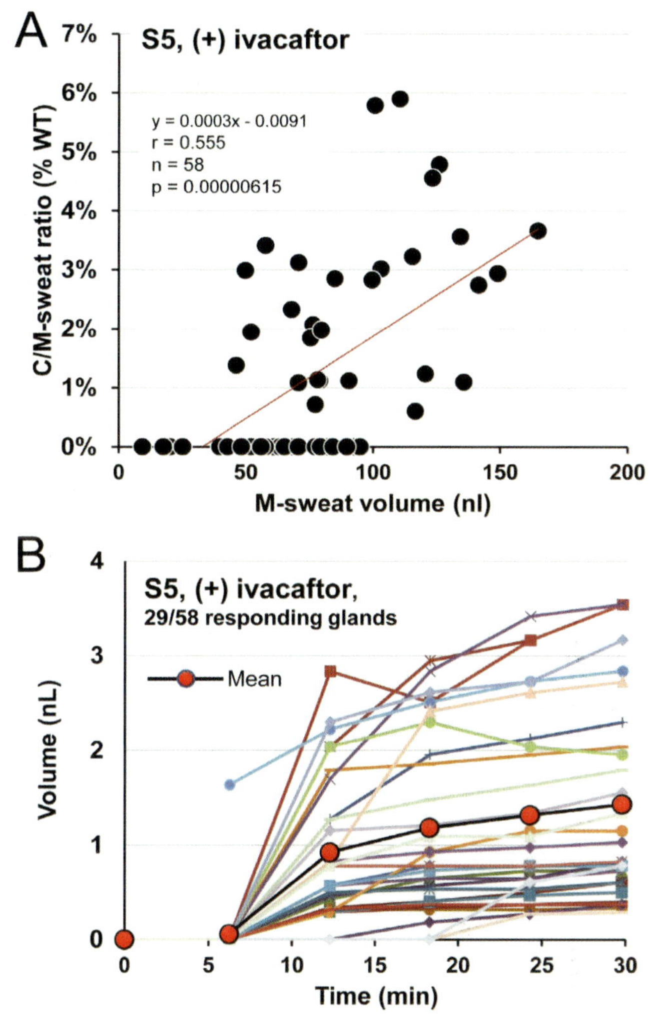

Figure 5. C-sweat secretion (+) ivacaftor in CF subject 5: male, F508del/G551D. S5 was tested only once, (+) ivacaftor. (A) Gland-by-gland correlations of M- and C-sweating using the same conventions as previously. M-sweating was measured in 58 glands. Of these, 29 (50%) also produced C-sweat, with C/M ratios of 0.6% to 5.9% of the mean WT ratio. (B) Volume vs. time plots for β-stimulated, C-sweating. β-adrenergic cocktail injected at time 0.

a test, and we use this probability as an alternative index of C-sweat production (see **Appendix S1**).

Note that this method is useful for testing statistical significance when many glands do not respond, the situation with CF subjects (−) ivacaftor, but becomes insensitive as the response rate increases and P(C-sweat) approaches 1. For example, WT and HZ both have P(C-sweat) ≈ 1, but C/M ratios of 1 and 0.5 respectively. The upper limit for the utility of this method is a function of CFTR functional levels and gland secretory capacity (M-sweat rate) and remains to be determined.

Results

For six CF subjects each carrying one G551D mutation, CFTR-independent M-sweating was imaged for 15 minutes, allowing us to identify 58–143 sweat glands per subject and measure the M-sweat rates for each gland. The same glands were then stimulated with the β-adrenergic cocktail to stimulate CFTR-dependent

C-sweating, which was imaged for 30 min. Two subjects were tested (+/−) ivacaftor, two only (+) ivacaftor and two only (−) ivacaftor (**Table 1**). Images of M-sweat and C-sweat bubbles are shown for each G551D CF subject in **Fig. 1**.

G551D subjects: within-subject comparisons (−) and (+) ivacaftor

Subject 1 (**S1**, male, F508del/G551D) was tested 3 times in each condition. (This is the preferred paradigm for testing, but it could not be used with all subjects because of limited subject availability.) M-sweat is considered to be CFTR-independent [16,17], but unexpectedly, S1's M-sweat rates were significantly larger (+) ivacaftor (78.0 versus 58.5 nl^{-gland}, p<.01; see **Fig. 2A**). Glands differed significantly in their typical M-sweat rates (p<.0001), but not in their sensitivity to ivacaftor (p>.38). Indeed,

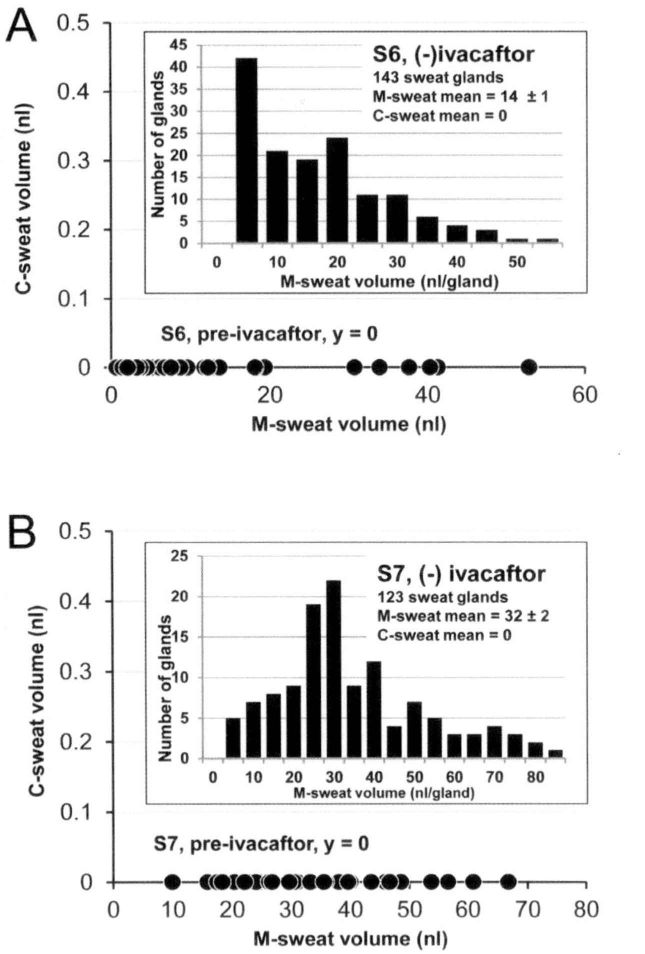

Figure 6. Absence of C-sweat secretion (−) ivacaftor in two G551D CF subjects. (A) S6: female, F508del/G551D. Each symbol in the main graph shows M-sweat volumes produced by a single sweat gland (x-axis) and C-sweat (truncated y axis, all C-sweat values were zero). The distribution of M-sweat volumes is shown in the inset. (B) S7: female, F508del/G551D. Same format as for S6.

M-sweating, presumably reflecting gland size, varied ~10 fold, as previously observed [10]. There was also significant variation in average M-sweat rates across weeks ($p<.05$); but in this subject the 6 tests were spread out across a 6 month period.

Ivacaftor caused a qualitative difference in C-sweating. No gland produced C-sweat in any of 3 tests (−) ivacaftor, but (+) ivacaftor 16–21% of the glands responded (**Table 1**) and produced an average of 0.1–0.15 nl^{-gland} on each of 3 tests (**Fig. 2B**). (Glands with zero C-sweat were included in the averages). As noted in **Appendix S1**, we dichotomized the C-sweat response, and then replaced by '1' one of the '0's (i.e., non-secretions) in the (−) ivacaftor condition. A logistic mixed model analysis of the minimally perturbed responses showed the effect of ivacaftor was significant [P(C-sweat) was estimated to be.1035 and.0009 in the (+) and (−) ivacaftor conditions, respectively, $p<.0005$]. Here too, glands ($p<.0001$), but not weeks ($p>.99$), differed significantly in the probability of a C-sweat response.

Fig. 2C presents data for S1 on a gland-by-gland basis, in which each point represents the joint mean values for C-sweat and M-sweat for a single gland. The top, truncated graph of **Fig. 2C** shows that no glands produced C-sweat in the absence of ivacaftor across the full range of M-sweat responses (0/231 = 0% response rate based on a mean of 2.35 measurements for each of 98 glands), hence all points are arrayed along the x axis according to their M-sweat responses. The bottom graph of **Fig. 2C** shows the results (+) ivacaftor. C-sweat responses were observed for 24 glands on at least one test with an overall response rate of 17.9% and C/M ratios 0%–4% of the average WT ratio. **Fig. 2C** also shows that the C/M ratio was not constant across the glands, but increased significantly as a function of the M-sweat rate ($r = 0.31$, $p<0.02$), see also [10]. The positive relationship between C/M and M, which was significant for all but one subject, was used to arrive at better estimates of the% of CFTR function restored by ivacaftor (see discussion).

As an additional means to estimate the level and significance of CFTR function that is restored by ivacaftor, we developed a prediction equation based on the gland's M-sweat response (+) ivacaftor, as discussed in **Appendix S1**. If the significant differences in P(C-sweat) across glands is due mainly to factors, e.g., gland size, that are reflected in the M-sweat response (+) ivacaftor, then one would expect that, when M-sweat response is included as a predictor, 'gland' would no longer be significant as a random effect. Similarly, to the extent that differences among weeks are reflected in the M-sweat response, 'week' would no longer be significant as a random effect. A logistic mixed model analysis showed that M-sweat response (on a log scale) was a significant predictor of P(C-sweat) ($b = 2.43$, $p<.0001$) in the (+) ivacaftor condition. Further, neither 'gland' ($p>.17$) nor 'week' ($p\approx 1$) was significant, suggesting that differences in CFTR function (i.e., in the CFTR-dependent C-sweat response) across glands and weeks can be adequately accounted for, or 'explained', by differences in the CFTR-independent M-sweat responses of the glands. On the log scale, M-sweat levels vary from 0 to 5.527, and the corresponding probabilities of a C-sweat response are.00006 and.23

Subject S2 (**S2**, female, F508del/G551D) was tested twice in each condition. Unlike S1, S2's M-sweat values did not differ between (+) and (−) ivacaftor (26.5 versus 25.3 nl^{-gland}, $p>.9$; see **Fig. 3A**). C-sweating for S2 was evaluated in the same way as for S1. **Fig. 3B** shows that no C-sweat volume was produced (−) ivacaftor, and only a tiny average volume (<20 pl^{-gland}) was produced (+) ivacaftor because only 1–4 out of 90 glands responded (**Fig. 3C, D**). A logistic mixed model analysis of the minimally perturbed responses showed a non-significant effect of ivacaftor ($p>.13$). Here too glands ($p<.0001$), but not weeks ($p>.99$), differed significantly in the probability of a C-sweat response. In predicting P(C-sweat) from M-sweat response (+) ivacaftor, a logistic mixed model analysis yielded unreliable estimates of the variances of the random effects for gland and week, most likely because less than 3% of glands yielded observable levels of
C-sweat. A simple logistic regression without random effects did show that M-sweat response (on a log scale) was a significant predictor of P(C-sweat) ($b = 3.88$, $p<.05$) (see discussion).

Two additional G551D subjects tested only (+) ivacaftor

Subject 3 (**S3**, female, F508del/G551D) was tested only once. M-sweating was measured for 90 glands, of which 21 (23%) produced measureable C-sweat with C/M ratios 0.3%–9% of the mean WT ratio (**Fig. 4A**). The average C/M for all glands was 0.41% WT. **Fig. 4B** plots volumes vs. time for C-sweat from each of the 21 responding glands. Most responding glands had long post-injection latencies, and many continued to increase throughout the 30 min period. This subject (or test) was unusual in that

Table 2. Summary of results for R117H-5T CF subjects and the healthy control.

			Gland numbers			Gland volumes/rates				Ratios			
ID	**G**	**Test Date**	**MCh glands (n)**	**Cktl glands (n)**	**C/M n glands (%)**	**MCh Avg. Final Vol. (nl/gland)**	**MCh Rate Estimate nl/gl/min**	**Cktl Avg Final Vol (pl/gl)**	**Cktl Rate (pl/gl/min)**	**C mean/ M mean**	**% WT**	**% WT (Highest 12 M-sweat)**	**% WT (Hi-12, Loss-Corrected)**
S4 G551D/R117H-5T (+) ivacaftor data													
S4	F	8/22/2012	37	8	22%	16.05	1.07	100	3.33	0.31%	1.22%	-	—
S4	F	11/6/2012	32	6	19%	10.66	0.69	30	1.00	0.14%	0.55%	-	—
S4	F	4/30/2013	37	11	30%	13.57	0.57	150	5.00	0.55%	2.16%	-	—
S4 (+) Averages			**35.33**	**8.33**	**23%**	**13.43**	**0.78**	**93**	**3.11**	**0.35%**	**1.31%**	**2.13%**	**7.83%**
S8 R117H/I508del (−) ivacaftor													
S8	M	1/31/2013	52	1	2%	46.76	3.12	6	0.19	0.01%	0.02%	—	—
S8	M	2/8/2013	54	1	2%	49.88	3.33	12	0.39	0.01%	0.04%	—	—
S8	M	2/15/2013	50	1	2%	59.51	3.97	4	0.14	0.00%	0.01%	—	—
S8 (−) Averages			**52**	**1**	**0%**	**52**	**3**	**7**	**0.24**	**0.01%**	**0.03%**	**0.06%**	**1.50%**
S8 R117H/I508del (+) ivacaftor													
S8	M	3/15/2013	53	28	53%	41.40	2.76	531	17.70	0.64%	2.42%	—	—
S8	M	3/22/2013	53	45	84%	54.35	3.62	766	25.55	0.71%	2.66%	—	—
S8	M	3/29/2013	49	42	86%	53.88	3.59	1146	38.20	1.06%	4.01%	—	—
S8	M	6/17/2013	53	43	81%	57.84	3.86	645	21.49	0.56%	2.10%	—	—
S8	M	6/24/2013	53	40	75%	53.85	3.59	474	15.80	0.44%	1.66%	—	—
S8 (+) Averages			**52.2**	**39.6**	**76%**	**52.26**	**3.48**	**712**	**23.75**	**0.68%**	**2.57%**	**4.51%**	**5.89%**
Healthy Control													
WT	F	3/14/2013	51	50	98%	35.94	2.40	9687	323	13%	51%	—	—
WT	F	3/25/2013	51	51	100%	36.98	2.47	9371	312	13%	48%	—	—
WT	F	3/28/2013	51	51	100%	28.81	1.92	11519	384	20%	75%	—	—
WT	F	5/2/2013	51	50	98%	36.48	2.43	10540	351	14%	54%	—	—
WT Averages			**51**	**50.5**	**99%**	**34.55**	**2.30**	**10279**	**343**	**15%**	**57%**	**60.65%**	**62.97%**

Table is arranged using same format as Table 1 and shows data for S8, S4 and the healthy control.

two glands with low M-sweat rates had high C-sweat rates, leading to unusually high C/M ratios and resulting in a non-significant association between C/M ratio and M-sweat rate ($r = 0.002$, $p = 0.98$). Excluding those two glands gave $r = 0.314$, $p = 0.003$).

Subject 5 (**S5**, male, F508del/G551D), was tested only once (+) ivacaftor. M-sweating was measured in 58 glands, of which 29 (50%) produced C-sweat, giving C/M ratios of 0.6% to 5.9% of the mean WT ratio (**Fig. 5A**). The time course of increases in C-sweat bubble volumes in this subject was similar to S4 (**Fig. 5B**). (Time courses of responding glands from S1 and S2 were similar to S3 and S5, data not shown). The C/M ratio increased significantly as a function of the M-sweat rate ($r = 0.555$, $p = 0.000006$).

In predicting P(C-sweat) from M-sweat response (+) ivacaftor, a logistic mixed model analysis showed that M-sweat response (on a log scale) was a significant predictor of P(C-sweat) (S3: $b = 1.43$, $p < .05$; S5: $b = 3.73$, $p < .01$).

Two additional G551D subjects tested only (−) ivacaftor

Two female G551D CF subjects, **S6** and **S7**, were each tested once only (−) ivacaftor. They did not return for repeat pre-testing or since starting ivacaftor. Each subject had abundant sweat glands, none of which responded to the β-adrenergic cocktail with any measureable C-sweat (0/266 glands, main graphs of **Fig. 6A, B**). The insets show the distribution of M-sweat volumes for these two subjects; note the prevalence of low-secreting glands for S6.

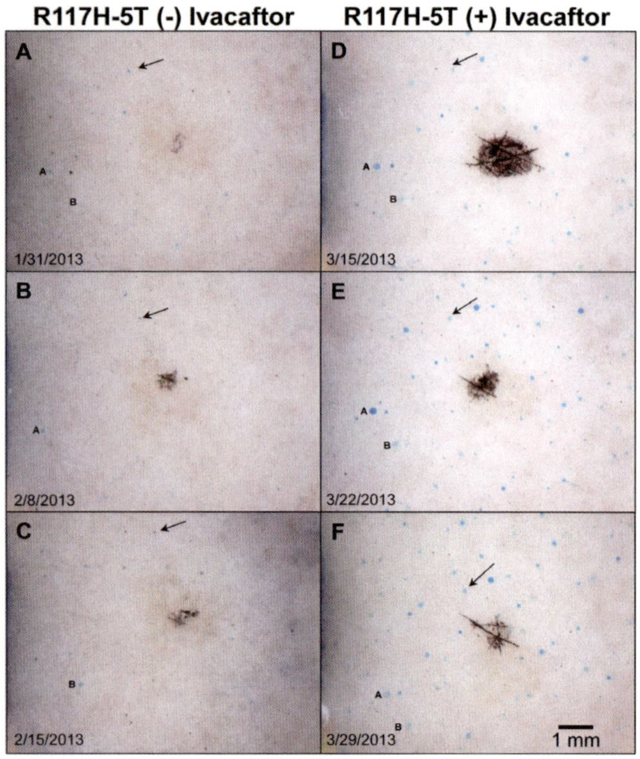

Figure 7. Images of C-sweat responses for CF subject 8: male, I507del/R117H-5T (±) ivacaftor (N of 1 trial). S8 was tested 3 times (−) ivacaftor and 5 times (+) ivacaftor. Only the first 3 (+) ivacaftor tests are shown. (A-C) (−) ivacaftor; (D-F) (+) ivacaftor. Each image shows the field 30 min after the cocktail injection. A light freckle served as the landmark, with an ink spot on the freckle to improve registration and focusing. For image (F) the ink spot was too high causing the field to shift down. In this pancreatic sufficient subject, a few glands marked as A, B, or arrows) produced small amounts of C-sweat (−) ivacaftor.

Within-subject study of an R117H-5T subject (−) and (+) ivacaftor

Subject 8 has genotype I507del/R117H-5T. The I507del mutation does not traffic [18,19] and so is predicted to be unresponsive to ivacaftor, allowing us to assess the *in vivo* effect of ivacaftor on the R117H-5T mutation in isolation. S8 was tested 3 times (−) ivacaftor and 5 times (+) ivacaftor **(Table 2)**. In the (−) ivacaftor condition, the C-sweat response to the β-adrenergic cocktail was not completely absent for this pancreatic sufficient subject. One gland (G43, arrows in **Fig. 7**) in the region of interest (ROI) and two glands outside the ROI (glands A, B in **Fig. 7A-C**) responded to cocktail in the (−) ivacaftor condition on all 3 tests. Using just the glands in the ROI gave a response rate of 3/153 (1.9%).

C-sweating increased unequivocally in the (+) ivacaftor condition (**Figs. 7, 8**). After starting ivacaftor, 53–85% of the glands responded on each test, with an average response rate of 75±15% (SD) across the 5 tests. **Fig. 8A** shows the mean final volumes of C-sweat for each of 8 tests. C-sweat volume (−) ivacaftor could be measured in only one gland so the average was almost undetectable (0.007 nl^{-gland} accumulated over the 30 min observation period), but in the presence of ivacaftor 53 glands produced an average of 0.71±0.04 nl^{-gland} during the 30 min period. The C/M-sweat ratio expressed as a% of the WT mean was 0.01% (−) ivacaftor and was 2.2±0.6% (SD) (+) ivacaftor (**Fig. 9B**). Mean responses for each of the 53 glands (±) ivacaftor are shown in **Fig. 9C, D** where each point is the mean of 5 M-sweat responses (x axis) and 5 C/M ratios as a% of the mean WT value (y axis). The response rate for 10 selected glands is shown in **Fig. 8E**.

As we did for S1 and S2, we performed an additional analysis by dichotomizing the C-sweat response before conducting a logistic mixed model analysis of the raw responses. The effect of ivacaftor was significant [P(C-sweat) was estimated to be.8065 and.0085 in the (+) and (−) ivacaftor conditions, respectively, $p<.0001$]. Like S2 but unlike S1, S8's M-sweat values did not differ between (+) and (−) ivacaftor (46.1 versus 46.0 nl^{-gland}, $p>.9$; see **Fig. 8F**). Consistent with the other subjects tested in this way, glands differed significantly from one another in their typical M-sweat rates ($p<.0001$), but not in their sensitivity to ivacaftor ($p>.45$). In predicting P(C-sweat) from M-sweat response (+) ivacaftor, M-sweat (on a log scale) was a significant predictor of P(C-sweat) ($b=2.00$, $p<.0001$), with M-sweat levels varying from −0.064 to 4.998, and P(C-sweat) levels from 0.0013 to 0.9711 (**Appendix S1**).

Study of a CF subject with two responsive mutations: G551D/R117H-5T

Subject 4 (**S4**, female, G551D/R117H-5T) has two mutations that are each expected to respond to ivacaftor. This led us to expect a greater response, but she also had the fewest glands and lowest M-sweat rate of any subject, which predicted a smaller C-sweat response as noted above. S4 was tested 3 times (+) ivacaftor (**Table 2**). We identified 40 glands; 2 are shown in (**Fig. 9A, B**). M-sweating was measured from 32–37 of these gland on each trial (the lowest number for any subject). Of these, 13 (40%) also produced C-sweat on at least one of the three tests. On average, 22% of glands (range 15–30%) in a given trial produced C-sweat. The C/M ratios for responding glands ranged from 0.7% to 11.4% of the mean C/M ratio for WT subjects (**Fig. 9C**); the average ratio for all glands was 1.31% WT. The response time course (**Fig. 9D**) was similar to other subjects, presumably reflecting the offsetting factors of a larger response to ivacaftor and a smaller M-sweat rate. The C/M ratio increased significantly as a function of the M-sweat rate ($r=0.61$, $p=0.00003$). M-sweat response (on a log scale) was a significant predictor of P(C-sweat) ($b=2.03$, $p<.0001$), with M-sweat levels varying from −0.60 to 3.78, and the P(C-sweat) levels from 0.0005 to 0.7876 (**Appendix S1**).

Responses of a control subject

As stated in methods, the comparison C/M ratio for the CF subjects in this study was the mean C/M ratio of 0.2651 obtained from 6 healthy control subjects in our initial report of the bioassay [10]. As an additional, contemporaneous control, we tested a female healthy control 4 times using an identical protocol. Summary results are shown in **Fig. 10** and **Table 2**). For this subject the ROI contained 51 identified glands. The mean M-sweat final volume for the 15 min test period was 33.9± 1.8 nl^{-gland} (51 glands, 4 tests); means for individual tests were: 35.9±2.0, 37.0±2.1, 28.8±1.8 and 36.5±3.2 $nl^{-gland-30\ min}$ (**Fig. 10A**, open columns). C-sweating was observed for all but one gland in one test. The mean final volume of C-sweat for the 30 min observation period was 10.24±0.77 nl^{-gland}; mean values for each of the four trials were: 9.7±0.7, 9.4±0.7 11.5±1.0 and 10.5±0.9 (**Fig 10A**, blue columns). The mean C/M ratio was 0.143±0.005; ratios for each test were: 0.129±0.006, 0.124±0.004, 0.203±0.015 and 0.178±0.016 (**Fig. 10B**). **Fig. 10C** plots the gland-by-gland comparison of C-sweating (as C/M ratio as a percent of the previously determined WT mean)

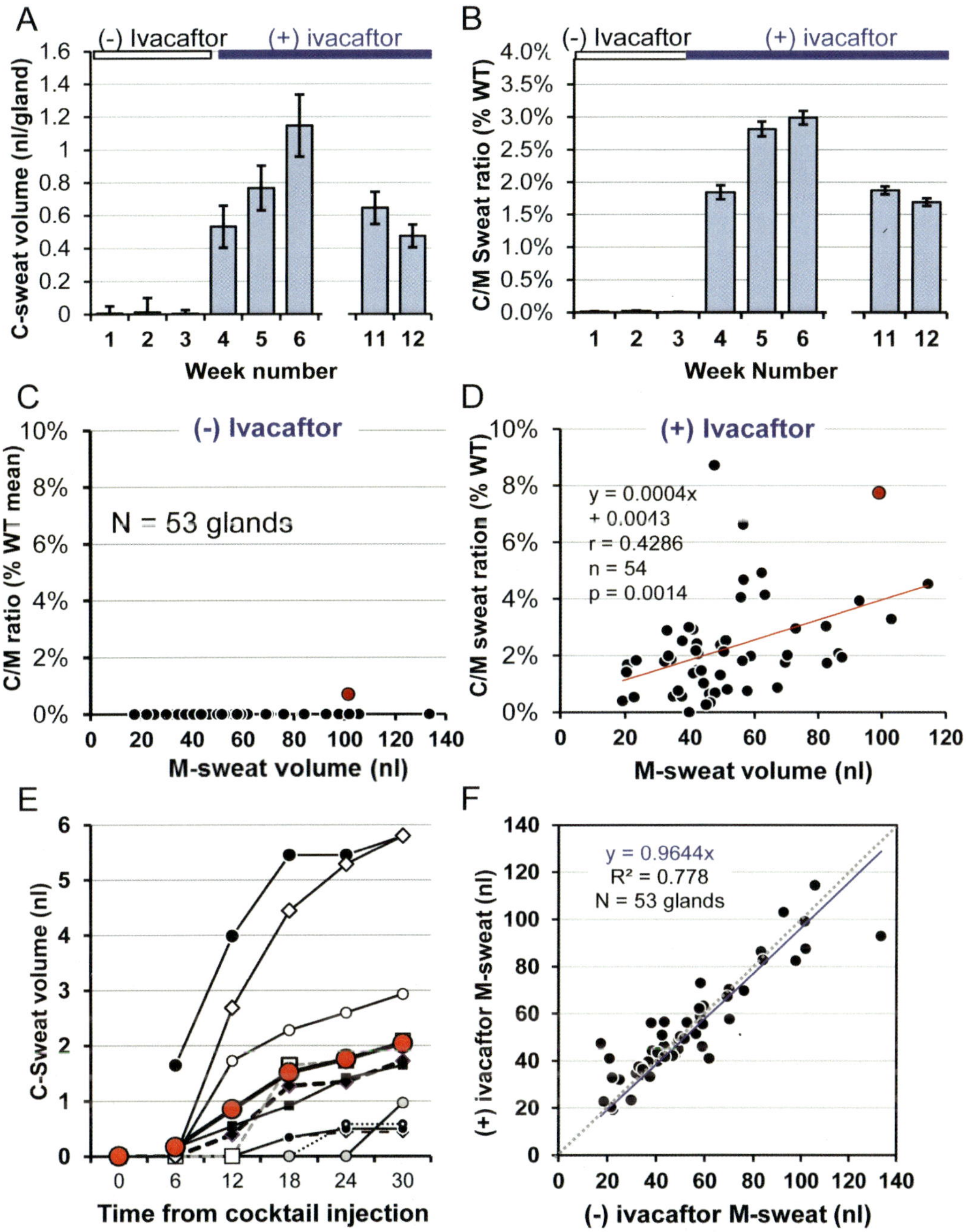

Figure 8. Summary data for S8, R117H-5T, (±) ivacaftor. (A) Mean ± SEM for the final (30 min) volume of C-sweat secretion per gland (50–53 glands measured for each test) (±) ivacaftor. (B) C-sweat/M-sweat ratios expressed as percent of the WT mean. Results are means ± SEM for 49–53 glands per test. (C-D) Gland-by-gland correlations of M-sweat and C-sweat responses in the absence (C), and presence (D) of ivacaftor. Each symbol represents a single gland and shows its average C/M ratio expressed as a% of the WT average (y-axis) vs. its mean M-sweat volume (x-axis). A single gland (G43) in the original ROI produced C-sweat (−) ivacaftor (red symbol); this gland had the second highest C/M ratio in the (+) ivacaftor condition (red symbol). In the (+) ivacaftor condition, 92% of the glands in the ROI produced C-sweat on at least one of the 3 trials, at C/M ratios 0.3%–8.7% of the mean WT C/M ratio. (E) C-sweat volume vs. time for 10 responding glands selected to represent the range of responses for S8 (+) ivacaftor. β-adrenergic cocktail injected at time 0. (F) Absence of ivacaftor effect on M-sweating in this subject. Each point represents a single identified sweat gland, and shows the average M-sweat volumes from 3 tests (−) ivacaftor (x-axis) and 5 tests (+) ivacaftor (y-axis). Dashed 45 degree line indicates equivalence; linear fit does not differ significantly from it.

vs. M-sweat. The overall C/M ratio for this control subject was 54±0.02% of the WT average, which is at the lower end of the range for the WT subjects (range: 52–142%). A significantly positive trend between the C/M ratio and M-sweat volumes was also observed in this WT subject; $r = 0.55$, $p = 0.00002$. The response time course for C-sweating of 11 selected glands from one test is shown in **Fig. 10D**; unlike the CF subjects, all glands had produced measureable C-sweat volumes by 12 min post-injection.

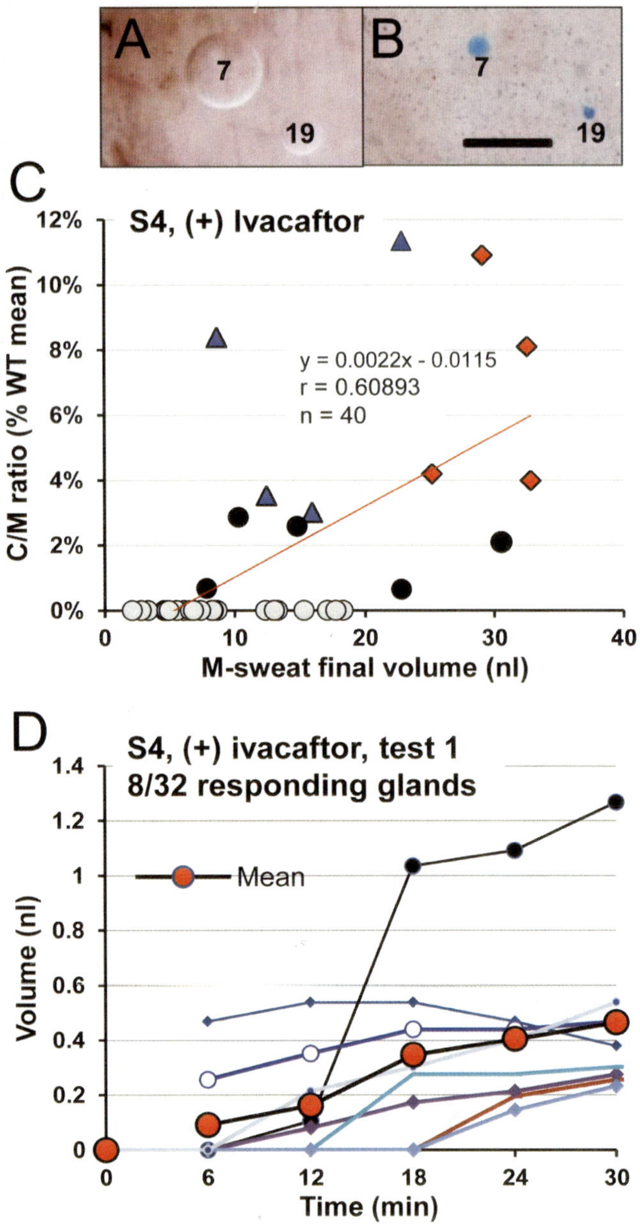

Figure 9. Summary data for S4, a female CF subject having two potentially responsive mutations: G551D & R117H-5T who was tested 3 times (+) ivacaftor. (A) Examples of M-sweat. (B) Examples of C-sweat. Calibration =0.5 mm. (C) Gland-by-gland correlations of M- and C-sweating using same conventions as previous figures. Symbols: Filled circles, C-sweat on 1/3 trials, blue triangles, 2/3 trials and red diamonds, 3/3 trials. (D) Volume vs. time plots for C-sweating from a single experiment (test 1). β-adrenergic cocktail injected at time 0.

Individual differences across subjects and sensitivity of the C/M ratio to sweat gland secretory capacity

Table 1 shows summary results for all 6 G551D CF subjects; **Table 2** has the summary results for the other subjects.

Fig. 11 provides summary data and analyses for all 6 CF subjects tested (+) ivacaftor. **Fig. 11A** plots the mean C/M ratios (left axis, blue columns) and M-sweat rates (right axis, red symbols that also indicate the subject's gender). Mean single gland M-sweat rates (probably determined mainly by gland size) varied widely and were larger for males. (The number [density] of glands also varies widely among individuals, but because we use individual glands as the units of analysis, this factor was not confounded with secretion rate, as it is in most sweat assays.) **Fig. 11B** plots the percentage of identified glands from each subject that produced measurable volumes of C-sweat. The G551D subjects differed significantly from one another in the proportion of glands that produced measureable C-sweat (ANOVA, $F = 54.8$, $p = 0.001$). **Fig. 11C** plots the C/M ratios after equating M-sweat rates. Because C-sweating is jointly dependent on M-sweating and CFTR function, we isolated CFTR's contribution by selecting a subset of glands from each subject such that the average M-sweat rates for the samples were nearly equivalent (**Fig. 11C**, right axis, red squares). The corresponding C/M ratios for these matched samples of glands (**Fig. 11C**, left axis, blue columns,) show that G551D subjects still differ widely: e.g. S5's ratio is ~7-fold >S1's. Even so, the differences within G551D subjects are overshadowed by the much higher C/M ratio seen in R117H-5T subject 8, and in S4, who, with two responsive mutations, had the highest C/M ratio after partially correcting for M-sweat rate.

A consistent result of this study is that the C/M ratio in subjects with low C-sweat rates is positively correlated with M-sweat rates (**Figs. 2C, 3C, 4A, 5A, 8D** and **9C** and **10A**). This relationship is summarized for all subjects in **Fig. 12A**. It was previously hypothesized that the positive correlation resulted from at least two subtractive processes: physical capacitance (filling of gland lumen before sweat emerges) and absorption of sweat volume in the duct [10]. These have negligible consequences at high sweat rates, but become progressively evident at lower sweat rates. If this hypothesis is correct, it follows that the larger values for each subject, rather than the average for all glands, should more accurately quantify CFTR function. Accordingly, **Fig. 13** (blue columns, left axis) plots for each subject the mean C/M (% WT) of the 12 glands having the highest M-sweat rates, which yielded C/M ratios from <1%–4.5% of the mean WT ratio. The red columns in **Fig. 13** are based on an additional correction that incorporates data from single channel measurements (see discussion).

Discussion

Our first goal in this study was to determine if this bioassay could detect improved CFTR function in CF subjects with G551D or R117H-5T mutations who were taking ivacaftor. We knew before starting that ivacaftor increases G551D CFTR function sufficiently to benefit health [4,5]. Therefore, the positive results with these subjects validate the assay rather than the compound. But no clinical data were available on ivacaftor treated R117H-5T subjects, so our finding of a strong ivacaftor effect for subjects with this compound allele provides *in vivo* support for the prediction that ivacaftor will be therapeutic in such patients [2].

A second goal was to determine if the assay could detect individual differences among the subjects. In fact, we observed large (~6-fold), inter-subject differences in C-sweat responses among the four G551D subjects taking ivacaftor, after correcting for M-sweat rates (**Fig. 11C**). Individual differences could arise from different G551D-CFTR expression levels, differences in transport processes affecting CFTR-dependent sweat secretion, drug pharmacokinetics/tissue distribution, different responses of the in trans F508del allele, and compliance. Such differences are expected to have clinical implications. We were blinded to results from clinical studies of these subjects, but it will be possible to compare the two data sets in the future.

A third goal was to determine if the assay could quantify the extent to which ivacaftor restored function to G551D and

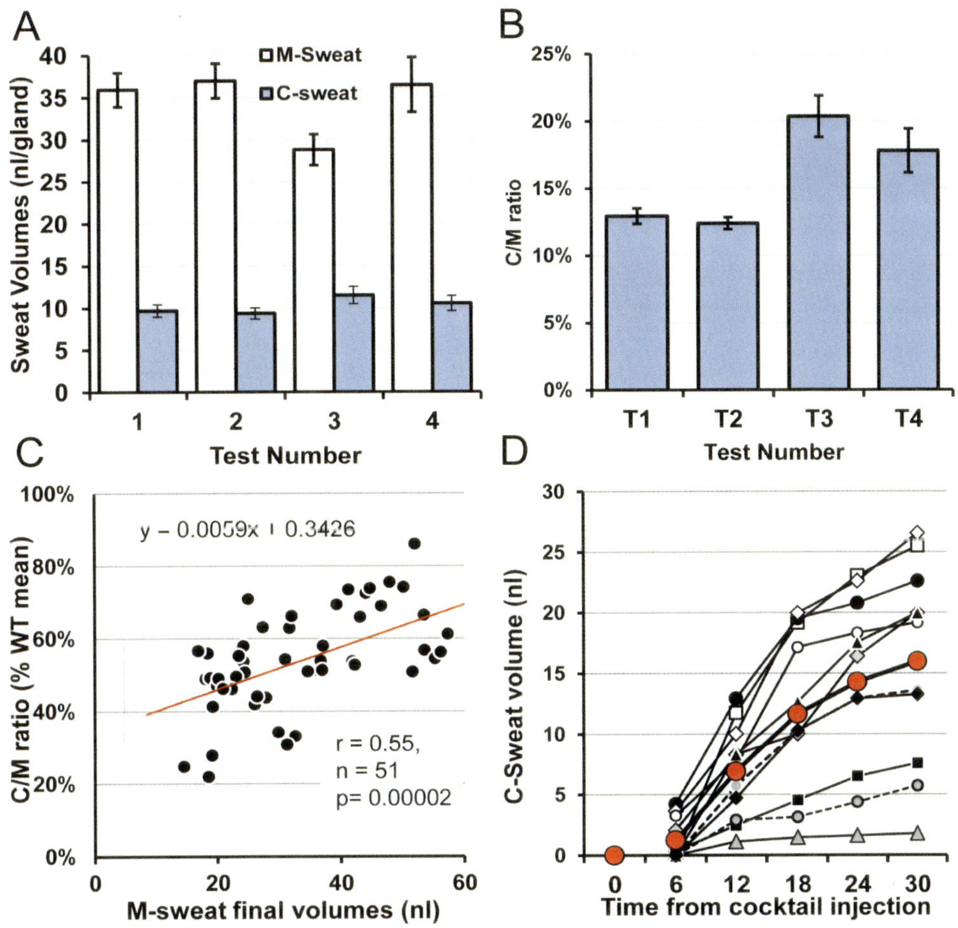

Figure 10. M- and C-sweating in a female, healthy control subject. (A) M-sweat and C-sweat responses for each of 4 tests (Mean ± SEM, n = 51 glands). Each open bar is the average final M-sweat volume in response to 15 min stimulation with MCh; each blue bar is the average final C-sweat volume in response to 30 min of β-adrenergic cocktail. (B) C-sweat/M-sweat ratios for each test. (C) Gland-by-gland correlation of mean C/M sweat ratios, expressed as a% of the WT average, vs. the mean M-sweat response. Each symbol represents mean values for a single gland based on ~4 tests. Responses for this subject were at the low end of the control range. (D) Time course of C-sweating in 11 responsive glands selected to cover the range of C-sweat secretion rates.

R117H-5T CFTR. We hypothesized that primary C-sweat (as elaborated in the secretory coil) provides an accurate readout of CFTR function [10], and that some primary secretion was occurring in most treated glands. However, because subtractive processes reduce the volume of primary C-sweat, uncorrected C-sweating underestimates CFTR function. Therefore, we used independent evidence about channel number and P_O to correct for the losses.

CF is caused by reductions in apical membrane conductance mediated by CFTR, which in turn is a function of channel number, open probability, and single channel conductance: $G_{CFTR} = nP_O\gamma$. The P_O of WT CFTR is ~0.4, e.g. ref. [2]. When considering channel number (n), it is necessary to take account of wide variations arising especially from the length of a polythymidine tract in intron 8 [13]. This tract is found as 3 variable repeat alleles of 9T, 7T or 5T, which in the non-CF population exist in proportions of ~9%, 80% and 11% respectively [20]. The tract length influences splicing of exon 9 such that as tract length shortens, exon 9 skipping increases, resulting in less functional CFTR [13]. With the 5T allele, only ~10% of full-length, functional CFTR is produced, *vs.* 50–100% with 7T and >95% with 9T [13]. Furthermore, a variable TG repeat also affects the number of functional CFTR transcripts [21]. Thus, healthy controls have a wide range of CFTR (n) and hence CFTR function. Importantly, this variation is seldom considered when assessing the operation of most organs with *in vivo* assays, because CFTR function is logarithmically related to most outputs (e.g. sweat chloride, **Fig. 14**) and hence is not rate limiting until it approaches zero (which is why CF is a recessive disease). However, CFTR *is* rate-limiting for C-sweating, which accounts for its linear output [10,22] and (**Fig. 14**). Thus, variation in CFTR (n) is expected to be expressed quantitatively in the C/M sweat ratio. Indeed, the C/M ratio varied 3-fold among 6 healthy controls tested with this method [10] and varied 4-fold among 19 controls in the original study of C/M ratios using a different method [22]. In both studies CF heterozygotes showed a similar dispersion around a mean C/M value half that of the healthy controls [10,22]. On average, healthy control subjects have 70% full length transcripts [13], which we used to set the average WT value for n in the following estimates of CFTR function, i.e. we assume that ~70% transcripts gave the mean C/M ratio of 0.265 for healthy controls [10]. With this background, we first consider results for the R117H-5T subject.

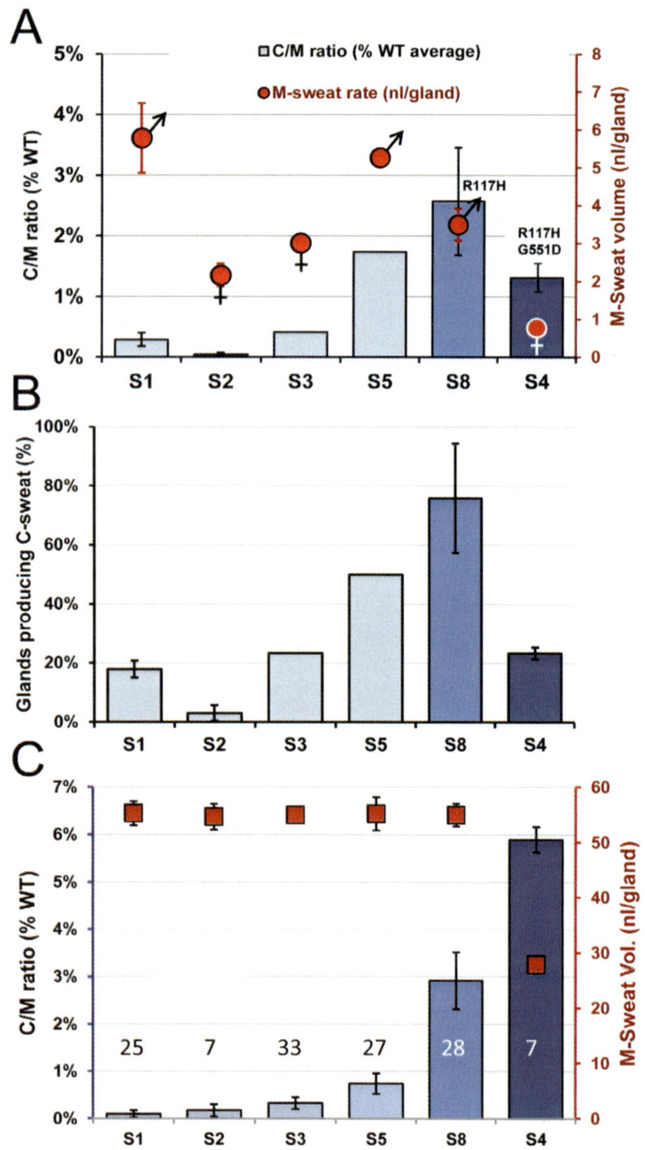

Figure 11. Summary of CFTR-dependent sweat secretion for six CF subjects (+) ivacaftor. (A) Columns (left axis) show C-sweat/M-sweat ratios (mean ± SEM) for each subject, expressed as% of mean WT value. Filled red gender signs (right axis) show M-sweat rates for each subject in the presence of ivacaftor (Mean ± SD). Error bars for S1, S4 and S8 are based on 3 tests, S2 on 2 tests. S1-S3 and S5 each has one G551D mutation, S8 has R117H-5T, and S4 has both. (B) Percentage of glands producing C-sweat in each subject (Mean ± S.D). For healthy control and CF heterozygote (carrier) subjects this value is 97–99±3% [10]. (C) C/M ratios (+) ivacaftor at equivalent M-sweat rates. Filled red squares (right axis) show M-sweat rates (mean ± S.D) for a sample of 7–33 glands from each subject chosen to give a mean M-sweat volume of ~55 nl^{-gland} (= 3.67 $nl^{-min-gland}$). Columns (left axis) show C/M ratios (mean ± SEM), expressed as% of mean WT value for the same sample of glands. Numbers indicate sample size for each subject. S4 had the fewest glands and the lowest M-sweat rates, which prevented matching her sample to the others.

Quantifying R117H-5T CFTR function in vivo and in vitro

R117H-5T CFTR retains partial function and confers pancreatic sufficiency when *trans* to a severe allele. Studies of heterologously expressed CFTR channels by Sheppard and colleagues [12] found that the whole-cell Cl^- conductance of R117H was reduced to 15% of WT, while single channel analysis found that both P_O and γ were reduced predicting ~24% WT CFTR channel function. In a male and a female each having R117H/R117H on a 7T/7T background, all clinical indices were normal except for CBAVD in the male, electrophysiological measurements of nasal and intestinal epithelia were also normal, and sweat chloride values were 34 mM for the male and 42 mM for the female [23]. However, when R117H-CFTR is in *cis* with a 5T allele, n = 0.1/0.7 = 14% WT, reducing R117H-5T function to 2.1–3.7% of WT function. If the other allele is nonfunctional, as it is in S8, the expected residual function will be 1.1%–1.85% of WT (average 1.5%). Remarkably then, <2% of CFTR function, if also found in the pancreas, appears to be sufficient to confer pancreatic sufficiency and to reduce sweat chloride levels from 100 to ~80 mM [24].

To estimate the amount of primary sweat in S8 that was lost in the (−) ivacaftor condition, we assigned a CFTR functional level = 1.5% WT to S8, based on the above analysis of R117H-5T function [12,13]. For S8's 12 glands with highest M-sweat rates, the predicted rate of C-sweating, if he were a WT subject, would be 1.59 $nl^{-min-gland}$, and 1.5% of that value = 0.024 $nl^{-min-gland}$. However, we observed only 0.001 $nl^{-min-gland}$, leading to a loss estimate of 0.023 $nl^{-min-gland}$. If ivacaftor restored normal P_O to R117H and left n and γ unchanged, it would increase R117H-5T CFTR function equivalent to 5T function on 1 allele, or 7% of WT. The C/M ratio for the top 12 glands of S8 (+) ivacaftor was 4.51% of WT (left axis, blue column, **Fig. 12B**). Correcting for the loss estimate increased the C/M ratio to 6.1% of WT (right axis, red column, **Fig. 12B**). Thus, in this R117H-5T subject, functional estimates based on patch-clamp [12] and mRNA transcript analysis [13] converged with those of based on C/M-sweat bubble analysis.

Quantifying G551D CFTR function in vivo and in vitro

The G551D mutation severely decreases P_O to near zero (~0.004) without a known effect on n or γ [15]. The calculations used above predict that this level of function is invisible to the sweat bubble test, consistent with the lack of any observed sweating in the 4 G551D subjects tested (−) ivacaftor. The P_O of G551D-CFTR (+)-ivacaftor has been measured as 0.04 [14] and 0.12 [2] or 10–30% of the WT value of 0.4. Subjects S1–S3 and S5 each have one G551D and one (nonfunctional) F508del allele, so their ivacaftor-potentiated CFTR function should have been half of those values or 5–15% of WT. C/M ratios from the top 12 M-sweat rate glands (**Fig. 12A, B**) gave values of 0.24% to 2.77%, and correcting for the loss estimate of 0.023 $nl^{-min-gland}$ gave 1.56% for S1 to 4.08% for S5. The highest value is similar to the estimate of ~5% CFTR function predicted from the ivacaftor-potentiated P_O value of 0.04 [**14**]. Based on all the data and on comparisons with the ivacaftor-treated R117H subject, we estimate ivacaftor-potentiated CFTR function in G551D/F508del subjects to be <5% WT.

Subject S4 has mutations R117H-5T and G551D. In the (+) ivacaftor condition, the data from patch clamp and transcript analysis predicts CFTR function of 2.6–5% function for R117H-5T, and up to 5% for G551D, or up to 10% function for the combination. The corrected C/M value for this subject was 7.7%, the highest value observed, consistent with an additive effect of ivacaftor acting on both mutations.

Does ivacaftor increase M-sweating?

The present experiments do not answer that question. Two of 3 subjects where M-sweating was tested (+/−) ivacaftor did not show a change. The increased M-sweating seen in S1 (+) ivacaftor occurred in tests that were run over a 6 month period, and two

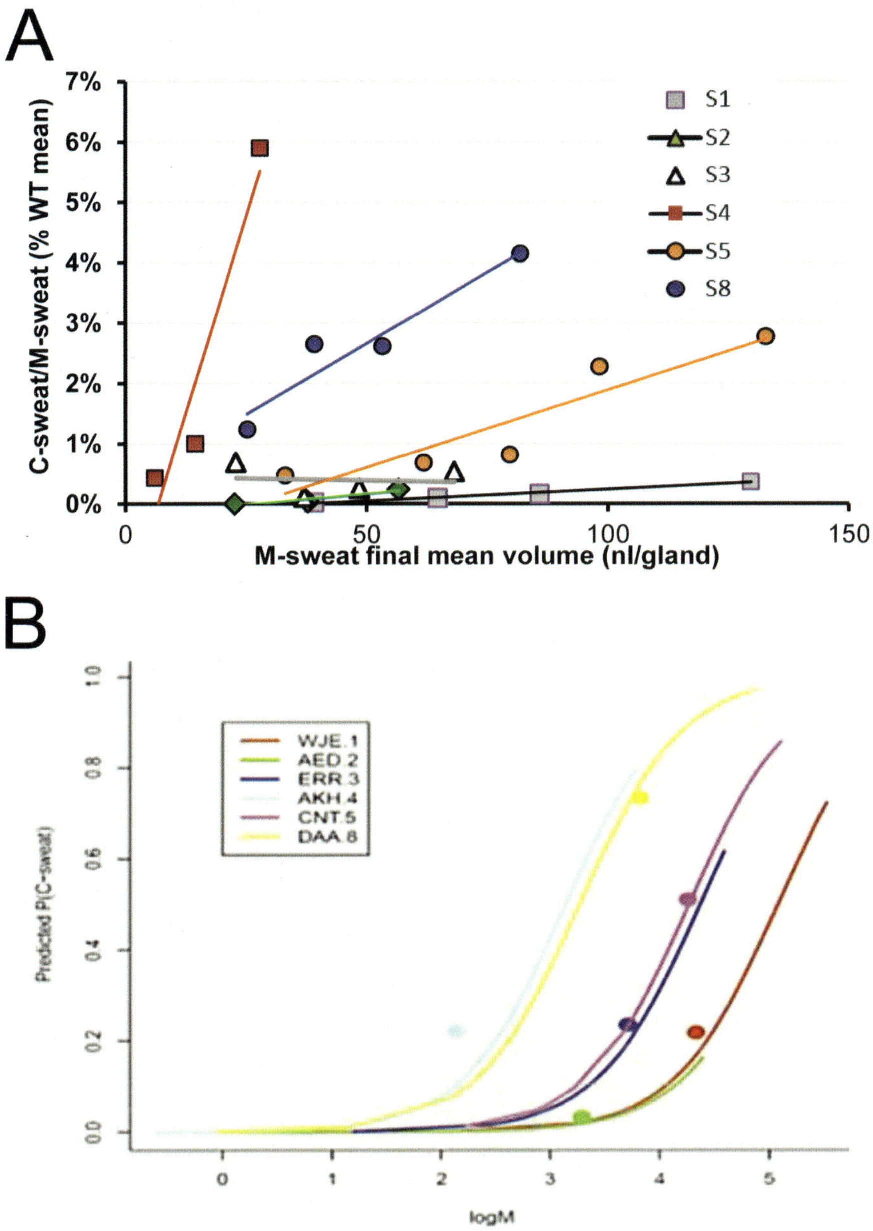

Figure 12. C-sweat values as a function of M-sweat rates. (A) Summary data showing dependence of C/M ratios to M-sweat rates for all 6 subjects tested (+) ivacaftor. For clarity, each subject's glands, glands were rank ordered according to their M-sweat rates and then divided into 3–5 bins according to their M-sweat rates (mean of 16.6 glands per bin). Each point plots the average M-sweat response on the x-axis and the average C/M ratio as a% of the WT mean on the y-axis for each bin; lines are linear fits. Each gland was measured 1–3 times, and the average number of glands included in each bin was 16.6 (range 5–26 glands). C/M vs. M-sweat correlations were significant for all subjects except S3. (B) C-sweat response is coded as 1, if some C-sweat is observed on a test, and 0, otherwise; and P(C-sweat) denotes the probability that C-sweat is observed. Then P(C-sweat) is also the average of the recoded 0/1 C-sweat response. We predicted P(C-sweat) as a function of log M-sweat using the combined data from all 6 CF subjects tested (+) ivacaftor. A logistic mixed model analysis showed that CF patients differed in their overall P(C-sweat) levels, but not in the within-patient effect of M-sweat response on P(C-sweat) across glands ($p > .57$), and that the average across patients of the within-patient effect of M-sweat was significantly positive ($b = 2.14$, $p < .0001$). The predicted P(C-sweat) levels are plotted for each patient. See methods and Appendix S1.

(−) ivacaftor tests in winter months gave lower values than any other tests. There was no opportunity to test again off-drug. M-sweating has been considered to be CFTR-independent because of its persistence in CF subjects [16,17], but CFTR contributes to cholinergically-mediated fluid secretion in several tissues and species [25,26,27,28,29,30,31]. Stimulation of M3 muscarinic receptors strongly activates CFTR when both are expressed in BHK cells [32], and apical UTP activates CFTR in primary human airway cells [33]. It is possible that CFTR is activated during M-sweating, but its contribution may be masked by a high apical conductance conferred by CaCC channels.

Limitations

Four limitations specific to the present study are that it was done open label, with a small number of subjects, the results could not be correlated with clinical or sweat chloride data because of

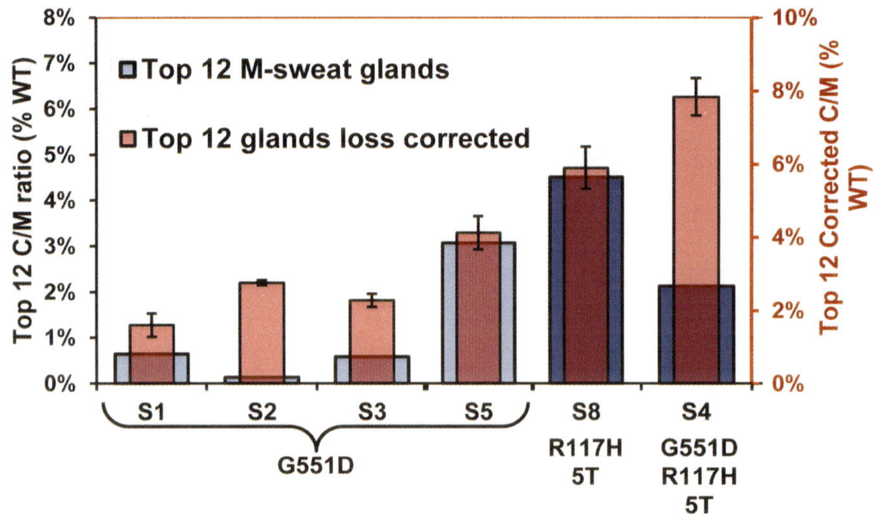

Figure 13. Loss-reduced and loss-corrected estimates of CFTR function in CF subjects (+) ivacaftor. Each blue column (left axis) shows mean C/M ratios (mean ± SEM) for the 12 glands with the highest M-sweat rates for each subject; higher sweat rates reduce C-sweat losses. Each transparent red column (right axis) shows the corrected C/M ratios (mean ± SEM) for the 12 fastest M-secreting glands, obtained by adding 0.029 $nl^{-min-gland}$ to the observed C-sweat secretion rates (see text).

ongoing studies, and only two subjects were tested with triplicate (±) ivacaftor tests. The inaccessibility of subjects for repeated (±) testing was our main concern, because the assay is well suited for n-of-1 studies where each subject (and each gland) serves as its own control [34,35,36,37]. It will be important to carry out more n-of-1 studies with ivacaftor in which this assay is one component of the assessment, and to establish the assay in other laboratories. Because of large and consistent individual differences in measurements of healthy controls, it will be important to expand the number control subjects and to correlate their results with genotype, sweat chloride, and CFTR transcript analysis.

Conclusions

Multiple measures of C-sweating and M-sweating from individual glands revealed that oral dosing with ivacaftor improved β-adrenergic cocktail-stimulated, CFTR-dependent sweating (C-sweating) in CF subjects with G551D or R117H-5T mutations. The C/M ratio across all measured glands was smaller than predicted based on patch clamp/transcript analyses. We hypothesize that this resulted from a proportionally larger loss of sweat volume via ductal absorption and gland capacitance at lower sweat rates. After correcting for these losses, estimated CFTR

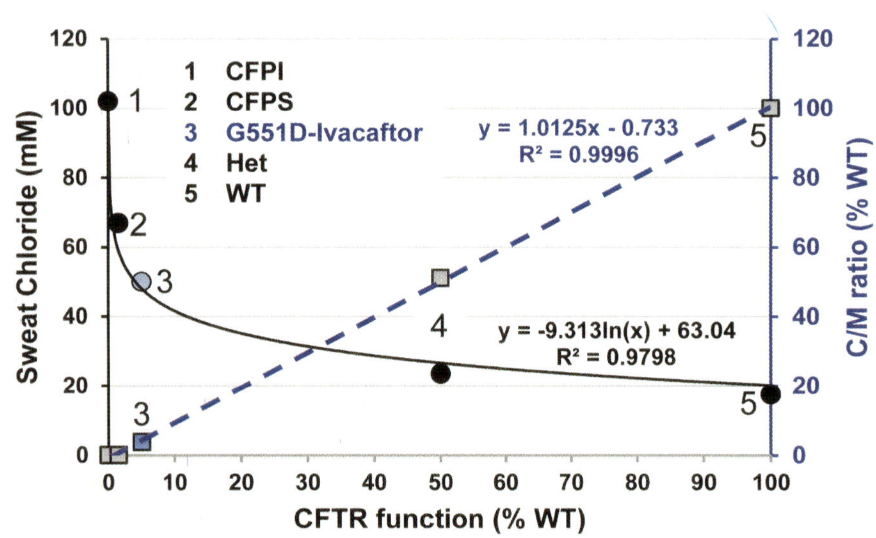

Figure 14. Two measures of CFTR function in the sweat gland. The sweat chloride concentration (left y axis,) is plotted (solid line) against CFTR function as a% of average WT values, plotted on the x axis. Sweat chloride is an inverse logarithmic function of CFTR function (n $P_O\,\gamma$) and hence is most sensitive at the lowest levels of CFTR function. The C-sweat/M-sweat ratio as% WT (right axis), is plotted (dashed line) against CFTR function as a% of average WT values, plotted on the x axis. The C/M ratio provides a direct readout of CFTR function and is linear over most of the range; the loss-reduced and loss-corrected values extend the linear range close to zero CFTR function. Sweat chloride point 3 is from ref. [5], the rest are from ref. [38]. C/M point 3 is from present paper, other points are from ref. [10]. CFTR values 0, 50 and 100 are defined, 1.5% and 5% function assigned by patch clamp and mRNA measures.

function was 2.66±1.06% of WT for the 4 G551D subjects, 6.1% for the R117H-5T subject, and 7.7% for the subject with both mutations. The finding that CFTR-dependent sweat secretion was greater in R117H-5T than in G551D subjects supports prior work suggesting that ivacaftor will be clinically useful for subjects with the R117H-5T mutation [6]. In sum, the corrected *in vivo* estimates of restored CFTR function overlap estimates based on patch clamp data, and suggest that excellent clinical responses can be expected by restoring less than 10% of CFTR function.

Acknowledgments

We are grateful to the subjects who participated in these trials and in previous trials required to develop this assay. We thank Dr. Iris Schrijver, Stanford Medical Center for genotyping the healthy control, and Jonathan Chen, Julie Desch, Nam Soo Joo, Franklin B. Krasne, Mauri Krouse, Sara E. Modlin, Olivia Peeps, Barkha Tiwana, and members of the Cystic Fibrosis Foundation Therapeutics Sweat Consortium for valuable assistance and discussions.

Author Contributions

Conceived and designed the experiments: JJW. Performed the experiments: JEC MHW HJC IHP JHJ JJW. Analyzed the data: JEC JJW MHW EACT. Contributed reagents/materials/analysis tools: EF EACT. Wrote the paper: JJW EACT RBM JEC. Recruited subjects: CD ZD CM. Supplied relevant clinical data: CD ZD CM. Discussed interpretations: CD ZD CM.

References

1. Sosnay PR, Siklosi KR, Van Goor F, Kaniecki K, Yu H, et al. (2013) Defining the disease liability of variants in the cystic fibrosis transmembrane conductance regulator gene. Nat Genet.
2. Yu H, Burton B, Huang CJ, Worley J, Cao D, et al. (2012) Ivacaftor potentiation of multiple CFTR channels with gating mutations. Journal of cystic fibrosis: official journal of the European Cystic Fibrosis Society 11: 237–245.
3. Van Goor F, Hadida S, Grootenhuis PD, Burton B, Cao D, et al. (2009) Rescue of CF airway epithelial cell function in vitro by a CFTR potentiator, VX-770. Proc Natl Acad Sci U S A 106: 18825–18830.
4. Accurso FJ, Rowe SM, Clancy JP, Boyle MP, Dunitz JM, et al. (2010) Effect of VX-770 in persons with cystic fibrosis and the G551D-CFTR mutation. N Engl J Med 363: 1991–2003.
5. Ramsey BW, Davies J, McElvaney NG, Tullis E, Bell SC, et al. (2011) A CFTR potentiator in patients with cystic fibrosis and the G551D mutation. The New England journal of medicine 365: 1663–1672.
6. Van Goor F, Yu H, Burton B, Huang C, Hoffman B (2012) Ivacaftor potentiates multiple mutant cystic fibrosis transconductance regulator (CFTR) forms. Pediatr Pulmonol 47: 233.
7. Drumm ML, Konstan MW, Schluchter MD, Handler A, Pace R, et al. (2005) Genetic modifiers of lung disease in cystic fibrosis. N Engl J Med 353: 1443–1453.
8. Guo X, Pace RG, Stonebraker JR, Commander CW, Dang AT, et al. (2011) Mucin variable number tandem repeat polymorphisms and severity of cystic fibrosis lung disease: significant association with MUC5AC. PLoS One 6: e25452.
9. Veeze HJ, Halley DJ, Bijman J, de Jongste JC, de Jonge HR, et al. (1994) Determinants of mild clinical symptoms in cystic fibrosis patients. Residual chloride secretion measured in rectal biopsies in relation to the genotype. The Journal of clinical investigation 93: 461–466.
10. Wine JJ, Char JE, Chen J, Cho HJ, Dunn C, et al. (2013) In Vivo Readout of CFTR Function: Ratiometric Measurement of CFTR-Dependent Secretion by Individual, Identifiable Human Sweat Glands. PLoS One 8: e77114.
11. Farber S (1945) Some organic digestive disturbances in early life. J Mich Med Soc 44: 587.
12. Sheppard DN, Rich DP, Ostedgaard LS, Gregory RJ, Smith AE, et al. (1993) Mutations in CFTR associated with mild-disease-form Cl- channels with altered pore properties. Nature 362: 160–164.
13. Chu CS, Trapnell BC, Curristin S, Cutting GR, Crystal RG (1993) Genetic basis of variable exon 9 skipping in cystic fibrosis transmembrane conductance regulator mRNA. Nat Genet 3: 151–156.
14. Jih KY, Hwang TC (2013) Vx-770 potentiates CFTR function by promoting decoupling between the gating cycle and ATP hydrolysis cycle. Proc Natl Acad Sci U S A 110: 4404–4409.
15. Bompadre SG, Sohma Y, Li M, Hwang TC (2007) G551D and G1349D, two CF-associated mutations in the signature sequences of CFTR, exhibit distinct gating defects. J Gen Physiol 129: 285–298.
16. Cooke RE, Gochberg SH (1956) Physiology of the sweat gland in cystic fibrosis of the pancreas. Pediatrics 18: 701–715.
17. Bijman J, Quinton PM (1984) Influence of abnormal Cl- impermeability on sweating in cystic fibrosis. Am J Physiol 247: C3–9.
18. Cheng SH, Gregory RJ, Marshall J, Paul S, Souza DW, et al. (1990) Defective intracellular transport and processing of CFTR is the molecular basis of most cystic fibrosis. Cell 63: 827–834.
19. Champigny G, Imler JL, Puchelle E, Dalemans W, Gribkoff V, et al. (1995) A change in gating mode leading to increased intrinsic Cl- channel activity compensates for defective processing in a cystic fibrosis mutant corresponding to a mild form of the disease. EMBO J 14: 2417–2423.
20. Friedman KJ, Heim RA, Knowles MR, Silverman LM (1997) Rapid characterization of the variable length polythymidine tract in the cystic fibrosis (CFTR) gene: association of the 5T allele with selected CFTR mutations and its incidence in atypical sinopulmonary disease. Hum Mutat 10: 108–115.
21. Cuppens H, Lin W, Jaspers M, Costes B, Teng H, et al. (1998) Polyvariant mutant cystic fibrosis transmembrane conductance regulator genes. The polymorphic (Tg)m locus explains the partial penetrance of the T5 polymorphism as a disease mutation. J Clin Invest 101: 487–496.
22. Behm JK, Hagiwara G, Lewiston NJ, Quinton PM, Wine JJ (1987) Hyposecretion of beta-adrenergically induced sweating in cystic fibrosis heterozygotes. Pediatr Res 22: 271–276.
23. de Nooijer RA, Nobel JM, Arets HG, Bot AG, van Berkhout FT, et al. (2011) Assessment of CFTR function in homozygous R117H-7T subjects. J Cyst Fibros 10: 326–332.
24. Wilschanski M, Zielenski J, Markiewicz D, Tsui LC, Corey M, et al. (1995) Correlation of sweat chloride concentration with classes of the cystic fibrosis transmembrane conductance regulator gene mutations. J Pediatr 127: 705–710.
25. Taylor CJ, Baxter PS, Hardcastle J, Hardcastle PT (1988) Failure to induce secretion in jejunal biopsies from children with cystic fibrosis. Gut 29: 957–962.
26. Berschneider HM, Knowles MR, Azizkhan RG, Boucher RC, Tobey NA, et al. (1988) Altered intestinal chloride transport in cystic fibrosis. Faseb J 2: 2625–2629.
27. Bijman J, Veeze H, Kansen M, Tilly B, Scholte B, et al. (1991) Chloride transport in the cystic fibrosis enterocyte. Adv Exp Med Biol 290: 287–294; discussion 294–286.
28. Salinas D, Haggie PM, Thiagarajah JR, Song Y, Rosbe K, et al. (2005) Submucosal gland dysfunction as a primary defect in cystic fibrosis. Faseb J 19: 431–433.
29. Joo NS, Cho HJ, Khansaheb M, Wine JJ (2010) Hyposecretion of fluid from tracheal submucosal glands of CFTR-deficient pigs. J Clin Invest 120: 3161–3166.
30. Cho HJ, Joo NS, Wine JJ (2011) Defective fluid secretion from submucosal glands of nasal turbinates from CFTR−/− and CFTR (DeltaF508/DeltaF508) pigs. PloS one 6: e24424.
31. Sun X, Sui H, Fisher JT, Yan Z, Liu X, et al. (2010) Disease phenotype of a ferret CFTR-knockout model of cystic fibrosis. J Clin Invest 120: 3149–3160.
32. Billet A, Luo Y, Balghi H, Hanrahan JW (2013) Role of tyrosine phosphorylation in the muscarinic activation of the Cystic Fibrosis Transmembrane conductance Regulator (CFTR). J Biol Chem.
33. Namkung W, Finkbeiner WE, Verkman AS (2010) CFTR-adenylyl cyclase I association responsible for UTP activation of CFTR in well-differentiated primary human bronchial cell cultures. Mol Biol Cell 21: 2639–2648.
34. Rochon J (1990) A statistical model for the "N-of-1" study. Journal of clinical epidemiology 43: 499–508.
35. Spiegelhalter DJ (1988) Statistical issues in studies of individual response. Scandinavian journal of gastroenterology Supplement 147: 40–45.
36. Barlow DH, Hersen M (1984) Single Case Experimental Designs MA, USA: Allyn and Bacon.
37. Kazdin AE (1982) Single-Case Research Designs: Methods for Clinical and Applied Settings. New York, USA: Oxford University Press.
38. Gonska T, Choi P, Stephenson A, Ellis L, Martin S, et al. (2012) Role of Cystic Fibrosis Transmembrane Conductance Regulator (CFTR) in patients with chronic sinopulmonary disease. Chest 142: 996–1004.

Multi-Country Estimate of Different Manifestations of Aspergillosis in Cystic Fibrosis

Joanne Armstead, Julie Morris, David W. Denning*

National Aspergillosis Centre, University Hospital South Manchester, The University of Manchester and Manchester Academic Health Science Centre, Manchester, United Kingdom

Abstract

Aspergillus spp. can lead to allergic bronchopulmonary aspergillosis (ABPA), *Aspergillus* sensitisation and *Aspergillus* bronchitis in CF. The relative frequencies of these entities have recently been ascertained in a large UK adult CF cohort. We have used this data to estimate the burden of aspergillosis and ABPA cases in adult CF patients in 30 countries reporting CF. National and international CF registry data was accessed and assessed for completeness and age distribution. Published proportions of ABPA (17.7%), *Aspergillus* sensitisation (14.6%) and *Aspergillus* bronchitis (30%) in CF were applied to those > 18 years and compared with notified ABPA cases. Of the 76,201 estimated CF patients worldwide (not including India), 37,714 were >18 years. The proportion of adults to children varied from 63% in Norway to 20% in Brazil. ABPA caseload in adults is anticipated to be 6,675 cases of which only 2,221 cases (33%) are currently recorded, indicating substantial underdiagnosis. The ABPA diagnosis rate compared with estimated rates varies by country from 101% (France) to 14.5% (Greece), although genetic variation could account for genuine differences compared with the UK. *Aspergillus* bronchitis is not currently recognised or recorded in CF registries but there are an anticipated 10,988 adult cases. *Aspergillus* sensitisation, associated with increased bronchiectasis and reduced FEV1, affects an anticipated 5,506 patients without ABPA or *Aspergillus* bronchitis. Together ABPA and *Aspergillus* bronchitis are estimated to affect 17,989 adults, 47.7% of the adult CF population. ABPA also occurs in children and teenagers and 984 cases were documented in registries. Diagnosed ABPA rates by age were available for the ECFS registry, USA, UK, Ireland, Belgium and Netherlands. The rate was <1% under 4 years, and increased throughout childhood and adolescence, with marked variation between countries. Newly published diagnostic criteria and methods should facilitate better recognition of aspergillosis in CF, allowing better CF disease control.

Editor: Dominik Hartl, University of Tübingen, Germany

Funding: This work was funded by the University Hospital of South Manchester. The funders had no role in study design, data collection and analysis, decision to publish, or preparation of the manuscript.

Competing Interests: The authors have read the journal's policy and have the following conflicts: Dr. Denning holds founder shares in F2G Ltd a University of Manchester spin-out company and has current grant support from the National Institute of Allergy and Infectious Diseases, National Institute of Health Research, the European Union and AstraZeneca. He acts as a consultant to Trinity group, T2 Biosystems, GSK, as well as other companies over the last 5 years including Pfizer, Schering Plough (now Merck), Astellas and Gilead. In the last 3 years, he has been paid for talks on behalf of Astellas, GSK, Gliead and Pfizer. Armstead and Morris have no conflicts to declare.

* E-mail: ddenning@manchester.ac.uk

Introduction

Cystic fibrosis (CF) is a recessive genetic disorder caused by the mutation of the cystic fibrosis trans membrane conductance regulator (CFTR) gene [1]. The CFTR protein plays a vital role in transporting salt and water across the surface of epithelia [2]. The abnormal function of this protein affects many organs of the body, especially the lung epithelia whereby the production of thick, sticky mucous often results in chronic lung infection and inflammation[2]. *Aspergillus* is a fungus present in both indoor and outdoor environments [3]; however it only tends to cause infection within susceptible individuals, such as those with CF.

Aspergillus fumigatus is the most common species of *Aspergillus* that causes morbidity in patients with CF. Colonisation of this fungus can manifest in various ways such as IgE-mediated sensitisation and allergic bronchopulmonary aspergillosis (ABPA). Varying prevalence of ABPA has frequently been reported since it was first diagnosed in 1965 by Mearns et al [4]. The Epidemiologic Registry of CF data involving 12,447 adult and children CF patients gathered from 224 CF centres within nine European countries was analysed and suggested 7.8% of patients had ABPA [5]. This figure varied between the countries, ranging from 2.1% in Sweden to 13.6% in Belgium. ABPA was also found to be less prevalent in patients below the age of 6 [5]. A similar study involving 14,210 patients from the Epidemiologic Study of CF reported a much lower prevalence of 2% [6]. Other smaller studies have found higher rates of up to 15% patients being diagnosed with ABPA [5,7,8]. There are increased ABPA rates within adolescent [6] and adult populations [9–12]. ABPA is often diagnosed late; on occasions as long as 10 years after presentation [13]. Generally the disease is under-diagnosed globally, and an estimated 4.8 million adults with asthma are affected [14]. Many in asthma cases are still misdiagnosed as pulmonary tuberculosis, [15] with some studies suggesting 17–50% of ABPA cases are misdiagnosed [16]. Early diagnosis would enable better management of aspergillosis and probably an improved prognosis in CF patients.

The proportion of CF patients with *A. fumigatus* colonisation in respiratory secretions ranges from 6% to 58% [16–18]. A retrospective cohort study involving 259 patients found 61 (24%)

were at least intermittently colonized with *A. fumigatus* between 2002 and 2007 [17]. Culture methods vary substantially between centres, and culture is an insensitive means of determining colonisation [19]. A colonised patient may or may not have ABPA or another manifestation of aspergillosis.

Baxter et al. recently developed a novel diagnostic classification system of aspergillosis in adult CF patients of *Aspergillus* hypersensitivity and colonisation beyond ABPA [19]. In this study sputum samples were collected from 130 patients not receiving azole therapy and analysed to detect *Aspergillus* using two new methods; real-time PCR (RT-PCR) and galactomannan (GM) antigen. These tests were combined with the standard serologic analysis to create a new classification system of aspergillosis in CF [19]. Latent class analysis of these samples demonstrated three distinct classes of aspergillosis in adults with CF and one non-diseased class. 49 patients (37.7%) were in class 1 which represents non-diseased CF patients with or without *Aspergillus* in sputum but negative GM and no immunologic response. 23 patients (17.7%) had ABPA and were placed in class 2 whereby the patient had all high immunologic markers, positive RT-PCR and positive GM. 19 patients (14.6%) were *Aspergillus* IgE-sensitised in class 3 with or without Aspergillus in sputum but negative *A. fumigatus* IgG and negative GM. Finally class 4 involved 39 patients (30.0%) with *Aspergillus* bronchitis (AB) who demonstrated negative IgE markers but positive *A. fumigatus* IgG, RT-PCR and GM. These data clearly need replication in other centres, but serve as a basis for an initial estimate of CF-associated aspergillosis burden.

This quantitative evidence base on which to diagnose ABPA, AB and AS is an improvement on the previous criteria for diagnosing ABPA. We therefore set out to estimate the prevalence of different forms of aspergillosis in CF in as many countries as possible based on the recent publication of the different phenotypes of aspergillosis in CF. Where pediatric data on ABPA frequency was available, we have included this, but not modelled *Aspergillus* sensitisation or bronchitis.

Methods

Literature search for ABPA rates

A literature search on published data on ABPA and *Aspergillus* colonisation frequency in CF was done using Medline, Embase, Scopus, Ovid and Google scholar in July 2013. Searches for the prevalence of ABPA in CF in different countries were also conducted. The quality of the study for epidemiologic purposes was evaluated by assessing the diagnostic criteria for ABPA and *Aspergillus* sensitisation, and separately for *Aspergillus* colonisation. In addition particular attention was paid to the denominator. Only papers that met the 2003 ABPA in CF consensus criteria [7] and provided appropriate denominators were included.

Annual data reports

We accessed the most recent annual reports published from those countries with National CF registries. Only reports that presented the number of CF patients stratified by age were used. Some of these reports also included the number of patients who had been diagnosed with ABPA, however very few stratified this finding by age.

We gained information regarding the number of individuals with CF from 2011 annual data reports for the UK [9], US [20], France [21], Germany [11], Canada [22], Australia [23], Ireland [10], the Netherlands [12] and New Zealand [24]. In addition 2010 annual data reports from Brazil [25] and Belgium [26] were also used. The locally diagnosed figures for ABPA are shown to provide a comparison with our estimates to indicate the possibility of underdiagnoses.

Registry data

The European CF Society (ECFS) provided additional patient registry data, expanding on their latest 2008–2009 ECFSPR report [27,28]. The ECFS includes data for Austria, Belgium, Czech Republic, Denmark, France, Germany, Greece, Hungary, Ireland, Israel, Italy, Latvia, The Netherlands, Portugal, Republic of Moldova, Serbia, Slovenia, Spain, Sweden and Switzerland [27,28].

We contacted representatives from all CF registries we could identify by email to ask for more specific data from each country. We requested information for the number of patients with CF, the age stratification of these patients- preferably in 5 year age blocks, the sex of these individuals and the number diagnosed with ABPA alongside their diagnostic criteria for this. Specific data requests were made in the UK, the Netherlands, Belgium, Latvia, US and Ireland. These representatives provided their data directly (personal communications). Many other contacted representatives explained that the ECFS annual report was the best way to get their information. Unfortunately some countries did not have representatives to email and some did not reply.

For countries without a national registry, data were scant and not included. We did not attempt to access information from countries or continents with a low Caucasian population such as Asia or Africa. If we gained two sets of information for a country we used the most recent and complete set.

Estimation method

We have used the percentage of individuals within each latent class from the work by Baxter et al [19]. This study only included individuals over the age of 18 therefore we are only representing the adult population for the various countries. We have extrapolated these percentages to show the estimated number of individuals in each category and added 95% confidence intervals to these percentages to provide a limited form of sensitivity analysis in the absence of other data on which to base our estimations. The figures we have used are shown in Table 1 below. Where country registry data was incomplete, but an estimate of the proportion of data is known, we have increased the estimates according to that proportion.

Age distribution of ABPA documented

We compared the age distribution of ABPA for the countries that had their data stratified into 5 year age blocks (ECFSPR data, US, Belgium, Ireland, and the Netherlands) (Figure 1). We used more up to date data than in the ECFSPR report for Belgium and Ireland that we gained directly from their national registries.

Results

We accessed sufficient data to estimate the prevalence of the different phenotypes of aspergillosis in 30 countries (Table 2). The ECFS provided data for Austria, Belgium, Switzerland, Czech Republic, Germany, Denmark, Spain, France, Greece, Hungary, Ireland, Israel, Italy, Latvia, Republic of Moldova, Portugal, Serbia, Sweden and Slovenia. The more recent data obtained for France, Germany, Ireland and Latvia superseded the ECFS report. We estimate 6,483 adults with ABPA compared with 1,564 (24%) recorded in registries, 10,988 with *Aspergillus* bronchitis and 5,347 who are sensitised to *Aspergillus fumigatus*.

The USA is the country with the biggest CF population (27,840 patients in 2013). Of these patients 13,657 were ≥18 years old (B.

Table 1. Percentages of patients in different classes of aspergillosis with 95% confidence intervals [19].

	Number of patients	Percentage (%)	95% Confidence Interval (%–%)
No aspergillosis	49	37.7	29.8–46.3
ABPA	23	17.7	12.1–25.2
Aspergillus sensitisation	19	14.6	9.6–21.7
Aspergillus Bronchitis	39	30.0	22.8–38.4
Total	130	100.0	

Marshall, pers. Comm.). We estimated that 5,149 (95% CI: 4,070–6,323) would have no disease; 2,417 (95% CI: 1,652–3,442) would have ABPA; 1,994 (95% CI: 1,311–2,964) would have AS and 4,097 (95% CI: 3,114–5,244) would have AB. Data registrations in the US showed 869 (6.4%) individuals >18 were diagnosed with ABPA and 854 (6%) of those <18 years old with CF (n = 14,183) had ABPA. The adult estimate is a third (34.6%) of our estimated number. [29] One review found prevalence rates of ABPA in various studies from the USA have ranged from 1.9% to 10.8% [30]. A large scale study in the USA involving 14,210 patients with CF found only 2.1% of patients to have been diagnosed with ABPA [6].

The UK has 8,679 CF patients registered with 4,933 over the age of 18. As this only represented 89% of the population we provide estimates based on 5,290 adults (Port CF, pers. comm.). There were 1,994 (95% CI: 1,576–2,449) patients likely to have no aspergillosis or sensitisation, 936 (95% CI: 640–1,333) with ABPA, 772(95% CI: 508–1,148) with AS and 1587 (95% CI: 1,206–2,031) with AB. Interestingly 582 individuals had been diagnosed with ABPA >18 years of age in 2011 within the UK (Port CF, Pers. comm.) Two very low prevalence rates of ABPA have been suggested in previous research of 5.8% [31] and 6.8% [32]. These studies are slightly dated and used relatively low sample sizes. In 2008 another small scale study was carried out that diagnosed

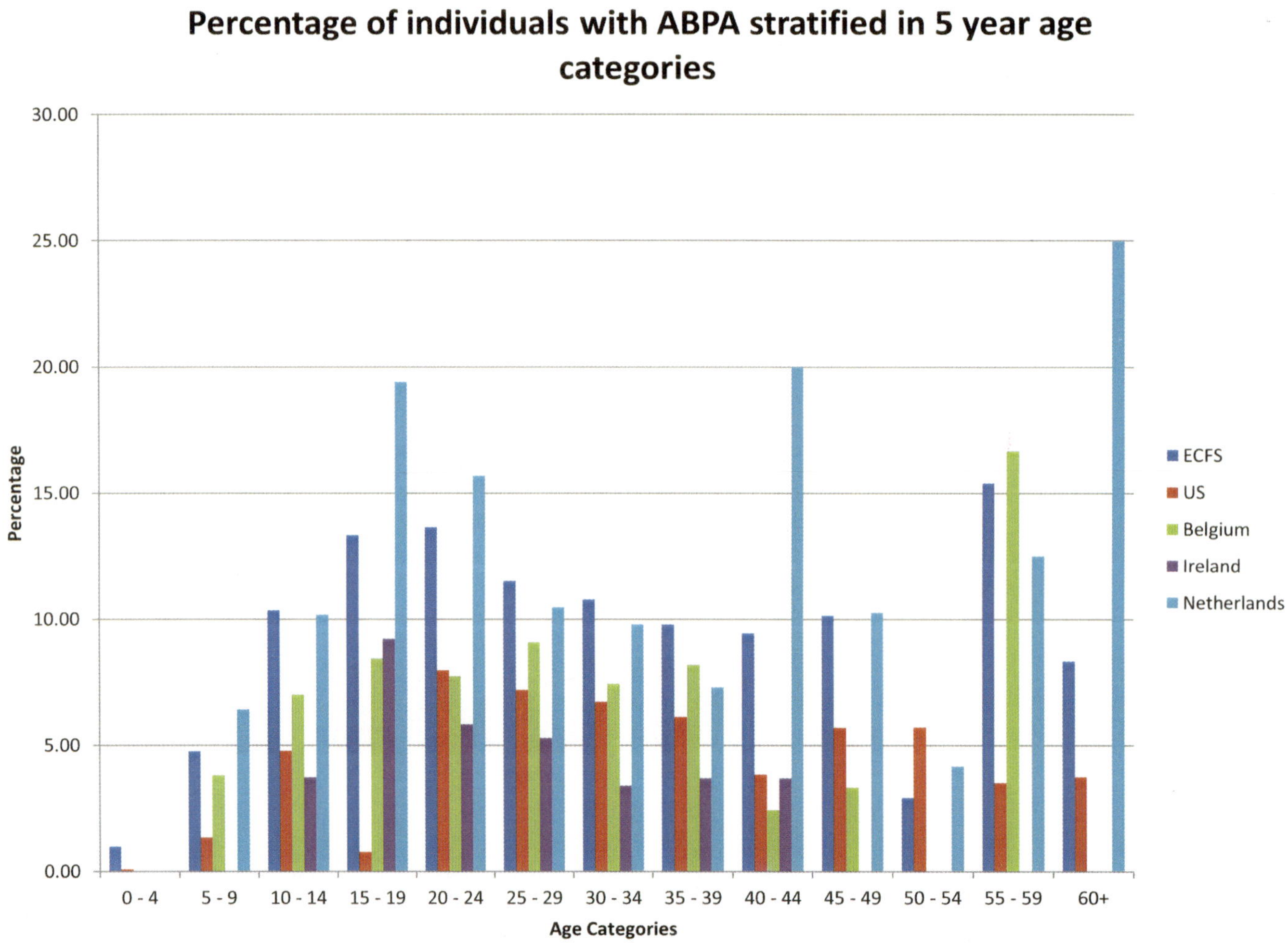

Figure 1. The percentage of individuals with CF stratified in 5 year age categories for numerous countries.

Table 2. Estimated and recorded prevalence of ABPA and estimated incidence of Aspergillus bronchitis and prevalence of Aspergillus sensitisation by country.

Country	Year	Est. CF pop. (>18 yrs)	None	Asp sensitisation	Asp bronchitis	ABPA	Documented ABPA (%)
United States	2013	13657	5347	2071	4255	2510	869(34.6%)
UK	2011	5290	1994	772	1587	936	654 (69.8%)
France	2009	2873	1083	420	862	509	514 (101.2%)
Germany	2009	2782	1049	406	835	492	204 (41.5%)
Canada	2011	2238	844	327	671	396	N/A
Italy	2009	2550	961	372	765	451	N/A
Australia	2012	1556	587	227	467	275	N/A
Spain	2009	977	368	143	293	173	43 (25.1%)
Brazil	2010	367	139	54	110	65	N/A
Netherlands	2011	768	290	112	230	136	69 (50.8%)
Poland	2007	354	133	52	106	63	N/A
Belgium	2010	602	227	88	181	107	N/A
Ireland	2011	559	211	82	168	99	25 (25.3%)
Austria	2009	210	79	31	63	37	13 (34.4%)
Switzerland	2009	75	28	11	23	13	8 (62.8%)
Sweden	2009	368	139	54	110	65	2 (3.5%)
Hungary	2009	223	84	33	67	40	N/A
Israel	2009	302	114	44	91	53	21 (39.5%)
Czech Republic	2009	216	81	32	65	38	N/A
Greece	2009	195	74	28	59	35	5 (14.5%)
Denmark	2009	259	98	38	78	46	N/A
Slovakia	2007	216	81	32	65	38	N/A
New Zealand	2011	205	77	30	62	36	N/A
Norway	2011	178	57	26	53	32	N/A
Portugal	2009	79	30	11	24	14	2 (17.1%)
Serbia	2009	37	14	5	11	7	2 (32.3%)
Slovenia	2009	19	7	3	6	3	4 (121%%)
Uruguay	2010	19	7	3	6	3	N/A
Republic of Moldova	2009	6	2	1	2	1	N/A
Latvia	2013	8	3	1	2	1	0
Estimated affected		**37714**	**14218**	**5506**	**11314**	**6675**	**1774**

8.75% of patients with ABPA [33]. Six adults with AB were identified in Leeds previously [34]. The number of children with ABPA in the UK is recorded as 324, (8.16% of children with CF.) Diagnosed ABPA rates in children and adolescents in the UK were 0.1% (0–3 yrs), 3.1% (4–7 yrs), 9.9% (8–11 yrs), 17.6% (12–15 yrs) and 15.7% (16–19 yrs) (Port CF, Pers. comm).

France has the third largest CF population documented (5,993 patients, 2,586>18years) [21] This only represented 90% of the total CF population in France therefore we based our results using an estimation of 2,873 adults. Our estimations placed 1,083 (95% CI: 856–1,330) patients in the no disease class, 509 (95% CI: 348–724) in the ABPA group, 420 (95% CI: 276–624) in AS group and 835 (95% CI: 634–1068) in the AB class. The 2009 ECFSPR had data for 5,640 individuals with CF, 2,586 were >18 years old and 463 had ABPA, representing 90% of an assumed total of 514 adults [28]. Therefore currently ABPA is probably fully captured by French CF physicians, a substantial improvement since 2000 which found the prevalence of ABPA in France to be just 3.9% [30]. Two recent studies apparently under-reported ABPA compared with notification: 8.9% [35] and 7.4% (95% CI: 6.5–8.4) of 2,935 CF patients had ABPA [5]. The number of children with ABPA documented in France is 277 (9.1%) [21].

Germany had 4,877 CF patients with data in 2011, with 2,504≥18 years old [11]. As this was only 90% of the CF population we used an adjusted total of 2,782 for our estimates. Our estimations suggested 1,049 (95% CI: 829–1,288) of these individuals would be in the non-disease class, 492 (95% CI: 337–701) to have ABPA, 406 (95% CI: 267–604) would be sensitised to Aspergillus and 835 (95% CI: 634–1,068) in the AB group. The annual data report suggested only 184 patients ≥18 years [11] had been diagnosed with ABPA. This is 7.3% of this adult population which is substantially lower than the 17.7% estimated by Baxter et al. Data from the Epidemiologic Registry of Cystic Fibrosis found 11.5% of 3,070 patients in Germany' population had ABPA [5]. The ECFSPR had data from 5,048 CF patients in Germany in 2009 and found 176 out of 2,619 individuals ≥18 years had ABPA; this is just 6.72% of this population which is once again dramatically lower than our estimates [28]. 117 children were documented to have ABPA in Germany, this is 4.81% of all Germany's children with CF [27].

Canada has 3,913 people affected by CF registered in 2011 with 2,234 ≥18years old [22]. Our estimation places 844 (95% CI: 667–1,036) without aspergillosis or sensitisation; 396 (95% CI: 271–564) in the ABPA group; 327 (95% CI: 215–486) with *Aspergillus* sensitisation and 671 (95% CI: 510–859) in the AB group. Geller et al. only found 1% of patients in Canada had ABPA in CF [6], however this is outdated research from 1999 and they may not have been using the correct diagnostic criteria, notably the 2003 ABPA in CF consensus criteria [7]. The Canadian annual data report only gave data regarding the number of patients with a positive culture of *Aspergillus*, which was 22% in 2011 [22]. A positive *Aspergillus* culture does not necessarily suggest an individual will have a disease related to that fungus, but is likely to represent either ABPA or AB.

Australia has 3,156 patients with CF registered with 1,556 of 18 years or more in their 2012 report [23]. Of the 1,556 adults with CF we estimate 587 (95% CI: 464–720) to be non-diseased; 275 (95% CI: 188–392) to have ABPA; 227 (95% CI: 149–338) to have AS and 467 (95% CI: 355–598) to have AB. One study found a lower ABPA prevalence rate in Australia of 4% [36]. The Australian annual data report does not include data about ABPA however they reported 25.2% of patients had *Aspergillus spp.* in their sputum in 2011 [23].

The Netherlands has 1,374 patients registered (2011 data) and 745 of these patients are 18 years or older [12]. The registered total is 97% of the total CF population so we based our estimated on 100% of the population (768 adults). Using the percentages of patients suspected in each latent class we estimate 290 (95% CI: 229–356) to have no disease; 136 (95% CI: 93–194) to have ABPA; 112 (95% CI: 74–167) to have AS and 230 (95% CI: 175–295) to have AB. The Netherlands has 67 patients over the age of 20 diagnosed with ABPA (V. Gulmans, personal communications) which is approximately 50% of the number suggested using Baxter's data. A European epidemiologic study of ABPA in CF found 6.8% (95% CI: 4.4%–9.9%) of patients in the Netherlands had ABPA [5]. The total number of CF patients documented to have ABPA was 128 (9.32%).

Belgium 2010 report documented 100% of their CF data that included 1,138 patients, 602 of these were ≥18 years old [26]. We estimate 227 (95% CI: patients to have no disease, 107 adults to have ABPA, 88 patients to have AS and 181 patients to have AB. Only 43 individuals >18 years had been diagnosed with ABPA in Belgium in 2010 (M. Thomas, pers. comm.) The ECFS 2009 had data for 1,129 individuals with CF in Belgium. 48 of the 581 individuals ≥18 years had ABPA [28]. These studies show 7.14% and 8.26% respectively would have ABPA; both are significantly lower than our estimate. Data from the ERCF found 13.6% (95% CI: 5.2–27.4) of CF patients in Belgium had ABPA [5] which is closer to our estimates. 32 (5.97%) children with ABPA were documented.

Ireland has a very high prevalence of CF. Ireland had 100% of data for CF patients with 559 of these aged 18 or older [10] from a population of 1073 patients. Of these 559 adults we estimate 211 (95% CI: 167–259) to not have disease, 99 (95% CI: 68–141) to have ABPA, 82 (95% CI: 54–121) to have AS and 168 (95% CI: 127–215) to have AB. In 2011, Ireland had 21 individuals over the age of 16 who have been diagnosed with ABPA [10] which is almost a fifth of our estimate despite including patients aged 16–18. The ERCF found 11.0% (95% CI: 8.6–13.7) to have ABPA in a population of 621 CF patients [5]. This figure is much greater than that from the annual data report and differs from the ECFSPR that found 2.32% of the 517 individuals with CF over 18 had ABPA [28]. The number of children in Ireland documented to have ABPA is just 15 (2.92%).

Data has also been published in a conference report for Hungary, Poland, Czech Republic and Slovakia for CF patients registered in these countries in 2007 [37]. This report documented information for 1,183 patients in Poland who have CF with 354 of these ≥18 years [37]. It is unknown whether this conference report involved 100% of CF patient data for Poland; therefore we used the numbers documented. We have estimated that 133 (95% CI: 105–164) have no disease; 63 (95% CI: 43–89) have ABPA; 52 (95% CI: 34–77) have AS and 106 (95% CI: 81–136) have AB. Unfortunately this report had no data for the number of these CF patients with ABPA to give a comparison. We had no other studies that estimated the number of individuals with ABPA in any of these countries.

Despite Brazil reporting 1,555 patients with CF in 2010 only 316 of these patients are 18 years or older [25]. These figures only represented 86% of the population therefore we based our results on 367 adults. We estimate 139 (95% CI: 109–170) of these adults will be classed as having no-disease, 65 (95% CI: 44–93) are in the ABPA group, 54 (95% CI: 35–80) classed with AS and 110 (95% CI: 84–141) to have AB. Brazil only had 15 individuals diagnosed with ABPA in 2010 out of the total 1,555 patients [25], again much lower than our estimate of 56 in the adult population. Amongst 74 individuals with CF in Bahia, Brazil, 2 (2.7%) were diagnosed with ABPA [38]. This study recognised the need to monitor these patients for ABPA as many were sensitised to *A. fumigatus*.

We had two sets of data for Hungary. 2007 data published in a conference report involved 576 patients with 238 of these ≥18 years old [37]. The ECFSPR register contains data for 555 CF patients from 2009, 201 of whom are ≥18 years old[27]. We used 223 adults to make our estimations as only 90% of the CF population was documented. We estimated 84 (95% CI: 67–103) would have no disease; 40 (95% CI: 27–56) would have ABPA; 33 (95% CI: 21–48) AS and 67 (95% CI: 51–86) would have AB. The ECFSPR did not have any data regarding the number of individuals currently diagnosed with ABPA [27].

Slovakia had similar figures to Hungary in the 2007 report with 416 individuals with CF, 216 who are >18 years old [37]. Of these 216 we estimated 81 (95% CI: 64–100) would have no disease; 38 (95% CI: 26–54) would have ABPA; 32 (95% CI: 21–47) would have AS and 65 (95% CI: 49–83) would have AB. There was no other research showing the number of people with ABPA in Slovakia.

New Zealand reported 100% of CF data in 2011 with 415 patients reported to have CF. There were 205 patients over 18 years of age [24]. We estimated that 77 (95% CI: 61–95) of these would have no disease; 36 (95% CI: 25–52) would have ABPA; 30 (95% CI: 20–44) would have AS and 62 (95% CI: 47–79) would have AB. The New Zealand 2011 annual data report gave details of the number of patients with a positive culture of *Aspergillus* age stratified in 5 year age blocks [24]. They found 22.1% of patients >16 years old were positive for *Aspergillus* [24]. A small study involving 277 Australasian (Australia and New Zealand) CF patients reported that 4% were diagnosed with ABPA in 2002 (criteria for diagnosis were in line with the 2003 criteria [7]) and 18.8% were colonised or infected with *Aspergillus* [36].

We gathered data for the Czech Republic from the 2007 conference report which involved 490 patients with CF and 190 adult CF patients (≥18 years old) [37]. The ECFSPR also had more recent data for the Czech Republic with 507 CF patients in 2009, 216 of which were ≥18 years [27]. 100% of CF patients data was documented and we therefore estimated that 81 (95% CI: 64–100) would have no disease; 38 (95% CI: 26–54) would have ABPA; 32 (95% CI: 21–47) would have AS and 65 (95% CI: 49–83) would have AB. The ECFSPR found that 10 people over the age of 18 were diagnosed with ABPA, however data was missing for 22 adults [27]. 16 children were documented to have ABPA; this is 5.5% of the total number of children with CF.

The Norway CF patient registry involved 100% of their CF patients data and shows 178 patients over 18 years in 2011 [39]. According to our estimates 67 (95% CI: 53–82) of these patients would have no disease; 32 (95% CI: 22–45) would have ABPA; 26 (95% CI: 17–39) would have AS and 53 (95% CI: 41–68) would have AB. Unfortunately this registry does not contain data regarding the number of individuals with ABPA.

The CF registry in Uruguay had 86 patients recorded with 19 over the age of 18 [40]. We were unsure as to the percentage of patients represented however using these figures we estimated 7 (95% CI: 6–9) would have no disease; 3 (95% CI: 2–5) would have ABPA; 3 (95% CI: 2–4) would have AS and 6 (95% CI: 4–7) would have AB. Once again no data was available for the number of CF patients with ABPA. The state social security institution in Uruguay (BPS) was giving treatment and following up 170 patients in 2012. They estimate that there are another 150 patients not diagnosed with CF in Uruguay. They suggest 29% of patients are over 18 years of age; therefore approximately 49 of those diagnosed patients would be adults. This suggests the CF registry in Uruguay underestimates the number of patients in their country with CF, therefore our aspergillosis estimates may be too low[41].

Finally we analysed the 2013 data sent from Latvia involving 38 patients, 8 of whom are older than 18 (K. Malina, pers. comm.) Of these 1 would have ABPA and 1 AS and 2 would have AB. No patients in Latvia are currently diagnosed with ABPA in the ECFR [5] or ECFSPR datasets (n = 28) [27].

The ECFSPR provided information for Spain. They had 740 patients registered with CF in 2009 and 293 were ≥18 years [27]. Only 30% of Spanish CF patients were included in the ECFSPR therefore we based our results on 977 adults (100%). We estimate that 368 (95% CI: 291–452) of these patients would have no disease; 173 (95% CI: 118–246) would have ABPA; 143 (95% CI: 94–212) would have AS and 293 (95% CI: 223–375) would have AB. Spain has only identified 13 individuals with ABPA over the age of 18 (4.44%); this is dramatically below our estimates. 12 (2.69%) children were documented to have ABPA [27]. Registro Europeo de FQ published data for Spain between 2008–2010 that noted 20 (3.2%) patients of all ages to have ABPA [12]. Another paper looking at the serious fungal infections that occur in Spain estimated 59,210 ABPA patients with asthma as their underlying diagnosis, a rate of 126 individuals per 100,000, although it not known how many are actually diagnosed [43].

The ECFSPR from 2009 had approximately 87.5% of the CF Swedish population recorded. There were 578 patients and 322 were 18 years or older [27]. Our estimations, based on 100% population (368 adults) found 139 (95% CI: 110–170) would have no disease; 65 (95% CI: 45–93) would have ABPA; 54 (95% CI: 35–80) would have AS and 110 (95% CI: 84–141) would have AB. Sweden only documented 2 people ≥18 years with ABPA (0.62%), however they did have 6<18 years with ABPA, this is 2.34% of children with CF [27]. This shows that it would be beneficial to extend this research to include both children and adults. Mastella et al. diagnosed ABPA in 2.1% out of 424 individuals of all ages with CF in 2000 [5].

Only 14% of CF patients' data are recorded by the ECFSPR for Italy. Of the 357 patients ≥ to 18 years [27] we estimated that if 100% of patients were documented there would be 2,550 adults. Using 2,550 we estimated 961 (95% CI:760 1181) of these patients would have no disease; 451 (95% CI: 309–643) would have ABPA; 372 (95% CI: 245–553) would have AS and 765 (95% CI:581–979) would have AB. Italy has no data published regarding ABPA prevalence; this may be partly due to the lack of a National Registry within this country.

All centres of Israel participate in the ECFSPR giving data for approximately 90% of the patients with CF. In this report there are 533 patients with CF, 272 are ≥18years of age [27]. We predicted that if 100% of data were present there would be 302 adult patients. Therefore we estimated: 114 (95% CI: 90–140) of these patients would have no disease; 53 (95% CI: 37–76) would have ABPA; 44 (95% CI: 29–66) would have AS and 91 (95% CI: 69–116) would have AB. Israel had reported 19 patients ≥18 to have ABPA in 2009 [27]. This is approximately 7% of the adult CF population, once again much lower than our estimation. Israel has 14 (5.36%) children documented with ABPA.

Denmark has a national CF registry with 100% of patients participating in the ECFSPR. In 2009 there were 451 patients registered, 259 of these patients were adults and included in our estimate [27]. We predicted 98 (95% CI: 77–120) of these patients would have no disease; 46 (95% CI: 31–65) would have ABPA; 38 (95% CI: 25–56) would have AS and 78 (95% CI: 59–99) would have AB. Denmark had no information registered regarding the number of patients with ABPA in the ECFSPR[27]. However some research was published in 2000 showing that 3.4% of patients in a sample of 353 patients with CF had CF [5]. This is dramatically below our estimated value; however the research is relatively dated and occurred prior to more modern diagnostic techniques and consensus criteria.

The ECFSPR had data for approximately 34% of the Austrian population with CF. There were 352 patients in the sample and 82 of these patients were adults therefore we estimated that in a 100% sample there would be 210 adults. Using this figure we found 79 (95% CI: 63–97) of these patients would have no disease; 37(95% CI: 25–53) would have ABPA; 31 (95% CI: 20–46) would have AS and 63 (95% CI: 48–81) would have AB The ECFSPR data described 5 people (6.1%) with ABPA [27]. Another epidemiology study of ABPA in CF in several countries found that 5.3% of 169 patients with CF in Austria had ABPA. [5] There were 6 individuals <18 years (2.22%) that were documented to have ABPA [27].

Switzerland also has a low percentage of CF patients in the ECFSPR with just 24% recorded (190 patients). Only 18 of these patients are in the adult population [27], however when adjusted to 100% there were 75 adults. We estimated 28 (95% CI: 22–35) of these patients would have no disease; 13 (95% CI: 9–19) would have ABPA; 11 (95% CI: 7–16) would have AS and 23 (95% CI: 17–29) would have AB. Two of the 18 adults (11%) were diagnosed with ABPA in the ECFSPR report. However 32 children were diagnosed with ABPA, this is 18.6% of the 172 children with CF [27]. We believe this data is incomplete as the number of patients in the >18 years category appears far too low.

Serbia had 122 patients recorded in the ECFSPR, which is approximately 95% of the total number of patients with CF. Serbia has a relatively low population of adults with CF, just 35 [27], 37 when adjusted to 100% providing estimates of 7 with ABPA, 5 with AS and 11 with AB. Two adults with ABPA were mentioned in the ECFSPR dataset. Only 1 child was documented to have ABPA [27].

Portugal does not have a national registry and therefore approximately 42% of data for CF patients in Portugal are within the ECFSPR report. Of the 117 patients with data 33 are 18 years or older [27] which we have estimated as 79 adults if 100% of data was present. We estimated that 30 (95% CI: 23–36) of these patients would have no disease; 14 (95% CI: 10–20) would have ABPA; 11 (95% CI: 8–17) would have AS and 24 (95% CI: 18–30) would have AB. Only 1 patient was reported to have ABPA in ECFSPR [27].

Greece has just 20% CF patient representation in the ECFSPR report. There are 92 patients in the registry and 39 of these are adults [27]. We estimated that 195 adults would be present if there was 100% documentation. Therefore we estimate 74 (95% CI: 58–90) of these patients would have no disease; 35 (95% CI: 24–49) would have ABPA; 28 (95% CI: 19–42) would have AS and 59 (95% CI: 44–75) would have AB. Only 1 patient had been diagnosed with ABPA [27].

The ECFSPR has only 66 patients registered for Slovenia (75% of the Slovenia CF population.) Fourteen patients are >18 years [27] (19 if 100% of data). Of these 19 patients, we estimated that 7 would have no disease; 3 would have ABPA; 3 would have AS and 6 would have AB. No patients in the adult population are diagnosed with ABPA. However 4 children were diagnosed with ABPA, this is 7.69% of the 52 children [27].

Finally the ECFSPR captured 100% of data for the Republic of Moldova CF patients, with only 41 patients [27]. Using the 6 adult patients within this cohort we calculated that one would have ABPA, one would have AS and 2 would have AB. There is currently no data available for the true number of patients who have been diagnosed with ABPA in the Republic of Moldova.

It was suggested that CF in the Indian diaspora in the UK may be in the 1 in 40,000 to 1 in 10,000 range [44]. In addition using the prevalence of F508del it has been suggested there may be 10,247 to 23,730 CF patients in India [45]. Unfortunately we were unable to involve India in our results as the estimates of the total number of patients are vague and there no figures for the number of adults (if any) with CF. In 1971 the first 3 cases of ABPA were reported in India [46]. The prevalence of ABPA in adults asthmatics in India may be substantially higher than in the rest of the world which has studied these rates [14] a substantial 27.2% in 564 adult asthmatics in North India [47].

We compared the number of individuals with CF who were <18 years and >18 years. This data provides insight into the success of care in each country as a larger proportion of their CF population >18 years would suggest better quality of care. The results are shown in Table S1 and Figure S1 which rank the countries from the highest to the lowest percentage of >18 years. We have not included New Zealand in this figure as we only have data for the number <16 and >16 years, or Switzerland because these data are notably incomplete.

The ECFSPR recorded the number of individuals across Europe with ABPA in 5 year intervals (figure 1). Out of 17,737 individuals, 2,203 had unknown/missing data, 14,244 had no ABPA in the year of follow up and 1,290 had ABPA [27]. Individuals aged 0–4 and 5–9 had a very low percentage of individuals with ABPA of 0.91% and 4.11% respectively. The percent with ABPA increased to 8.51% of 10–14 year olds and plateaued at ~10.3% of 15–19 and 20–24 year olds. Of the 1,290 individuals with ABPA, 1,024 (79%) were between the ages of 10 and 34. After 34 years, the number of people with CF in Europe decreases and the percentages of individuals with ABPA is generally around 7% [27], perhaps indicating earlier death (or transplantation). As these data are derived from a very large population it is clear that CF patients aged 15 to 24 are most at risk of ABPA, despite the likely problems of under diagnosis.

We compared this ECFSPR with data from US, Belgium, Ireland and the Netherlands (Figure 1). Similar trends were found, such as the number of children with ABPA was <1% under 4 years and the percentages tended to increase in adolescent years and those in their 20s. The high percentage of ABPA in Netherlands in those older than 60 reflects a small number of individuals with CF in that age range. Exact data for the number of individuals with CF in each age band and the number diagnosed with ABPA are shown in Table S2. As we have not modelled aspergillosis rates in people under the age of 18 further research involving all age categories and the different classes of aspergillosis would be beneficial.

Discussion

In this study of the majority of the world's CF adult population, we estimate there to be 6,675 adults with ABPA, compared with 2,221 (33%) recorded in registries, 11,314 with *Aspergillus* bronchitis and 5,506 who are sensitised to *Aspergillus fumigatus*. Our estimations suggest many countries need to revise their methods of screening for and diagnosing ABPA and Aspergillus bronchitis which together may affect nearly 50% of patients. We argue that the ABPA estimates have real validity because of the match with recorded cases in France. We have provided 95% confidence intervals as a limited form of sensitivity analyses, in the absence of alternative data on which to base estimations. It is highly likely that even with excellent diagnostics applied systematically across whole cohorts, that there will be variations, perhaps substantial variations, from these estimates. Variations could arise for genetic, environmental, seasonality, clinical practice, patients switching between aspergillosis phenotypes and other undefined reasons. The ranges of estimates provided for each country may cover most of the variation, but until national studies are done, this will not be known. Studies are required in many countries to determine the prevalence rates of ABPA, AS and AB using these new diagnostic methods. These confirmatory epidemiological studies could be extremely beneficial to improving the management of patients with CF across the world.

Clinically, ABPA is difficult to recognise due to its similar clinical presentation to CF exacerbations related to many pathogens. Wheezing, exercise intolerance, change in pulmonary function and increased sputum production are not specific to ABPA. Serology (notably *Aspergillus* specific IgE and *Aspergillus* IgG) and/or detection of high quantities of *A. fumigatus* in the airways are required to establish the diagnosis. In 2003 Stevens et al proposed the minimum criteria required for diagnosis. These criteria consisted of clinical deterioration; total serum IgE concentrations >500 IU/ml; immediate cutaneous reactivity to *Aspergillus* in a skin prick test; and another serological marker or chest radiography or CT scan showing recent abnormalities [7]. Our work suggests that these criteria should be revised, but the principle remains that screening for ABPA is important.

An *Aspergillus*-specific IgE (sIgE) >5.7 KUA/L has 100% sensitivity and 94% specificity to distinguish ABPA from all over forms of aspergillosis and normal [19]. Values of sIgE > 3.75 KUA/L and <5.7 KUA/L denote *Aspergillus* sensitisation without ABPA (sensitivity 94% and specificity 100%). While replication of these data and cut-offs is required in another similar study, these values can be used to confirm or refute our estimates in other adult CF populations.

Aspergillus bronchitis is a newly recognised entity in CF [48] and as such the high proportion of patients with this condition was and remains a surprise. A two year reduction in FEV1 associated with *Aspergillus* bronchitis, which may or may not be reversible with antifungal therapy (possibly combined with targeted antibiotic therapy) is clearly a new target for intervention in CF with a reasonable prospect of significant clinical improvement. We have demonstrated excellent and partial responses to antifungal therapy in patients with Aspergillus bronchitis without CF [49]. Some patients with ABPA also have high Aspergillus IgG titres, one of the cardinal features of *Aspergillus* bronchitis in CF, and these ABPA patients may also have *Aspergillus* bronchitis. We haven't modelled this.

It is not clear currently that each Aspergillus phenotype is completely discrete. Experience alongside our data indicates that patients may switch phenotypes (19) and some may have overlap or two syndromes. For example, patients with extensive bronchiectasis and ABPA may also have AB. This needs further evaluation, and in particular non-overlapping diagnostic tests. Therefore the estimates here can only be approximate and represent a cross-sectional analysis, not a longitudinal one.

ABPA often manifests in late childhood in CF, as amply demonstrated by the registry data. Overall 984 children with ABPA were documented with rates in the paediatric population varying from a low of <1% in Serbia to 9.1% (France), 9.3% (Netherlands) and 18.6% (Switzerland). It is likely that ABPA is underdiagnosed in most countries, but diagnostic criteria in children are barely studied and so the variation could reflect differing criteria for defining cases.

Acute exacerbations of ABPA are treated with corticosteroids which are partially effective but carry a substantial penalty in CF of more frequent diabetes and osteoporosis, both significant clinical problems in CF. Antifungal therapy with itraconazole is only occasionally effective because of poor bioavailability in many, despite elevated doses and use of the oral solution. Voriconazole is more reliably bioavailable, but is often not tolerated and has long term adverse events such as photosensitivity, skin cancer, periostitis due to excess fluoride and peripheral neuropathy. Furthermore *A. fumigatus* has recently shown increasing resistance to these triazoles [50,51] [52]. Appropriate use and therapeutic drug monitoring is therefore essential for these agents in CF. But assuming good exposure, the potential impact for patients with ABPA and possibly for Aspergillus is large.

Aspergillus sensitisation is of uncertain significance. It has been shown to be associated with reduced FEV_1 in individuals with CF [53–55], but it is not clear if this is a causal relationship or an epiphenomenon. It is also not clear if it is amenable to antifungal therapy or any immunomodulatory treatment, or whether reduced FEV1 would be reversible or progressive loss reduced. It is also not clear if it is a precursor to ABPA or a separate distinct aspergillosis phenotype within CF.

We postulate there are two alternative models of the development of ABPA, *Aspergillus* sensitisation or *Aspergillus* bronchitis (Figure 2). Model 1 depicts the sequential development of ABPA after *Aspergillus* sensitisation [56] and *Aspergillus* bronchitis after the development of bronchiectasis and persistent colonisation. Model 2 depicts alternative pathways, perhaps genetically determined, without sequential development of different manifestations. This model suggests the four different disease patterns are not interdependent.

We created boxplots using the Baxter et al data and found no significant different in the ages of the individuals in the latent classes (figure 3). This finding is consistent with model 2 (Figure 2), although 17% of patients re-evaluated over a 9 month period moved between classes during follow-up. Clearly this area requires more longitudinal studies.

We have based our estimates on Model 2. The median age of the ABPA group was younger than that of the AS group, 22 years and 28 years respectively. If model 1 was proven to be correct the estimated national burdens for each class may differ. Another small scale study involving 80 paediatric patients also found the ABPA population to be younger than those who were *Aspergillus* sensitised, again making model 1 highly unlikely [33]. Hutcheson et al carried out a 12 year longitudinal study using 118 patients from a CF clinic at Cardinal Glennon Children's Hospital in St. Louis. Throughout this time they studied the development of 5 *in vivo* and *in vitro* immune parameters of *A. fumigatus* sensitisation with the aim of determining the parameters which could predict those patients who were likely to be diagnosed with ABPA in the future. They found no link between those with *Aspergillus* sensitisation and those who developed ABPA and in many cases found there was often a reduction in the positive parameters over time [57]. This finding was supported by another longitudinal study in 147 patients aged 5 to 43 years. They also found fluctuations in the levels of IgE and IgG specific to *Aspergillus* and a marked decline in total IgE over time despite ABPA status [58]. This once again suggests there is no link between AS and ABPA and therefore supports Model 2 that we have used in our estimations.

Unfortunately many countries do not have complete data sets for the number of patients with CF. This may be due to several reasons, such as the lack of a national registry; poor diagnosis of CF or many countries with a low population of Caucasians have a low prevalence rate of CF leading to late recognition. We were unable to identify any population data for countries in Africa, Asia, the Middle East, the Arctic Region or Latin America, with the exception of Brazil and Uruguay. In addition we were regrettably unable to obtain data for the following European countries:

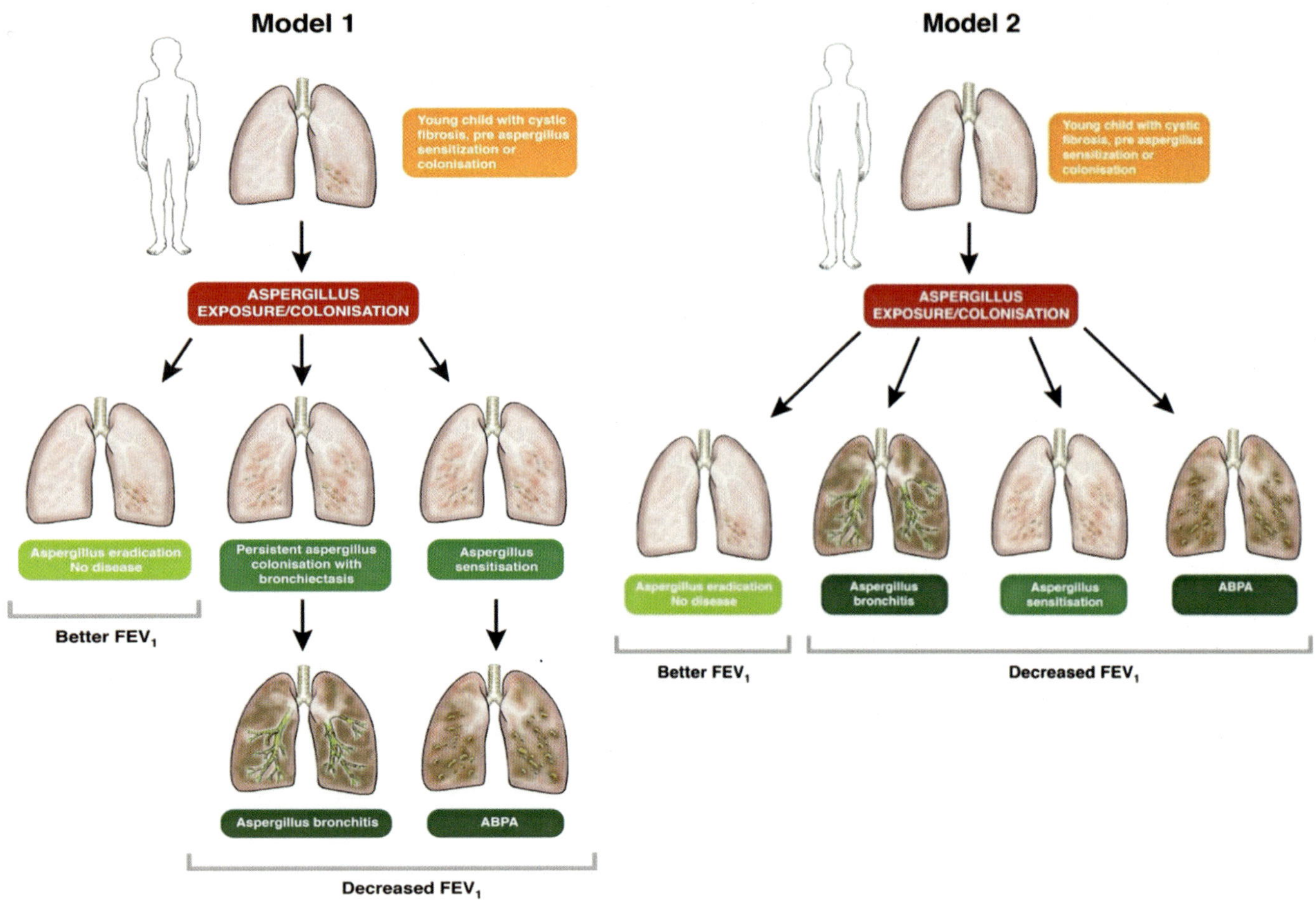

Figure 2. Alternative models of the development of ABPA, *Aspergillus* sensitisation or *Aspergillus* bronchitis.

Bulgaria, Croatia, Cyprus, Estonia, Finland, Lithuania, Luxembourg, Malta, Romania, Iceland, Montenegro, Turkey, Albania, Bosnia and Herzegovina and Kosova.

Some countries without national registries did not have full data sets within the European Cystic Fibrosis Society report of 2008–2009. The 2009 estimated coverage for Austria is 39%, for Greece is 20%, Italy 14%, Portugal 42%, Slovenia 75%, Spain 30%, 85–90% in Sweden and 24% in Switzerland. We have compensated for these by assuming that the unrecorded patients are similar to those that are recorded, which may be a fallacious assumption.

The aspergillosis cases that are recorded in the registries were varied. Some just reported the number of patients with any species of *Aspergillus* detected in sputum samples (Australia [23], Canada [22], New Zealand [24]) which is likely to represent ABPA or AB, but may represent occasional colonisation. Germany's data annual report presented the number of individuals diagnosed with ABPA for both <18 and >18 [11] and the UK and Irish data shows the number of individuals >16 years old with ABPA [9,10]. In addition following a data request the ECFS, the Netherlands, US, UK, Belgium and Latvia sent their data regarding the number of individuals with ABPA stratified in 5 year age groups. Belgium [26] and Brazil [25] only documented the total number of individuals with ABPA without any age stratification. France released data regarding the number of individuals treated for aspergillosis in 5 year age categories [21]. Some countries did not release any data regarding *Aspergillus* or ABPA such as the US [20], Poland [37], Uruguay [40], Slovakia [37], Norway [27,39], Czech Republic [27,37] and Hungary [37].

A key issue for the future is whether ABPA, AB and AS could be prevented. *Aspergillus* species are ubiquitous moulds found in organic debris and are common indoor moulds especially in areas with lots of dust for example the curtains, floor mats and the attic [59]. There is some evidence to show that the prevalence of ABPA increases with increasing concentrations of *A. fumigatus*, for example there is more ABPA in agricultural conditions [60] and where there is *A. fumigatus* in the immediate outside environment [61]. Manifestations of ABPA are a complex interaction between the patient's immune response and the number and virulence of the organisms [62]. It is highly likely that ABPA is a multi-genic disorder, given multiple genetic associations with ABPA [56] and so complete avoidance is unlikely to be a successful prevention strategy. Immunisation, aggressive eradication in genetically susceptible individuals and long term suppressive antifungal therapy, possibly combined with (as yet undefined) immunomodulatory therapy are likely to be the most successful prevention and management strategies for the future.

Summary

In summary we have estimated the number of patients with ABPA, *Aspergillus* sensitisation and *Aspergillus* bronchitis in many countries based on a recent publication that used established serological techniques combined with RT-PCR and GM to

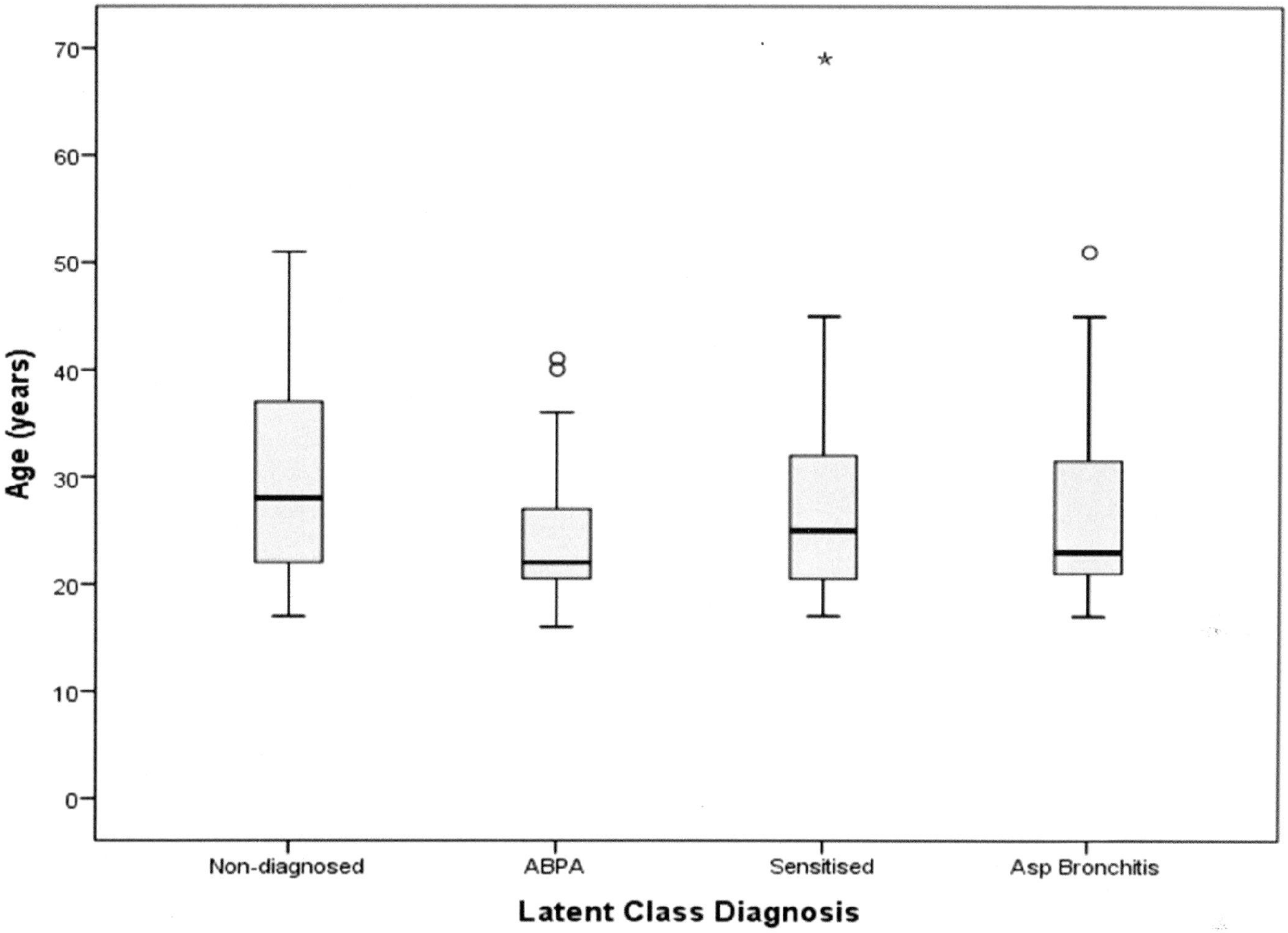

Figure 3. Boxplot to show the difference in ages between the different diagnostic groups of aspergillosis.

reclassify aspergillosis in adult patients with CF. Further epidemiological studies are required using these new techniques to determine the prevalence of these different classes of aspergillosis within various countries globally and within the paediatric population.

Supporting Information

Figure S1 The percentage of cystic fibrosis patients under and over 19 years of age in numerous countries.

Table S1 The number of individuals with CF <18 and >18 years in numerous countries.

Table S2 Numbers of patients with recorded ABPA by age bands in different countries.

Acknowledgments

- Steering Group of the Dutch CF registry for 2011 data of the Netherlands
- Port CF for 2011 data for the UK
- Godfrey Fletcher CEO Cystic Fibrosis Registry of Ireland for 2011 data
- V. Gulmans for Germany's 2011 data
- M. Thomas for 2010 data in Belgium
- Karīna Mahļina Latvia for 2013 data regarding Latvia
- European Cystic Fibrosis Society Steering Group.
- Helen Carruthers- medical illustrations (figure 1 and figure 2)
- Caroline Baxter for the age distribution of patients in her cohort of 130.
- Bruce Marshall for 2013 data for the US.

Author Contributions

Conceived and designed the experiments: JA DWD. Performed the experiments: JA. Analyzed the data: JA JM DWD. Wrote the paper: JA DWD.

References

1. Riordan JR, Rommens JM, Kerem B, Alon N, Grzelczak Z, et al. (1989) Identification of the cystic fibrosis gene: cloning and characterization of complementary DNA. Science 245: 1066–1072.
2. Grubb BR, Boucher RC (1999) Pathophysiology of gene-targeted mouse models for cystic fibrosis. Physiological Reviews 79: S193–214.
3. Hedayati MT, Mayahi S, Denning DW (2010) A Study on *Aspergillus* species in houses of asthmatic patients from Sari City, Iran and a brief review of the health effects of exposure to indoor *Aspergillus*. Environmental Monitering and Assessment 168: 481–487.
4. Mearns M, Young W, Batten J (1965) Transient pulmonary infiltrations in cystic fibrosis due to allergic aspergillosis. Thorax 20: 385–392.

5. Mastella G, Rainisio M, Harms HK, Hodson ME, Koch C, et al. (2000) Allergic bronchopulmonary aspergillosis in cystic fibrosis. A European epidemiological study. European Respiratory Journal 16: 464–471.
6. Geller DE, Kaplowitz H, Light MJ, Colin AA (1999) Allergic bronchopulmonary aspergillosis in cystic fibrosis: reported prevalence, regional distribution, and patient characteristics. Scientific Advisory Group, Investigators, and Coordinators of the Epidemiologic Study of Cystic Fibrosis. Chest 116: 639–646.
7. Stevens DA, Moss RB, Kurup VP, Knutsen AP, Greenberger P, et al. (2003) Allergic Bronchopulmonary Aspergillosis in Cystic Fibrosis—State of the Art: Cystic Fibrosis Foundation Consensus Conference. Clinical Infectious Diseases 37: S225–264.
8. Greenberger PA (2001) Clinical aspects of allergic bronchopulmonary aspergillosis. Frontiers in bioscience: a journal and virtual library 8: s119–s127.
9. UK CF Registry (2013) Annual Data Report 2011. Kent, UK.
10. The Cystic Fibrosis Registry of Ireland (2011) Annual Report.
11. Sens B, Stern M (2011) Qualitätssicherung Mukoviszidose 2011. Hanover, Germany.
12. Dutch Cystic Fibrosis Registry (2012) Annual Data Report 2011. Netherlands.
13. Kirsten D, Nowak D, Rabe KF, Magnussen H (1993) Diagnosis of bronchopulmonary aspergillosis is often made too late. Medizinische Klinik (Munich) 88: 353–356.
14. Denning DW, Plevry A, Cole DC (2013) Global burden of allergic bronchopulmonary aspergillosis with asthma and its complication chronic pulmoary aspergillosis in adults. Medical mycology 51: 361–370.
15. Chakrabarti A, Sethi S, Raman DS, Behera D (2002) Eight year study of allergic bronchopulmonary aspergillosis in an Indian teaching hospital. Mycoses 45: 295–299.
16. Milla CE, Wielinski BS, Regelmann WE (1996) Clinical significance of the recovery of *Aspergillus species* from the respiratory secretions of cystic fibrosis patients. Pediatric Pulmonology 21: 6–10.
17. Vrakrijker AMM, van der Ent CK, van Berkhout FT, Stellato RK, Willems RJL, et al. (2010) *Aspergillus fumigatus* colonization in cystic fibrosis: implications for lung function? Clinical Microbiology and Infection 17: 1381–1386.
18. Amin R, Dupuis A, Aaron S, Ratjen F (2010) The Effect of Chronic Infection with *Aspergillus fumigatus* on Lung Function and Hospitalization in Patients with Cystic Fibrosis. Chest 137: 171–176.
19. Baxter CG, Dunn G, Jones AM, Webb K, Gore R, et al. (2013) Novel immunologic classification of aspergillosis in adult cystic fibrosis. The Journal of Allergy and Clinical Immunology 132: 560–566.
20. Cystic Fibrosis Foundation Patient Registry Annual Data Report 2011.
21. Vaincre la Mucoviscidose, Ined French Cystic Fibrosis Registry- Annual Data Report 2011.
22. Cystic Fibrosis Canada (2013) The Canadian Cystic Fibrosis Registry 2011 Annual Report. Toronto, Canada.
23. Cystic Fibrosis Australia(2012) Cystic Fibrosis in Australia 2011: 14th Annual Report from the Australian Cystic Fibrosis Data Registry. Baulkham Hills, Australia.
24. Cystic Fibrosis Association of New Zealand (2011) Port CFNZ 2011 National Data Registry. New Zealand.
25. Grupo Brasileiro De Estudos De Fibrose Cistica (2010) Registro Brasileiro de Fibrose Cistica Ano 2010. Brazil.
26. Belgische Mucoviscidose Register, Registre Belge de la Mucoviscidose, Scientific Institute of Public Health, (2010) The Belgian Cystic Fibrosis Registry Summary Report. Belgium.
27. Viviani L, Zolen A, Olesen HV (2012) European Cystic Fibrosis Society Patient Registry Annual Data Report 2008–2009 data. Denmark. 1– 102 p.
28. European Cystic Fibrosis Society (2009) European Cystic Fibrosis Society Patient Report for aspergillosis.
29. Marshall B (2013) United States Cystic Fibrosis Foundation patient data for ABPA.
30. Pihet M, Carrere J, Cimon B, Chabasse D, Delhaes L, et al. (2009) Occurrence and relevance of filamentous fungi in respiratory secretions of patients with cystic fibrosis- a review. Medical mycology 47: 387–397.
31. Simmonds EJ, Littlewood JM, Evans EG (1990) Cystic fibrosis and allergic bronchopulmonary aspergillosis. Archives of Disease in childhood 65: 507–511.
32. Marchant JL, Warner JO, Bush A (1994) Rise in total IgE as an indicator of allergic bronchopulmonary aspergillosis in cystic fibrosis. Thorax 49: 1002–1005.
33. Barton RC, Hobson RP, Denton M, Peckham D, Brownlee K, et al. (2008) Serologic diagnosis of allergic bronchopulmonary aspergillosis in patients with cystic fibrosis through the detection of immunoglobulin G to Aspergillus fumigatus. Diagnostic Microbiology and Infectious Disease 62: 287–291.
34. Shoseyov D, Brownlee KG, Conway SP ea (2006) Aspergillus bronchitis in cystic fibrosis. Chest 130: 222–226.
35. Paugam A, Baixench MT, Demazes-Dufeu N, Burgel PR, Sauter E, et al. (2010) Characteristics and consequences of airway colonization by filamentous fungi in 201 adult patients with cystic fibrosis in France. Medical Mycology 48: S32–S36.
36. Skov M, McKay K, Koch C, Cooper PJ (2005) Prevalence of allergic bronchopulmonary aspergillosis in cystic fibrosis in an area with a high frequency of atopy. Respiratory medicine 99: 887–893.
37. Kopacz E, Ras I, Sonik B (2009) Konferencia V4-CF Zborník prednášok. wordpress.
38. Carneiro AC, Lemos AC, Arruda SM, Santana MA (2008) Prevalence of allergic bronchopulmonary aspergillosis in patients with cystic fibrosis in the state of Bahia, Brazil. Jornal Brasileiro de Pneumologia 34: 900–906.
39. Av Norsk senter for cystisk fibrose Oslo universitetssykehus (2011) Cystisk fibrose: Populasjonen i Norge pr 01.01.11 Oslo universitetssykehus.
40. Spagna F, Cabeza S (2010) La fibrosis quistica en Uruguay. Uruguay.
41. State Social Security Institution Uruguay (BPS) (2012) Fibrosis Quistica en Uruguay: situacion y perspectivas. montevideo.
42. Cordero CV (2008–2010) Registro Europeo de FQ. Datos españoles.
43. Juan Luis Rodriguez Tudela, Manuel Cuenca-Estrella, Cristóbal León, Jose Maria Miro, Asunción Nuñez Boluda, et al. (2013) Burden of serious fungal infections in Spain.
44. Prasad R, Sharma H, Kaur G (2010) Molecular Basis of Cystic Fibrosis Disease: An Indian Perspective Indian journal of clinical biochemistry 25: 335–341.
45. Kapoor V, Shastri SS, Kabra M, Kabra SK, Ramachandran V, et al. (2006) Carrier frequency of F508del mutation of cystic fibrosis in Indian population. Journal of Cystic Fibrosis 5: 43–46.
46. Shah JR (1997) Allergic pulmonary aspergillosis. Journal of associated physicians India 19: 835–841.
47. Agarwal R, Gupta D, Aggarwal AN, Behera D, Jindal SK (2006) Allergic Bronchopulmonary Aspergillosis: Lessons From 126 Patients Attending a Chest Clinic in North India. Chest Journal 130: 442–448.
48. Shoseyov D, Brownlee KG, Conway SP, Kerem E (2006) Aspergillus bronchitis in cystic fibrosis. Chest 130: 222–226.
49. Chrdle A, Mustakim S, Bright-Thomas RJ, Baxter CG, Felton T, et al. (2012) Aspergillus bronchitis without significant immunocompromise. Annals of the New York Academy of Sciences 1272: 73–85.
50. Mellado E, Garcia-Effron G, Alcazar-Fuoli L, Melchers WJ, Verweij PE, et al. (2007) A new *Aspergillus fumigatus* resistance mechanism conferring in vitro cross-resistance to azole antifungals involves a combination of cyp51A alterations. Antimicrobial Agents Chemother 2007 51: 1897–1904.
51. Howard SJ, Arendrup MC (2011) Acquired antifungal drug resistance in Aspergillus fumigatus: epidemiology and detection. Medical Mycology 49: S90–S95.
52. Burgel PR, Baixench MT, Amsellem M, Audureau E, Chapron J, et al. (2012) High Prevalence of Azole-Resistant Aspergillus fumigatus in Adults with Cystic Fibrosis Exposed to Itraconazole. Antimicrobial Agents and Chemotherapy 56: 869–874.
53. Kanthan S, Bush A, Kemp M, Buchdahl R (2007) Factors effecting impact of Aspergillus fumigatus sensitization in cystic fibrosis. Pediatric Pulmonology 42: 785–793.
54. Wojnarowski C, Eichler I, Gartner C, Götz M, Renner S, et al. (1997) Sensitization to Aspergillus fumigatus and lung function in children with cystic fibrosis. American journal of respiratory and critical care medicine 155: 1902–1907.
55. Fillaux J, Brémont F, Murris M, Cassaing S, Rittié JL, et al. (2012) Assessment of Aspergillus sensitization or persistent carriage as a factor in lung function impairment in cystic fibrosis patients. Scandinavian Journal of Infectious Diseases 44: 842–847.
56. Agarwal R, Chakrabarti A, Shah A, Gupta D, Meis JF, et al. (2013) Allergic bronchopulmonary aspergillosis: review of literature and proposal of new diagnostic and classification criteria. Clinical and Experimental allergy: Journal of the British Society for Allergy and Clinical Immunology 43: 850–873.
57. Hutcheson PS, Knutsen AP, Rejent AJ, Slavin R G (1996) A 12-year longitudinal study of Aspergillus sensitivity in patients with cystic fibrosis. Chest 110: 363–366.
58. el-Dahr JM, Fink R, Selden R, Arruda LK, Platts-Mills TA, et al. (1994) Development of immune responses to Aspergillus at an early age in children with cystic fibrosis. American jounrnal of respiratory and critical care medicine 150: 1513–1518.
59. Woodcock A, Steel N, Moore CB, Howard SJ, Custovic A, et al. (2006) Fungal contamination of bedding. Allergy 61: 140–142.
60. Henderson AH (1968) Allergic aspergillosis: review of 32 cases. Thorax 23: 501–512.
61. Beaumont F, Kauffman HF, Sluiter HJ, De Vries K (1984) Environmental aerobiological studies in allergic bronchopulmonary aspergillosis. Allergy 39: 183–193.
62. Agarwal R, Chakrabarti A (2010) Epidemiology of Allergic Bronchopulmonary Aspergillosis. Aspergillosis: From Diagnosis to Prevention pp. 671–688.

12

IFN-γ Stimulates Autophagy-Mediated Clearance of *Burkholderia cenocepacia* in Human Cystic Fibrosis Macrophages

Kaivon Assani[1], Mia F. Tazi[2], Amal O. Amer[2], Benjamin T. Kopp[1,3]*

1 Center for Microbial Pathogenesis, The Research Institute at Nationwide Children's Hospital, Columbus, Ohio, United States of America, **2** Department of Microbial Infection and Immunity and the Department of Internal Medicine, The Ohio State University, Columbus, Ohio, United States of America, **3** Section of Pediatric Pulmonology, Nationwide Children's Hospital, Columbus, Ohio, United States of America

Abstract

Burkholderia cenocepacia is a virulent pathogen that causes significant morbidity and mortality in patients with cystic fibrosis (CF), survives intracellularly in macrophages, and uniquely causes systemic infections in CF. Autophagy is a physiologic process that involves engulfing non-functional organelles and proteins and delivering them for lysosomal degradation, but also plays a role in eliminating intracellular pathogens, including *B. cenocepacia*. Autophagy is defective in CF but can be stimulated in murine CF models leading to increased clearance of *B. cenocepacia,* but little is known about autophagy stimulation in human CF macrophages. IFN-γ activates macrophages and increases antigen presentation while also inducing autophagy in macrophages. We therefore, hypothesized that treatment with IFN-γ would increase autophagy and macrophage activation in patients with CF. Peripheral blood monocyte derived macrophages (MDMs) were obtained from CF and non-CF donors and subsequently infected with *B. cenocepacia*. Basal serum levels of IFN-γ were similar between CF and non-CF patients, however after *B. cenocepacia* infection there is deficient IFN-γ production in CF MDMs. IFN-γ treated CF MDMs demonstrate increased co-localization with the autophagy molecule p62, increased autophagosome formation, and increased trafficking to lysosomes compared to untreated CF MDMs. Electron microscopy confirmed IFN-γ promotes double membrane vacuole formation around bacteria in CF MDMs, while only single membrane vacuoles form in untreated CF cells. Bacterial burden is significantly reduced in autophagy stimulated CF MDMs, comparable to non-CF levels. IL-1β production is decreased in CF MDMs after IFN-γ treatment. Together, these results demonstrate that IFN-γ promotes autophagy-mediated clearance of *B. cenocepacia* in human CF macrophages.

Editor: Erich Gulbins, University of Duisburg-Essen, Germany

Funding: This work was supported by funds provided by the Public Health Preparedness for Infectious Diseases program (phpid.osu.edu) (BK, AA) and Nationwide Children's Hospital institutional funds (BK). The funders had no role in study design, data collection and analysis, decision to publish, or preparation of the manuscript.

Competing Interests: The authors have declared that no competing interests exist.

* E-mail: Benjamin.Kopp@NationwideChildrens.org

Introduction

Cystic fibrosis (CF) is an inherited, life-limiting disease that causes multi-organ dysfunction characterized by progressive respiratory infections with inspissated mucous [1,2]. Patients with CF can be infected by a variety of pathogens, including the rapidly transmissible *Burkholderia cenocepacia* [3–6]. *B. cenocepacia* is a unique CF pathogen that causes either a distinct clinical phenotype of systemic fatal septicemia or hastened chronic respiratory deterioration with diminished long term survival [7,8]. Therapeutic options are severely limited due to multi-drug resistance and near universal exclusion from lung transplant eligibility due to poor post-transplant survival in chronically infected patients [9–13].

Macrophages are a first-line defense against pathogens including *B. cenocepacia*. The vital role of macrophages in CF pathogen interactions, in addition to airway epithelial cells, has been highlighted by several groups [14–19]. Bacteria survive in CF macrophages despite successful phagocytosis due to links between CF transmembrane conductance regulator (CFTR) dysfunction and impaired phagolysosomal killing [17,20,21]. *B. cenocepacia* is also specifically able to evade degradation in CF macrophages leading to severe and persistent inflammation [19,22,23]. Additionally, in model systems *B. cenocepacia* replicates inside of macrophages prior to dissemination [24].

In conjunction with macrophage defects, CF leads to deficient autophagy through inflammatory mediated cross-linking of the essential beclin-1 autophagy initiator interactome [25]. Autophagy is a physiologic process that normally augments innate responses to intraphagosomal pathogens and may relate to macrophage clearance defects. Deficient autophagy prevents destruction of engulfed *B. cenocepacia* in murine CF macrophages [22,26]. Autophagy stimulation by rapamycin reduces murine CF bacterial burden and inflammation [22]. Autophagy stimulation with rapamycin also enhances clearance of other major CF pathogens such as *Pseudomonas aeruginosa* [27] and *Staphylococcus aureus* [28], but autophagy has not been studied in human CF macrophages. Restoration of functional autophagy with an anti-inflammatory peptide, IDR-1018, decreases inflammation in CF cells [29], and may globally alleviate CF symptoms by releasing sequestered essential autophagy molecules, such as the autophagy adaptor molecule P62/SQSTM1 (p62)[30]. Relief of sequestered autophagy molecules enabled protein aggregate clearance and improved CFTR trafficking, lending benefits of autophagy-stimulated pathogen clearance [25].

Although rapamycin was effective in murine CF studies, systemic side effects of rapamycin in CF [31] and increased development of interstitial lung disease [32] prevent clinical trials. Additionally, autophagy stimulation by immununologics, such as rapamycin, raises questions how this would affect other microorganisms in the lungs of CF patients. Alternatively, IFN-γ has been shown to increase macrophage clearance of apoptotic cells in chronic granulomatous disease (CGD) [33], and is used prophylactically in CGD patients to prevent acquisition of severe infections such as *Burkholderia* species [34,35]. CGD, the only other known clinical disease commonly affected by *Burkholderia* species, also has known phagocytic killing defects [36,37] and was recently shown to have deficient autophagic responses to *B. cenocepacia*[*38*]. Furthermore, IFN-γ treatment enhances the autophagy response in macrophages derived from non-CGD patients resulting in clearance of pathogens that evade typical phagocytic degradation [39]. IFN-γ therapy is well tolerated in CGD patients who have altered immune functions and polymicrobial infections similar to CF [34,40]. Although a trial of inhaled IFN-γ in CF patients with mild to moderate disease did not prove effective in altering lung function [41], IFN-γ has never been studied systemically in CF, or specifically in *B. cenocepacia* infected patients, who may require more than local lung treatment.

We hypothesize that due to known defects in CF macrophage autophagy, IFN-γ will reduce *B. cenocepacia* burden in human CF macrophages through more effective killing and enhanced autophagy that degrade *B. cenocepacia* in nascent vacuoles.

Materials and Methods

Bacterial Strains and Culture

Burkholderia cenocepacia strain k56-2 is a clinical isolate of the ET12 lineage originally isolated from a CF patient's sputum. The strain was tagged dsRED and grown in Luria-Bertani (LB) broth at 37°C overnight with high amplitude shaking. The *B. cenocepacia* MHK1 strain is derived from k56-2 and has a mutation in an antibiotic efflux pump that confers gentamicin sensitivity, but does not alter the trafficking of the mutant in macrophages [42]. For colony forming unit (CFU) analysis, 50 μg/ml gentamicin (Invitrogen, 3564) was added for 0.5 hours as described previously [43]. To enumerate intracellular bacteria, infected macrophages were lysed with ice-cold PBS (Invitrogen, 14190) at designated times. Extracellular bacteria were enumerated directly from cell supernatants during macrophage viability assays. Recovered bacteria were quantified by plating serial dilutions on LB agar plates and counting colonies using the Acolyte Colony Counter, 5710/SYN.

Human Monocyte-Derived Macrophages (MDMs) –Ethics Statement

Human subjects underwent written informed consent for blood donation at the Nationwide Children's Hospital as approved by the Institutional Review Board of Nationwide Children's Hospital. Written consent from legal guardians of minors was obtained as well as written assent from minors aged 9 to 17 years. Blood was drawn in heparinized tubes. Exclusion criteria included history of *B. cepacia* complex culture positivity, chronic immunosuppression, CFTR modulator use, and history of transplantation. Chronic azithromycin was the only immunomodulatory medicine taken by some subjects during the study period. Peripheral blood mononuclear cells (PBMCs) were isolated from 27 CF and 27 non-CF healthy controls. Monocytes were separated using a Ficol gradient via Lymphocyte Separation Medium (Corning, 25-072-CV). Isolated monocytes were re-suspended in RPMI (Gibco, 22400-089) and 10% human AB serum (Lonza, 14-490E) to a concentration of 2×10^6 cells/mL and incubated for 5 days at 37°C to derive macrophages. Macrophages were then infected with *B. cenocepacia* strain k56-2 at a multiplicity of infection (MOI) ranging from 2–10 over the stated times.

Reagents

IFN-γ (eBioscience, 14-8319-80) was used at a concentration of 200 ηg/ml based upon effectiveness in trial experiments. Rapamycin (LC laboratories, AY-22989) was added to the cells at a concentration of 25 μg/ml. Treatments were added 1 hour post infection and the cells were allowed to incubate for 2, 4, and 24hours before obtaining results. Two mM 3-methyladenine (3MA, M9281) and 10 nM Bafilomycin (Sigma-Aldrich, B1793) were added one hour prior to infection in inhibitor experiments.

Immunoblotting

Macrophage supernatants were removed post treatment and the cells were washed twice with phosphate buffered saline (PBS). The cells were lysed in lysis buffer and primed with a protease inhibitor (Roche Applied Science, 10-519-978-001). Then, 30 ug of protein was separated by SDS-PAGE and transferred onto polyvinylidene difluoride (PVDF) membranes. Membranes were immunoblotted for LC3 (Sigma-Aldrich, L8918), p62 (Sigma-Aldrich, P0067), beclin-1 (Abcam, ab51031), actin (Abcam, ab8226-100), IFNGR1 (Abcam, ab61179), IFNGRbeta (Abcam, ab84524), and calreticulin (Stressgen, #SPA-600). Protein bands were detected with HRP-conjugated secondary antibodies visualized using enhanced chemiluminescent (ECL) reagents (Life Sciences, RPN2106).

Table 1. Patient Demographics.

	non CF patients (n = 27)	CF patients (n = 27)
Mean age (years ± st. dev.)	33.5±9.2	30.4±11.5
Males	30%	59%
Caucasian	100%	100%
Mean FEV1 (% predicted)	N/A	57.1±21.4
Pseudomonas colonization	N/A	81%
MRSA colonization	N/A	48%

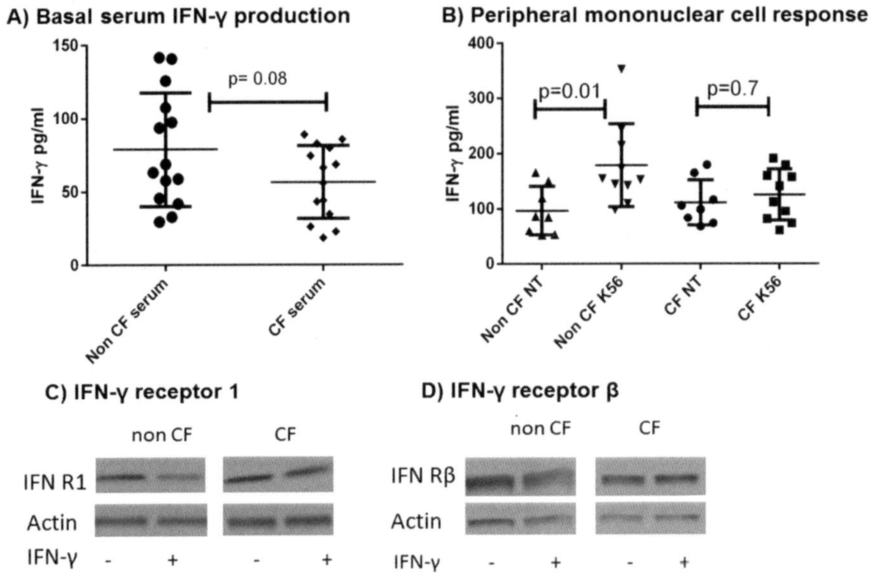

Figure 1. IFN-γ is deficiently produced in CF PBMCs in response to *B. cenocepacia.* 1A) IFN-γ levels from the serum of 14 non-CF and 14 CF patients at the time of blood donation, p = 0.056, n = 14 subjects for each condition, Mann-Whitney testing. 1B) IFN-γ production from PBMC 24 hour cell supernatants from CF and non-CF patients. NT represents uninfected cells, and k56 were infected with *B. cenocepacia* k56-2. n = 8 subjects for NT and 10 subjects k56, Mann-Whitney testing. 1C) Immunoblot for IFN-receptor 1 from cell lysates of MDMs infected with k56-2+/− treatment with IFN-γ. 1D) Immunoblot for IFN-receptor β from cell lysates of MDMs infected with k56-2+/− treatment with IFN-γ.

Enzyme-Linked Immunosorbent Assay (ELISA)

MDM culture supernatants were clarified and stored at −20°C until assayed for cytokine content. MDMs were infected for 4 and 24 hours with k56-2. The quantification of IL-1β, IFN-γ, and IL-10 in supernatants was determined by sandwich ELISA following the manufacturer's protocol (R&D system Inc, DY285) as previously described [43].

Cytotoxicity

MDMs were infected with k56-2 for 4 and 24hours and the culture supernatants were collected and centrifuged. Histone-associated DNA fragments were detected using a cytotoxicity detection photometric assay kit according to the manufacturer's protocol (Roche Applied Science, 11 644 793 001). All experiments were performed in at least triplicate. Additionally, macrophage viability was assessed via naphthol staining. MDMs were plated in 24-well plates, infected for 1 h, then treated for 24 h. Cells were washed and treated with 1% Cetavlon in 0.1 M citric acid with 0.05% Napthol blue black (Sigma-Aldrich), pH 2.2, for 15 min at room temperature. Stained nuclei were enumerated on a haemacytometer using phase-contrast microscopy.

Confocal Microscopy

Confocal microscopy sample were analyzed with an Olympus FV10i Spectral Confocal microscope. Two million MDMs were cultured on 12 mm glass cover slips in 24-well tissue culture plates and infected synchronously with k56-2 at an MOI of 2 or 10. Nuclei were stained with the nucleic acid dye 4′,6′-diamino-2-phenylindole (DAPI) blue for imaging. LC3 stained green with a cleaved LC3 antibody detection (Abgent, AP1805a). Lysosomes were stained green with Lysotracker Green (Invitrogen, L7526). p62 was detected with a green fluorescent ligand (BD Bioscience, 610832). At least one hundred macrophages were scored for each condition with scoring verified by independent study members. All experiments were performed in at least triplicate.

Transmission Electron Microscopy

TEM Images were obtained using a FEI Technai G2 Spirit transmission electron microscope (FEI, USA), Macrofire (Optronics) digital camera and AMT image capture Software with assistance from the Campus Microscopy and Imaging Facility (CMIF) at The Ohio State University. MDMs were isolated and infected with k56-2 at an MOI of 10 for 1 hour prior to 24 hour experimental treatments. Cells were cultured on Permanox (Lab-Tek) chamber slides and fixed with 2.5% gluteraldehyde in 0.1 M phosphate buffer with 0.1 M sucrose. Slides were post fixed with 1% osmium tetroxide in phosphate buffer then en bloc stained with 2% uranyl acetate in 10% ethanol, dehydrated in a graded series of ethanols and embedded in Eponate 12 epoxy resin (Ted Pella Inc., USA). Ultrathin sections were cut on a Leica EM UC6 ultra microtome (Leica microsystems, Germany), collected on copper grids, and then stained with lead citrate and uranyl acetate.

Statistical Analysis

Statistical analysis was performed using GraphPad Prism software (version 6.0). Statistical significance was determined with a two-tailed $p<0.05$. Mann-Whitney was used for non-parametric measurements, and ANOVA was used where appropriate.

Results

Patient Demographics

Subject demographics are described in Table 1. CF and non-CF subjects were similar in terms of ethnicity (100% Caucasian) and mean age (30.4±11.5 years vs. 33.5±9.2 years, p = 0.53). Subjects with CF had a mean forced expiratory volume in one second (FEV1) % predicted of 57.1%, indicative of moderately severe lung function at the time of sampling. 81% of CF patients had chronic respiratory cultures positive for *P. aeruginosa*, and 48% had methicillin resistant *S. aureus* (MRSA). Importantly, 48% of subjects were on chronic azithromycin prophylaxis, and this treatment was not noted to influence the experiments below.

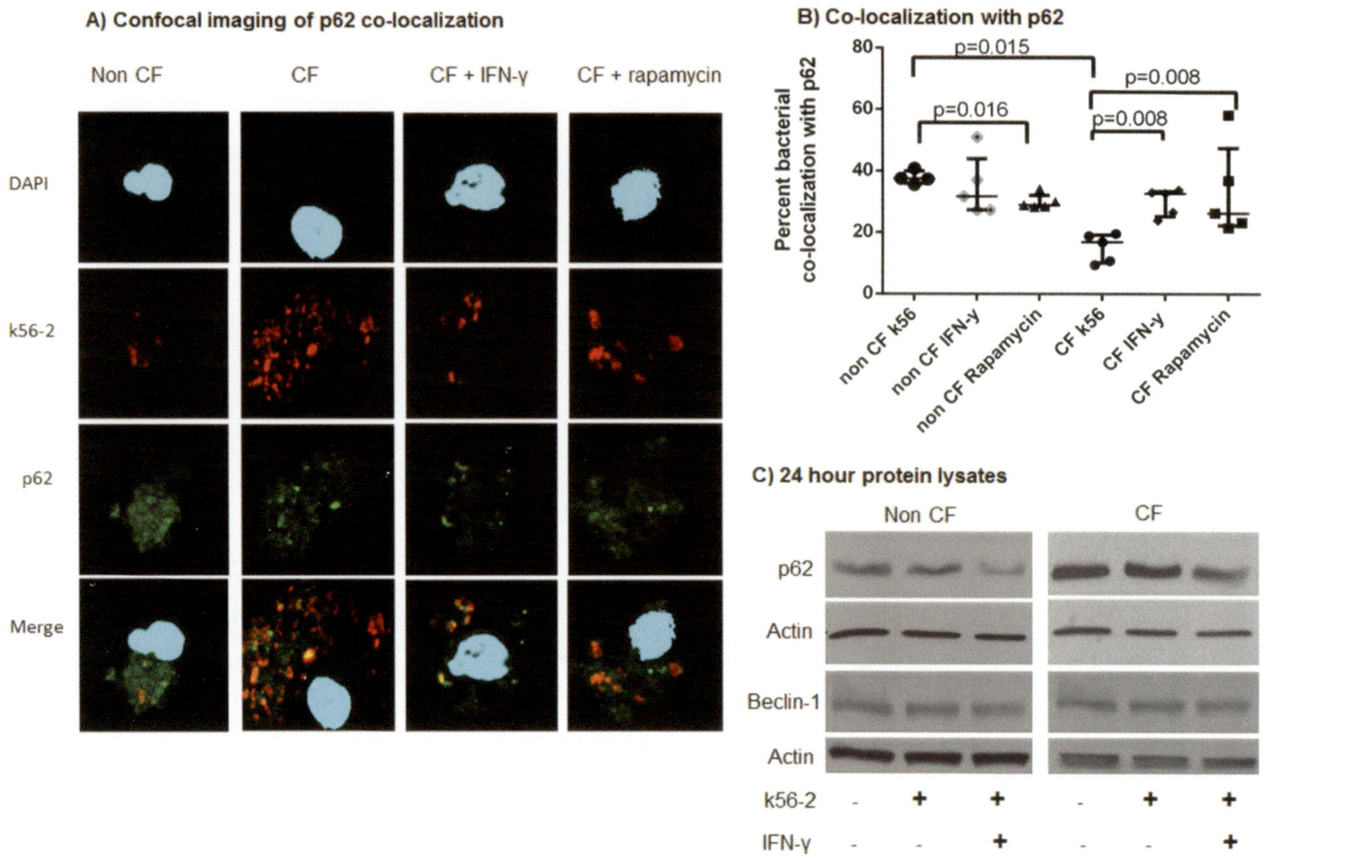

Figure 2. IFN-γ increases *B. cenocepacia* co-localization with p62 and decreases p62 accumulation in CF. 2A) Confocal microscopy for non-CF and CF macrophages infected with m-RFP expressing k56-2. IFN-γ or rapamycin treatment was administered after 1 hour of infection for a 24 hour treatment period. p62 is stained green, and macrophage nuclei are stained blue with DAPI. Co-localization of bacteria with p62 is noted in yellow in the bottom panel. 2B) The percentage of bacterial co-localization with p62 was scored for over 100 macrophages per condition, n = 5 subjects per condition, Mann-Whitney testing. 2C) Immunoblot for non-CF and CF macrophages demonstrating p62 accumulation in CF with reduction during IFN-γ therapy, representative of 5 subjects. Immunoblot of beclin-1 levels for non-CF and CF macrophages from cell lysates of control (NT) and MDMs infected with k56-2+/− treatment with IFN-γ, n = 4.

Azithromycin has been show to block autophagy in CF macrophages in vitro [44], but CF Patient Registry data does not support an increased risk of mycobacterial infections for those on chronic azithromycin as proposed in the study by Renna and colleagues[45]. Cell cultures in our experiments were not further treated with azithromycin.

IFN-γ Production is Reduced in CF PBMCs

IFN-γ effectively stimulates autophagic responses in macrophages [46,47]. However, CF cells insufficiently produce IFN-γ in response to another pathogen, *P. aeruginosa* [48]. To determine if IFN-γ is differentially produced in CF in response to *B. cenocepacia*, IFN-γ was measured in the serum of CF and non-CF subjects prior to macrophage isolation and in PBMC culture supernatants with and without 24 hour *B. cenocepacia* infection. Mean serum levels of IFN-γ were non-significantly lower in CF versus non-CF subjects (56.6±6.6 vs. 78.9±10.4, $p = 0.08$, Figure 1A). Infected non-CF PBMC supernatants displayed significantly higher IFN-γ levels compared to uninfected, whereas there was no change in IFN-γ production between uninfected and infected CF PBMCs (Figure 1B). Uninfected CF and non-CF PBMC IFN-γ levels were both slightly higher than serum levels. There was no difference in IFN-γ production between CF patients on azithromycin therapy and those not (figure S1A). Additionally, there was no difference in IFN-γ receptor expression during infection between IFN-γ treated and non-treated MDMs as measured by immunoblotting (Figures 1C, 1D). Our results are consistent with studies from *P. aeruginosa* [48], suggesting a defective host CF IFN-γ response to multiple pathogens in CF.

IFN-γ Increases *B. cenocepacia* Co-localization with p62

p62 is an essential intracellular protein that targets cargo for autophagy as well as regulates signaling pathways involved in cell survival and/or death [49]. This docking molecule is required for targeting *B. cenocepacia* to autophagosomes in a murine model[26], however its mechanism of action in human cells infected with *B. cenocepacia* is unknown. Using confocal microscopy, we investigated how p62 targets *B. cenocepacia* in human CF macrophages by examining MDMs for co-localization of bacteria with p62 after a 24 hour infection. MDMs were stimulated with rapamycin or IFN-γ for the duration of infection. Untreated CF macrophages demonstrated significantly less median co-localization with p62 compared to non-CF macrophages (16.8% (10.1–19.1) vs. 37.0% (34.9–40.0), $p = 0.016$, Figures 2A, B). IFN-γ or rapamycin treatment significantly increased median bacterial co-localization with p62 in CF human MDMs (CF IFN-γ 32.7% (25.2–33.4),

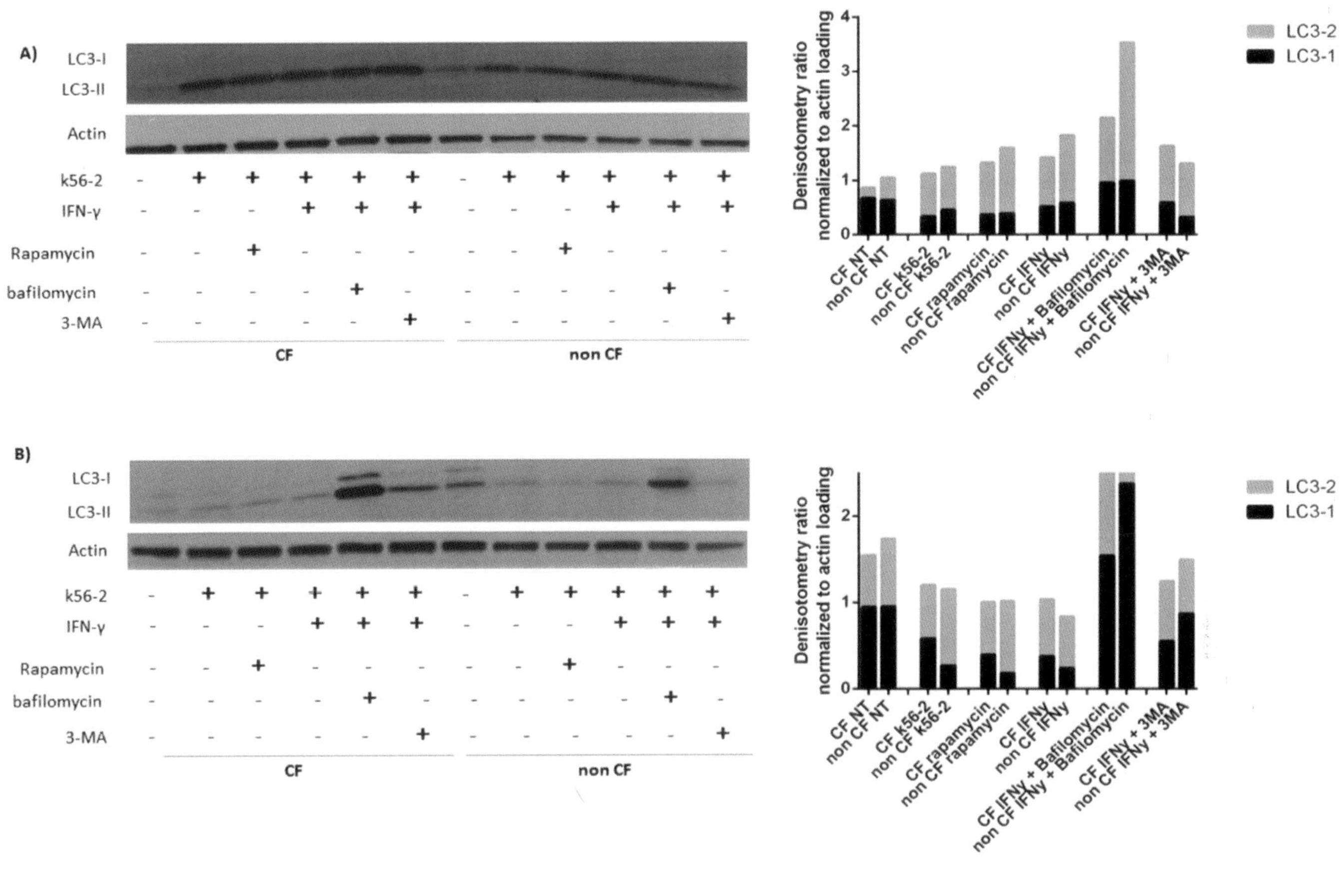

Figure 3. Autophagic flux is decreased in CF. 3A) Representative immunoblot of 4 hour treatment protein lysates for LC3-1 and LC3-2 from non-CF and CF macrophages, with corresponding summed band densitometries normalized to loading control. All lanes are marked with a "+" if the corresponding treatments were added: *B. cenocepacia* infection (k56-2), autophagy stimulators (IFN-y, Rapamycin) and autophagy inhibitors (Bafilomycin, 3-MA). Inhibitors were added one hour prior to infection. Autophagy stimulators were added one hour after infection for a total of 4 hours of treatment. Data is representative of 3 independent experiments. 3B) Representative immunoblot of 24 hour treatment protein lysates for LC3-1 and LC3-2 from non-CF and CF macrophages with corresponding summed band densitometries normalized to loading control. All lanes are marked with a "+" if the corresponding treatments were added: *B. cenocepacia* infection (k56-2), autophagy stimulators (IFN-y, Rapamycin) and autophagy inhibitors (Bafilomycin, 3-MA). Inhibitors were added one hour prior to infection. Autophagy stimulators were added one hour after infection for a total of 24 hours of treatment. Data is representative of 3 independent experiments.

p = 0.006, CF rapamycin 26.3% (22.4–47.4), p = 0.008, Figures 2A,B) nearing non-CF levels. p62 levels detected by western blotting are increased in uninfected and infected CF MDMs compared to non-CF MDMs (Figure 2C). Twenty-four hour IFN-γ treatment of non-CF and CF MDMs resulted in a decrement in p62 accumulation (Figure 2C). To ensure that initiation of the beclin-1 interactome was not influencing p62 expression, beclin-1 was measured via immunoblotting and confocal microscopy after 24 hour infection. There was no difference in beclin-1 levels between CF and non CF MDMs (Figure 2C, confocal not shown). Altogether, this data suggested that p62 is either sequestered or inefficiently utilized by human CF MDMs, and IFN-γ can alleviate this undesirable phenotype in CF cells.

Autophagic Flux is Enhanced by IFN-γ in CF MDMs

Autophagic flux is deficient in CF cells [25,30]. Microtubule-associated proteins 1A/1B light chain 3A (LC3) can be monitored to assess autophagosome formation and flux. During the autophagic process, cytosolic LC3 (LC3-I) is conjugated to phosphatidylethanolamine to form LC3-II, which is then recruited to the autophagosomal membrane. We analyzed LC3 concentrations by immunoblotting to monitor the conversion of LC3-I to LC3-II, as well as depletion/accumulation of the proteins to assist in determination of turnover of proteins. During basal, uninfected conditions (NT), CF macrophages demonstrated persistence of increased LC3-1 over 24 hours compared to non CF as evidence by high proportion of LC31 relative to total LC3 (Figures 3A, 3B). Infection with k56-2 leads to persistently elevated LC3-1 levels in CF by 24 hours compared to non CF, but to a lesser extent than basal conditions (Figure 3B). LC31 levels are seen to decrease in CF similar to non CF levels by 24 hours with the use of either IFN-γ or rapamycin (Figure 3B). Specific autophagy inhibitors were used to monitor treatment effects. The addition of bafilomycin to inhibit autophagolysosomal fusion via inhibiting vacuolar H+ ATPase (V-ATPase) caused an increase in LC3-1 in CF at 4 and 24 hours (Figures 3A,3B), reversing the effects of IFN-γ. The addition of 3-methyladenine (3-MA) to block autophagosome formation via inhibiting type III Phosphatidylinositol 3-kinases had a similar, but lesser effect in CF on LC3 conversion compared to bafilomycin. Combining data from 4 and 24 hour time points suggests a deficit in autophagic flux in CF macrophages, with enhancement through autophagy stimulators such as IFN-γ that are increasing autophagosome formation.

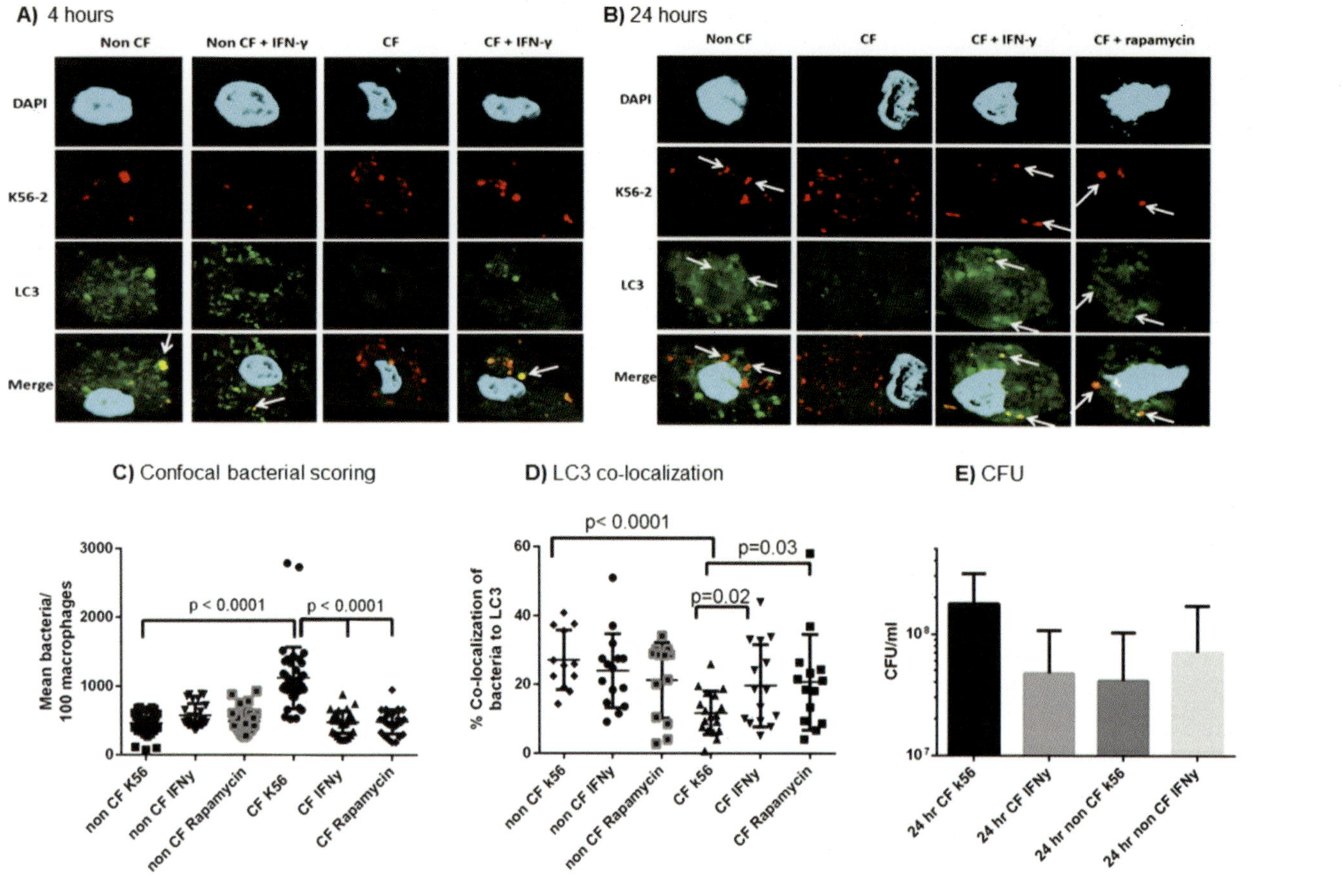

Figure 4. IFN-γ increases autophagosome formation. 4A) Confocal microscopy for non-CF and CF macrophages infected with m-RFP expressing k56-2. IFN-y treatment was administered after 1 hour of infection for a 4 hour treatment period. LC3 is stained green, and macrophage nuclei are stained blue with DAPI. Co-localization of bacteria with LC3 is noted in yellow in the bottom panel as noted by white arrows. 4B) 24 hour IFN-γ and rapamycin treatments similar to 4A. 4C) Summary of scored bacteria per 100 macrophages from individual subjects for the confocal microscopy experiments from 4B, n = 17 subjects, with 2 replicates per subject, unpaired t-test. 4D) The percentage of bacterial co-localization with LC3 was scored for over 100 macrophages per condition from 4B, n = 17 subjects, with 2 replicates per subject, unpaired t-test. 4E) CFU counts for non-CF and CF macrophages infected with MHK1 for 24 hours (n = 6).

Autophagy Stimulation Increases Bacterial Clearance in CF

B. cenocepacia infection causes increased bacterial burden in human and murine CF cells, indicating an innate defect in clearing the pathogen in CF [19,22]. Persistent bacterial loads can lead to systemic involvement and/or heightened inflammation. Because autophagy regulates pathogen clearance, we stimulated autophagy in MDMs with IFN-y or rapamycin for 4 and 24 hours and assessed bacterial clearance by confocal microscopy and CFU. Twenty-four hours is an expected clinical dosing regimen of IFN-γ, and 4 hours was chosen to ensure sufficient autophagosome formation, as murine studies have shown that even in wild type macrophages *B. cenocepacia* requires at least 2 hours to traffic to autophagosomes. There is no difference in bacterial counts at 2 hours (figure S2). At 4 hours of treatment, there were significantly higher bacterial counts in both autophagy-stimulated and unstimulated CF macrophages compared to non-CF macrophages (Figures 4A). However, CF macrophages treated with IFN-γ for 4 hours had a higher proportion of bacterial co-localized with autophagosomes as marked by LC3 compared to untreated CF macrophages (Figure 4A). A 24 hour treatment of IFN-γ or rapamycin markedly reduced bacterial counts in the CF macrophages compared to untreated CF macrophages (Figures 4B, 4C, 4E). These reductions mirror bacterial levels in non-CF macrophages. There was no difference in bacterial counts between CF patients on azithromycin therapy and those not (Supplemental Figure 1B). 24 hour extracellular bacterial counts were not reduced (Figure S2). There is a sustained increase in the co-localization of bacteria with LC3 after 24 hours of autophagy stimulation in CF macrophages compared to untreated CF macrophages ($p = 0.02$, Figures 4B, 4D). Electron microscopy confirmed these confocal findings. Untreated non-CF macrophages contained double membrane vacuoles surrounding *B. cenocepacia*, indicative of autophagosome formation (Figure 5A). Untreated CF macrophages displayed only single membrane bound vacuoles (5C), but when stimulated with IFN-γ, CF macrophages displayed double membrane vacuoles similar to the non-CF (5D). This observation suggests autophagosome formation is stimulated upon IFN-γ treatment in the CF MDMs. Additionally, IFN-γ had no direct effects on bacterial growth when added to bacteria in media devoid of MDMs, with no difference in bacterial growth over 24 hours between media with k56-2 alone, and media with k56-2 plus IFN-γ (Figure S3). In summation, these results indicate that IFN-γ effectively stimulates early autophagic targeting of *B. cenocepacia* to autophagosomes, thus allowing enhanced clearance after 24 hours.

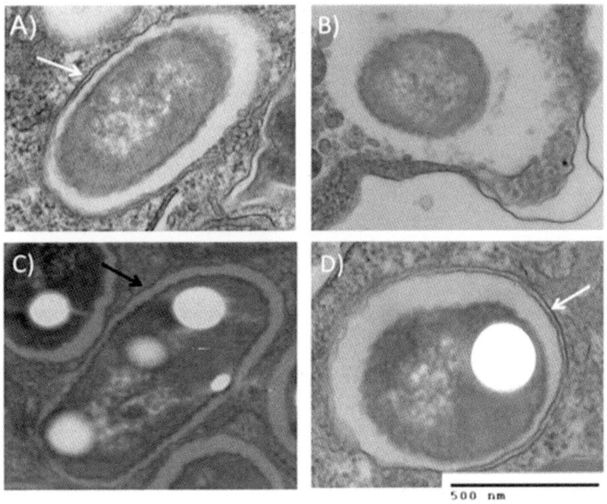

Figure 5. IFN-γ stimulates double-membrane autophagosome formation. 5A) Electron microscopy of non-CF macrophage infected with k56-2 only for 24 hours. White arrow indicates double membrane formation indicative of autophagosomes. 5B) EM of non-CF macrophage treated with IFN-γ for 24 hours. 5C) EM of CF macrophage infected with k56-2 only. Black arrow indicates single membrane vacuole. 5D) EM of CF macrophage treated with IFN-γ for 24 hours. White arrow indicates double membrane formation. Pictures are marked with 500 nm marker.

Lysosome Targeting is Increased in Autophagy Stimulated CF MDMs

Rapamycin increases lysosomal degradation of *B. cenocepacia* in CF murine macrophages by promoting phagosome-lysosome fusion via autophagy [22]. Human CF macrophages also demonstrate decreased co-localization of *B. cenocepacia* with lysosomes[19]. We examined the extent to which IFN-γ enhances autophagosome fusion with lysosomes by infecting human MDMs with *B. cenocepacia* for 1 hour and then treating with IFN-γ for 2 and 24 hours. We then scored co-localization of a fluorescent lysotracker with bacteria using confocal microscopy. After 2 hours of infection, untreated CF macrophages exhibited very little co-localization of bacteria with lysosomes (11.5±3.2%, Figures 6A, B) compared to non-CF macrophages (29.9±8.5%, Figures 6A, B). However, CF macrophages treated with IFN-γ demonstrate increased lysosomal co-localization of bacteria (26.5±.5%, $p < 0.0001$, Figures 6A, B). After 24 hours of IFN-γ therapy CF macrophages demonstrated a sustained lysosomal co-localization of remaining bacteria, similar to what was observed in non-CF macrophages (34.8±5.4% vs. 37.0±9.5%, $p = 0.5$, Figures 6C, D). Untreated CF macrophages have significantly less lysosomal co-localization compared to treated CF macrophages at 24 hours. (25.1±9.4%, $p = 0.038$, Figures 6C, D). Together, the results demonstrate delayed lysosomal targeting of *B. cenocepacia* in CF MDMs. Combined with prior results, IFN-γ treatment increases autophagosome formation in CF macrophages, enhancing lysosomal targeting of *B. cenocepacia*.

IL-1β Production is Decreased with Autophagy Stimulation

CF macrophages excessively produce the pro-inflammatory cytokine IL-1β in response to *B. cenocepacia* infection [19,50]. Human bronchial epithelial cells do not produce IL-1β in response to *B. cenocepacia* [51]. During *B. cenocepacia* infection pyrin inflammasome activation results in IL-1β release from mononuclear cells [52]. Therefore, we measured IL-1β production in human CF macrophages after autophagy stimulation as a primary source of excess inflammatory cytokine production during infection. MDMs were infected with *B. cenocepacia* and treated with IFN-γ or rapamycin for 4 and 24 hours and cell supernatants were examined by ELISA for IL-1β production. After 4 hours of autophagy stimulation, IL-1β levels were similar between treated and untreated CF macrophages, but CF macrophages had significantly more IL-1β than non-CF macrophages ($p = 0.0012$, Figure 7A). However, in CF macrophages treated with IFN-γ, IL-1β levels diminished by 24 hours of treatment ($p = 0.045$), while untreated CF macrophages infected with *B. cenocepacia* perpetuate elevated IL-1β production (Figure 7B). There was no difference in IL-1β production between CF patients on azithromycin therapy and those not (figure S1C). IL-10 was also measured as it can directly impair IFN-γ signaling pathways and its production can correlate with inflammatory cytokines such as IL-1β. There was no difference in IL-10 production in 24 hour supernatants between uninfected, infected, and IFN-γ treated CF and non-CF macrophages (Figure 7C). These results demonstrate autophagy induction plays a role in reducing IL-1β production in macrophage responses to *B. cenocepacia*.

Cell Death is Decreased by IFN-γ Treatment during *B. cenocepacia* Infection

B. cenocepacia promotes increased cell death in human CF macrophages [19]. Autophagy has an interconnected role with apoptosis and necrosis in the regulation of cell death [53]. We examined MDMs for LDH release at 4 and 24 hours after infection to assess cell death as a result of autophagy stimulation in CF macrophages infected with *B. cenocepacia*. After 4 hours of infection IFN-γ treated CF MDMs trended towards higher cell death compared to untreated CF MDMs (Figure 8A). All CF macrophages had higher cell death than non-CF macrophages (Figure 8A). After 24 of infection CF macrophages remained with slightly higher cell death than non-CF, except for IFN-γ treated CF MDMs. There was also no difference among autophagy stimulated CF macrophages compared to un-stimulated CF macrophages (Figures 8B). Macrophage viability was additionally assessed at 24 hours of infection via a naphthol blue/black assay. At 24 hours there was no difference in macrophage viability between CF and non CF macrophage (Figure 8C). Macrophage viability was not decreased with IFN-γ treatment (Figure 8c). Taken together, this data suggests that autophagic clearance of *B. cenocepacia* in CF macrophages decreases cell death in a human model after IFN-γ treatment.

Discussion

The discovery of new therapeutic classes or novel utilization of existing therapeutics is imperative for CF patients infected with *B. cenocepacia* due to its devastating impact on morbidity and mortality. Here, we demonstrate the effectiveness of autophagy stimulation as a therapeutic class, specifically IFN-γ in clearing *B. cenocepacia* from human CF macrophages. This is a crucial finding considering the mounting evidence for CFTR dysfunction in monocyte-pathogen interactions in CF[54], as well as the ability of *B. cenocepacia* to replicate within macrophages [24,55]. By improving the clearance of *B. cenocepacia* from macrophages, we can minimize the chances of overwhelming bacteremia as well as reduce continued pro-inflammatory signaling. Our work is aligned well with a recent study from Al-Khodor and colleagues in CGD macrophages [38], and importantly demonstrates the effectiveness of a post infection therapeutic intervention. Autophagy stimulation

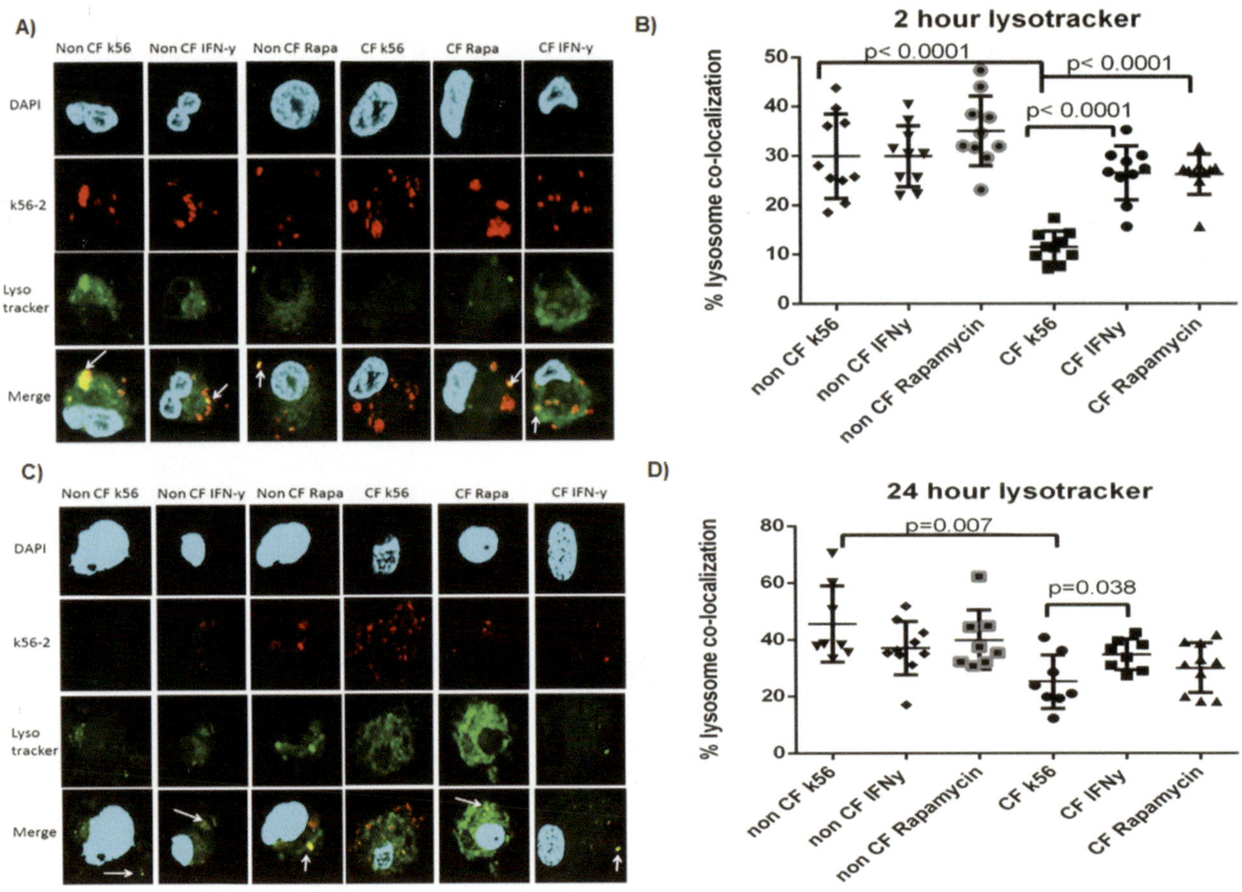

Figure 6. Lysosomal co-localization is increased with IFN-γ in CF. 6A) Confocal microscopy for non-CF and CF macrophages infected with k56-2. Macrophages were labeled with green lysotracker and bacterial co-localization to lysosomes was measured after a 2 hour infection. Macrophage nuclei are stained blue with DAPI. Co-localization of bacteria with lysotracker is noted in yellow by white arrows. 6B) Quantitative scoring of % bacterial co-localization with lysosomes from 6A, n = 8 subjects, Mann Whitney testing. 6C) 24 hour k56-2 infection with lysotracker staining. 6D) Bacterial co-localization with lysotracker quantitative scoring for 5C, n = 8 subjects, Mann-Whitney testing.

also holds the promise of clearing other pathogens in CF besides *B. cenocepacia* [27,28,56], as well as facilitating CFTR trafficking [30].

IFN-γ has numerous signaling effects in the body including host defense, autoimmunity, inflammatory responses, and is a major activator of macrophages [57]. Importantly, we found deficient production of IFN-γ with adequate receptor expression in CF PBMCs in response to *B. cenocepacia* compared to non-CF PBMCs, suggesting a natural defect in CF macrophage priming/pathogen

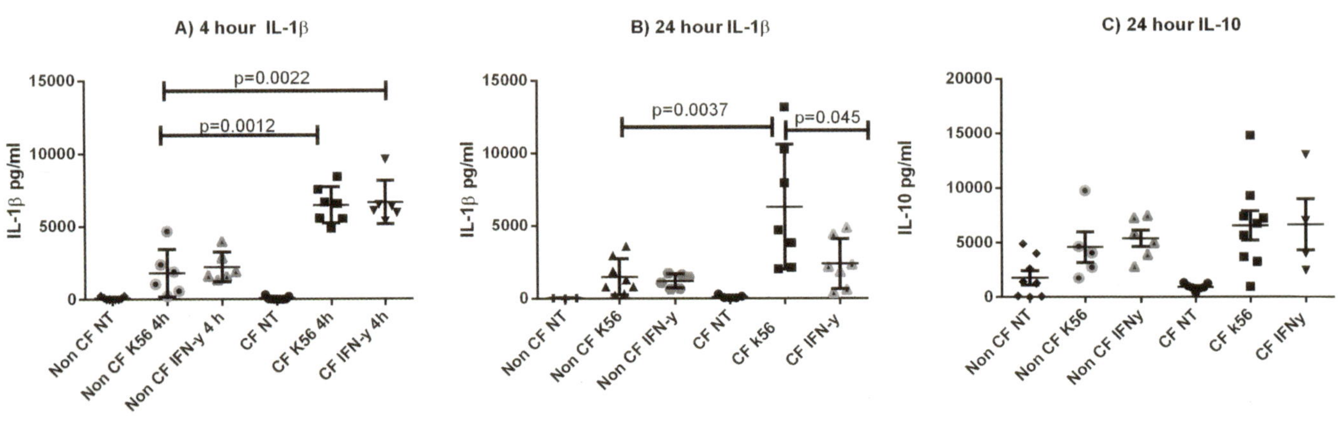

Figure 7. IL-1β is decreased with IFN-γ treatment in CF. IL-1β levels in macrophage supernatants after infection with k56-2 and either a 4 hour treatment with IFN-γ or a control diluent (7A) or a 24 hour IFN-γ treatment (7B), n = 7 subjects, Mann-Whitney analysis. 7C) IL-10 levels in macrophage supernatants after infection with k56-2 and a 24 hour treatment with IFN-γ or a control diluent, n = 7 subjects, Mann-Whitney analysis. Significant differences are noted.

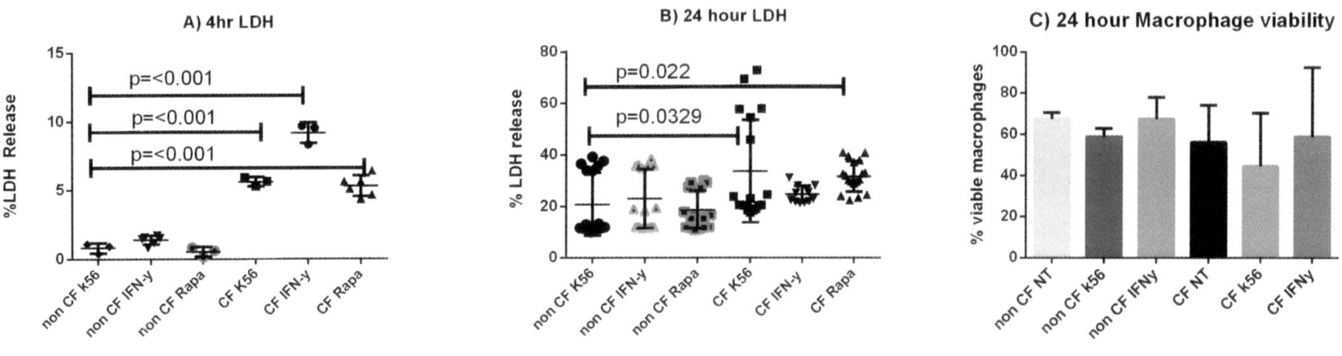

Figure 8. Cell death is decreased with autophagy stimulation in CF. Percent LDH release from MDM supernatants treated with autophagy stimulators IFN-γ or Rapamycin for 4 hours (8A) or 24 hours (8B), n = at least 6 subjects per condition, Mann-Whitney testing. 8c) Percent of macrophages deemed viable per naphthol staining after a 24 hour infection, n = 2.

response. This was in contrast to our previous work with the J2315 strain [19], however our previous study may have been affected by the different strain as well as negligible baseline IFN-γ from pure macrophage cultures. IFN γ has been previously studied in CF as an inhalational therapy in patients without *Burkholderia* infections, demonstrating no significant effects on lung function, sputum bacterial density, or inflammatory sputum markers [41]. However, in that study only 2 of the 48 treated patients had detected serum IFN-γ levels, and they did not measure lower airway IFN-γ levels to monitor deposition efficacy. Furthermore, the effective aerosol deposition of IFN-γ is low in several non-CF studies, which questions the efficacy of the aforementioned CF study as alveolar macrophages would not be affected by upper airway deposition. A 2004 study of aerosolized IFN-γ in TB patients demonstrated greater upper airway deposition of IFN-γ than lower airway, with a mean lower airway deposition of only 35.8 μg of a 500 ug dose [58]. Recent studies in patients with idiopathic pulmonary fibrosis demonstrated only 65% lower airway deposition using a Philips Respironics I-neb [59]. Based on the sputum density of CF patients it is reasonable to assume that nebulized concentrations of IFN-γ would be even lower in CF patients' lower airways, necessitating systemic IFN-γ use in situations such as *B. cenocepacia* septicemia or worsening patient progression until improved aerosol deposition can be achieved. Prior studies in CF murine models of *P. aeruginosa* infection effectively utilized IFN-γ as a systemic therapy [60], and patients with CGD inject IFN-γ subcutaneously to prevent infections with species including *Burkholderia* [34]. Known side effects of IFN-γ administration are fever, headaches, myalgias, fatigue, irritability, and flulike syndromes, but overall it has been safely used in CGD [61]. The effects of IFN-γ on the total CF microbiome still remain to be characterized, but on individual pathogens such as *B. cenocepacia* and *P. aeruginosa*, there is a demonstrable benefit on bacterial clearance.

Autophagy stimulation is also known to reduce inflammasome mediated IL-1β production [62] and attenuates hyperinflammatory responses from CF cells [29] independent of *B. cenocepacia*. We demonstrated that IFN-γ was effective in reducing the exaggerated IL-1β production that is observed in response to *B. cenocepacia* in CF macrophages. This result was not unexpected given the possibility of inflammasome dependent IFN-γ signaling [63], as well as the observed reduction in bacteria with IFN-γ treatment in the CF macrophages. Therefore, our results suggest the reductions in IL-1β are likely due to both the reduced burden observed and dampened inflammasome activation. IL-10 was unchanged with treatment, but was not significantly different between CF and non CF prior to treatment, and therefore not likely to be reduced with IFN-γ therapy. Importantly, IL 10 was not significantly overproduced in response to therapy.

In addition to reductions in bacteria and inflammatory cytokines, autophagy stimulation was effective in increasing autophagosome formation and trafficking of *B. cenocepacia* to lysosomes. *B. cenocepacia*-containing vacuoles have been shown to have prolonged arrest phases [64], and the ability to correctly utilize otherwise sequestered autophagic machinery may be key in overcoming this delay. Electron microscopy confirmed the presence of single membrane vacuoles containing *B. cenocepacia* in untreated CF macrophages that were effectively converted to double membrane autophagosomes upon IFN-γ stimulation. This process was marked by decreased p62 accumulation and decreased LC3-I accumulation, suggesting effective autophagic flux, allowing for early autophagolysosomal fusion and subsequent bacterial clearance.

This study is limited by the use of a single pathogen model, which was necessary to accurately follow *B. cenocepacia* trafficking as well as cytokine production. Future studies will examine multi-pathogen models to examine more closely effects on pathogen interactions. Further work is also needed *in vivo* to determine the benefits in human subjects. *B. cenocepacia* also possesses several quorum sensing systems that may affect its activity in humans and during a 24 hour infection model [65–67]. This will be important to consider in future multi-pathogen studies. Additionally, we tried to overcome inherent human subject differences in cell signaling and baseline medications through the use of multiple subjects. Importantly, we did not see differences in *B. cenocepacia* clearance by CF patients chronically on azithromycin, but samples did not receive further supplementation with azithromycin during any of the experiments.

In summary, CF macrophages have a deficient IFN-γ response to *B. cenocepacia*, ineffective utilization of the autophagy cargo molecule p62, decreased autophagosome formation, and delayed lysosomal uptake. IFN-γ treatment increased autophagy mediated clearance of *B. cenocepacia* in human CF macrophages via increased autophagosome formation and lysosomal trafficking, and was associated with decreased inflammatory cytokine production. The use of IFN-γ or autophagy stimulating drugs is promising for treating life-threatening or chronic infections from *B. cenocepacia* in patients with CF, but further study is needed to determine their efficacy outside of cell culture models.

Supporting Information

Figure S1 Chronic azithromycin use has no effect on CF MDMs. S1A) Serum (n = 7) and infected PBMC (k56, n = 5) IFN-γ levels from CF and non-CF patients separated by patients with (+azithromycin) and without chronic azithromycin prophylaxis. S1B) Summary of scored bacteria per 100 macrophages from individual subjects for the confocal microscopy experiments from 4B and separated by patients with (+azithromycin) and without chronic azithromycin prophylaxis. S1C) IL-1β levels in macrophage supernatants after infection with k56-2 and either a 24 hour treatment with IFN-γ or a control diluent and separated by patients with (+azithromycin) and without chronic azithromycin prophylaxis.

Figure S2 No difference in 2 hour or supernatant CFUs. CFU counts for non-CF and CF macrophages infected with MHK1 for 2 (n = 3) and 24 hour supernatants (n = 3) with or without IFN-γ treatment.

Figure S3 IFN-γ has no effect on bacterial growth in media devoid of MDMs. Optical density (OD) of bacteria cultured in LB broth alone (k56-2) versus LB + IFN-γ (IFN-γ) was compared over 24 hours during normal growth conditions at 37° with high amplitude shaking. Inset shows negligible difference at 24 hours in OD.

Acknowledgments

Thank you to Richard Montione from the CMIF at The Ohio State University for aiding with TEM processing. Thank you to Anwari Akhter and Kyle Caution for editing and experimental input. Thanks to Don Hayes Jr. for his editorial comments. Dr. Miguel Valvano kindly donated the MHK strain.

Author Contributions

Conceived and designed the experiments: KA AOA BTK. Performed the experiments: KA MFT BTK. Analyzed the data: KA MFT AOA BTK. Contributed reagents/materials/analysis tools: AOA BTK. Wrote the paper: KA BTK.

References

1. Grasemann H, Ratjen F (2013) Early lung disease in cystic fibrosis. Lancet Respir Med 1: 148–157.
2. Kreda SM, Davis CW, Rose MC (2012) CFTR, mucins, and mucus obstruction in cystic fibrosis. Cold Spring Harb Perspect Med 2: a009589.
3. Govan JR, Brown PH, Maddison J, Doherty CJ, Nelson JW, et al. (1993) Evidence for transmission of Pseudomonas cepacia by social contact in cystic fibrosis. Lancet 342: 15–19.
4. Sun L, Jiang RZ, Steinbach S, Holmes A, Campanelli C, et al. (1995) The emergence of a highly transmissible lineage of cbl+ Pseudomonas (Burkholderia) cepacia causing CF centre epidemics in North America and Britain. Nat Med 1: 661–666.
5. Walsh NM, Casano AA, Manangan LP, Sinkowitz-Cochran RL, Jarvis WR (2002) Risk factors for Burkholderia cepacia complex colonization and infection among patients with cystic fibrosis. J Pediatr 141: 512–517.
6. Drevinek P, Mahenthiralingam E (2010) Burkholderia cenocepacia in cystic fibrosis: epidemiology and molecular mechanisms of virulence. Clin Microbiol Infect 16: 821–830.
7. Jones AM, Dodd ME, Govan JR, Barcus V, Doherty CJ, et al. (2004) Burkholderia cenocepacia and Burkholderia multivorans: influence on survival in cystic fibrosis. Thorax 59: 948–951.
8. Isles A, Maclusky I, Corey M, Gold R, Prober C, et al. (1984) Pseudomonas cepacia infection in cystic fibrosis: an emerging problem. J Pediatr 104: 206–210.
9. Alexander BD, Petzold EW, Reller LB, Palmer SM, Davis RD, et al. (2008) Survival after lung transplantation of cystic fibrosis patients infected with Burkholderia cepacia complex. Am J Transplant 8: 1025–1030.
10. De Soyza A, Meachery G, Hester KL, Nicholson A, Parry G, et al. (2010) Lung transplantation for patients with cystic fibrosis and Burkholderia cepacia complex infection: a single-center experience. J Heart Lung Transplant 29: 1395–1404.
11. Egan TM, Detterbeck FC, Mill MR, Bleiweis MS, Aris R, et al. (2002) Long term results of lung transplantation for cystic fibrosis. Eur J Cardiothorac Surg 22: 602–609.
12. Murray S, Charbeneau J, Marshall BC, LiPuma JJ (2008) Impact of burkholderia infection on lung transplantation in cystic fibrosis. Am J Respir Crit Care Med 178: 363–371.
13. Olland A, Falcoz PE, Kessler R, Massard G (2011) Should cystic fibrosis patients infected with Burkholderia cepacia complex be listed for lung transplantation? Interact Cardiovasc Thorac Surg 13: 631–634.
14. Brennan S, Sly PD, Gangell CL, Sturges N, Winfield K, et al. (2009) Alveolar macrophages and CC chemokines are increased in children with cystic fibrosis. Eur Respir J 34: 655–661.
15. Bruscia EM, Zhang PX, Ferreira E, Caputo C, Emerson JW, et al. (2009) Macrophages directly contribute to the exaggerated inflammatory response in cystic fibrosis transmembrane conductance regulator−/− mice. Am J Respir Cell Mol Biol 40: 295–304.
16. Bruscia EM, Zhang PX, Satoh A, Caputo C, Medzhitov R, et al. (2011) Abnormal trafficking and degradation of TLR4 underlie the elevated inflammatory response in cystic fibrosis. J Immunol 186: 6990–6998.
17. Del Porto P, Cifani N, Guarnieri S, Di Domenico EG, Mariggio MA, et al. (2011) Dysfunctional CFTR alters the bactericidal activity of human macrophages against Pseudomonas aeruginosa. PLoS One 6: e19970.
18. Hartl D, Gaggar A, Bruscia E, Hector A, Marcos V, et al. (2012) Innate immunity in cystic fibrosis lung disease. J Cyst Fibros 11: 363–382.
19. Kopp BT, Abdulrahman BA, Khweek AA, Kumar SB, Akhter A, et al. (2012) Exaggerated inflammatory responses mediated by Burkholderia cenocepacia in human macrophages derived from Cystic fibrosis patients. Biochem Biophys Res Commun 424: 221–227.
20. Vandivier RW, Richens TR, Horstmann SA, deCathelineau AM, Ghosh M, et al. (2009) Dysfunctional cystic fibrosis transmembrane conductance regulator inhibits phagocytosis of apoptotic cells with proinflammatory consequences. Am J Physiol Lung Cell Mol Physiol 297: L677–686.
21. Di A, Brown ME, Deriy LV, Li C, Szeto FL, et al. (2006) CFTR regulates phagosome acidification in macrophages and alters bactericidal activity. Nat Cell Biol 8: 933–944.
22. Abdulrahman BA, Khweek AA, Akhter A, Caution K, Kotrange S, et al. (2011) Autophagy stimulation by rapamycin suppresses lung inflammation and infection by Burkholderia cenocepacia in a model of cystic fibrosis. Autophagy 7: 1359–1370.
23. Kotrange S, Kopp B, Akhter A, Abdelaziz D, Abu Khweek A, et al. (2011) Burkholderia cenocepacia O polysaccharide chain contributes to caspase-1-dependent IL-1beta production in macrophages. J Leukoc Biol 89: 481–488.
24. Vergunst AC, Meijer AH, Renshaw SA, O'Callaghan D (2010) Burkholderia cenocepacia creates an intramacrophage replication niche in zebrafish embryos, followed by bacterial dissemination and establishment of systemic infection. Infect Immun 78: 1495–1508.
25. Luciani A, Villella VR, Esposito S, Brunetti-Pierri N, Medina D, et al. (2010) Defective CFTR induces aggresome formation and lung inflammation in cystic fibrosis through ROS-mediated autophagy inhibition. Nat Cell Biol 12: 863–875.
26. Abdulrahman BA, Khweek AA, Akhter A, Caution K, Tazi M, et al. (2013) Depletion of the ubiquitin-binding adaptor molecule SQSTM1/p62 from macrophages harboring cftr DeltaF508 mutation improves the delivery of Burkholderia cenocepacia to the autophagic machinery. J Biol Chem 288: 2049–2058.
27. Yuan K, Huang C, Fox J, Laturnus D, Carlson E, et al. (2012) Autophagy plays an essential role in the clearance of Pseudomonas aeruginosa by alveolar macrophages. J Cell Sci 125: 507–515.
28. Schnaith A, Kashkar H, Leggio SA, Addicks K, Kronke M, et al. (2007) Staphylococcus aureus subvert autophagy for induction of caspase-independent host cell death. J Biol Chem 282: 2695–2706.
29. Mayer ML, Blohmke CJ, Falsafi R, Fjell CD, Madera L, et al. (2013) Rescue of Dysfunctional Autophagy Attenuates Hyperinflammatory Responses from Cystic Fibrosis Cells. J Immunol 190: 1227–1238.
30. Luciani A, Villella VR, Esposito S, Gavina M, Russo I, et al. (2012) Targeting autophagy as a novel strategy for facilitating the therapeutic action of potentiators on DeltaF508 cystic fibrosis transmembrane conductance regulator. Autophagy 8: 1657–1672.
31. Hardinger KL, Cornelius LA, Trulock EP, 3rd, Brennan DC (2002) Sirolimus-induced leukocytoclastic vasculitis. Transplantation 74: 739–743.
32. Chhajed PN, Dickenmann M, Bubendorf L, Mayr M, Steiger J, et al. (2006) Patterns of pulmonary complications associated with sirolimus. Respiration 73: 367–374.
33. Fernandez-Boyanapalli R, McPhillips KA, Frasch SC, Janssen WJ, Dinauer MC, et al. (2010) Impaired phagocytosis of apoptotic cells by macrophages in chronic granulomatous disease is reversed by IFN-gamma in a nitric oxide-dependent manner. J Immunol 185: 4030–4041.

34. (1991) A controlled trial of interferon gamma to prevent infection in chronic granulomatous disease. The International Chronic Granulomatous Disease Cooperative Study Group. N Engl J Med 324: 509–516.
35. Errante PR, Frazao JB, Condino-Neto A (2008) The use of interferon-gamma therapy in chronic granulomatous disease. Recent Pat Antiinfect Drug Discov 3: 225–230.
36. McPhail LC, DeChatelet LR, Shirley PS, Wilfert C, Johnston RB Jr, et al. (1977) Deficiency of NADPH oxidase activity in chronic granulomatous disease. J Pediatr 90: 213–217.
37. Sanmun D, Witasp E, Jitkaew S, Tyurina YY, Kagan VE, et al. (2009) Involvement of a functional NADPH oxidase in neutrophils and macrophages during programmed cell clearance: implications for chronic granulomatous disease. Am J Physiol Cell Physiol 297: C621–631.
38. Al-Khodor S, Marshall-Batty K, Nair V, Ding L, Greenberg DE, et al. (2014) Burkholderia cenocepacia J2315 escapes to the cytosol and actively subverts autophagy in human macrophages. Cell Microbiol 16: 378–395.
39. Gutierrez MG, Master SS, Singh SB, Taylor GA, Colombo MI, et al. (2004) Autophagy is a defense mechanism inhibiting BCG and Mycobacterium tuberculosis survival in infected macrophages. Cell 119: 753–766.
40. Holland SM (2010) Chronic granulomatous disease. Clin Rev Allergy Immunol 38: 3–10.
41. Moss RB, Mayer-Hamblett N, Wagener J, Daines C, Hale K, et al. (2005) Randomized, double-blind, placebo-controlled, dose-escalating study of aerosolized interferon gamma-1b in patients with mild to moderate cystic fibrosis lung disease. Pediatr Pulmonol 39: 209–218.
42. Hamad MA, Skeldon AM, Valvano MA (2010) Construction of aminoglycoside-sensitive Burkholderia cenocepacia strains for use in studies of intracellular bacteria with the gentamicin protection assay. Appl Environ Microbiol 76: 3170–3176.
43. Akhter A, Gavrilin MA, Frantz L, Washington S, Ditty C, et al. (2009) Caspase-7 activation by the Nlrc4/Ipaf inflammasome restricts Legionella pneumophila infection. PLoS Pathog 5: e1000361.
44. Renna M, Schaffner C, Brown K, Shang S, Tamayo MH, et al. (2011) Azithromycin blocks autophagy and may predispose cystic fibrosis patients to mycobacterial infection. J Clin Invest 121: 3554–3563.
45. Binder AM, Adjemian J, Olivier KN, Prevots DR (2013) Epidemiology of nontuberculous mycobacterial infections and associated chronic macrolide use among persons with cystic fibrosis. Am J Respir Crit Care Med 188: 807–812.
46. Al-Zeer MA, Al-Younes HM, Lauster D, Abu Lubad M, Meyer TF (2013) Autophagy restricts Chlamydia trachomatis growth in human macrophages via IFNG-inducible guanylate binding proteins. Autophagy 9: 50–62.
47. Matsuzawa T, Kim BH, Shenoy AR, Kamitani S, Miyake M, et al. (2012) IFN-gamma elicits macrophage autophagy via the p38 MAPK signaling pathway. J Immunol 189: 813–818.
48. Moser C, Kjaergaard S, Pressler T, Kharazmi A, Koch C, et al. (2000) The immune response to chronic Pseudomonas aeruginosa lung infection in cystic fibrosis patients is predominantly of the Th2 type. APMIS 108: 329–335.
49. Komatsu M, Kageyama S, Ichimura Y (2012) p62/SQSTM1/A170: physiology and pathology. Pharmacol Res 66: 457–462.
50. McKeon S, McClean S, Callaghan M (2010) Macrophage responses to CF pathogens: JNK MAP kinase signaling by Burkholderia cepacia complex lipopolysaccharide. FEMS Immunol Med Microbiol 60: 36–43.
51. Gillette DD, Shah PA, Cremer T, Gavrilin MA, Besecker BY, et al. (2013) Analysis of human bronchial epithelial cell proinflammatory response to Burkholderia cenocepacia infection: inability to secrete il-1beta. J Biol Chem 288: 3691–3695.
52. Gavrilin MA, Abdelaziz DH, Mostafa M, Abdulrahman BA, Grandhi J, et al. (2012) Activation of the Pyrin Inflammasome by Intracellular Burkholderia cenocepacia. J Immunol 188: 3469–3477.
53. Jain MV, Paczulla AM, Klonisch T, Dimgba FN, Rao SB, et al. (2013) Interconnections between apoptotic, autophagic and necrotic pathways: implications for cancer therapy development. J Cell Mol Med 17: 12–29.
54. Van de Weert-van Leeuwen PB, Van Meegen MA, Speirs JJ, Pals DJ, Rooijakkers SH, et al. (2013) Optimal complement-mediated phagocytosis of Pseudomonas aeruginosa by monocytes is cystic fibrosis transmembrane conductance regulator-dependent. Am J Respir Cell Mol Biol 49: 463–470.
55. Sajjan SU, Carmody LA, Gonzalez CF, LiPuma JJ (2008) A type IV secretion system contributes to intracellular survival and replication of Burkholderia cenocepacia. Infect Immun 76: 5447–5455.
56. Junkins RD, Shen A, Rosen K, McCormick C, Lin TJ (2013) Autophagy enhances bacterial clearance during P. aeruginosa lung infection. PLoS One 8: e72263.
57. Farrar MA, Schreiber RD (1993) The molecular cell biology of interferon-gamma and its receptor. Annu Rev Immunol 11: 571–611.
58. Condos R, Hull FP, Schluger NW, Rom WN, Smaldone GC (2004) Regional deposition of aerosolized interferon-gamma in pulmonary tuberculosis. Chest 125: 2146–2155.
59. Diaz KT, Skaria S, Harris K, Solomita M, Lau S, et al. (2012) Delivery and safety of inhaled interferon-gamma in idiopathic pulmonary fibrosis. J Aerosol Med Pulm Drug Deliv 25: 79–87.
60. Johansen HK, Hougen HP, Rygaard J, Hoiby N (1996) Interferon-gamma (IFN-gamma) treatment decreases the inflammatory response in chronic Pseudomonas aeruginosa pneumonia in rats. Clin Exp Immunol 103: 212–218.
61. Marciano BE, Wesley R, De Carlo ES, Anderson VL, Barnhart LA, et al. (2004) Long-term interferon-gamma therapy for patients with chronic granulomatous disease. Clin Infect Dis 39: 692–699.
62. Shi CS, Shenderov K, Huang NN, Kabat J, Abu-Asab M, et al. (2012) Activation of autophagy by inflammatory signals limits IL-1beta production by targeting ubiquitinated inflammasomes for destruction. Nat Immunol 13: 255–263.
63. Mitchell AJ, Yau B, McQuillan JA, Ball HJ, Too LK, et al. (2012) Inflammasome-dependent IFN-gamma drives pathogenesis in Streptococcus pneumoniae meningitis. J Immunol 189: 4970–4980.
64. Lamothe J, Valvano MA (2008) Burkholderia cenocepacia-induced delay of acidification and phagolysosomal fusion in cystic fibrosis transmembrane conductance regulator (CFTR)-defective macrophages. Microbiology 154: 3825–3834.
65. Subramoni S, Sokol PA (2012) Quorum sensing systems influence Burkholderia cenocepacia virulence. Future Microbiol 7: 1373–1387.
66. Aubert DF, O'Grady EP, Hamad MA, Sokol PA, Valvano MA (2013) The Burkholderia cenocepacia sensor kinase hybrid AtsR is a global regulator modulating quorum-sensing signalling. Environ Microbiol 15: 372–385.
67. O'Grady EP, Viteri DF, Sokol PA (2012) A unique regulator contributes to quorum sensing and virulence in Burkholderia cenocepacia. PLoS One 7: e37611.

Improvement of Chloride Transport Defect by Gonadotropin-Releasing Hormone (GnRH) in Cystic Fibrosis Epithelial Cells

Nathalie Benz[1,2], Sophie Le Hir[1,3], Caroline Norez[4], Mathieu Kerbiriou[1,5], Marie-Laure Calvez[1,5], Frédéric Becq[4], Pascal Trouvé[1]*, Claude Férec[1,3,5,6]*

1 Institut National de la Santé et de la Recherche Médicale, UMR1078, Brest, France, **2** Association Gaetan Saleun, Brest, France, **3** C.H.U. Brest, Hôpital Morvan, Laboratoire de Génétique Moléculaire, Brest, France, **4** Institut de Physiologie et Biologie Cellulaires, Centre national de la recherche scientifique FRE 3511, Université de Poitiers, Poitiers, France, **5** Université de Bretagne Occidentale, Faculté de Médecine et des sciences de la santé, Brest, France, **6** Etablissement Français du Sang - Bretagne, Brest, France

Abstract

Cystic fibrosis (CF), the most common autosomal recessive disease in Caucasians, is due to mutations in the CFTR gene. F508del, the most frequent mutation in patients, impairs CFTR protein folding and biosynthesis. The F508del-CFTR protein is retained in the endoplasmic reticulum (ER) and its traffic to the plasma membrane is altered. Nevertheless, if it reaches the cell surface, it exhibits a Cl^- channel function despite a short half-life. Pharmacological treatments may target the F508del-CFTR defect directly by binding to the mutant protein or indirectly by altering cellular proteostasis, and promote its plasma membrane targeting and stability. We previously showed that annexine A5 (AnxA5) directly binds to F508del-CFTR and, when overexpressed, promotes its membrane stability, leading to the restoration of some Cl^- channel function in cells. Because Gonadotropin-Releasing Hormone (GnRH) increases AnxA5 expression in some cells, we tested it in CF cells. We showed that human epithelial cells express GnRH-receptors (GnRH-R) and that GnRH induces an AnxA5 overexpression and an increased Cl^- channel function in F508del-CFTR cells, due to an increased stability of the protein in the membranes. Beside the numerous physiological implications of the GnRH-R expression in epithelial cells, we propose that a topical use of GnRH is a potential treatment in CF.

Editor: Dominik Hartl, University of Tübingen, Germany

Funding: The authors thank the association Gaëtan Salaün, the SFR Scinbios (Brest) and the French foundation "Vaincre la Mucoviscidose" for their financial support. The funders had no role in study design, data collection and analysis, decision to publish, or preparation of the manuscript.

Competing Interests: The authors have declared that no competing interests exist.

* E-mail: pascal.trouve@univ-brest.fr (PT); claude.ferec@univ-brest.fr (CF)

Introduction

Cystic fibrosis (CF) is the most common autosomal recessive disease in Caucasians. It is caused by mutations in the gene encoding the cystic fibrosis transmembrane conductance regulator (CFTR) protein [1]. CFTR which is a member of the ATP-binding cassette (ABC) transporter superfamily, functions as an ion channel [1,2]. It is mostly expressed in the apical membrane of epithelial cells and helps to maintain the fluid and electrolyte balance across the cell membrane. CFTR comprises two membrane-spanning domains (MSDs), two nucleotide-binding domains (NBDs) and a regulatory domain (RD). The CFTR protein undergoes a complex biosynthetic pathway in the endoplasmic reticulum (ER) in which molecular chaperones and co-chaperones are involved [3]. Wild-type CFTR (Wt-CFTR) biogenesis initiates in the ER where the protein is core-glycosylated, leading to an immature precursor form known as band B (~145 KDa). It further undergoes maturation and glycosylation through the Golgi, originating a complex mature form (band C, ~170-kDa) [4]. Only 25% to 70% of the precursor Wt-CFTR matures, depending on the cell type [5]. The remaining part undergoes ubiquitination and degradation by the proteasomal pathway [6,7]. In membranes, once phosphorylated by protein kinase A (PKA) in the R domain, CFTR functions as an ATP-gated chloride (Cl^-) channel [8].

Among the 1930 described mutations in the CFTR gene (http://www.genet.sickkids.on.ca/cftr/app), the deletion of phenylalanine at position 508 (F508del) is the most common one, associated with ~70% of CF alleles [9]. The F508del mutation causes a protein folding defect, the nascent protein beeing retained in the ER. As a result, most of the F508del-CFTR channels are degraded intracellularly and very little is targetted to the plasma membrane [10–13]. Nevertheless, in the plasma membrane it exhibits a Cl^- channel activity despite an open probability 15 times lower than that of Wt-CFTR [14–16]. Furthermore, the F508del-CFTR protein has a faster turnover at the cell surface than Wt-CFTR [17].

In order to overcome the F508del-CFTR defects and provide a potential treatment for CF, potentiators aimed to correct the channel's activity and correctors of the F508del-CFTR trafficking defect have been developed. Potentiators that increase the mutated CFTR's channel activity when it is phosphorylated function via direct binding to modulate the NBDs dimerization or to increase ATP binding and hydrolysis [18–20]. Correctors may act indirectly or by a direct binding to F508del-CFTR. Indirect correctors such as 4-phenylbutyrate [21], glycerol [22], low temperature [23] and miglustat [24] act upon folding, ER retention, degradation and F508del-CFTR trafficking. To date, only few correctors that act specifically on F508del-CFTR by a direct binding and called pharmacological chaperones, are reported. These are VRT325, Corr4a, VRT532 and benzo[*c*]quinolizinium compounds [25–27]. Among potential proteins that bind to CFTR, we demonstrated that annexin A5 (AnxA5) binds directly to Wt- and F508del-CFTR when the channel is in the plasma membrane of cells. Indeed, we showed that AnxA5 is associated with the NBD1 of CFTR and using a siRNA and overexpression approach, we showed that CFTR's channel function and membrane localization were dependent on AnxA5 expression [28].

Because our previous results showed that raised AnxA5 expression induced an augmented function of F508del-CFTR due to increased membrane localization [29], the aim of the present study was to highlight a mean to increase AnxA5 expression in F508del-CFTR expressing cells, using a drug with no side effect upon cell survival. Because it was previously showed that AnxA5 is synthesized in gonadotropes and in various cell types under the effect of gonadotropin-releasing hormone (GnRH) or some of its analogs, through mitogen activated protein kinase (MAPK), we tested the hypothesis that GnRH could increase AnxA5 expression in a human epithelial cell line and subsequently induce an increased F508del-CFTR function [30–32]. Using PCR, western blottings, iodide (I^-) efflux experiments and patch-clamp experiments we show here that human epithelial cells express GnRH- receptors (GnRH-R) and that GnRH induces an AnxA5 overexpression and subsequently an increased Cl^- channel function of F508del-CFTR, likely due to an increased localization of the protein in membranes.

In conclusion, we show here that human epithelial cells do express GnRH-R, which has numerous physiological implications. We also propose that a topical use of GnRH is a potential treatment for CF.

Methods

Cell Culture

The 16HBE14o$^-$ and the CFBE41o$^-$ airway epithelial cell lines were obtained from Professor D. Gruenert [33,34]. The 16HBE14o− cell line was originally developed from human bronchial epithelium to study CFTR and retains many features of differentiated bronchial epithelial cells [33]. The CFBE41o- respiratory epithelial cell line was derived from the bronchus of a patient with cystic fibrosis and immortalized with SV40. Cell culture media and supplements were purchased from Lonza (Basel, Switzerland) and PAA (Pasching, Austria). The transduced CFBE41o$^-$ cell lines (CFBE41o$^-$/corrected called CFBE41o−/corr and CFBE41o$^-$/F508del) used in experiments were cultured as described previously [35]. CFBE41o$^-$/corr and CFBE41o$^-$/F508del cells were obtained by wild-type and F508del-CFTR cDNA stably introduction into CFBE41o$^-$ cells, harbouring therefore the same genetic background [34,36]. Cells were treated with 10^{-9} M synthetic GnRH ([Gly-OH10]-LH-RH) from Sigma-Aldrich (Saint-Louis, MO, USA) for 30, 60, 120, 180 and 310 min.

Transfection

For GnRH-R overexpression and inhibition, cells were transfected using Lipofectamine 2000 (Life Technologies Corporation, Carlsbad, CA, USA), according to the manufacturer's instructions, with either the human cDNA clone pCMV6-XL5/GNRH-R (OriGene Technologies Inc., Rockville, MD, USA) or the human GnRH-R siRNA (5′-GGAAUUUGGUAUUGGUUUG-3′, siGENOME individual duplex (Thermo Fisher Scientific Inc., Waltham, MA, USA). The scrambled control siRNA was siGENOME Non-Targeting (Thermo Fisher Scientific Inc.).

RNA Extraction and Quantitative Real-time PCR

Quantitative Real-Time PCR was performed to assess the basal GnRH-R and AnxA5 mRNA expression in cells and to study their modulation after GnRH treatment. Cultured medium was removed and cells were washed twice with phosphate-buffered saline (PBS). RNA was extracted using RNeasy Plus mini kit (QIAGEN, Mississauga, ON, Canada) according to the manufacturer's instructions. Extracted RNA was eluted in RNase-free water and the concentration was determinated using a nanophotometer (Implen GmbH, München, Germany). Relative quantification of the transcripts was assessed in a two steps format (RT and qPCR). Real-Time PCR was performed using a QuantiTect® SYBR® Green PCR kit (QIAGEN, Mississauga, ON, Canada), according to the manufacturer's instructions. A Chromo 4™ System (Bio-Rad Laboratories Inc., Hercules, CA, USA) was used to amplify cDNAs and detect emitted fluorescence. The following primers were used: GnRH-R (319 pb), forward 5′-GACCTTGTCTGGAAAGATCC-3′ and reverse 5′-CAGGCTGATCACCACCATCA-3′; AnxA5 (149 pb), forward 5′-TTCTCAGAGGCACTGTGACTGACT-3′ and reverse 5′-GATTTCCTGGCGCTGAGCATTACT-3′; G3PDH (121 pb), forward 5′-CCCATGTTCGTCATGGGTGTGAAC-3′ and reverse 5′-CAAAGTTGTCATGGATGACCTTGGC-3′. Reactions were carried out with the following parameters: enzyme activation at 95°C for 15 min, denaturation at 95°C for 30 sec, annealing at 57°C for 30 sec, extension at 72°C for 30 sec and a final extension at 72°C for 10 min. 30 and 35 cycles were used for AnxA5 and GnRH-R, respectively. For negative controls (NTC), cDNA was replaced by sterile RNase free water. Poly-A^+ mRNA from human breast adenocarcinoma (MCF 7 cells) and Poly-A^+ mRNA from human pituitary gland (both from Clontech, Member of Takara Bio Inc., Shigan, Japan) were used as positive controls.

Protein Extraction and Western Blot Analysis

Untreated cells and GnRH treated cells were washed twice with cold PBS and were lyzed in RIPA buffer (25 mM Tris, 150 mM NaCl, 1% Triton X-100, 1% Na-Deoxycholate, 0.1% SDS, 10 mM iodoacetamide, 100 µM PMSF; pH = 7.5) in the presence of Complete Protease Inhibitor Cocktail (Roche, Basel, Switzerland). Total protein concentrations were determined using Lowry's methodology using bovine serum albumin as a standard [37]. Samples were resolved by SDS-PAGE (7.5 to 10%) and transferred onto a PVDF membrane (GE Healthcare, Chalfont St Giles, UK). After blotting, membranes were blocked with 5% (w/v) non-fat dried skimmed milk in PBS-0.1%Tween 20 or TBST (Tris-buffered saline plus 0.1% Tween 20). Blots were probed overnight at 4°C with mouse monoclonal antibody anti-GnRH-R (1:150, LH-RH Receptor Ab-3, clone GNRH03, MM France, Francheville, France) or goat polyclonal antibody anti-AnxA5 (1:400, clone R-20, Santa Cruz Biotechnology, CA, USA). Blots were further incubated with HRP-conjugated secondary antibodies [1:20000, anti-mouse and anti-goat secondary antibody were from Santa Cruz Biotechnology and Abcam (Cambridge, UK), respectively] and visualized by enhanced chemiluminescence. ECL Plus and Forte chemiluminescence detection kits were from GE Healthcare and Merk Millipore (Billerica, MA, USA),

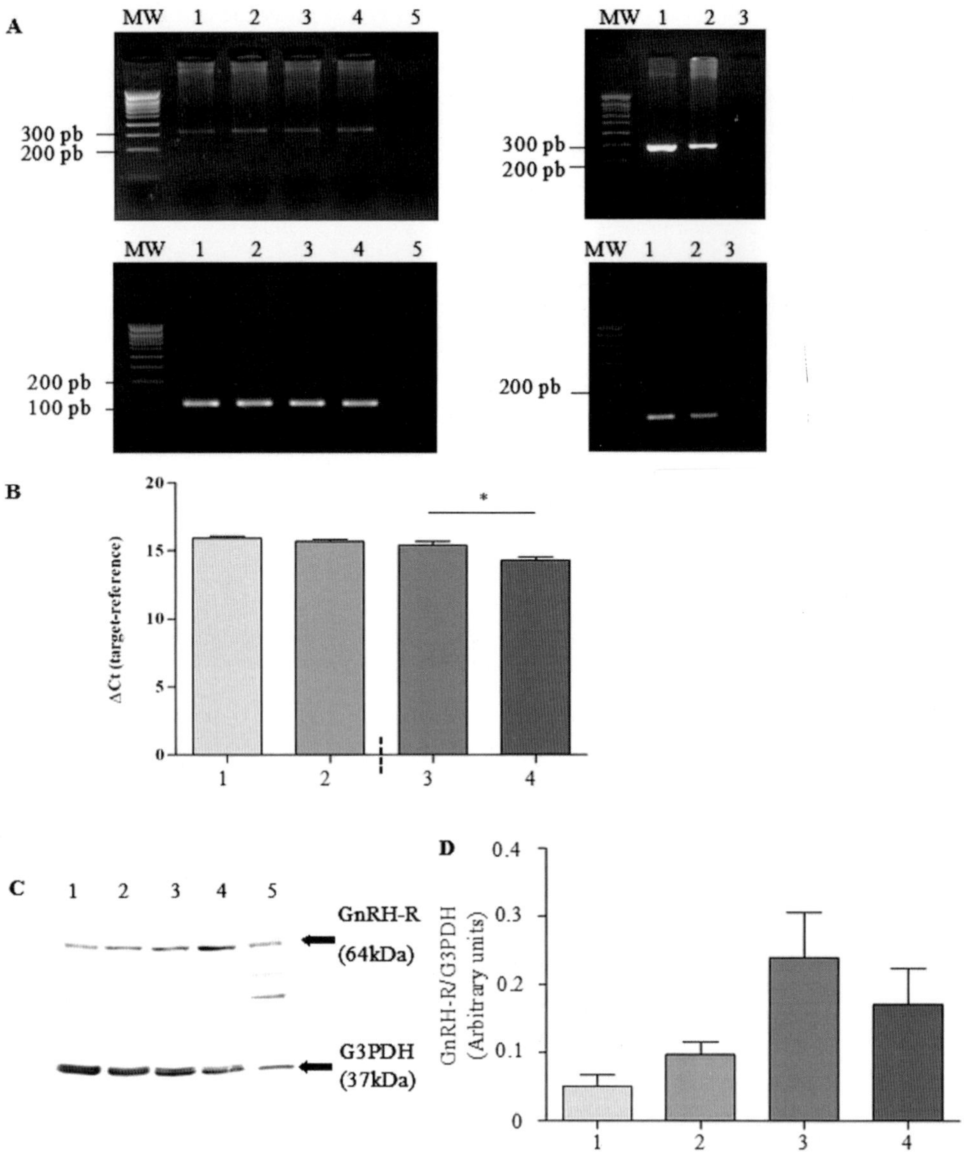

Figure 1. Basal mRNA and protein expression of GnRH-R. A. The upper left panel shows representative PCR bands for GnRH-R (319 bp) after separation (2% agarose gel). A single band is observed in 16HBE14o$^-$ (lane 1), CFBE41o$^-$ (lane 2), CFBE41o$^{-/}$corr (lane 3) and CFBE41o$^{-/}$F508del (lane 4) cells. No signal is observed in the negative control (lane 5). The upper right panel shows positive controls (human pituitary gland and human MCF7cell line, lanes 1 and 2, respectively) for the detection of GnRH-R. cDNAs were from the human pituitary gland and the human MCF7cell line (breast adenocarcinoma), respectively. The mRNA expression of G3PDH (121 bp) is shown lower panel for the same samples. MW is the molecular weight given in base pairs (bp). **B.** The quantitative analysis (n = 5) of the mRNA of GnRH-R. Ct is the Cycle Threshold. A hight Ct correspond to **low mRNA** abundance because more PCR cycles are needed to detect it. Endogenous control has a lower Ct than the target mRNA. Therefore, a low ΔCt (= Ct gene – Ct control) correspond to high mRNA abundance **C.** Upper panel shows representative immunoblots of GnRH-R (64 kDa) and lower panel shows representative immunoblots of G3PDH (37 kDa). A protein expression is observed in 16HBE14o$^-$ (lane 1), CFBE41o$^-$ (lane 2), CFBE41o$^{-/}$corr (lane 3) and CFBE41o$^{-/}$F508del (lane 4) cells. A positive control (lane 5) was used for the detection of GnRH-R (human breast duct carcinoma (T-47D) whole cell lysate). G3PDH was used for further normalization. **D.** The densitometric analysis of GnRH-R expression (n = 6) did not show any difference between cell lines.

respectively. The relative intensity of each band was estimated by densitometry using BIO-1D software (BioRad). Each value was normalized to the amount of G3PDH in the same lane which was assessed on the same immunoblots probed with mouse monoclonal antibody anti-G3PDH (1:30000, clone 6C5, Interchim SA, Montluçon, France). Positive controls for GnRH-R and AnxA5 were a whole cell lysates of human breast duct carcinoma (T-47D, Tebu-Bio, Le-Perray-en-Yvelines, France) and pure AnxA5 from human placenta (33 kD, Sigma-Aldrich), respectively.

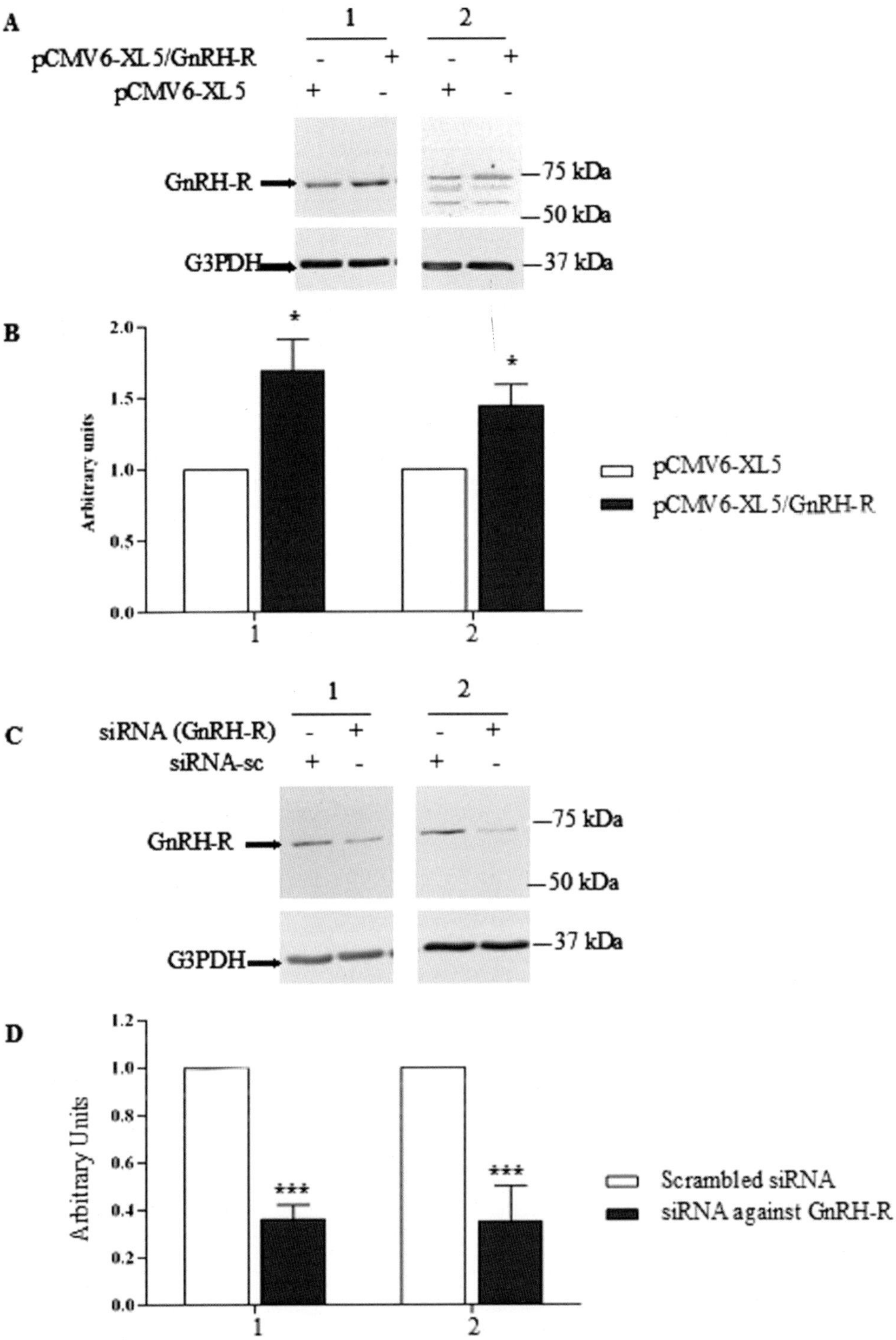

Figure 2. Validation of the detection of GnRH-R in immunoblots. A. Representative immunoblots of GnRH-R detection (upper panel) after 48 h transfection with the Human cDNA clone pCMV6-XL5/GNRH-R in 16HBE14o$^-$ (1) and CFBE41o$^-$ (2) cells. pCMV6-XL5 empty plasmid was used as a control. **B.** The densitometric analysis after normalization by G3PDH expression and comparison with the controls, indicate that the GnRH-R expression in significantly increased, (n = 5). **C.** Representative immunoblots of GnRH-R detection after 72 h transfection with a siGENOME individual duplex targeting GnRH-R in 16HBE14o$^-$ (1) and CFBE41o$^-$ (2) cells. siGENOME Non-Targeting was used as control. A decreased expression of GnRH-R is observed in both cell types. **D.** The densitometric analysis after normalization by G3PDH expression and comparison with the controls, indicate that the GnRH-R expression is significantly decreased in 16HBE14o$^-$ (1) and CFBE41o$^-$ (2) cells (n = 7) in the presence of siRNA.

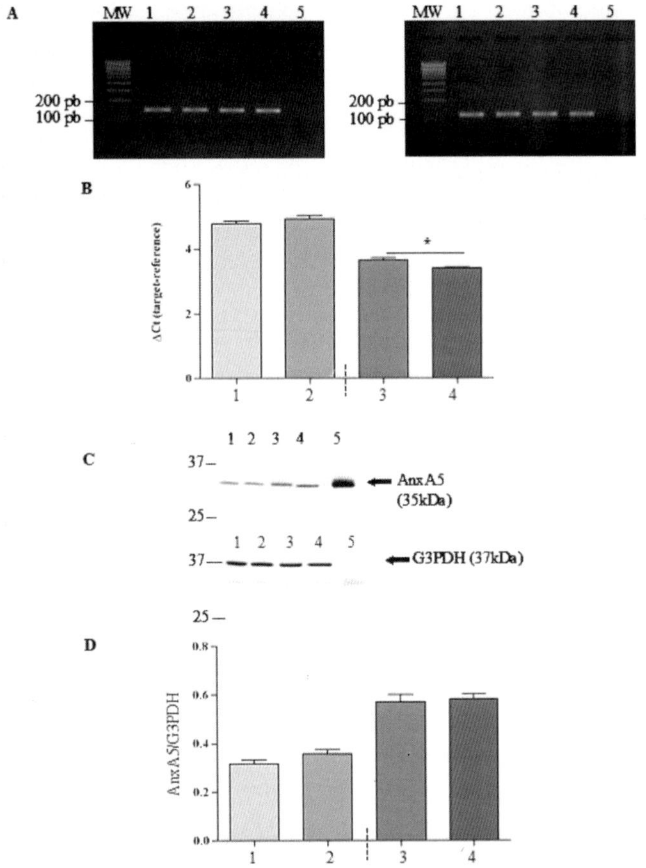

Figure 3. Basal mRNA and protein expression of AnxA5. A. The left image shows representative PCR bands for AnxA5 (149 bp) and the right image shows representative PCR bands for G3PDH (121 bp, 2% agarose gel). A single band is observed in 16HBE14o$^-$ (lane 1), CFBE41o$^-$ (lane 2), CFBE41o$^-$/corr (lane 3) and CFBE41o$^-$/F508del (lane 4) cells. No signal is observed in the negative control (lane 5). MW is the molecular weight given in base pairs (bp). B. The gene expression of AnxA5 was determined by quantitative Real-Time PCR in each cell line and data were analyzed by using ΔCt (target – reference). Comparison between CFBE41o$^-$/corr (3) and CFBE41o$^-$/F508del (4) cells show a higher expression in CF cells. C. The upper image shows a representative immunodetection of AnxA5 protein (35 kDa) and the lower image shows the immunodetection of G3PDH (37 kDa) protein expression in 16HBE14o$^-$ (lane 1), CFBE41o$^-$ (lane 2), CFBE41o$^-$/corr (lane 3) and CFBE41o$^-$/F508del (lane 4) cells. Pure AnxA5 was used as a positive control (lane 5). G3PDH was detected to show that the loading was identical in each lane and for further normalization. D. Statistical analysis of AnxA5 expression (n = 6) indicate that the expression of AnxA5 does not vary among cell lines although it tends to be higher in CFBE41o$^-$/corr and CFBE41o$^-$/F508del cells than in 16HBE14o$^-$ or CFBE41o$^-$ cells.

I^- Effluxes Experiments

Cells were cultured in 24-well microplates for 3 to 7days. Confluent monolayers were used, and iodide effluxes were assayed as previously described [38]. Briefly, the F508del-CFTR Cl^- channel activity was assayed by measuring the rate of iodide (^{125}I) efflux from cells and time-dependent rates of ^{125}I efflux were calculated from the following: ln (^{125}I t1/^{125}It2)/(t1– t2), where ^{125}It is the intracellular ^{125}I at time t, and t1 and t2 successive time points. Curves were constructed by plotting rates of ^{125}I versus time. All comparisons were based on maximal values for the time-dependent rates (k = peak rates, min^{-1}), excluding the points used to establish the baseline (k peak-k basal, min^{-1}). Activators were included in the efflux buffer from time 3 min, and collection continued at 1-min intervals for an additional 7 min in the continued presence of tested compounds (for other details, [38])). To test the effect of GnRH exposure on halide permeability, CF and non-CF cells monolayers were incubated with 0.1 to 100 nM GnRH for 1 h before the efflux experiment.

Patch-clamp Experiments

Patch-clamp experiments were performed with an automatic Nanion's electrophysiology workstations Port-a-Patch (Nanion Technologies GmbH, Germany) coupled to an external amplifier unit HEKA EPC-10 [39]. Whole-cell patch-clamp recordings were performed at room temperature (20–25°C) on isolated CFBE41o–/corr and CFBE41o–/F508del cells, with and without GnRH treatment. Before recording, the culture medium was replaced by the external solution contained the following (in mM): 140 NaCl, 2 CaCl2, 1 MgCl2, 10 Hepes, 5 D-glucose monohydrate. Its final pH value was adjusted to 7.4 with NaOH and its osmolarity was 298 mOsmol. The internal solution contained the following (in mM): 50 CsCl, 10 NaCl, 60 Cs-Fluoride, 20 EGTA, 10 Hepes/CsOH, and 5 Mg-ATP (Mg salt); pH 7.2; 285 mOsmol. CFTR-inhibitor solution (10 µM CFTRinh172, Sigma) and CFTR-activator solution (10 µM forskolin and 30 µM genistein both from Sigma) were added to the external solution to inhibit or activate CFTR, respectively. Voltage-clamp pulses were generated and data were captured using the Patchmaster program (Nanion Technologies GmbH, Germany). Voltage-dependent properties were assessed by applying voltage steps of 100 ms duration from a holding potential of -80 mV to test potentials ranging from −80 to +80 mV with 10 mV increments. Series resistance was compensated. For graphic representations of I/V relationship currents were normalized by membrane capacitances to remove variability due to differences in cell sizes.

Cell Surface Biotinylation

Cells were grown in serum-free medium overnight before GnRH incubation. Culture medium was then removed and cells were washed three times with PBS plus 0.1 mM CaCl2 and 1 mM MgCl2 (pH 7.4) and once with PBS (pH 8). Cells were exposed to sulfo-NHS-SS-biotin for 30 min on ice, rinsed twice with BSA quenching buffer (1% BSA in PBS, pH 7.4) and incubated 10 min in the same buffer. Cells were scraped in PBS, pH 7.4 and centrifuged at 2400 rpm (6 min, 4°C). Cell pellets were suspended in RIPA buffer plus anti-proteases and incubated for 30 min on ice. The resulting lysates were centrifuged at 16000 g for 15 min at 4°C and total cellular protein content was determined using Lowry's method. The supernatants were incubated with streptavidin beads (Novagen/EMD Chemicals, Madison, WI, USA) overnight at 4°C. After a brief centrifugation, supernatants were removed and the beads were washed four times in RIPA. Biotinylated proteins were eluted from streptavidin beads using 5X sample buffer containing 2-mercaptoethanol to cleave the NHS-SS-biotin and western blots were probed overnight at 4°C with a mouse monoclonal anti-CFTR antibody (1:500, clone M3A7, Merk Millipore). For normalization, Na^+/K^+-ATPase expression was assessed on the same blots probed with a mouse monoclonal antibody (1:200, clone 9-A5, Santa Cruz Biotechnology). A positive control was used to assess the mature band of CFTR (T84, human colorectal carcinoma whole cell lysate).

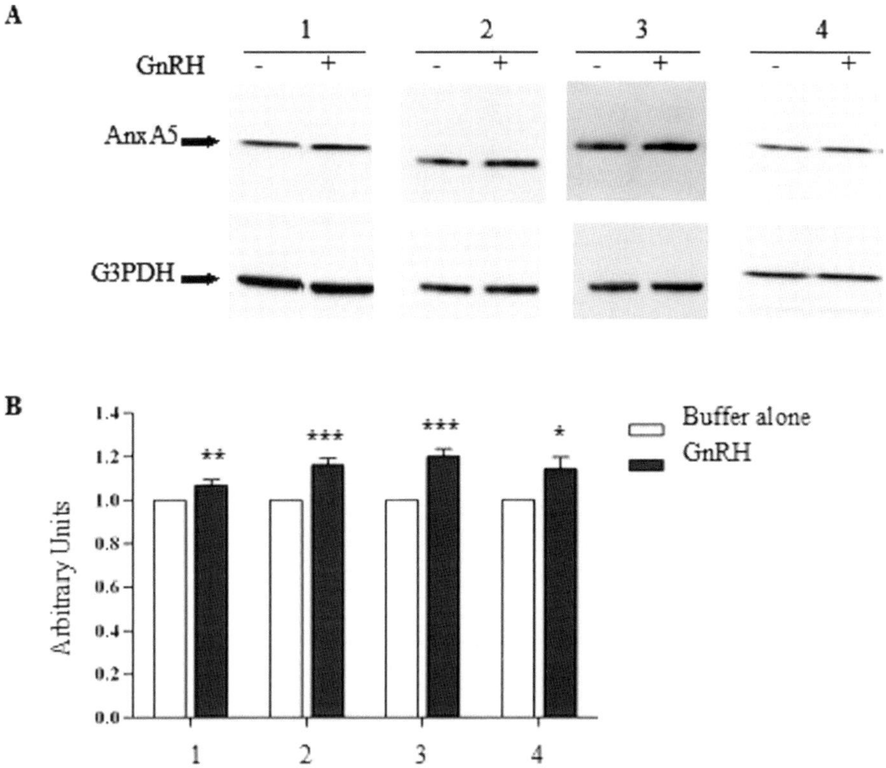

Figure 4. AnxA5 expression when cells are treated for 60 min with GnRH. A. Representative immunoblots showing AnxA5 and G3PDH expression in 16HBE14o$^-$ (1), CFBE41o$^-$ (2), CFBE41o$^{-/}$corr (3) and CFBE41o$^{-/}$F508del (4) cells after 60 min of treatment by GnRH (10^{-9} M). An increased expression is observed in all cell types. **B.** Densitometric analysis of AnxA5 expression. Data are normalized by G3PDH. AnxA5 protein expression is presented as mean ± S.E.M (7 independent experiments with n ≥2 for each experiment). For each cell line, the statistical analysis was performed by comparing the normalized amount of AnxA5 between cells incubated with buffer alone (white bars adjusted to 1) and cells incubated with GnRH (black bars).

Confocal Microscopy

CFBE41o$^{-/}$corr and CFBE41o$^{-/}$F508del cells were plated on 18-mm diameter glass coverslips at low density and maintained in culture at 37°C for 24 to 48 h before exposure to GnRH. Cells were rinsed in TBS, fixed (3% paraformaldehyde in TBS, 20 min, room temperature), rinsed in TBS, permeabilized (0.10% Triton X-100 in TBS) and rinsed again. The samples were then stained by indirect immunofluorescence. After fixation, non-specific sites were blocked with 0.5% bovine serum albumin (BSA) in TBS (60 min at room temperature). The cells were then stained with primary antibody (anti-CFTR antibody 24-1, 1:50, RD Systems, Minneapolis, MN, USA) for 90 min at room temperature and rinsed four times in TBS containing 0.5% BSA. Next, samples were incubated with the goat anti-mouse secondary antibody conjugated to Cy3 (1:400, Jackson Immunoresearch Laboratories, West Grove, PA, USA) for 60 min at room temperature. After final washes, samples were mounted in VectaShield plus DAPI (VECTOR Laboratories Inc., Burlingame, CA, USA), dried, and viewed with a confocal laser-scanning microscope (LSM 780, Axio Observer, Plan-Apochromat 63X/1.40 oil; Carl Zeiss GmbH, Jena, Germany). Negative controls in which primary antibody was omitted was performed.

Statistics

Results are expressed as the means ± S.E.M of n observations. Data were compared using the Student's t test analysis with STATGRAPHICS version 4.1 (SIGMA PLUS, Levallois-Perret, France) and differences were considered statistically significant when $p<0.001$ (***); $p<0.01$ (**) and $p<0.05$ (*).

Results

Basal Expression of GnRH-R

Basal mRNA and protein expression of GnRH-R was assessed in 16HBE14o$^-$, CFBE41o$^-$, CFBE41o$^{-/}$corr and CFBE41o$^{-/}$F508del cells. As shown in Fig. 1A, a single PCR band for GnRH-R (319 bp) was observed in the four cell lines whereas no signal was observed in the negative control. cDNAs from human pituitary gland and human MCF7 cell line (breast adenocarcinoma), were used as positive controls. The mRNA expression of G3PDH (121 bp) in the same samples showed no variation of the signal intensity. The mRNA expression of GnRH-R was quantified (Fig. 1B). Because the genetic background is only comparable between CFBE41o−/corr and CFBE41o−/F508del cells, statistical analysis was only performed for these cells and a higher mRNA expression was observed in CFBE41o−/F508del cells. Western blots were performed to detect GnRH-R (64 kDa) and G3PDH (37 kDa) in the cell lines (Fig. 1C), using a whole cell lysate of human breast duct carcinoma (T -47D) as a control. The results indicate that the GnRH-R is present in all the samples. The densitometric analysis of the signals (Fig. 1D) did not show any difference between CFBE41o−/corr and CFBE41o−/F508del cells.

To assess the GnRH-R antibody's specificity, the GnRH-R's expression was modulated before immunodetection. First,

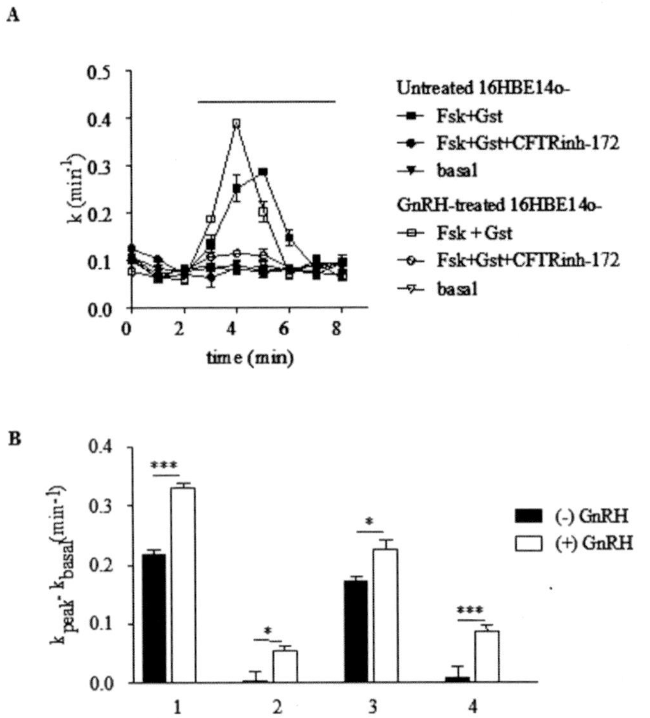

Figure 5. Activation of wild-type and F508del-CFTR chloride channel activity in cells treated by GnRH. A. Example of mean traces showing the restoration of an iodide efflux in 16HBE14o- cells untreated or treated 1 h with 1 nM GnRH and stimulated by 10 µM forskolin and 30 µM genistein. **B.** Bar graph showing the enhancement of the chloride channel function of CFTR in 16HBE14o$^-$, CFBE41o$^-$, CFBE41o$^{-/}$corr and CFBE41o$^{-/}$F508del cells (1, 2, 3 and 4, respectively) using iodide efflux experiments. Histograms show the mean relative rate of iodide efflux in each cell type, with and without GnRH treatement. A significant increase is observed in the presence of GnRH (n = 4).

16HBE14o$^-$, CFBE41o$^-$ cells were transfected with a GnRH-R expression vector in which the cDNA encoding GnRH-R was ligated. As shown in Fig. 2A, the immunoblots indicated that the transfection induced an increased expression of the receptor. The control cells were transfected with the empty vector and G3PDH was detected for further normalization. The quantitative analysis of the blots (Fig. 2B) showed that the transfection of the expression vector induced an increased expression of GnRH-R of 70% and 44% in 16HBE14o$^-$, CFBE41o$^-$ cells, respectively, when compared to the control cells. Second, a siRNA directed against GnRH-R was used and a decreased expression of the protein was observed in both cell types (Fig. 2C). The quantitative analysis of the blots (Fig. 2D) showed that the siRNA induced an decrease expression of GnRH-R of 64% and 65% in 16HBE14o$^-$, CFBE41o$^-$ cells, respectively, when compared to the control cells which were transfected with a scrambled siRNA.

Basal Expression of AnxA5

Basal mRNA and protein expression of AnxA5 was assessed in 16HBE14o$^-$, CFBE41o$^-$, CFBE41o$^{-/}$corr and CFBE41o−/F508del cells. As shown in Fig. 3A, AnxA5 mRNA (149 bp) was detected in all cell lines whereas, no signal was observed in the negative control. The gene expression of AnxA5 was quantified in cells using Real-Time PCR. Analysis of the data (Fig. 3B) between CFBE41o−/corr and CFBE41o−/F508del cells showed a higher expression in the cells expressing the mutated CFTR. AnxA5 expression was further assessed by western blottings (Fig. 3C). The statistical analysis (Fig. 3D) indicated that AnxA5 expression does not vary within cell lines. Nevertheless, the amount of AnxA5 protein tended to be higher in CFBE41o−/corr and CFBE41o$^{-/}$F508del cells than in 16HBE14o$^-$ or CFBE41o$^-$ cells.

AnxA5 Expression in Cells Submitted to GnRH Treatment for 60 min

In order to determine whether GnRH modulates AnxA5 expression and to determine the shortest time to be used for GnRH treatment, 16HBE14o$^-$, CFBE41o$^-$, CFBE41o$^{-/}$corr and CFBE41o$^{-/}$F508del cells were treated with 10^{-9} M GnRH for 30, 60, 120, 180 and 310 min (not shown). At each time point, the protein expression of AnxA5 was evaluated and normalized with that of G3PDH. The AnxA5 expression was compared to that of cells incubated with buffer alone used as a control. Fig. 4A shows an example of the obtained western blots at the 60 min time point. An increased intensity of the AnxA5 band was observed in all cell types. Densitometry of the bands, normalization using G3PDH and quantification were performed (Fig. 4B). It was concluded that a 60 min treatment led to a significant increase of AnxA5 expression in the four cell types.

Increased Endogenous F508del-CFTR's Function by GnRH Treatment

To test the activity of CFTR channels under GnRH treatment in 16HBE14o$^-$, CFBE41o$^-$, CFBE41o$^{-/}$corr and CFBE41o-/F508del cells, functional analysis was performed by measuring the cAMP regulated and CFTR-dependent iodide efflux after 1 h incubation at 37°C with GnRH (10^{-9} M). The activity of CFTR was stimulated by a mixture of adenylate cyclase activator forskolin (Fsk, 10 µM) plus isoflavone genistein (Gst, 30 µM) or inhibited by the thiazolidinone specific CFTR blocker CFTRinh-172 (10 µM). Example of mean traces showing an increased iodide efflux in 16HBE14o$^-$ cells, untreated or treated with GnRH is shown in Fig. 5A. This example shows that after adding Fsk/Gst, the rate of iodide efflux increased at a maximum rate (peak value) after 4 min and that the peak was higher in the presence of GnRH. Experiments were conducted for all cell types and the results are represented as bar graphs in Fig. 5B. Statistical analysis indicated that in the presence of GnRH, the rates of iodide efflux were significantly increased in 16HBE14o$^-$, CFBE41o$^-$, CFBE41o$^{-/}$corr and CFBE41o$^{-/}$F508del cells when compared to untreated cells, indicating that CFTR and F508del-CFTR's function are increased by GnRH. The concentration-response effect of GnRH was further determined in the presence or absence of Fsk and Gst (Fig. 6). Calculated an EC50 in 16HBE14o$^-$, CFBE41o$^-$, CFBE41o$^{-/}$corr and CFBE41o$^{-/}$F508del cells were 0.6±1.4 nM, 0.8±1.2 nM, 0.9±1.3 nM and 2.2±1.4 nM, respectively.

CFTR's function in CFBE41o−/corr and CFBE41o_/F508del cells was also assessed by patch-clamp experiments in the whole cell configuration ((n = 5 to 9 cells from different cell cultures, Fig. 7). Mean cell capacitances were 21.4 and 18.66 pF for CFBE41o−/corr and CFBE41o_/F508del cells, respectively. Fig. 7A (upper panel) show the normalized I/V curve obtained when CFBE41o−/corr cells were treated or not with GnRH for 1 hour, with activators and with the CFTR inhibitor. It can be observed that activation and inhibition were efficient in both cases showing the specificity of the recordings. It was also observed that GnRH treatment of the cells induced an increased current density.

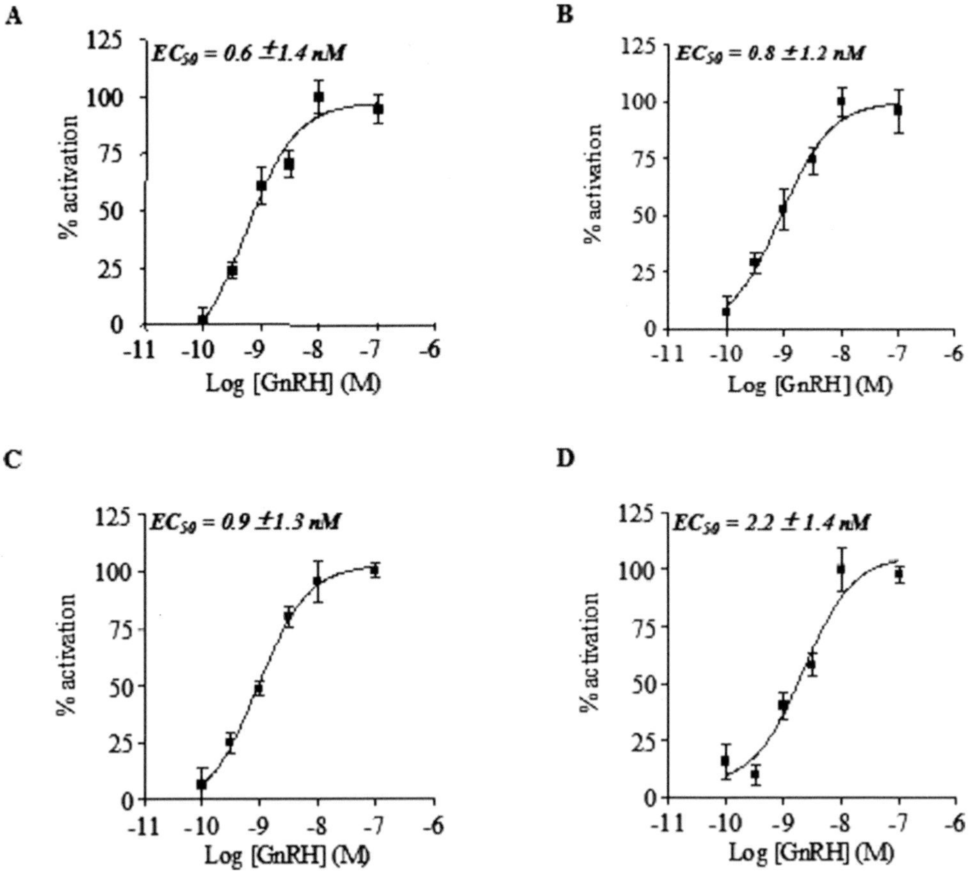

Figure 6. Concentration-dependent effect of GnRH. Concentration-dependent enhancement of CFTR's function by GnRH in 16HBE14o$^-$ (A), CFBE41o$^-$ (B), CFBE41o$^{-/}$corr (C) and CFBE41o$^{-/}$F508del (D): CFTR activity was assessed with the iodide effluxes technique in the presence of forskoline (10 μM) plus genistein (30 μM) after 1h of incubation. Results are expressed as normalized means (± SEM, n = 4).

Statistical analysis was further performed and presented as a bar graph (Fig. 7A, lower panel). In untreated cells inhibition and activation of CFTR were significantly efficient whereas in treated cells only inhibition led to a significant decreased current density. When untreated cells were compared to treated cells, solely the basal current densities were significantly increased by GnRH. The absence of activation by Fsk/Gst in GnRH treated cells could be explained by the fact that the concentration of the activators was the same in both treated and untreated cells and because the basal current density was higher in the presence of GnRH. The drawn conclusion is that GnRH induces an increased current density in CFBE41o−/corr cells. I/V curves obtained with CFBE41o_/F508del cells in the same conditions as for CFBE41o−/corr cells are shown in Fig. 7B (upper panel). As in Fig. 7A, basal normalized currents, as well as modulated currents by activation and inhibition were higher in the presence of GnRH. Statistical analysis and bar graphs (Fig. 7B, lower panel) showed a basal current in untreated CFBE41o_/F508del cells, likely due to the presence of Mg-ATP in the internal solution, activating the weak quantity of CFTR within membranes. The use of Fsk/Gst and CFTRinh-172 was inefficient upon the mutated CFTR's function. In treated cells, the basal current density was close to 5 times higher than in untreated cells. This difference was highly significant despite being lower than in CFBE41o−/corr cells. In these conditions, Fsk/Gst and CFTRinh-172 were efficient as in corrected cells. Therefore, F508del-CFTR's function under GnRH treatment exhibited the same pattern as Wt-CFTR, with a much lower intensity (in the range of 100 pA).

Increased Membrane Expression of CFTR after GnRH Treatment

The presence of CFTR within membranes after 1 hour treatment by GnRH was assessed by biotinylation experiments. Cells were biotinylated with Sulfo-NHS-SS-biotin, pulled-down with streptavidin-agarose and subjected to 7.5% SDS-PAGE. Total cell lysates were used as controls. Representative immunoblots showing the detection of CFTR in biotinylated surface proteins from 16HBE14o$^-$ and CFBE41o$^{-/}$corr cells are shown in Fig. 8A and 8B, respectively. CFTR was present in total lysates and in pulled down samples. The densitometric analysis of CFTR's cell surface expression was performed and normalized with the biotinylated Na^+/K^+-ATPase level. The statistical analysis clearly indicates that the amount of biotinylated CFTR is higher after GnRH treated cells (Fig. 8C). An increased amount of CFTR in membranes of 33 and 36% was observed in 16HBE14o$^-$ and CFBE41o$^{-/}$corr cells, respectively. Whereas CFTR was detected in controls, we failed to detect it in biotinylated surface proteins from CFBE41o$^-$ and CFBE41o$^{-/}$F508del cells (not shown).

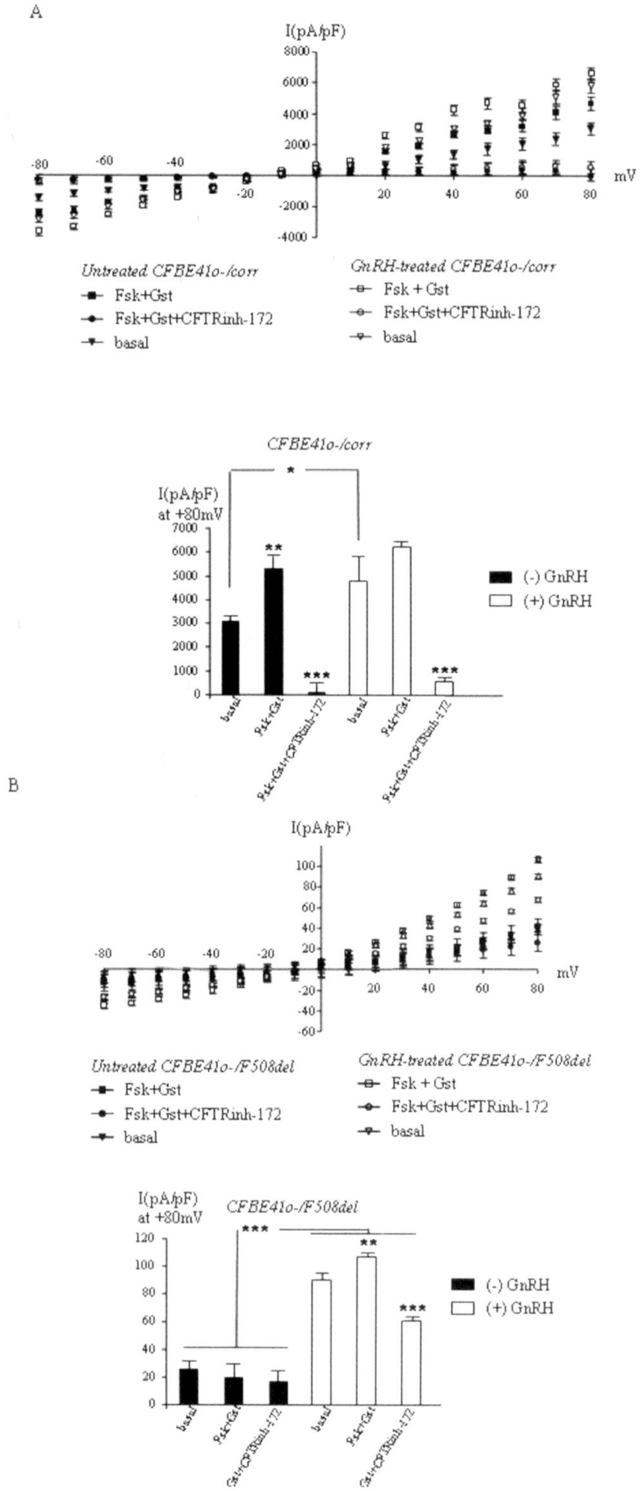

Figure 7. Activation of CFTR current in CFBE41o−/corr and CFBE41o−/F508del cells by patch -clamp experiments. A. Upper panel shows I/V curves (normalized by cell capacitance pF, mean±SEM) for CFTR current in CFBE41o−/corr cells in the whole cell configuration. Basal condition is with MgATP in the intracellular buffer. CFTR was activated by forskolin plus genistein and inhibited by CFTR inhibitor 172. Curves obtained with and without GnRH treatment (1 hour) were plotted. The lower panel shows the statistical analysis of the currents noted at +80 mV. **B.** Same as in A for CFBE41o−/F508del cells.

Increased Membrane Localization of CFTR after GnRH Treatment

Because we failed to detect CFTR in CFBE41o$^-$ and CFBE41o$^-$/F508del cells due to the poor expression of the protein, membrane localization of CFTR in CFBE41o$^-$/F508del cells was assessed by confocal microscopy, in the absence (Fig. 9A) and in the presence (Fig. 9B) of a GnRH treatment (120 min). Without any treatment, CFTR was mainly observed around the nuclei of the cells. We therefore speculated that it was present in the ER. When cell were treated with GnRH, CFTR had a more spread localization and it was observed at the periphery of the cells, looking like the plasma membrane, as shown in Fig. 9B by white arrows. Controls performed without CFTR antibody showed no labelling (not shown).

Comparison of the Effect of Miglustat and GnRH

The time-dependent effects of miglustat and GnRH were assessed and compared in CFBE41o$^-$ and CFBE41o$^-$/F508del cells (Fig. 10). CFTR's function was assessed by the iodide effluxes technique in the presence of 1 nM GnRH or 100 µM miglustat. As shown in Fig. 10A, miglustat induced an increased iodide efflux in CFBE41o$^-$ cells after 1 hour treatment. The increase was higher at the 2 hours time point. GnRH also induced an increased iodide efflux but the effect was lower, but significant, and did not increase after 2 hours of treatment. In CFBE41o$^-$/F508del cells (Fig. 10B), the same time-dependent effect as in CFBE41o$^-$ cells was observed.

Discussion

The most common mutation causing CF, F508del-CFTR, is known for more than 20 years [1]. The F508del-CFTR nascent protein is recognized by the cellular quality control machinery and is degraded. A very small amount succeeds in trafficking to the cell membrane where it functions as a Cl^- channel. Many efforts were performed in order to identify molecules that could correct the trafficking defect. Indeed, it is estimated that the required correction to ameliorate the symptoms in CF patients is between 10% and 30% of wild-type CFTR function [40,41].

Among proteins that directly bind to CFTR, we previously showed that AnxA5 binds to NBD1 and, when over expressed, may restore some Cl^- channel function due to an increased stabilization of CFTR in membranes [28,29]. AnxA5 belongs to the annexin family which is characterized by calcium-dependent phospholipid binding. Annexins are found in a wide variety of species, from plants to human [42–44]. They are known to inhibit PLA2, PKC, and blood coagulation [42]. Under specific conditions, AnxA5 can also form a calcium channel [45]. Despite these molecular characteristics, their physiological role within cells remains unclear.

Whereas the CFTR/AnxA5 interaction as well as the augmented Wt-CFTR whole-cell currents, due to over-expression of AnxA5, was further confirmed, it was not seen in F508del-CFTR expressing cells [46]. The discrepancy with our previous results and within the referred study is likely due to the used cell system. These authors suspect that AnxA5 does not interact specifically with CFTR. This discrepancy is likely due to the use of a non specific AnxA5 antibody [46]. Because it is suggested that some CFTR is expressed at the apical membrane in epithelial cells from CF patients [47], despite a reduced level when compared to non-CF cells, and because we found a positive effect of AnxA5, our aim was to highlight a non toxic mean to increase AnxA5 expression in F508del-CFTR expressing cells. Some previous results clearly demonstrate that GnRH stimulation induces the

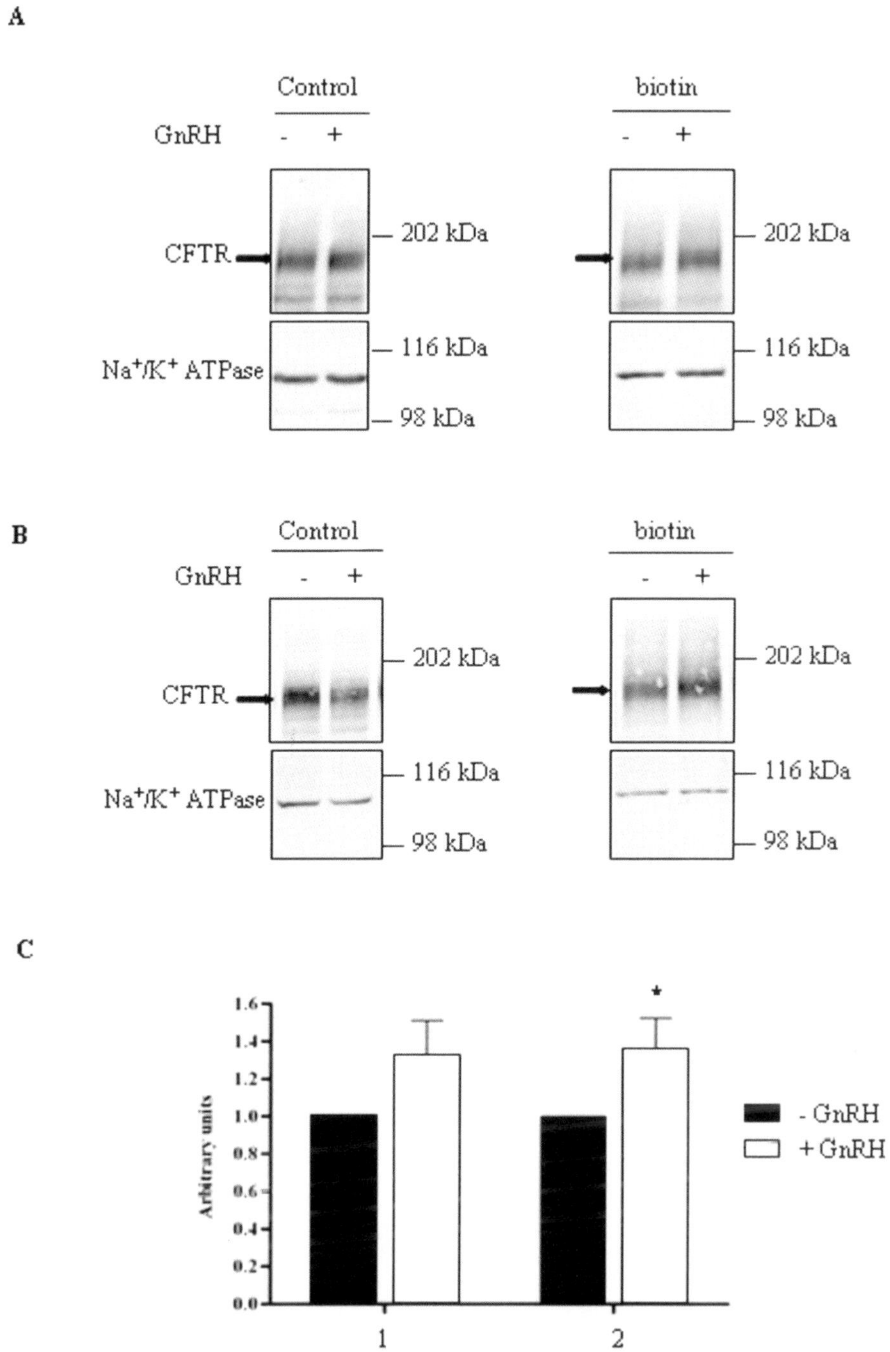

Figure 8. Membrane expression of CFTR after GnRH treatment. The presence of CFTR within membranes was detected by biotinylation experiments. **A.** Representative immunoblots showing the detection of CFTR in biotinylated surface proteins from 16HBE14o^{-} cells. CFTR is present in total proteins (left) and in biotinylated surface proteins (right) after GnRH treatment (10^{-9} M) for 60 min. The arrowheads indicate the fully glycosylated (180 kDa) CFTR. B. Same image as in A. with CFBE41o$^{-/}$corr cells. C. Histograms of the densitometric analysis of CFTR's cell surface expression (n = 4) in 16HBE14o^{-} (1) and CFBE41o$^{-/}$corr (2) cells The biotinylated CFTR level is normalized to the biotinylated Na^{+}/K^{+}-ATPase level. Cells incubated with buffer alone are referred as 1 arbitrary unit.

expression of AnxA5 in the gonadotropes, luteal cells and other cell types [30–32]. Therefore, we tested the hypothesis of an AnxA5 increased synthesis in response to GnRH stimulation in human epithelial cells of the airways.

GnRH is secreted by GnRH neurons in the hypothalamus and is transported to the gonadotropes of the anterior pituitary gland. It is a decapeptide involved in the control of reproduction and binds to a specific G protein-coupled receptor to allow gonadotropin secretion. GnRH and its receptor are reported to be expressed in human tissues outside of the hypothalamus, such as liver, heart, skeletal muscle and kidney where its functions are unclear [48].

The first step of the present work was to assess the expression of GnRH-R and AnxA5 in human epithelial cells (Fig. 1 to 3).

A

B

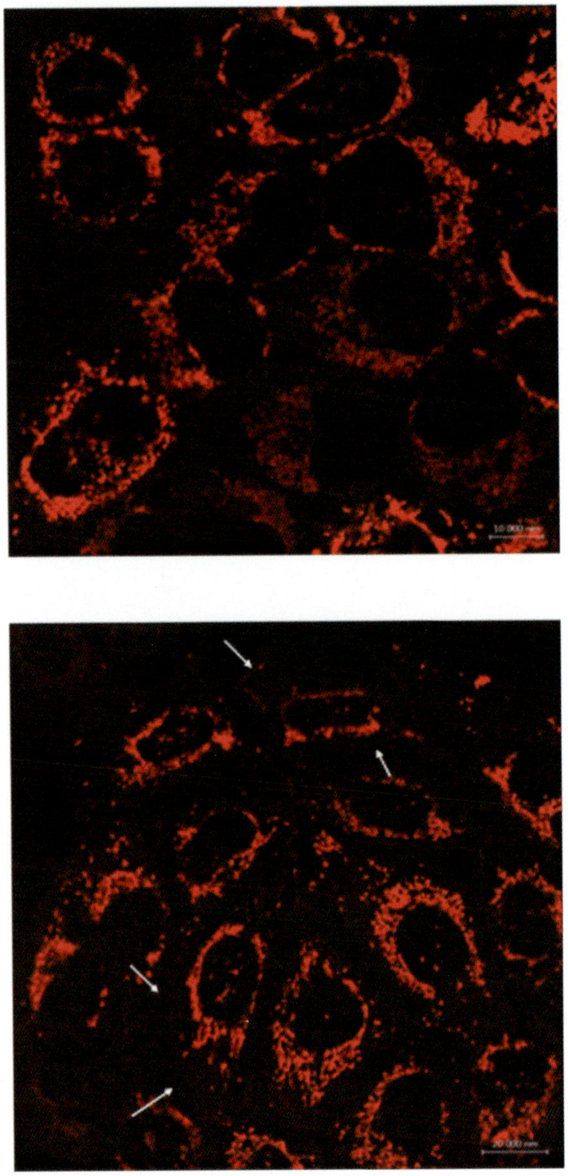

Figure 9. Immunolocalization of CFTR in CFBE41o−/F508del cells after GnRH treatment. A. Representative confocal photomicrographs of the localization of F508del-CFTR in cells without any treatment. CFTR is likely observed around the nuclei, in the endpoplasmic reticulum. B. Representative confocal photomicrographs of the localization of F508del-CFTR in cells after GnRH treatment. CFTR is likely observed in the endpoplasmic reticulum but also in membranes.

A

B

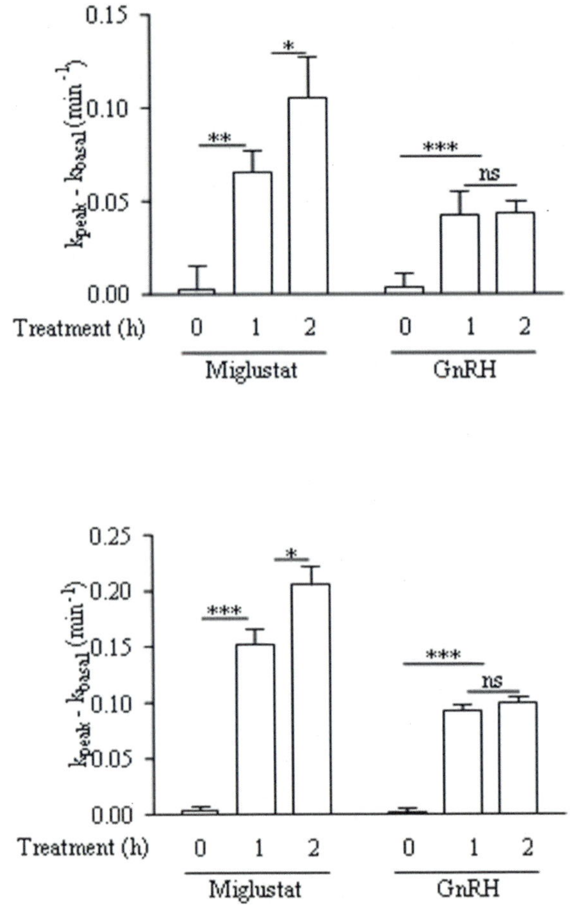

Figure 10. Comparison of the effect of miglustat and GnRH. Comparison of the time-dependent effect of GnRH or miglustat upon F508del-CFTR function in CFBE41o- cells (A) and in CFBE41o^{-}/F508del cells (B). CFTR activity was assessed with the iodide effluxes technique in the presence of forskolin (10 µM) plus genistein (30 µM) after 1 nM GnRH or 100 µM miglustat incubation (n = 4).

16HBE14 o^{-}, CFBE41o^{-} and the transduced CFBE41o^{-} airway epithelial cell lines CFBE41o^{-}/corr and CFBE41o^{-}/F508del were used [35]. Using PCR and western blottings, we observed an AnxA5 and GnRH-R expression in these cells. Because the genetic background of 16HBE14o^{-}, CFBE41o^{-} cells are different, their GnRH-R expression was not compared. The GnRH-R expression (protein) did not vary between CFBE41o^{-}/corr and CFBE41o^{-}/F508del cells. Because anti-GnRH-R antibodies are debated, we decided to assure us of the results. For this, GnRH-R expression was modulated (increased and decreased) before immunodetection and we showed that the observed band was indeed GnRH-R. The GnRH-R expression in airway epithelial cells is in accordance with previous results showing its expression in extrapituitary tissues. A high expression level of the mRNA was found in prostate, thymus, and kidney. In heart, brain, placenta, lung, liver, skeletal muscle, pancreas, colon, ovary, small intestine, spleen, and testis the mRNA was also detected [49]. The presence and localization of GnRH-R in airway epithelial cells (Calu-3) was also shown using immunochemical methods [49,50]. Here, we present for the first time the GnRH-R expression in 16HBE14o^{-}, CFBE41o^{-} and the transduced CFBE41o^{-} airway epithelial cell lines, using immunoblots. AnxA5 expression was studied in our cell models at the mRNA and protein level and we found that it is also expressed. This result is in accordance with previous results [51]. Therefore, GnRH-R and AnxA5 expression being shown, further experiments were conducted.

The second step of the work was to study AnxA5 expression under GnRH treatment and the effect of the hormone on the function of CFTR (Fig. 4 to 6). The four cell types were treated with GnRH (10^{-9} M) for 30, 60, 120, 180 and 310 min (not shown) and western-blottings were performed. A significant increased AnxA5 expression was observed at the 60 min time point and remained stable until 310 min. This increased expression of AnxA5 under GnRH treatment was previously

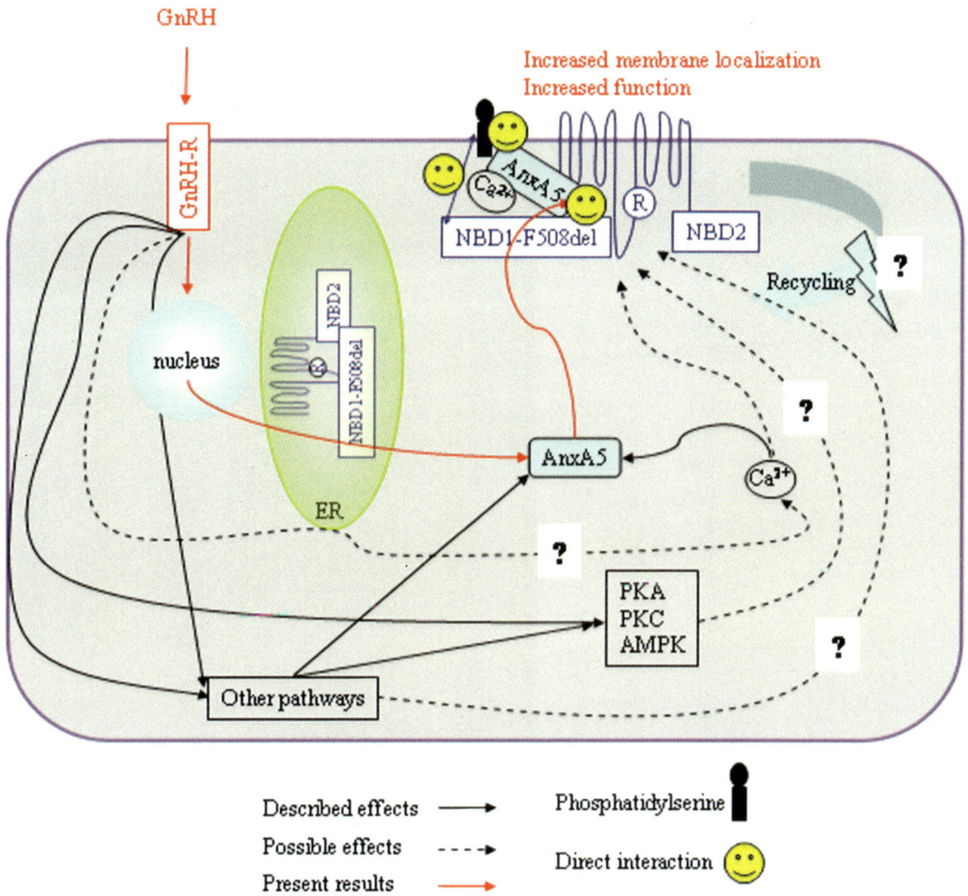

Figure 11. Schematic representation of the GnRH's effect on F508del-CFTR function. We found that F508del-CFTR's membrane localization and function are increased under GnRH treatment, associated with an increased expression of AnxA5 (red lines). Nevertheless, according to previous results, AnxA5 over expression is likely not the solely event triggered in cells by GnRH. Described events are summarized in black lines and their possible involvement upon F508del-CFTR activity are shown in dotted black lines.

described. Indeed, a continuous exposure to GnRH driving a specific gene expression of AnxA5 without desensitization was reported [32]. Nevertheless, our further experiments were conducted at 60 min of GnRH treatment, corresponding to a significant increased AnxA5 expression in 16HBE14o$^-$, CFBE41o$^-$, CFBE41o$^{-/}$corr and CFBE41o$^{-/}$F508del cells. Functional analysis was performed by measuring the CFTR-dependent iodide efflux in the absence and in the presence of GnRH. Statistical analysis indicated that with GnRH, the rates of iodide efflux were significantly increased in 16HBE14o$^-$, CFBE41o$^-$, CFBE41o$^{-/}$corr and CFBE41o$^{-/}$F508del cells when compared to untreated cells. EC_{50} were relatively low (2.2 nM in CFBE41o$^{-/}$F508del cells). To provide further evidence of an increased channel function of CFTR in CFBE41o−/F508del cells, whole-cell patch-clamp experiments were performed with and without GnRH treatment of the cells. The main conclusion drawn from these experiments is that in CFBE41o−/corr as well as in CFBE41o−/F508del cells, current densities via CFTR are increased in the presence of GnRH, corroborating the results obtained in iodide efflux experiments. In CFBE41o−/F508del cells, GnRH also lead to a regulation of CFTR by Fsk/Gst and CFTRinh-172, what was not observed in untreated cells. Therefore, GnRH increases sufficiently the chloride channel function of the mutated CFTR to lead to the observation of its modulation.

Our third step was to give some potential explanations to the observed increased Cl^- channel function of CFTR in the presence of GnRH. We assessed a possible increased anchoring of CFTR within membranes by biotinylation and confocal microscopy (Fig. 8, 9). According to our previous work [28,29], we found that the presence of F508del-CFTR was increased in membranes. Our results showing in the CFBE41o−/F508del cells an increased CFTR membrane localization after GnRH treatment could not be related to the additional plasmid inserted in the CFBE41o- cells because in biotinylation experiments without GnRH, the amount of CFTR in 16HBE14o- cells is not different than in CFBE41o−/corr cells. Nevertheless, the observed increased Cl^- channel function of CFTR in the presence of GnRH is likely not only due to the weak AnxA5 overexpression. The presence of CFTR within membranes after treatment was difficult to detect and due to the pleiotropic effects of GnRH, we hypothesize that the increased AnxA5 expression in likely not the only reason for this effect. Indeed, the expression of AnxA5 is directly stimulated by GnRH, probably through protein kinase C, MAKP and calcium pathways which are also involved in the regulation and in the targeting of CFTR in membranes [30–32,38,52–54]. A schematic representation of our findings together with known effects of GnRH is presented in Fig. 11. The involved pathways explaining the increased membrane localization of F508del-CFTR when cells are stimulated by GnRH, as well as the involvement of calcium are under investigation in our laboratory. Interestingly, the rapid and sustained action of GnRH seems different of the action of correctors or potentiators. We found of interest to compare the action of the well known corrector miglustat [24] with that of GnRH (Fig. 10). Time dependant effects of miglustat and GnRH were different. Whereas, miglustat induced a continuous increased iodide efflux until 2 hours, the GnRH effect observed at the 1 hour time point remained stable until the 2 hours. This observation permit to say that actions are likely different and reinforce the hypothesis that GnRH does not act as a corrector. Miglustat permits F508del-CFTR to escape the ER whereas GnRH maintains it in membranes. The association of both miglustat and GnRH will be further explored in primary cultures. Nevertheless, beside miglustat, several classes of F508del-CFTR correctors have been identified and could be tested. Indeed, despite many efforts to identify potentiators (such as VX-770) and correctors (such as VX-809), and, recently, a class of compounds with dual potentiator and corrector activities, much work remain to find out new molecules with beneficial effects on F508del-CFTR defects (for review [55]). The study of a combined effect of GnRH together with recently described compounds would be of interest to assess the benefit of the association of such molecules.

In conclusion, we show here for the first time that GnRH-R are expressed in the used airway epithelial cells at the protein level and we propose that GnRH restores some Cl^- channel function in CF cells. Because some GnRH analogs such as leuprolide, buserelin and goserelin are already used in medical practice as nasal sprays, we intend to test these medications in human primary cells.

Acknowledgments

We thank the association Gaëtan Salaün, the SFR Scinbios (Brest) and the French foundation "Vaincre la Mucoviscidose". We also thank Dr Mohamed Keir (Nanion Technology, Germany) as well as Dr Gérard Sinquin and Dr Philippe Elies of the PIMM facility (Université de Brest, France).

Author Contributions

Conceived and designed the experiments: PT CF. Performed the experiments: NB SLH CN MLC PT. Analyzed the data: PT NB MK CN FB. Contributed reagents/materials/analysis tools: NB SLH CN MLC. Wrote the paper: PT.

References

1. Riordan JR, Rommens JM, Kerem B, Alon N, Rozmahel R et al. (1989) Identification of the cystic fibrosis gene: cloning and characterization of complementary DNA. Science 245: 1066–1073.
2. Bear CE, Li CH, Kartner N, Bridges RJ, Jensen TJ et al. (1992) Purification and functional reconstitution of the cystic fibrosis transmembrane conductance regulator (CFTR). Cell: 68: 809–818.
3. Amaral MD (2004) Cftr and chaperones: Processing and degradation. J MolNeurosci 23: 41–48.
4. Cheng SH, Gregory RJ, Marshall J, Paul S, Souza DW et al. (1990) Defective intracellular transport and processing of cftr is the molecular basis of most cystic fibrosis. Cell 63: 827–834.
5. Lukacs GL, Mohamed A, Kartner N, Chang XB, Riordan JR et al. (1994) Conformational maturation of cftr but not its mutant counterpart (delta f508) occurs in the endoplasmic reticulum and requires atp. EMBO J 13: 6076–6086.
6. Jensen TJ, Loo MA, Pind S, Williams DB, Goldberg AL et al. (1995) Multiple proteolytic systems, including the proteasome, contribute to cftr processing. Cell 83: 129–135.
7. Ward CL, Omura S, Kopito RR (1995) Degradation of cftr by the ubiquitin-proteasome pathway. Cell 83: 121–127.
8. Hwang TC, Sheppard DN (2009) Gating of the CFTR Cl^- channel by ATP-driven nucleotide-binding domain dimerisation. J Physiol 587: 2151–2161.
9. Zielenski J, Tsui LC (1995) Cystic fibrosis: genotypic and phenotypic variations. Annu Rev Genet 29: 777–807.
10. Cheng SH, Gregory RJ, Marshall J, Paul S, Souza DW et al. (1990) Defective intracellular transport and processing of CFTR is the molecular basis of most cystic fibrosis. Cell 63: 827–834.
11. Denning GM, Anderson MP, Amara JF, Marshall J, Smith AE et al. (1992) Processing of mutant cystic fibrosis transmembrane conductance regulator is temperature-sensitive. Nature 358: 761–764.
12. Sato S, Ward CL, Krouse ME, Wine JJ, Kopito RR (1996) Glycerol reverses the misfolding phenotype of the most common cystic fibrosis mutation. J Biol Chem 271: 635–638.
13. Welsh MJ, Denning GM, Ostedgaard LS, Anderson MP (1993) Dysfunction of CFTR bearing the delta F508 mutation. J Cell Sci. Suppl. 17: 235–239.
14. Dalemans W, Barbry P, Champigny G, Jallat S, Dott K et al. (1991) Altered chloride ion channel kinetics associated with the ΔF508 cystic fibrosis mutation. Nature 354: 526–528.
15. Ostedgaard LS, Rogers CS, Dong Q, Randak CO, Vermeer DW et al. (2007) Processing and function of CFTR-ΔF508 are species-dependent. Proc Natl Acad Sci USA 104: 15370–15375.
16. Miki H, Zhou Z, Li M, Hwang TC, Bompadre SG (2010) Potentiation of disease-associated cystic fibrosis transmembrane conductance regulator mutants by hydrolyzable ATP analogs. J Biol Chem 285: 19967–19975.
17. Lukacs GL, Chang XB, Bear C, Kartner N, Mohamed A et al. (1993) The delta F508 mutation decreases the stability of cystic fibrosis transmembrane conductance regulator in the plasma membrane. Determination of functional half-lives on transfected cells. J. Biol. Chem. 268: 21592–21598.
18. Hwang TC, Wang F, Yang IC, Reenstra WW (1997) Genistein potentiates wild-type and delta F508-CFTR channel activity. Am. J. Physiol. 273: C988–C998.
19. Cai Z, Sheppard DN (2002) Phloxine B interacts with the cystic fibrosis transmembrane conductance regulator at multiple sites to modulate channel activity. J. Biol. Chem. 277: 19546–19553.
20. Vergani P, Lockless SW, Nairn AC, Gadsby DC (2005) CFTR channel opening by ATP-driven tight dimerization of its nucleotide-binding domains. Nature 433: 876–880.
21. Rubenstein RC, Egan ME, Zeitlin PL (1997) In vitro pharmacologic restoration of CFTR-mediated chloride transport with sodium 4-phenylbutyrate in cystic fibrosis epithelial cells containing delta F508-CFTR. J. Clin. Invest. 100: 2457–2465.
22. Brown CR, Hong-Brown LQ, Biwersi J, Verkman AS, Welch WJ (1996) Chemical chaperones correct the mutant phenotype of the delta F508 cystic fibrosis transmembrane conductance regulator protein. Cell Stress Chaperones 1: 117–125.
23. Denning GM, Anderson MP, Amara JF, Marshall J, Smith AE et al. (1992) Processing of mutant cystic fibrosis transmembrane conductance regulator is temperature-sensitive. Nature 358: 761–764.
24. Norez C, Noel S, Wilke M, Bijvelds M, Jorna H et al. (2006) Rescue of functional delF508-CFTR channels in cystic fibrosis epithelial cells by the alpha-glucosidase inhibitor miglustat. FEBS Lett. 580: 2081–2086.
25. Wang Y, Bartlett MC, Loo TW, Clarke DM (2006) Specific rescue of cystic fibrosis transmembrane conductance regulator processing mutants using pharmacological chaperones. Mol. Pharmacol. 70(1): 297–302.
26. Wang Y, Loo TW, Bartlett MC, Clarke DM (2007) Correctors promote maturation of cystic fibrosis transmembrane conductance regulator (CFTR)-processing mutants by binding to the protein. J. Biol. Chem. 282: 33247–33251.
27. Becq F, Mettey Y, Gray MA, Galietta LJ, Dormer RL et al. (1999) Development of substituted Benzo[c]quinolizinium compounds as novel activators of the cystic fibrosis chloride channel. J. Biol. Chem. 274: 27415–27425.
28. Trouvé P, Le Drévo MA, Kerbiriou M, Fichou Y, Gillet D et al. (2007) Annexin V is directly involved in cystic fibrosis transmembrane conductance regulator's chloride channel function. Biochim Biophys Acta. 1772: 1121–1133.
29. Le Drévo MA, Benz N, Kerbiriou M, Gioux M, Pennec JP et al. (2008) Annexin A5 increases the cell surface expression and the chloride channel function of the ΔF508-Cystic Fibrosis Transmembrane Regulator. Biochim Biophys Acta 1782: 605–614.
30. Kawaminami M, Etoh S, Miyaoka H, Sakai M, Nishida M et al. (2002) Annexin 5 messenger ribonucleic acid expression in pituitary gonadotropes is induced by gonadotropin-releasing hormone (GnRH) and modulates GnRH stimulation of gonadotropin release. Neuroendocrinology 75(1): 2–11.
31. Yao B, Kawaminami M (2008) Stimulation of annexin A5 expression by gonadotropin releasing hormone (GnRH) in the Leydig cells of rats. J Reprod Dev 54(4): 259–264.
32. Kawaminami M, Uematsu N, Funahashi K, Kokubun R, Kurusu S (2008) Gonadotropin releasing hormone (GnRH) enhances annexin A5 mRNA expression through mitogen activated protein kinase (MAPK) in LbetaT2 pituitary gonadotrope cells. Endocr J. 55(6): 1005–1014.
33. Cozens AL, Yessi MJ, Kunzelmann K, Ohrui T, Chin L et al. (1994) CFTR expression and Chloride secretion in polarized immortal human bronchial epithelial cells. Am J Respir Cell Mol Biol 10: 38–47.
34. Bruscia E, Sangiuolo F, Sinibaldi P, Goncz KK, Novelli G et al. (2002) Isolation of CF cell lines corrected at DeltaF508-CFTR locus by SFHR-mediated targeting. Gene Ther. 9: 683–685.

35. Illek B, Maurisse R, Wahler L, Kunzelmann K, Fischer H et al. (2008) Cl transport in complemented CF bronchial epithelial cells correlates with CFTR mRNA expression levels. Cell. Physiol. Biochem. 22: 57–68.
36. Bebok Z, Collawn JF, Wakefield J, Parker W, Li Y et al. (2005) Failure of cAMP agonists to activate rescued deltaF508 CFTR in CFBE41o- airway epithelial monolayers. J. Physiol. 569: 601–615.
37. Lowry OH, Rosebrough NJ, Farr AL, Randall RJ (1951) Protein measurement with the Folin phenol reagent. J. Biol. Chem. 193: 265–275.
38. Norez C, Antigny F, Becq F, Vandebrouck C (2006) Maintaining Low Ca2+ Level in the Endoplasmic Reticulum Restores Abnormal Endogenous F508del-CFTR Trafficking in Airway Epithelial Cells. Traffic 7: 562–573.
39. Farre C, Stoelzle S, Haarmann C, George M, Brüggemann A et al. (2007) Automated ion channel screening: patch clamping made easy. Expert Opin Ther Targets 11(4): 557–65.
40. McKone EF, Emerson SS, Edwards KL, Aitken ML (2003) Effect of genotype on phenotype and mortality in cystic fibrosis: a retrospective cohort study. Lancet 361: 1671–1676.
41. Zhang L, Button B, Gabriel SE, Burkett S, Yan Y et al. (2009) CFTR delivery to 25% of surface epithelial cells restores normal rates of mucus transport to human cystic fibrosis airway epithelium. PLoS Biol. 7 e1000155.
42. Gerke V, Moss SE (2002) Annexins: from structure to function. Physiol Rev 82: 331–371.
43. Crompton MR, Moss SE, Crumpton MJ (1988) Diversity in the lipocortin/calpactin family. Cell 55: 1–3.
44. Moss SE, Morgan RO (2004) The annexins. Genome Biol 5: 219.
45. Rojas E, Pollard HB, Haigler HT, Parra C, Burns AL (1990) Calcium-activated endonexin II forms calcium channels across acidic phospholipid bilayer membranes. J Biol Chem 265: 21207–21215.
46. Faria D, Dahimène S, Alessio L, Scott-Ward T, Schreiber R et al. (2011) Effect of Annexin A5 on CFTR: regulated traffic or scaffolding? Mol Membr Biol. 28(1): 14–29.
47. Borthwick LA, Botha P, Verdon B, Brodlie MJ, Gardner A et al. (2011) Is CFTR-delF508 really absent from the apical membrane of the airway epithelium? PLoS One 6(8): e23226.
48. Kakar SS, Jennes L (1995) Expression of gonadotropin-releasing hormone and gonadotropin-releasing hormone receptor mRNAs in various non-reproductive human tissues. Cancer Lett. 98(1): 57–62.
49. Tieva A, Stattin P, Wikström P, Bergh A, Damber JE (2001) Gonadotropin-releasing hormone receptor expression in the human prostate. Prostate 47(4): 276–284.
50. Koushik K, Bandi N, Sundaram S, Kompella UB (2004) Evidence for LHRH-Receptor Expression in Human Airway Epithelial (Calu-3) Cells and Its Role in the Transport of a LHRH Agonist. Pharmaceutical Research 21(6): 1034–1046.
51. Reutelingsperger CP, van Heerde W, Hauptmann R, Maassen C, van Gool RG et al. (1994) Differential tissue expression of Annexin VIII in human. FEBS Lett. 349(1): 120–124.
52. Kawaminami M, Tsuchiyama Y, Saito S, Katayama M, Kurusu S et al. (2002) Gonadotropin-releasing hormone stimulates annexin 5 messenger ribonucleic acid expression in the anterior pituitary cells. Biochem Biophys Res Commun. 291(4): 915–920.
53. Alzamora R, King JD Jr, Hallows KR (2011) CFTR regulation by phosphorylation. Methods Mol Biol. 741: 471–488.
54. Baudouin-Legros M, Hinzpeter A, Jaulmes A, Brouillard F, Costes B et al. (2005) Cell-specific posttranscriptional regulation of CFTR gene expression via influence of MAPK cascades on 3'UTR part of transcripts. Am J Physiol Cell Physiol 289(5): C1240–C1250.
55. Rowe SM, Verkman AS (2013) Cystic fibrosis transmembrane regulator correctors and potentiators. Cold Spring Harb Perspect Med. 3(7): a009761.

14

A New Method to Improve the Clinical Evaluation of Cystic Fibrosis Patients by Mucus Viscoelastic Properties

Giovanna Tomaiuolo[1,2*], Giulia Rusciano[3], Sergio Caserta[1,2], Antonio Carciati[1], Vincenzo Carnovale[4], Pasquale Abete[4], Antonio Sasso[3], Stefano Guido[1,2]

1 Dipartimento di Ingegneria Chimica, dei Materiali e della Produzione Industriale, Università di Napoli Federico II, Napoli, Italy, **2** CEINGE-Advanced Biotechnologies, Napoli, Italy, **3** Dipartimento di Fisica, Università di Napoli Federico II, Complesso Universitario M.S. Angelo, Napoli, Italy, **4** Dipartimento di Scienze mediche Traslazionali - Unità di Fibrosi Cistica dell'adulto, Università di Napoli Federico II, Napoli, Italy

Abstract

In cystic fibrosis (CF) patients airways mucus shows an increased viscoelasticity due to the concentration of high molecular weight components. Such mucus thickening eventually leads to bacterial overgrowth and prevents mucus clearance. The altered rheological behavior of mucus results in chronic lung infection and inflammation, which causes most of the cases of morbidity and mortality, although the cystic fibrosis complications affect other organs as well. Here, we present a quantitative study on the correlation between cystic fibrosis mucus viscoelasticity and patients clinical status. In particular, a new diagnostic parameter based on the correlation between CF sputum viscoelastic properties and the severity of the disease, expressed in terms of FEV1 and bacterial colonization, was developed. By using principal component analysis, we show that the types of colonization and FEV1 classes are significantly correlated to the elastic modulus, and that the latter can be used for CF severity classification with a high predictive efficiency (88%). The data presented here show that the elastic modulus of airways mucus, given the high predictive efficiency, could be used as a new clinical parameter in the prognostic evaluation of cystic fibrosis.

Editor: Deepak Shukla, University of Illinois at Chicago, United States of America

Funding: Financial support from the Italian Ministry of Research under PRIN 2008 program is gratefully acknowledged. http://prin.miur.it/index.php?pag=2008. The funders had no role in study design, data collection and analysis, decision to publish, or preparation of the manuscript.

Competing interests: The authors have declared that no competing interests exist.

* E-mail: g.tomaiuolo@unina.it

Introduction

Cystic fibrosis (CF) is the most frequent life-limiting genetic disease in Caucasian populations, among whom it occurs in approximately 1 in 3000 births [1]. It is caused by mutations in a gene that encodes CF transmembrane conductance regulator (CFTR) protein which regulates the exchange of chloride and sodium ions across epithelial membranes [2-4]. The defect results in inflammation [5], infection and in thick, viscous mucoid secretions in multiple organs [6-9]. In healthy conditions, mucus is a complex fluid containing immunoglobulins, antiseptic enzymes, inorganic salts, proteins, glycoproteins known as mucins, and water. It is secreted by mucous cells and it has different functions, the most important one being acting as defense barrier against infectious agents [10,11]. From the rheological point of view, mucus is a dense, viscoelastic gel-like material, characterized by the presence of a large number of entanglements between glycoproteins and other mucosal components, stabilized by hydrogen bonding and electrostatic and hydrophobic interactions [12]. In CF patients, airways mucus, containing less water than normal, and a rather high amount of cellular debris, shows an increased viscoelasticity due to the increased concentration of high molecular weight components, especially DNA, and associated physical entanglements at the molecular level [12]. Such mucus thickening leads to abnormal mucus clearance and, finally, to bacterial overgrowth [10]. From the clinical point of view, the altered rheological behavior of mucus results in lung chronic infection and inflammation, which causes most of the cases of morbidity and mortality, despite the CF complications affect other organs as well [13]. In light of such pathological relevance, the rheological characterization of body fluids such as blood [14-17], amniotic fluid, synovial fluid [18] and mucus [10,19] have been the subject of a number of studies. Regarding mucus, two main approaches have been followed so far: i) microrheology, that is based on a magnetic microrheometer, an elegant technique for measuring rheological properties [20] of small volume of mucus [21-23], as well as multiple particle tracking [12] and dynamic light scattering [24]; the drawbacks of these techniques are related to mucus heterogeneity [12]; ii) macrorheology, where classical

Table 1. Data on Age, Colonization, Sub-colonization, and FEV1 values of 33 CF donors.

# ID	Age	Colonization	Sub colonization	FEV 1 %
SA1	24	Staphiloccocus aureus	Haemophilus Influenzae	97
SA2	26	Staphiloccocus aureus	Pseudomonas aeruginosa	79
SA3	21	Staphiloccocus aureus	Haemophilus Influenzae	70
SA4	32	Staphiloccocus aureus	Haemophilus Influenzae	69
SA5	26	Staphiloccocus aureus	Haemophilus Influenzae	64
SA6	26	Staphiloccocus aureus	Haemophilus Influenzae	43
PA1	25	Pseudomonas aeruginosa	Staphiloccocus aureus	81
PA2	33	Pseudomonas aeruginosa	Staphiloccocus aureus	61
PA3	39	Pseudomonas aeruginosa	Staphiloccocus aureus	57
PA4	48	Pseudomonas aeruginosa	Staphiloccocus aureus	43
PA5	32	Pseudomonas aeruginosa	Staphiloccocus aureus	48
PA6	56	Pseudomonas aeruginosa	Haemophilus Influenzae	40
PA7	28	Pseudomonas aeruginosa	Staphiloccocus aureus	62
PA8	31	Pseudomonas aeruginosa	Staphiloccocus aureus	44
PA9	28	Pseudomonas aeruginosa	Staphiloccocus aureus	49
PA10	26	Pseudomonas aeruginosa	Staphiloccocus aureus	68
PA11	27	Pseudomonas aeruginosa	Escherichia Coli	18
PA12	28	Pseudomonas aeruginosa	Staphiloccocus aureus	34
PA13	44	Pseudomonas aeruginosa	Haemophilus Influenzae	36
PA14	23	Pseudomonas aeruginosa	Staphiloccocus aureus	32
PA15	34	Pseudomonas aeruginosa	Staphiloccocus aureus	21
PA16	34	Pseudomonas aeruginosa	Staphiloccocus aureus	59
PA17	25	Pseudomonas aeruginosa	Staphiloccocus aureus	25
PA18	27	Pseudomonas aeruginosa	Staphiloccocus aureus	68
PA19	35	Pseudomonas aeruginosa	Staphiloccocus aureus	23
PA20	57	Pseudomonas aeruginosa	Haemophilus Influenzae	40
BC1	25	Burkholderia Cepacia	Haemophilus Influenzae	40
BC2	28	Burkholderia Cepacia	Pseudomonas aeruginosa	34
BC3	40	Burkholderia Cepacia	Pseudomonas aeruginosa	25
BC4	30	Burkholderia Cepacia	Pseudomonas aeruginosa	17
SM1	24	Pseudomonas aeruginosa	Stenotrophomonas maltophilia	20
SM2	28	Pseudomonas aeruginosa	Stenotrophomonas maltophilia	23
SM3	40	Stenotrophomonas maltophilia	Pseudomonas aeruginosa	31

rotational viscometers are used [25], either under continuous and oscillatory shear [19,26].

In this work, we investigate the correlation between CF sputum viscoelastic properties and disease severity, in terms of FEV1% and bacterial colonization. FEV1% is defined as the ratio of the Forced Expiratory Volume in 1 second (FEV1) to the Forced Vital Capacity (FVC). The FVC is the volume of air which can be forcibly and maximally exhaled out of the lungs until no more can be expired and is usually expressed in liters, thus FEV1% indicates what percentage of the total FVC has been expelled from the lungs during the first second of forced exhalation. In the following, FEV1% is represented by just FEV1. FEV1 is typically measured by spirometry, an highly patient cooperation-dependent maneuver, that shows several disadvantages, such as reproducibility. Here, we show that CF mucus elasticity and viscosity are strictly related with bacterial colonization, and can be used as diagnostic tools in addition to (and/or replacement of) FEV1, being independent on patient cooperation.

Materials and Methods

CF samples

Sputum samples were provided by the Dipartimento di Scienze Mediche Traslazionali - Unità di Fibrosi Cistica dell'adulto, following a procedure approved by the Ethics Committee of the Istituto Superiore di Sanità. Written informed consent was obtained from each individual. Sputum samples were collected in sterile containers from 33 patients (Table 1) affected by CF by voluntary expectoration during a routine clinical visit. The patients were categorized either as a function of bacterial colonization, i.e. i) Staphilococcus aureus; ii) Pseudomonas aeruginosa; iii) Burkholderia cepacia and Stenotrophomonas maltophilia, and of FEV1 value, i.e. i) FEV1 > 50% mild and moderate; ii) 30%<FEV1<50% severe; iii) FEV1 < 30% very severe. Freezing or homogenization of the sputum was not performed to avoid breakdown of structures.

Rheological measurements on CF sputum

Rheological measurements were performed using a Bohlin Instruments CVO 120 controlled-stress rheometer [27,28] operating either in continuous shear and in dynamic oscillatory mode using a 60 mm smooth stainless steel cone-plate geometry (cone angle 0.0175 rad). The sample was loaded on the plate center and possible air bubbles were removed. A steel cylindrical cage enveloping the cone-plate system has been used to prevent sample drying [29]. All the measurements were performed at room temperature to reduce sample degradation (no significant difference was found by setting the temperature to 37°C). Continuous shear tests were performed in a range of stress equal to 0.01-40 Pa, going from low stresses to high stresses and back to low values, to evaluate the possible presence of hysteresis loop. The delay time has been set equal to 4 seconds and the integration time was 20 seconds. Concerning oscillatory test, amplitude sweeps were performed to determine a stress (0.05-6 Pa) at which the response of the elastic modulus (*G'*) and loss modulus (*G''*) was within the linear viscoelastic region of the sample. Finally, frequency sweeps (0.1-50 rad/s) were performed to determine *G'* and *G''* behavior. Data obtained from the rheological measurements were used to calculate useful parameters such as the magnitude of the complex modulus *G** (equal to the absolute value of the sum of *G'* and *G''*) and loss tangent, or *tan* δ (equal to the ratio between *G''* and *G'*) at low (1 rad/s) and high (10 rad/s) oscillation frequency. Two derivative parameters that predict mucus clearability by ciliary and cough mechanism are the Mucus Clearability index (*MCI*) and the Cough Clearability index (*CCI*) and are calculated by using the value of G* and tan δ at low and high oscillation frequency respectively, as in the following formulas [23]:

$$MCI = 1.62 - \left(0.22 \cdot \log G^*\big|_{1rad/s}\right) - \left(0.77 \cdot \tan\delta\big|_{1rad/s}\right)$$

$$CCI = 4.44 - \left(1.07 \cdot \log G^*\big|_{10rad/s}\right) + \left(0.89 \cdot \tan\delta\big|_{10rad/s}\right)$$

Principal Component Analysis

Principal Component Analysis (PCA) is a statistical tool, widely used in many fields of sciences, for the analysis of multidimensional data sets [30,31]. It is used to condense the information contained in an set of eventually correlated variables (e.g. the observables associated to a physical state), into a set of uncorrelated variables called Principal Components (PCs). PCs are obtained as linear combination of the original variables. The procedure of data transformation involves the diagonalization of the correlation matrix of the initial data; as a result, the PCs are uncorrelated data, and carry the most relevant information to differentiate among the initial data. The order of the PCs denotes their importance in highlighting differences within the dataset, with PC1 describing the highest amount of variation, PC2 the second highest, and so on. The coefficients of the combination of PCs in terms of the original variables are named loadings and express the weight of each original observable to the global variance of data. The coordinates of the original data sets in the PCs space are instead referred as scores. Usually, the first 3 PCs are able to condensate more than 90% of the initial information; therefore, each set of the original data can be represented by a point in a low dimensional space (score-plot). Ideally, when plotted in the score space, points corresponding to similar data set should cluster together.

Results and Discussion

Rheological tests

An important property of mucus is its ability to maintain an unstirred layer of mucus adjacent to epithelial surfaces despite the vigorous shearing actions of coughing, and it does this by being a shear-thinning material that forms a lubricating plane between sliding surfaces [32]. In this work, CF sputum samples were subjected to steady state deformations of controlled shear stress to reproduce the *in vivo* conditions and study the behavior of sputum viscosity in continuous shear. The shear-thinning behavior of CF sputum is shown in Figure 1, where the average viscosity of CF sputum sample is shown as a function of the shear stress at which the sample is sheared, either for the level of severity (mild/moderate, severe and very severe depending on FEV1 values, as showed in Figure 1a) and for the type of bacterial colonization (S. aureus, P. aeruginosa, and B. cepacia and S. maltophila (Figure 1b)). As can be seen in the log-log plot, mucus viscosity shows an initial plateau zone followed by a shear-thinning region as shear stress increases: this behavior is probably due to the decreasing adhesive interaction between mucin fibers with increasing shear stress. The shear stress value at the end of the plateau (i.e., at the onset of shear thinning) is associated with a characteristic relaxation time of the material and it is different for the three cases. The classification of the CF sputum samples based on FEV1 values (Figure 1a) is not full-scale, the viscosity of very severe data (gray circle) being significantly lower than the one of severe data (white circle). In Figure 1b it is evident, instead, that classifying mucus sample using bacterial colonization, allows to distinguish the CF severity. It is known, in fact, that B. cepacia and S. matophilia lungs colonization increases the possibility of morbidity and mortality, being associated with a rapid decline in pulmonary function, more than P. aeruginosa and S. aureus [33-35]. In fact, the B. cepacia and S. maltophila set of data (grey triangle) is significantly higher than the S. aureus one (black triangle), while the P. aeruginosa set shows a halfway trend, being close to the S. aureus data at low and medium shear stress (below 10 Pa) and overcoming the B. cepacia and S. maltophila data at high shear stress. Error bars (such as in the following figures) represent the standard deviation of the measurements, which is mainly due to the quantity of saliva present in the sample that it was no possible to extract without damaging the samples. The t-test, on absolute values, was used to assess whether there is a statistically significant difference between the groups. For the mild-moderate and severe couple of data set the t-test passed for viscosities below 10 Pa both for FEV1 and bacterial colonization with $P<0.05$. For the severe and very severe couple of data set the t test did not pass.

In Figure 1c a hysteresis loop of CF sputum is shown. This curve is obtained by increasing and subsequently decreasing the imposed shear stress. This behavior is typical of a time

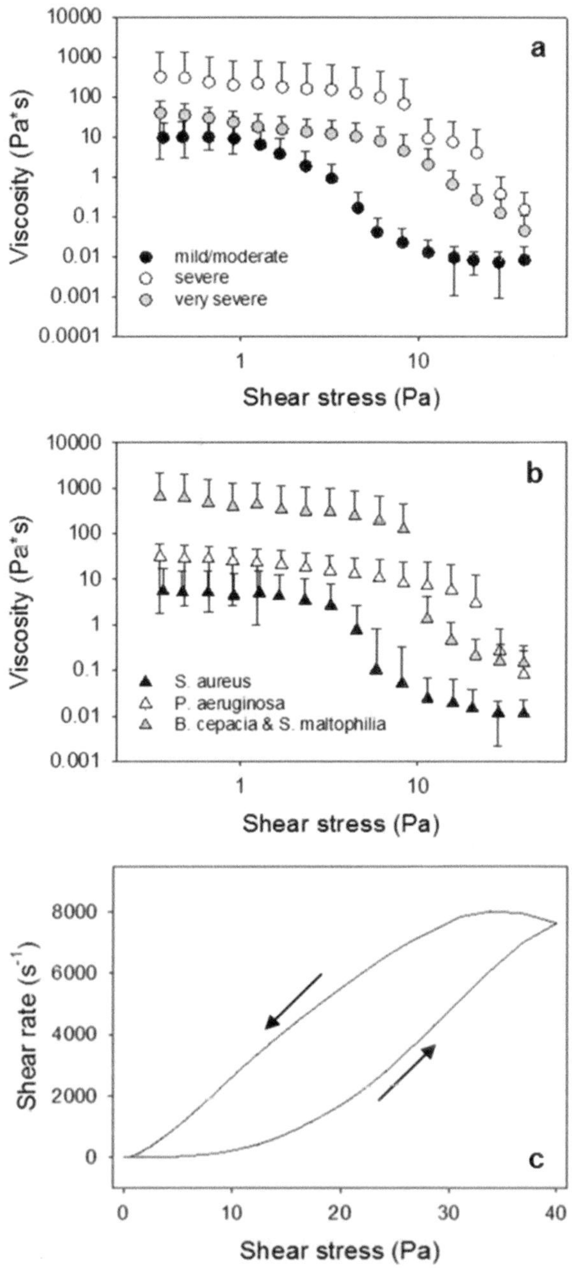

Figure 1. The steady state viscosity of CF sputum sample from 33 donors. a) Average viscosity from donors with different values of FEV1 (grey circle: very severe; white circle: severe; and black circle: mild/moderate) and b) Average viscosity from donors with different bacterial colonization (grey triangle: B. cepacia and S. maltophila, white triangle: P. aeruginosa and black triangle: S. aureus). Both for FEV1 and bacterial colonization, there is a significative difference between S. aureus and P. aeruginosa ($P<0.05$) at viscosity values below 10 Pa. c) Hysteresis loop of CF sputum.

dependent material and it is found when an irreversible breakdown of microstructure is elicited by the action of shear flow, the material being then unable to reform its original structure in the time scale of the measurement. The first part of the up-curve (marked with an arrow going from left to right) presents an horizontal region where shear rate is around 0. The last point of this region (ca 2 Pa) corresponds to the yield value of the material, i.e. the shear stress threshold above which the material is able to flow. Below the yield point the viscosity of the material is very high. The viscoelasticity of CF sputum was characterized by applying oscillatory deformations to the samples. *G'* is the *elastic* (or *storage*) *modulus*, which is

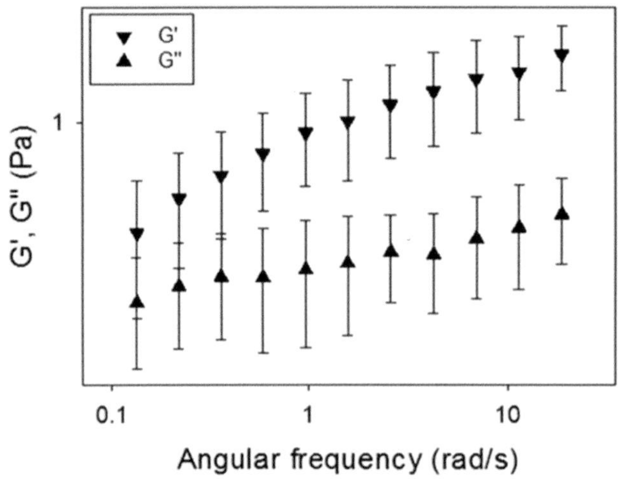

Figure 2. *G' and G'' as a function of angular frequency.* *G'* and *G''* are almost parallel lines, typical of a cross-linked gel.

a measure of stored energy and represents the elastic component of the material *G"* is the *viscous* (or *loss*) *modulus*, is a measure of the energy dissipated in the material and represents the viscous component of the material. Both the elastic modulus *G'* and the viscous modulus *G''* increase with frequency over a range of 0.1-50 rad/s. The elastic modulus *G'* of CF sputum predominates over the viscous modulus *G''* across the entire tested range of frequency, as shown in Figure 2, where *G'* and *G''* are plotted as a function of angular frequency. The *G'* predominance as well as the very similar dependence of *G'* and *G''* on frequency (*G'* and *G''* are almost parallel lines) are typical features of a cross-linked gel. In Figures 3a and 3b, *G'* and *G''* as a function of angular frequency are respectively shown for three levels of FEV1, corresponding to mild/moderate, severe and very severe. Both the elastic and viscous moduli grow with the reduction of the lungs activity and thus with the disease severity. The t-test was used to prove if there is a statistically significant difference between the groups. For the mild-moderate and severe couple of data set the t-test passed for *G'* at low and high values of angular frequency (0.1 and 10 rad/s), with P=0.043 and 0.048 respectively, while for *G''* it passed only for high values of angular frequency (10 rad/s) with P=0.019, this remarking the fact that the elastic contribution is the one that mostly correlates with disease severity. Concerning the correlation with bacterial colonization, *G'* and *G''* are respectively shown in Figures 3c and 3d as a function of angular frequency for S. aureus, P. aeruginosa and B. cepacia and S. maltophila. Also in this case, both the elastic and viscous moduli grow with the reduction of the lungs activity and thus with the disease severity. The t-test confirms that there is a statistically significant difference between the groups: in fact, it passed either for *G'* and *G''* at each value of angular frequency. For example, for *G'* at 1 rad/s, P=0.041 for S. aureus and P. aeruginosa data sets and at 10 rad/s P=0.008 for S. aureus and B. cepacia and S. maltophila, while for *G''* for S. aureus and B. cepacia and S. maltophila data sets P=0.028 and P=0.043 at 1 rad/s and 10 rad/s respectively. It is evident that the classification based on bacterial colonization works better than the one based on FEV 1. Thus, here, we propose a method to classify CF severity based on *G'* values at 1 rad/s and on the most diffused bacterial colonization. In particular, $G'<1.2$ Pa corresponds to S. aureus, 1.2 Pa$<G'<$4 Pa corresponds to P. aeruginosa and $G'>4$ Pa corresponds to B. cepacia and S. maltophila. The advantage of this classification is that, in principle, it would be possible to identify the type of bacterial colonization in few minutes, avoiding the long time and the big cost requested by microbiological measurements. Moreover, it would be possible to isolate patient with B. cepacia, that is very aggressive in person-to-person spread.

In Figure 4 a plot of loss modulus $G''(\omega)$ against storage modulus $G'(\omega)$ for the three FEV1 level of severity (Figure 4a) and for the different families of colonization (Figure 4b) is reported. As it can be seen in Figure 4a, the three sets of data classified by using the FEV1 values, nearly collapse into a single curve. This indicates that the rheological behavior of these samples, in terms of microstructure, is independent on FEV1 severity. Once again, this plot shows that the values of *G'* are higher than the ones of *G''* (see the scales of the axes), indicating that the elastic response of the material prevails on the viscous one. In Figure 4b, instead, the three sets of data classified by using the bacterial colonization, lie on curves of different slopes, indicating that the rheological behavior of these samples, in terms of microstructure, is dependent on colonization. For an elastic network the complex modulus and both its components depend on material parameters such as the number of elastically active entanglements and the concentration of high molecular weight species. The different slopes in Figure 4b show a different sensitivity of the moduli on such material parameters depending on disease severity. Indeed, one can distinguish three zones in the plot in Figure 4b: i) low *G'* and *G''* values, where S. aureus data are found; ii) high *G'* and *G''* values, where there are B. cepacia and S. maltophila data and iii) intermediate values of *G'* and *G''*, where

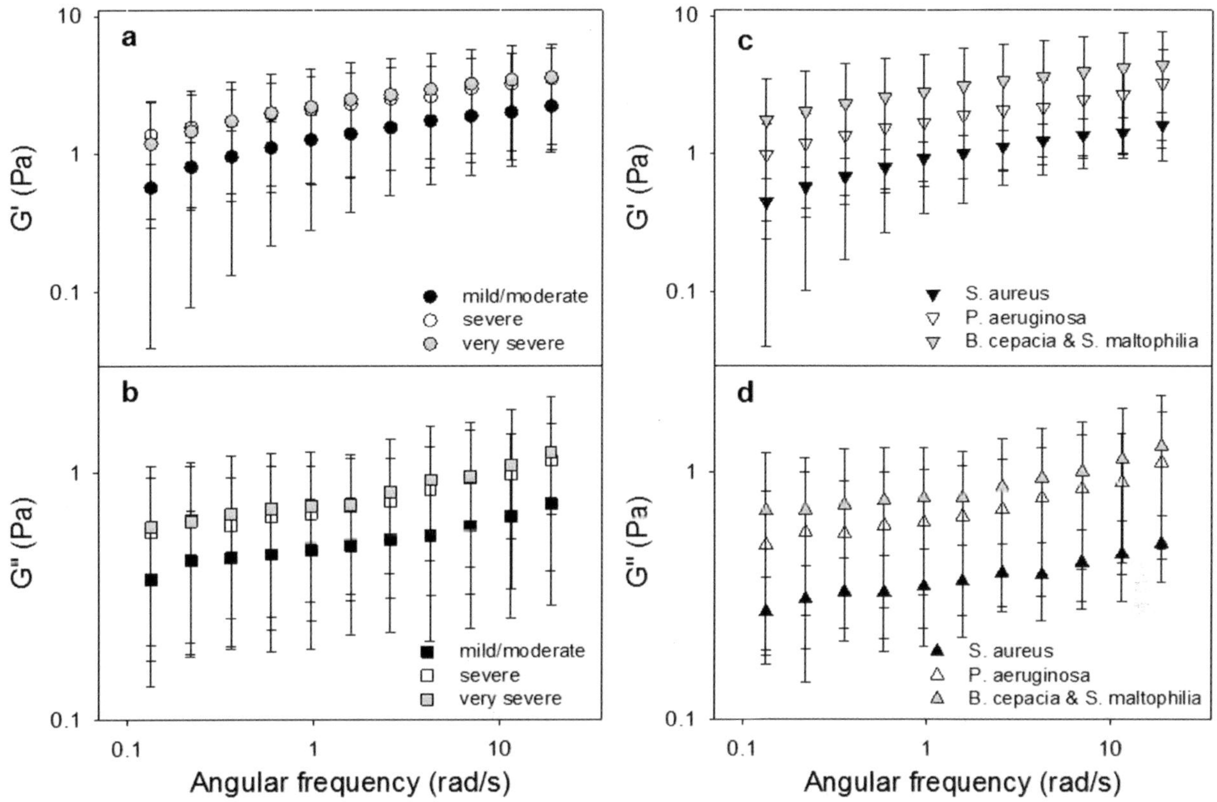

Figure 3. The elastic and loss modulus of CF sputum sample from 33 donors. a) *G*' and b) *G*'' as a function of angular frequency for the three levels of CF severity (i.e. FEV1 values corresponding to mild/moderate, severe and very severe level); c) *G*' and d) *G*'' as a function of angular frequency for different types of bacterial colonization (i.e. S. aureus, P. aeruginosa and B. cepacia and S. maltophila).

P. aeruginosa data are found. Thus, a classification of the type of bacterial colonization can be based on this plot.

Two more viscoelastic parameters were considered, in agreement with the literature: tan δ (loss tangent) and *G** (magnitude of complex modulus), each measured at 1 rad/s. The former, *tan* δ, being the ratio of *G*'' to *G*', represents the ratio of the viscous part to the elastic part (energy loss/energy stored) of the materials, and it is an useful quantifier of the presence and extent of elasticity in a fluid. A material that presents high (>> 1) tan δ deforms permanently when subjected to a stress and thus behaves as a liquid-like material; on the other hand, a material with low (<< 1) tan δ recoils or snaps back after the stress is removed and shows a solid-like behavior. The latter, *G**, is defined by *G**=*G*'+*iG*'', where *i* is the imaginary unit. The magnitude of *G** is given by $|G^*|=\sqrt{(G')^2+(G'')^2}$ and represents the overall resistance to deformation of a material, regardless of whether that deformation is recoverable (elastic) or non-recoverable (viscous). Here, the magnitude of *G** is represented by just *G**. In Figure 5a and 5b the comparison between the classification of patients by FEV1 and by colonization are respectively shown for *tan δ* and *log G**: *tan δ* (Figure 5a) is almost constant with FEV1 severity, but decreases with the bacterial colonization (from S. aureus to B. cepacia and S. maltophila) indicating that lung malfunction is caused by the increased elasticity of mucus. *log G**, in Figure 5b, is significantly increased in B. cepacia and S. maltophila samples as respect to S. aureus (P=0.018 and P=0.035 respectively) and this is another sign that elasticity governs mucus rheology in CF patients. For calculations of the mucociliary clearance index (*MCI*) and of the cough clearance index (*CCI*), *G*' and *G*'' at low frequency (0.1 rad/s) and at high frequency (10 rad/s) have been used. The low and high frequencies approximate the time scales in the airways due to ciliary beat and cough, respectively. In Figure 6a, the *MCI* shows a weak decrement with the severity of the disease either for FEV1 and bacterial colonization, while the *CCI* (Figure 6b) is significantly decreased in the case of bacterial colonization for in B. cepacia and S. maltophila samples as respect to S. aureus (P=0.014).

Statistical analysis

As final step, we analyzed our rheological data by PCA. This analysis was carried out in order to: *i*) test the effectiveness of our data in assessing the differences between the considered

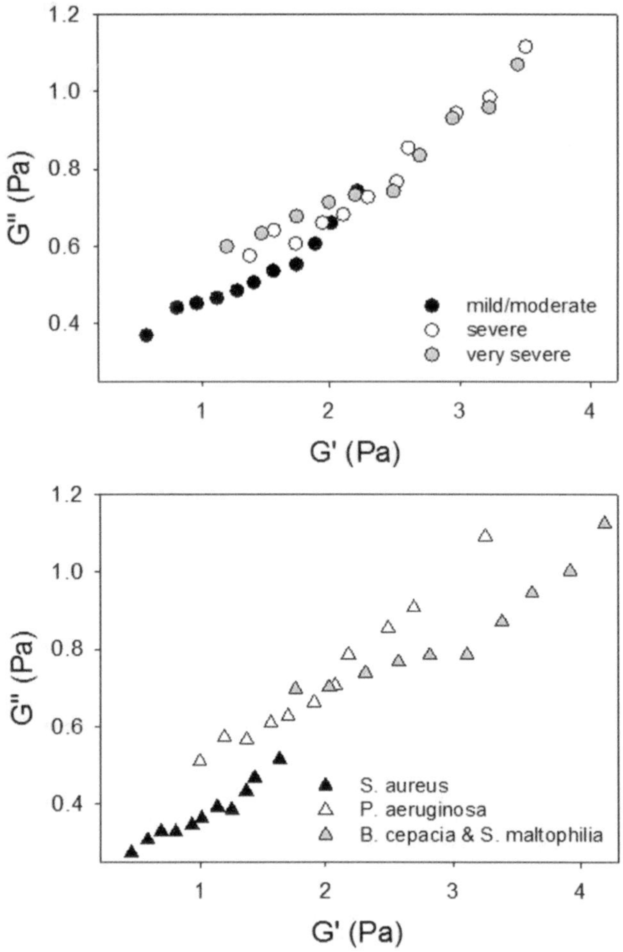

Figure 4. The loss modulus $G''(\omega)$ *vs* the elastic modulus $G'(\omega)$. ω values range from 0.134 rad/s to 18.7 rad/s. G'' vs G' for a) FEV1 (grey circle: very severe; white circle: severe; black circle: mild/moderate) and b) bacterial colonization (grey triangle: B. cepacia and S. maltophila; white triangle: P. aeruginosa; black triangle: S. aureus).

patients classes and *ii*) fully understand the relative importance of the different rheological data to classify patients. At this purpose, we associated to each of the 33 CF patients an array A_i of 11 selected rheological data (the so called observables), defined in Table 2. Therefore, these data were assembled in a 33x11 matrix A_{ij}, with *i* running on the patients and *j* on the observables. PCA was therefore performed on this matrix by using a custom-made Matlab routine, decomposing A_{ij} in PCs. The PCA routine includes mean centering and standardization of the original raw data. Figure 7 reports the loading of the first two PCs, which globally take into account 98.2 % of the total data variability. It is interesting to note that the weight of the original rheological observables in the definition of PC1 is dominated by *G'* values (observables 1,3,5), while the contribution of *G''* values is strongly reduced. Moreover, the contribution of *G'* increases with the frequency. Both results evidently confirm the experimental outcomes shown in the previous sections. Less trivial is the interpretation of PC2 loading. As for PC1, also PC2 loading shows an oscillating behavior between the *G'* and *G''* values; however, PC2 loading seems to suggest a contribution of MCI and CCI observables, whose values are enhanced with respect to PC1 loading. Figure 8 shows, instead, the scores of these PCs for each A_n, colored according to FEV class (Figure 8a) or to the patient bacterial colonization (Figure 8b). As it is possible to see from this figure, PCA analysis suggests some degree of correlation of rheological data with both patients infections and FEV1 values. In the case of bacterial colonization, points relative to S. aureus- and P. aeruginosa tend clearly to clusterize in the low PC1-score region, while B. cepacia- and S. maltophila points tend to occupy the high PC1-score region. Globally, a rough divisions of patients is provided by the dashed line depicted in Figure 8b, which efficiently separates points corresponding to these two groups of patients. This suggests that there is a high correlation between the patient bacterial infection and the new rheological observables defined by PC1 and PC2. As shown in Figure 8b, points present some clusterization in the PC1-PC2 plane also according to their

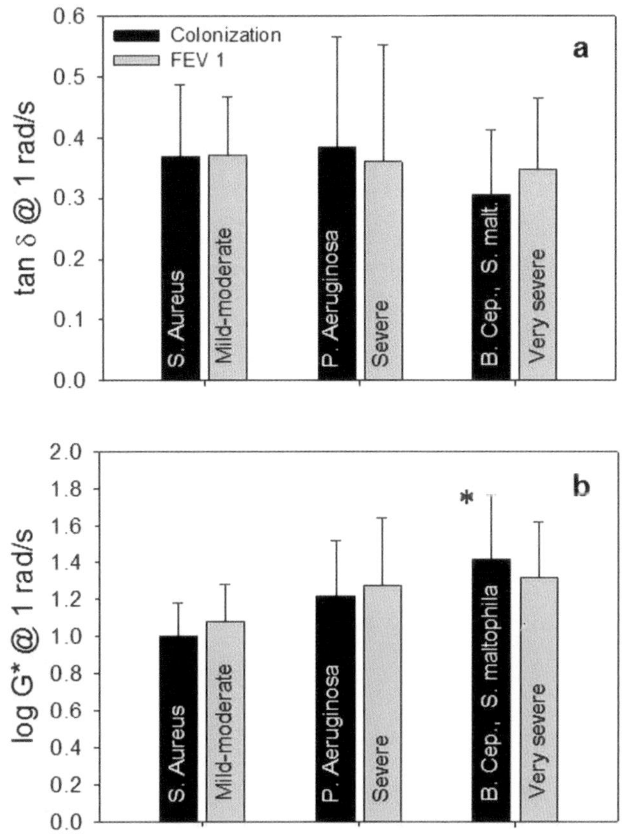

Figure 5. The loss tangent *tan* δ and the log value of the magnitude of the complex modulus *log G as a function of bacterial colonization and FEV1.** a) *tan* δ (mean±SD) at 1 rad/s as a function of bacterial colonization (black) and FEV1 severity (grey). In both cases the three set of data are not significantly different one from each other; b) *log G** (mean±SD) at 1 rad/s as a function of bacterial colonization (black) and FEV1 severity (grey). Regarding FEV1, the three set of data are not significantly different one from each other, while for bacterial colonization there is a significative difference between S. aureus and B. cepacia and S. maltophila (P=0.035).

FEV1 class, with mild/moderate and very severe patients presenting the lowest and the highest PC1 score, respectively. Moreover, mild/moderate patients exhibit also a slight clusterization along the PC2-score coordinate, while very severe patients present a wider spread along PC2-score axis. As for bacterial colonization, it is possible to define a line separating moderate/severe patients from the very-severe one (see continuous line in Figure 8b). Interestingly, two of the four apparently misclassified patients (BC2 and SM3) presents a FEV1 value which is border-line between the severe and very-severe FEV class (34 and 31, respectively). To test the effective reliability of PCA in discriminating CF patients according to both their bacterial infection and/or FEV1 class, we used the leave-one-out cross validation procedure (LOOCV) [36].

The results of this analysis were used to calculate the so called 'confusion matrix', in which all the correct guesses are located on the diagonal of the matrix (true positive, TP and true negative, TN), while misclassified data (false positive, FP and false negative, FN) are represented by the off-diagonal elements. From this matrix, the accuracy A=(TP +TN)/(TP+TN +FP+FN) was calculated.

The confusion matrices for the two cases analyzed herein are reported below (Table 3 and 4). From their analysis it is possible to estimate a classification efficiency of about 88% in both cases. This is a quite good result, considering the rather limited number of patients analyzed in this study, and it holds promise for the development of an high efficient algorithm for CF patients classification only based on the measurement of objective rheological parameters.

Conclusions

Rheological properties of mucus secretions from 33 Cystic Fibrosis patients were measured both under steady and oscillatory flow regime. The main finding is a strong correlation of the elastic component of the rheological response, as expressed by *G'*, with bacterial colonization and FEV1 values. Such correlation was found to be statistically significant by an advanced statistical analysis based on the PCA method,

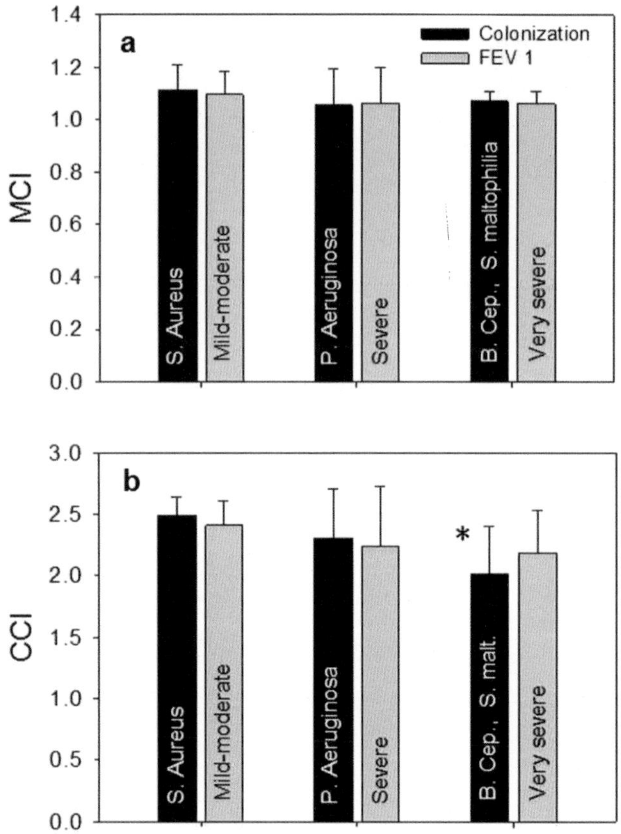

Figure 6. ***MCI* (mucociliary clearance index) and *CCI* (cough clearance index) as a function of bacterial colonization and FEV1.** a) *MCI* (mean±SD) at 1 rad/s as a function of bacterial colonization (black) and FEV1 severity (grey). In both cases the three set of data are not significantly different one from each other; b) *CCI* (mean±SD) at 10 rad/s as a function of bacterial colonization (black) and FEV1 severity (grey). Regarding FEV1, the three set of data are not significantly different one from each other, while for bacterial colonization there is a significative difference between S. aureus and B. cepacia and S. maltophila (P=0.014).

Table 2. Rheological observables used for PCA.

1	2	3	4	5	6	7	8	9	10	11
G'0.1	G"	G'	G"	G'	G"	η	Log G*	tan δ	MCI	CCI
rad/s	0.1 rad/s	1 rad/s	1 rad/s	10 rad/s	10 rad/s	10 Pa	1 rad/s	1 rad/s		

More specifically, the $\bar{j}^{th}$ column of this table defines the observable of the column $\bar{j}$ of the matrix of data A_{ij} ($j=\bar{j}$, i running on the [1-33] interval).

showing that the types of colonization and FEV1 classes are significantly correlated to the elastic modulus. The latter can be used for CF severity classification with a high predictive efficiency (88%). We therefore propose rheological measurements of mucus elasticity as a new way of CF patient classification, which could be applied as an additional tool for prognostic purposes together with the FEV1 index. Compared to FEV1, rheological tests have the advantage of being less patient dependent, since they are based on measurements of mucus samples with well-established scientific methodology, cheaper and less time consuming. Since a rheometer is not typically available in a clinical laboratory, a further possible application of this work is in the design of a device to measure mucus elasticity. Such a device could be disposable, user-friendly and cheap, and would allow one to use rheological parameters as a prognostic tool in the routine clinical tests.

Moreover, rheological characterization could allow to monitor the effect of pharmacological treatments (DNase, antibiotic, mucolytic, anti-inflammatory) *in vitro*. Many studies revealed that the high density mucus secretion in CF, and in other pulmonary diseases, has a detrimental effect on drugs delivery, due to their hindered diffusion through the highly viscous

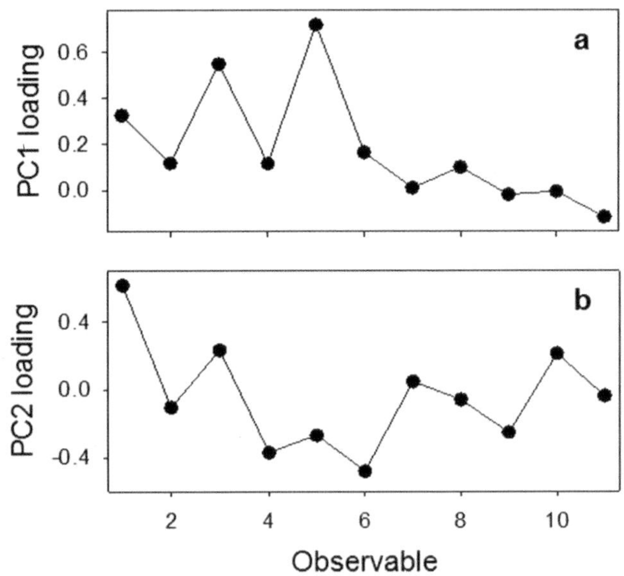

Figure 7. Loading plot for the first two PCs, taking globally into account 98.2% of data variability.

mucous layer. The rheological characterization proposed in this work could guide the development of new ways of administering therapeutics with increased local drug concentration in patients with reduced functionality of the CFTR protein [37,38].

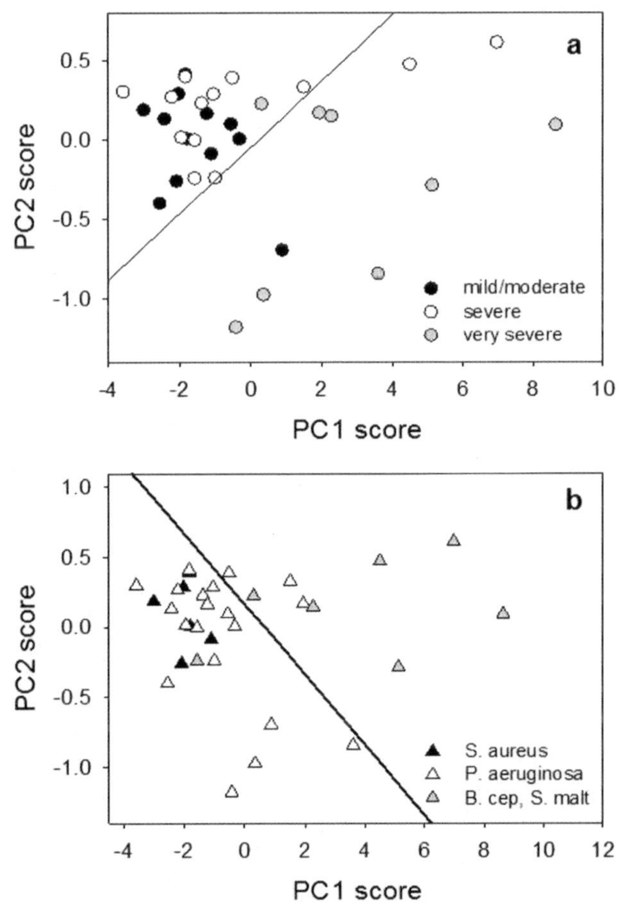

Figure 8. Principal Components Scatter Plot for the first two PCs. Points corresponding to the different patients are colored according to the patient bacterial colonization (a) or FEV1 class (b).

Table 3. Confusion matrix for CF-patients, classified according to their bacterial colonization.

TRUE CLASSIFICATION	PREDICTED CLASSIFICATION		
		S. aureus, P. aeruginosa	B. cepacia, S. maltophilia
	S. aureus, P. aeruginosa	23	3
	B. cepacia, S. maltophilia	1	6

Table 4. Confusion matrix for CF-patients, classified according to their FEV 1 class.

TRUE CLASSIFICATION	PREDICTED CLASSIFICATION		
		Mild/Moderate, Severe	Very severe
	Mild/Moderate, Severe	22	3
	Very severe	1	7

Acknowledgements

The authors wish to thank Prof. Giuseppe Marrucci for helpful discussion, Dr Rossella Tomaiuolo for fruitful suggestions, Speranza Esposito and Giuseppe Zeno for help in the experimental part. This study is related to the activity of the European network action COST MP1106 “Smart and green interfaces - from single bubbles and drops to industrial, environmental and biomedical applications".

Author Contributions

Conceived and designed the experiments: GT SG. Performed the experiments: GT AC. Analyzed the data: GT GR. Contributed reagents/materials/analysis tools: VC PA. Wrote the manuscript: GT GR SG. Performed the statistical analysis: GR. Supervised some of the rheological measurements: SC. Supervised the statistical analysis: AS. Revised the paper: SG AS. Mentored the authors during the development of the project: SG.

References

1. O'Sullivan BP, Freedman SD (2009) Cystic fibrosis. Lancet 373: 1891-1904. doi:10.1016/S0140-6736(09)60327-5. PubMed: 19403164.
2. Davis PB, Drumm M, Konstan MW (1996). Journal of Cystic Fibrosis - Am J Respir Crit Care Med 154: 1229-1256. doi:10.1164/ajrccm.154.5.8912731.
3. Davis PB (2001). Journal of Cystic Fibrosis - Pediatr Rev 22: 257-264.
4. Vij N, Downey GP (2013) The Yin and Yang of Cystic Fibrosis Transmembrane Conductance Regulator Function. Am J Respir Crit Care Med 187: 120-122. doi:10.1164/rccm.201211-2011ED. PubMed: 23322792.
5. Maiuri L, Luciani A, Giardino I, Raia V, Villella VR et al. (2008) Tissue transglutaminase activation modulates inflammation in cystic fibrosis via PPARgamma down-regulation. J Immunol, 180: 7697-7705. PubMed: 18490773.
6. Voter KZ, Ren CL (2008) Diagnosis of Cystic Fibrosis. Clin Rev Allergy Immunol 35: 100-106. doi:10.1007/s12016-008-8078-x. PubMed: 18506640.
7. Sheppard MN, Nicholson AG (2002) The pathology of cystic fibrosis. Curr Diagn Pathol 8: 50-59. doi:10.1054/cdip.2001.0088.
8. Amato F, Bellia C, Cardillo G, Castaldo G, Ciaccio M, et al. (2012) Extensive molecular analysis of patients bearing CFTR-related disorders. J Mol Diagn. United States: 2012 American Society for Investigative Pathology and the Association for Molecular Pathology. Published by Elsevier Inc. pp. 81-89
9. Tomaiuolo R, Fausto M, Elce A, Strina I, Ranieri A et al. (2011) Enhanced frequency of CFTR gene variants in couples who are candidates for assisted reproductive technology treatment. Clin Chem Lab Med 49: 1289-1293. PubMed: 21679131.
10. Lai SK, Wang Y-Y, Wirtz D, Hanes J (2009) Micro- and macrorheology of mucus. Adv Drug Deliv Rev 61: 86-100. doi:10.1016/j.addr.2008.09.012. PubMed: 19166889.
11. Lai SK, Wang YY, Cone R, Wirtz D, Hanes J (2009) Altering mucus rheology to "solidify" human mucus at the nanoscale. PLOS ONE 4: e4294. doi:10.1371/journal.pone.0004294. PubMed: 19173002.
12. Dawson M, Wirtz D, Hanes J (2003) Enhanced Viscoelasticity of Human Cystic Fibrotic Sputum Correlates with Increasing Microheterogeneity in Particle. Transport - J Biol Chem 278: 50393-50401.
13. Stenbit AE, Flume PA (2011) Pulmonary exacerbations in cystic fibrosis. Curr Opin Pulm Med 17: 442-447. PubMed: 21881509.
14. Tomaiuolo G, Barra M, Preziosi V, Cassinese A, Rotoli B et al. (2011) Microfluidics analysis of red blood cell membrane viscoelasticity. Lab Chip 11: 449-454. doi:10.1039/c0lc00348d. PubMed: 21076756.
15. Tomaiuolo G, Guido S (2011) Start-up shape dynamics of red blood cells in microcapillary flow. Microvasc Res 82: 35-41. doi:10.1016/j.mvr.2011.03.004. PubMed: 21397612.
16. Tomaiuolo G, Rossi D, Caserta S, Cesarelli M, Guido S (2012) Comparison of two flow-based imaging methods to measure individual red blood cell area and volume. Cytometry A 81: 1040–7. PubMed: 23081807.
17. Tomaiuolo G, Lanotte L, Ghigliotti G, Misbah C, Guido S (2012) Red blood cell clustering in Poiseuille microcapillary flow. Phys Fluids 24: 051903-051908. doi:10.1063/1.4721811.
18. Livak-Dahl E, Lee J, Burns MA (2013) Nanoliter droplet viscometer with additive-free operation. Lab Chip 13: 297-301. doi:10.1039/c2lc41130j. PubMed: 23192296.
19. Davis SS, Dippy JE (1969) The rheological properties of sputum. Biorheology 6: 11-21. PubMed: 5806400.
20. Jonás A, De Luca AC, Pesce G, Rusciano G, Sasso A et al. (2010) Diffusive mixing of polymers investigated by Raman microspectroscopy and microrheology. Langmuir 26: 14223-14230. doi:10.1021/la101498h. PubMed: 20681558.
21. King M, Macklem PT (1977) Rheological properties of microliter quantities of normal mucus. J Appl Physiol Respir Environ Exerc Physiol 42: 797-802. PubMed: 142075.
22. King M, Dasgupta B, Tomkiewicz RP, Brown NE (1997) Rheology of cystic fibrosis sputum after in vitro treatment with hypertonic saline alone and in combination with recombinant human deoxyribonuclease

I. Am J Respir Crit Care Med 156: 173-177. doi:10.1164/ajrccm.156.1.9512074. PubMed: 9230743.
23. Feng W, Garrett H, Speert DP, King M (1998) Improved clearability of cystic fibrosis sputum with dextran treatment in vitro. Am J Respir Crit Care Med 157: 710-714. doi:10.1164/ajrccm.157.3.9703059. PubMed: 9517580.
24. Celli J, Gregor B, Turner B, Afdhal NH, Bansil R et al. (2005) Viscoelastic properties and dynamics of porcine gastric mucin. Biomacromolecules 6: 1329-1333. doi:10.1021/bm0493990. PubMed: 15877349.
25. Minale M, Caserta S, Guido S (2010) Microconfined shear deformation of a droplet in an equiviscous non-newtonian immiscible fluid: experiments and modeling. Langmuir 26: 126-132. doi:10.1021/la902187a. PubMed: 20038166.
26. Serisier DJ, Carroll MP, Shute JK, Young SA (2009) Macrorheology of cystic fibrosis, chronic obstructive pulmonary disease & normal sputum. Respir Res 10: 63-. PubMed: 19580650.
27. Caserta S, Simeone M, Guido S (2008) Shear Banding in Biphasic Liquid-Liquid Systems. Phys Rev Lett 100: 137801. doi:10.1103/PhysRevLett.100.137801. PubMed: 18517998.
28. Caserta S, Guido S (2012) Vorticity banding in biphasic polymer blends. Langmuir 28: 16254-16262. doi:10.1021/la303232w. PubMed: 23134311.
29. Caserta S, Sabetta L, Simeone M, Guido S (2005) Shear-induced coalescence in aqueous biopolymer mixtures. Chemical Engineering Sciences 60: 1019-1027. doi:10.1016/j.ces.2004.09.076.
30. Jolliffe IT (2002) Principal Component Analysis. Berlin: Springer Verlag.
31. Vandenginste BGM, Massart DL, Buydens LMC, de Jong S, Lewi P et al. (1998) Handbook of Chemometrics and Qualimetrics B Amsterdam. Elsevier.
32. Cone RA (2009) Barrier properties of mucus. Adv Drug Deliv Rev 61: 75-85. doi:10.1016/j.addr.2008.09.008. PubMed: 19135107.
33. Gilligan PH (1991) Microbiology of airway disease in patients with cystic fibrosis. Clin Microbiol Rev 4: 35-51. PubMed: 1900735.
34. Harrison F (2007) Microbial ecology of the cystic fibrosis lung. Microbiology 153: 917-923. doi:10.1099/mic.0.2006/004077-0. PubMed: 17379702.
35. Waters V, Yau Y, Prasad S, Lu A, Atenafu E et al. (2011) Stenotrophomonas maltophilia in Cystic Fibrosis. Am J Respir Crit Care Med 183: 635-640. doi:10.1164/rccm.201009-1392OC. PubMed: 20889901.
36. de Jong BWD, Bakker Schut TC, Maquelin K, van der Kwast T, Bangma CH et al. (2006) Discrimination between Nontumor Bladder Tissue and Tumor by Raman. Spectroscopy - Anal Chem 78: 7761-7769.
37. Amato F, Seia M, Giordano S, Elce A, Zarrilli F et al. (2013) Gene Mutation in MicroRNA Target Sites of CFTR Gene: A Novel Pathogenetic Mechanism in Cystic Fibrosis? PLOS ONE 8: e60448. doi:10.1371/journal.pone.0060448. PubMed: 23555973.
38. Giordano S, Amato F, Elce A, Monti M, Iannone C et al. (2013) Molecular and Functional Analysis of the Large 5' Promoter Region of CFTR Gene Revealed Pathogenic Mutations in CF and CFTR-Related. Disorders - J Mol Diagn 15: 331-340. doi:10.1016/j.jmoldx.2013.01.001.

15

Advances toward the Elucidation of Hypertonic Saline Effects on *Pseudomonas aeruginosa* from Cystic Fibrosis Patients

Anne-Laure Michon[1,2]*, Estelle Jumas-Bilak[1,3], Raphaël Chiron[4], Brigitte Lamy[1,2], Hélène Marchandin[1,2]

1 UMR 5119 ECOSYM, Equipe Pathogènes et Environnements, U.F.R. des Sciences Pharmaceutiques et Biologiques, Université Montpellier 1, Montpellier, France, **2** Laboratoire de Bactériologie, Hôpital Arnaud de Villeneuve, Centre Hospitalier Régional Universitaire de Montpellier, Montpellier, France, **3** Laboratoire d'Hygiène hospitalière, Centre Hospitalier Régional Universitaire de Montpellier, Montpellier, France, **4** Centre de Ressources et de Compétences pour la Mucoviscidose, Hôpital Arnaud de Villeneuve, Centre Hospitalier Régional Universitaire de Montpellier, Montpellier, France

Abstract

Objectives: Nebulized hypertonic saline (HTS) has beneficial effects including reducing pulmonary exacerbations in Cystic Fibrosis (CF) patients. Several mechanisms may explain these effects but antimicrobial activity of NaCl remains largely unexplored. We aimed to measure the antimicrobial effect of NaCl on *Pseudomonas aeruginosa* isolated from the respiratory tract in CF patients.

Methods: NaCl minimal inhibitory concentration (MIC) and minimal bactericidal concentration (MBC) were determined for strains characterized for mucoidy, antimicrobial resistance, and ability to form biofilm using 0,9% to 15% NaCl solutions. NaCl effects on biofilm formation, preformed biofilm, and mobility were evaluated. Kinetics of antimicrobial effects was studied.

Results: The growth of all isolates (n = 85) from 34 patients was inhibited by 6% NaCl solution. A 10% concentration had a bactericidal activity on 90% of the isolates. Mucoid and multidrug resistant (MDR) isolates displayed lower MICs compared to non-mucoid and to non-MDR isolates, respectively. Time-kill kinetics showed that NaCl exhibited a rapid, dose and growth phase dependent bactericidal effect. Three percent or more of NaCl inhibited biofilm formation for 69% of strongly adherent isolates. A dose-dependent decrease of preformed biofilm viability and an inhibitory activity on bacterial motility were observed.

Conclusions: NaCl inhibited the growth of all isolates and killed 38% of tested isolates within concentration range currently used in therapeutics. Our results suggest that anti-pseudomonal activity is another mechanism of action of HTS to add to those already established. Clinical trials are needed to compare diverse HTS conditions of use (rhythm, dose and mode of delivery) to obtain efficient and optimized anti-*P. aeruginosa* effects. More generally, NaCl effect on other opportunistic pathogens as well as on global microbiotae recovered during polymicrobial diseases warrants further investigations.

Editor: Michael Tunney, Queens University Belfast, Ireland

Funding: This work was supported by the Ministère de l'enseignement supérieur et de la recherche, France. The funders had no role in study design, data collection and analysis, decision to publish, or preparation of the manuscript.

Competing Interests: The authors have declared that no competing interests exist.

* E-mail: al-michon@chu-montpellier.fr

Introduction

Cystic fibrosis (CF) is the most common inherited disease in Caucasians. The disorder is initiated by a defect in the CF transmembrane conductance regulator (CFTR) gene coding for an apical membrane chloride channel mediating transepithelial salt and liquid movement [1]. CF lung disease is characterized by a persistent inflammation and polymicrobial infectious disease evolving throughout life [2]. The chronic persistence of *Pseudomonas aeruginosa* is linked to lung function decline [3]. The consequences of hydro-electrolytic imbalance in the lung have been controversial in the past [1]. Currently, the volume of the airway surface liquid hypothesis suggesting that CFTR defect leads to water loss related to sodium chloride (NaCl) depletion in the mucus remains the main hypothesis [1,4]. According to this hypothesis, immotile dehydrated plugs are formed leading to inefficient mucociliary clearance that allows bacteria to cause lung infection [4]. This mechanism suggested that hypertonic saline (HTS) nebulization could favor mucociliary clearance [5]. Clinical trials confirmed beneficial effects on lung function and rate of pulmonary exacerbations but no effect on bacterial density was observed [6–11]. Testing HTS on a large population of *P. aeruginosa* CF isolates should elucidate the anti-microbial effect of NaCl.

The aim of this study was to characterize the effects of NaCl on 85 *P. aeruginosa* isolates from CF respiratory tract in 34 patients. Results were interpreted according to strains characteristics, i.e., mucoidy, multidrug resistance, and biofilm biomass formation.

Materials and Methods

Bacterial strains and collected data

Eighty-five clinical isolates of *P. aeruginosa* have been retrospectively studied (Pa1 to Pa85). Four reference strains, *P. aeruginosa* ATCC 27853, *P. aeruginosa* ATCC 15442, *P. aeruginosa* ATCC 9027, and *P. aeruginosa* CIP A22 were included in the study. Clinical isolates have been recovered over a 6-year period (from 2006 to 2011) from 36 respiratory tract samples in 34 CF patients attending our local CF center (Centre de Ressources et de Compétences de la Mucoviscidose) of Montpellier, France. Patient age ranged from two-month to 61-year old (median, 19 year-old). Chronic colonization was noted for 19 patients with a median period of colonization of 5 years (1 to 14 years). A single isolate was included for 12 patients and multiple colonial morphotypes, i.e., two to six isolates collected either from one or two samples, were tested for 22 patients. Species identification, mucoid status, and antimicrobial susceptibility were retrieved from routine bacteriological sputum analysis. A multidrug-resistant isolate was defined according to the Cystic Fibrosis Consensus Conference of 1994 as an organism resistant to all of the agents in at least of the following groups of antibiotics (ß-lactam agents, amino-glycosides, fluoroquinolones) [12]. HTS nebulization during the study period was noted for each patient.

Dilution methods used for bacteriostatic and bactericidal activity testing of NaCl

Inoculums for bacteria in stationary and logarithmic growth phases were prepared from MH agar and broth cultures, respectively, by visual comparison to MacFarland standards followed by dilution steps depending on the assay as previously recommended [13]. Minimal Inhibitory Concentration (MIC) determination was performed by 2 different methods, agar (MICa) and microbroth (MICb) dilution methods with bacteria in stationary phase. For MICa, Mueller-Hinton (MH) plates containing 0%, 0.9%, 1%, 2%, 3%, 4%, 5%, 6%, 7%, 8%, 9%, 10%, 12%, and 15% of NaCl were inoculated with a final inoculum of 10^4 colony forming units (CFU) per spot and incubated one night at 37°C as described previously [13] before reading. For MICb, MH broth containing 0%, 0.9%, 1%, 2%, 3%, 4%, 5%, 6%, 7%, 8%, 9% and 10% of NaCl were inoculated with a final inoculum of $5*10^5$ CFU/ml and incubated one night at 37°C as described previously [13] before reading. Minimal Bactericidal Concentration (MBC) corresponding to the lowest antimicrobial concentration reducing the inoculum by 99.99% within 24 h was determined from MICb assay by subculturing wells, which had no visible growth and the growth control well as described previously [14]. Each inoculum was confirmed by colony count and all assays were performed in duplicate. When different results were obtained in the two independent tests, the higher MIC or MBC value was taken as the result. Time-kill kinetic study of NaCl was performed with a macrobroth dilution method using final inoculum of $5*10^5$ CFU/ml with bacteria in stationary and/or in logarithmic growth phases according to the assay. Inoculation of NaCl-containing broth was performed as described previously [13]. The final test volume was 10 ml of MH and bacterial suspension loads were determined by subculturing serial dilutions of the inoculum after different incubation periods, i.e., 10 min, 30 min, 1 h, 2 h, 3 h, and 24 h, at 4°C or 37°C according to the assay.

Biofilm formation

The ability to form biofilm biomass was tested according to the crystal violet method [15] and strains were categorized as non-adherent, weakly, moderately, or strongly adherent [15,16]. The measurement of HTS effect on biofilm biomass formation was performed as described above using a final bacterial inoculum of $5*10^5$ CFU/ml in MH broth containing 0%, 0.9%, 1%, 2%, 3%, 4%, 5%, 6%, 7%, 8%, 9% and 10% of NaCl. All tests were carried out at least three times and results were averaged. The reduction in biofilm biomass formation and hypertonic saline activity on preformed biofilm were evaluated according to the modified method of Pompilio and colleagues [17].

Evaluation of bacterial motility

Motility of strains in presence of different concentrations of NaCl was globally estimated from diameter of spotted cultures on MH plates used for MICa. A strain was considered as motile when overnight cultures had increased diameter compared to the spot initial size. Motility has been estimated for all isolates for NaCl concentrations lower than MICs obtained by the agar dilution method.

Statistical analysis

MIC, MBC, and killing quotient (KQ) distributions were analyzed according to the mucoid status, the multidrug resistance, and the ability to produce biofilm. Differences between groups were assessed by Mann-Whitney's test, with the exception of the evaluation depending on biofilm producer groups, assessed by the Kruskal-Wallis' test and Spearman correlation coefficient when Kruskal-Wallis' test was positive. Data were analyzed at the total population level and at a restricted level defined by one isolate type per patient to avoid biased results due to possible clonal relatedness of isolates in a patient because strains have not been genotyped in this study. Statistical analysis of results was done with R project software (http://www.r-project.org). A P value ≤ 0.05 was considered to reflect significance.

Ethics statements

This in vitro study required neither the agreement of the ethical committee of our institution nor the patient informed consent because it involved only bacterial strains. The study does not involve the sample collection or patient data, and no patient intervention occurred with the obtained results. Only general data patients (age, type of colonization by P. aeruginosa) were reported but no patient-related data were analyzed. No primary human sample materials were used, only bacterial isolates from routine diagnostic procedures or strain collections. All analyzed clinical strains were acquired during routine diagnostic procedures. Accordingly, no acquisition of patient samples for the study was undertaken. We did not conduct research outside of our country of residence.

Results

Antibacterial effect of NaCl on the *P. aeruginosa* population

MIC and MBC results are presented in Table 1. Intra and inter-method variability is given in Table S1. For the 85 CF isolates, MIC values ranged from 0.9 to 6%. Depending on the method considered, MIC_{50} and MIC_{90} values were 4 or 5% and 5 or 6%, respectively. The growth of all the isolates was inhibited after a 24 h-incubation with 6% NaCl solution whatever the method considered. Moreover, NaCl displayed a bactericidal effect, 38% of the CF isolates being killed by a 7% NaCl solution, concentration currently used in therapeutics, 50% and 90% of the isolates being killed by 8% and 10% of NaCl, respectively. The effect of NaCl varied depending on the isolate, differences between

MICb and MBC value observed for a strain ranging from 1% to up to 7%. No correlation between MICb and MBC values was observed, some isolates displaying low MIC values of 1 or 3% and high MBC values of 7% or 10%, respectively and conversely (data not shown). This resulted in KQ values < 4 for the 83 strains exhibiting MBC values within tested range supporting a bactericidal activity of NaCl on a large majority of strains (Table 1).

NaCl activity varied according to relevant sub-populations of *P. aeruginosa*

Considering strains recovered in patients with multiple isolates, differences between MICb and/or MBC values ranging from 0 to 3% were observed. Variable response to NaCl with MICb and/or MBC values differing by 3% of NaCl were observed for the isolates recovered from four patients.

Table 2 exhibits MIC, MBC and KQ values of relevant sub-populations. MICb values obtained for mucoid CF isolates were significantly lower than the ones obtained for non-mucoid isolates when the total population ($P<0.0001$) and a subgroup defined by one isolate type, mucoid and/or non-mucoid, per patient ($P=0.0003$) were considered. MBC distribution did not significantly differ between mucoid and non-mucoid isolate groups when the subpopulation defined by one isolate type per patient was considered ($P=0.07$) but did when the whole population (n = 85) was considered ($P=0.01$), which may be related to a lower statistical power in relation to a limited number of strains in the subpopulation (n = 48). KQs for mucoid isolates were consequently higher than those for non-mucoid isolates ($P=0.0002$ and $P=0.0008$ for the whole population and the defined subpopulation, respectively) (Table 2). Twenty-two isolates recovered from eleven samples obtained from eleven patients were multidrug resistant (MDR). Considering the whole population (n = 85), non-MDR isolates displayed significantly higher MICb than did the MDR isolates ($P=0.0005$) while no difference was observed for MBC values. Consequently, KQs were higher for MDR isolates than for non-MDR isolates ($P=0.002$). A similar trend was observed when considering one randomly selected isolate type, MDR and/or non-MDR, per patient (n = 40) (MICb: $P=0.005$, KQ: $P=0.001$) (Table 2).

Five strains were recovered (Pa17 to Pa21) from one patient under 6% HTS treatment administered once or twice daily for 4 years. These isolates displayed low MICb values (3%, 3%, 2%, 3%, and 3%, respectively) and high MBC values (>10%, >10%, 8%, >10%, and >10%, respectively).

NaCl mechanism of action

Time-kill kinetics. Time-kill kinetics was performed on two strains selected for divergent phenotype, i.e., strain Pa1 (mucoid, MICb of 3%, MBC of 7%) and strain Pa71 (non-mucoid, MICb of 2%, MBC of 5%). Inoculum in logarithmic phase of growth was tested for isolate Pa71 against various concentrations of NaCl (Figure 1). Time-kill curves highlighted that a rapid decrease in inoculum size was observed from 30 min and before 3 h of contact with NaCl. NaCl antibacterial activity under *in vitro* conditions was shown to be both concentration- and time-dependent. Impact of both growth phase and temperature on time-kill kinetics of NaCl was evaluated on isolate Pa1 (Figure 2). The Pa1-time-kill curve also showed a rapid NaCl effect when bacteria in logarithmic phase of growth were incubated at 37°C in presence of NaCl at the MBC. With bacteria in stationary phase of growth tested in the same conditions, the killing effect was also observed but was drastically delayed (Figure 2) and the bactericidal effect of 4-log reduction of the inoculum was absent within 24h when the assay was performed at 4°C (Figure 2). Altogether, these results suggested that anti-*P. aeruginosa* activity of NaCl might be different than a mere osmotic effect because it depended on temperature conditions and physiological bacterial state.

Effects of NaCl on biofilm. All reference strains were able to form biofilm biomass, being either strongly, moderately, or weakly adherent. The majority of the 85 CF *P. aeruginosa* isolates were able to form biofilm biomass (n = 76) but most of these isolates were weakly adherent (n = 42) (Table 2). Most mucoid isolates were weakly adherent (Table 2). Among the 22 patients colonized by two or more *P. aeruginosa* colony types, five harbored isolates showing a unique adherence type and 13 had isolates showing two adherence types. More rarely, isolates recovered from a same patient may present three or four adherence types (two patients each).

We found that MICb values were correlated to the ability to form biofilm biomass, the strongly adherent isolates being associated with higher MICb values when both the whole population and a subgroup defined by one randomly selected isolate per type per patient were considered ($P<0.0001$ and $P=0.0004$, respectively) (Table 2). There was no significant trend between the MBC value and the level of adherence ($P=0.14$ and 0.12 respectively) (Table 2).

A reduction of at least 25% of biofilm biomass formation was highlighted for 23% to 69% of strongly adherent strains depending on the NaCl concentration with a dose-dependent effect, and for 27% to 53% of moderately adherent isolates (Figure 3). Twenty percent of weakly adherent isolates showed a decrease in their ability to form biofilm biomass independently of the NaCl concentration tested. With 2 and 3% of NaCl, rates of isolates

Table 1. NaCl Minimal Inhibitory Concentration (MIC), Minimal Bactericidal Concentration (MBC) and Killing quotient (KQ) distributions for the 85 CF isolates and the 4 reference strains of *P. aeruginosa*.

	NaCl MIC values (in %)											
	Agar dilution method			Broth dilution method			NaCl MBC values (in %)			Killing quotient (KQ)[a]		
Strains or isolates (n)	MIC_{50}	MIC_{90}	Range	MIC_{50}	MIC_{90}	Range	MBC_{50}	MBC_{90}	Range	KQ_{50}	KQ_{90}	Range
All strains (n = 89)	4	5	2–6	5	6	0.9–6	8	10	4->10	1.8	2.7	1.2–7.8
Reference strains (n = 4)	5	5	5	5	6	5–6	7	9	7–9	1.4	1.6	1.4–1.6
CF isolates (n = 85)	4	5	2–6	4	6	0.9–6	8	10	4->10	1.8	3	1.2–7.8

MIC_{50} and MIC_{90} values were defined as the lowest concentration of NaCl at which 50% and 90% of the isolates were inhibited, respectively.
[a]Only isolates exhibiting MBC values within tested range were considered.

Table 2. Comparison of NaCl Minimal Inhibitory Concentration (MIC), Minimal Bactericidal Concentration (MBC) and Killing quotient (KQ) distributions for subgroups of *P. aeruginosa* CF isolates according to mucoid characteristic, antimicrobial susceptibility pattern, ability to form biofilm and patient under HTS treatment.

			NaCl MIC values (in %)															
			Agar dilution method				Broth dilution method				NaCl MBC values (in %)				Killing quotient (KQ)[a]			
Population	Subgroup	Isolate type (n)	MIC_{50}	MIC_{90}	Range	*P* value [d]	MIC_{50}	MIC_{90}	Range	*P* value [d]	MBC_{50}	MBC_{90}	Range	*P* value[d]	KQ_{50}	KQ_{90}	Range	*P* value [d]
Total CF isolates	Mucoid characteristic	Mucoid (25)	3	4	2–4	**<0.0001**	3	5	0.9–5	**<0.0001**	7	9	6–>10	**0.01**	2.3	3.5	1.4–7.8	**0.0002**
		Non-mucoid (60)	5	5	2–6		5	6	2–6		8	10	4–>10		1.6	2.3	1.2–4	
	Antimicrobial susceptibility pattern	Multidrug resistance (22)	3	4	2–5	**<0.0001**	3	5	2–5	**0.0005**	8	>10	7–>10	0.3	2.3	3.5	1.4–4	**0.002**
		Non-multidrug resistance (63)	4	5	2–6		5	6	0.9–6		8	9	4–>10		1.8	2.3	1.2–7.8	
	Ability to form biofilm	No (9 of which 3 mucoid)	3	5	2–5	**<0.0001 Rs = 0.44**	3	5	2–5	**<0.0001 Rs = 0.48**	7	9	4–9	0.14	2.3	4	1.4–4	**0.0009 Rs = −0.37**
		Weak (42 of which 16 mucoid)	4	5	2–5		4	5	0.9–6		8	10	5–>10		1.8	3.5	1.2–7.8	
		Moderate (18 of which 3 mucoid)	5	5	2–5		5	6	2–6		8	>10	7–>10		1.8	2.3	1.2–3.5	
		Strong (16 of which 3 mucoid)	5	6	3–6		5	6	3–6		8	9	6–10		1.5	2	1.2–2.7	
	Patient under HTS treatment	Yes (5) [b]	2	3	2–3	ND	3	3	2–3	ND	>10	>10	8–>10	ND	ND	ND	ND	ND
		No (80)	4	5	2–6		5	6	0.9–6		8	9	4–>10		1.8	2.7	1.2–7.8	
One isolate per type, per patient [c]	Mucoid characteristic	Mucoid (18)	3	4	2–4	**<0.0001**	3	5	2–5	**0.0003**	7	9	7–>10	0.07	2.3	3.5	1.4–4.5	**0.0008**
		Non-mucoid (30)	5	5	2–6		5	6	2–6		8	9	5–>10		1.5	2.3	1.2–3.3	
	Antimicrobial susceptibility pattern	Multidrug resistance (11)	3	4	2–5	**0.002**	3	5	2–5	**0.005**	8	10	7–>10	0.6	2	3.5	1.6–3.5	**0.001**
		Non-multidrugresistance (29)	5	5	2–6		5	6	0.9–6		8	9	5–>10		1.5	2.3	1.2–7.8	
	Ability to form biofilm	No (7 of which 1 mucoid)	3	5	2–5	**<0.0001 Rs = 0.5**	3	5	2–5	**0.0004 Rs = 0.46**	7	9	4–9	0.12	2.3	4	1.4–4	0.056
		Weak (24 of which 8 mucoid)	4	5	2–5		4	6	2–6		8	10	5–>10		1.6	2·5	1.3–3.5	
		Moderate (15 of which 3 mucoid)	5	5	2–5		5	6	2–6		8	>10	7–>10		1.8	2·3	1.3–3.5	
		Strong (11 of which 2 mucoid)	5	6	4–6		5	6	4–6		9	9	7–10		1.5	2	1.3–2	
	Patient under HTS treatment	Yes (1)	ND	ND	2	ND	ND	ND	3	ND	ND	ND	>10	ND	ND	ND	ND	ND
		No (33)	5	5	2–6		5	6	2–6		8	9	5– >10		1.6	2.5	1.2–3.5	

MIC_{50} and MIC_{90} values were defined as the lowest concentration of NaCl at which 50% and 90% of the isolates were inhibited, respectively.
[a]Only isolates exhibiting MBC values within tested range were considered.
[b]5 isolates recovered in one patient.
[c]isolates were randomly selected.
[d]Comparison of MIC, MBC and KQ distribution between subgroups was performed with Mann-Whitney's test, with the exception of the evaluation depending on biofilm producer groups, assessed by the Kruskal-Wallis' test, and Spearman correlation coefficient (Rs) when Kruskal-Wallis' test was positive. A *P* value ≤0.05 was considered to reflect significance and was indicated in bold type.
ND, not determined either because only one isolate or one patient was included in the sub-population, or because one isolate exhibiting a MBC value within the tested range.

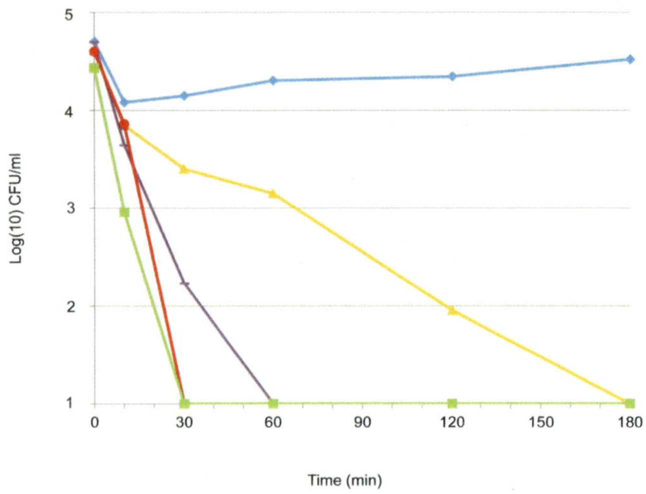

Figure 1. Time-kill kinetics of different NaCl concentrations against *P. aeruginosa* isolate Pa71. 3% NaCl solution (orange line, filled triangles), 5% NaCl solution - corresponding to the MBC value (violet line, dash), 7% NaCl solution (red line, filled circles), and 10% NaCl solution (green line, filled squares). Control (blue line, filled lozenges) was not exposed to NaCl. Time-kill curves of 15% (not shown) and 10% NaCl solution were similar.

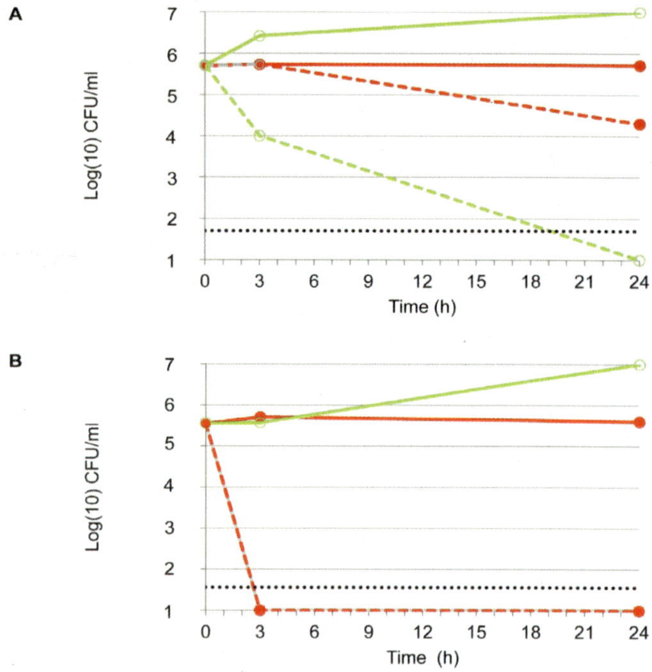

Figure 2. Time-kill kinetics of NaCl against *P.aeruginosa* Pa1 according to bacterial phase of growth and incubation temperature. Inoculum in stationary phase of growth (A) and in logarithmic phase of growth (B) for Pa1 (NaCl MBC: 7%). Bacterial suspension in NaCl at the MBC value were incubated at 37°C (green dotted line, open circles) or 4°C (red dotted line, filled circles). Controls (full lines) were not exposed to NaCl and were incubated at 37°C (green line, open circles) or 4°C (red line, filled circles). The horizontal dotted line indicates a 4-log reduction in viability. B: dotted green (open circles) and red (filled circles) lines are superposed.

showing reduction in biofilm biomass formation increased with the adherence level. Analysis conducted on subgroups defined by one isolate per type of adherence per patient showed similar results (data not shown).

In vitro activity of NaCl solution (7% and 10%) was evaluated on preformed biofilm for Pa28, Pa29, and Pa31, three strongly adherent, non-mucoid, non-MDR isolates with identical MICb and MBC values (MICb = 6%, MBC = 9%) recovered from three patients. Biofilm viability was reduced and this appeared to be dose dependent (Figure 4).

Time-kill kinetics showed a killing effect on preformed biofilm resulting in at least a 10^{-3} decrease in bacterial load and occurring between 1 h and 4 h of contact with 10% of NaCl (Figure 5).

Evaluation of NaCl activity on motility. For NaCl concentration above 2%, none of the 46 isolates displaying motility in the absence of NaCl were motile anymore (Figure 6), suggesting that NaCl inhibited isolate motility at concentrations lower than those inhibiting bacterial growth.

Discussion

Short-term and long-term clinical randomized trials in CF patients showed beneficial effects of HTS nebulization on lung function in reducing exacerbations or on the perception of effectiveness of chest physiotherapy [6,8,9,11]. Positive effects were explained by mucus rehydration and mucociliary clearance improvement, anti-inflammatory activity and indirect effects by activation of antimicrobial peptides [4,5,18]. No report investigated antimicrobial activity of NaCl as a possible explanation supporting beneficial effects of such a treatment.

We proposed the first study evaluating *in vitro* NaCl activity on a large population of *P. aeruginosa* isolated from CF patients. Multiple antimicrobial effects of NaCl on CF *P. aeruginosa* are demonstrated with NaCl concentrations used in therapeutics. Indeed, we showed that: i) 6% NaCl solution inhibits bacterial growth for all the tested isolates, ii) a killing effect was observed from 4% NaCl solution, and iii)10% NaCl solution had a bactericidal activity on 90% of the isolates. We also demonstrated that NaCl had effects on bacterial biofilm being able to alter biofilm biomass formation of strongly adherent isolates at sub-inhibitory concentrations and to have a killing effect on preformed biofilm. However, according to

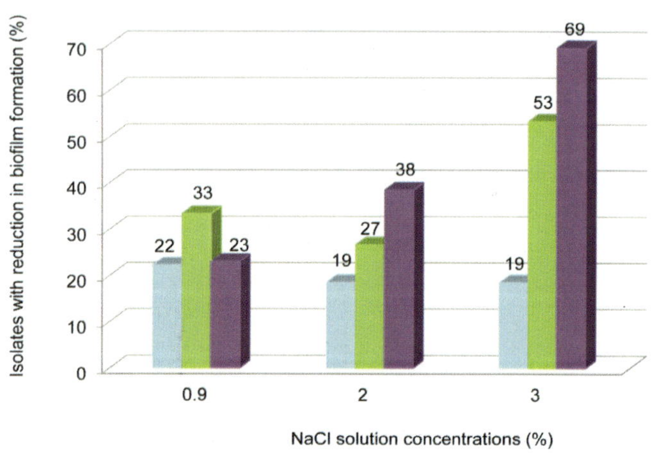

Figure 3. Effect of three sub-inhibitory concentrations of NaCl against *P. aeruginosa* CF isolate biofilm biomass formation. Tested for 55 adherent CF isolates of *P. aeruginosa* with MIC values > 3% distributed as follows: strongly adherent (n = 13, violet bars), moderately adherent (n = 15, green bars), weakly adherent phenotype (n = 27, blue bars). Prevention of biofilm biomass formation is presented as percentage of strains for which ability to form biofilm biomass was decreased by at least 25% compared to controls (not exposed).

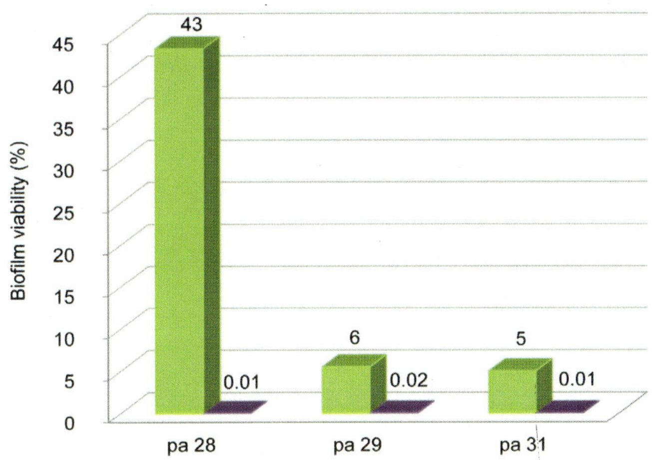

Figure 4. Activity of 7% and 10% NaCl solution against preformed biofilm for three strongly adherent isolates. 7% (green bars) and 10% (violet bars) NaCl solution was tested against preformed biofilm for the three *P. aeruginosa* CF isolates Pa28, Pa29, and Pa31. Results are expressed as percentage of biofilm viability compared to non-exposed control after 24 h of NaCl exposure.

MIC values, isolates with strong biofilm biomass production abilities were more resistant to NaCl action suggesting that the mature biofilm acts as a protection against inhibitory effect of NaCl. Finally, although the method used in this study did not allow study of the type of motility, i.e., swarming, swimming or twitching motility, affected by NaCl, we showed that NaCl inhibited the strain global motility as previously suggested for four *P. aeruginosa* strains [19]. Since bacterial motility and loss of motility are known to play a role in biofilm formation by *P. aeruginosa* [20], the specific impact of the motility inhibition by NaCl on biofilm formation has still to be evaluated. Time kill kinetics evaluated *in vitro* for 2 selected isolates suggested that NaCl antibacterial activity was both concentration- and time-dependent. Of note, these results were observed even though using the most stringent definition of the MBC, i.e., the lowest antimicrobial concentration reducing the inoculum by 99.99% within 24 h and bacterial growth conditions, i.e., bacteria in stationary phase of growth, which could have led to overestimation of MBC for some isolates. Of particular interest is the higher susceptibility to NaCl observed for clinically relevant subpopulations of *P. aeruginosa*, i.e., mucoid and/or multidrug resistant isolates. We found that the growth of mucoid isolates was inhibited by significantly lower NaCl concentrations than the one of non-mucoid isolates, as described for a *mucA22* mutant that was significantly more sensitive to osmotic stress than the isogenic parental *P. aeruginosa* PAO1 strain [21]. These results suggested that the reduction in exacerbation rate following prolonged treatment with HTS nebulization resulted from a population shift from mucoid to non-mucoid *P. aeruginosa* [21,22]. MICs were also significantly lower for MDR isolates than non-MDR isolates. Although not further investigated here, this could be related to a fitness cost of multidrug resistance [23] that could impair osmotic stress response. Altogether, active antimicrobial activity of NaCl against CF *P. aeruginosa* isolates might contribute to the *in vivo* global positive effect of HTS treatment. In addition, indirect effects may also enhance NaCl antimicrobial effect *in vivo* like disruption of inhibitory interactions between glycosaminoglycans present within the mucus and antimicrobial peptides [24].

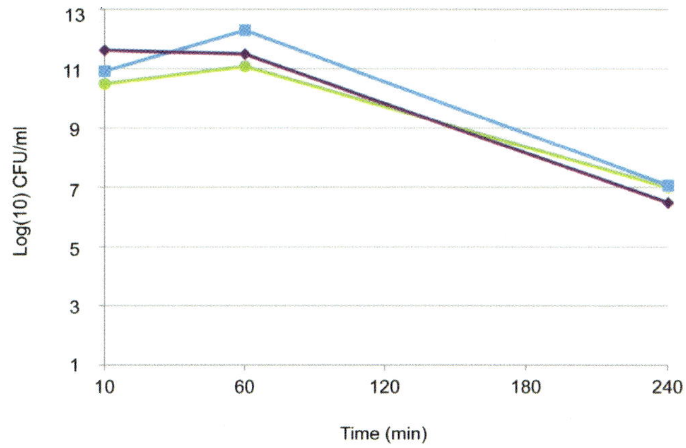

Figure 5. Time-kill kinetics of 10% NaCl solution against preformed biofilm for three strongly adherent CF isolates. *P. aeruginosa* CF isolates: Pa28 (green line, filled circles), Pa29 (blue line, filled squares), Pa31 (violet line, filled lozenges).

HTS treatment is currently not standardized and varies according to the study in the volume of aerosolized HTS (4, 5, or 10 ml), the rhythm of administration (twice or four times daily), the mode of administration (via jet or positive expiratory pressure nebulizers), and the HTS concentration (5.85%, 6%, or 7%) [6,8,9,11,25]. The effect of HTS appeared to be both dose-dependent [26] and time-dependent [27]. Considering the absence of significant change in the density of *P. aeruginosa* observed in a previous study [6], it could be assumed that the conditions of treatment, i.e., 4 ml of 7% HTS twice daily, were not bactericidal but only inhibitory against *P. aeruginosa in vivo*. Our results open important areas of research by suggesting that optimization of HTS conditions of use (rhythm, dose, mode of delivery) in CF may contribute to enhance anti-*P.aeruginosa* effects and thereby treatment clinical efficacy. However, studies that use *in vivo* models and randomized clinical trials are needed to evaluate the performances of diverse HTS administration conditions and to determine the more appropriate and efficient conditions of HTS use in CF patients. More largely our study highlights the potential use of NaCl as a basic but important component of the therapeutic arsenal used in the management of infectious diseases. Hyperosmotic stress is known for reducing biofilm growth and for being bactericidal on *Escherichia coli*, *P. aeruginosa*, and *Enterococcus faecalis*

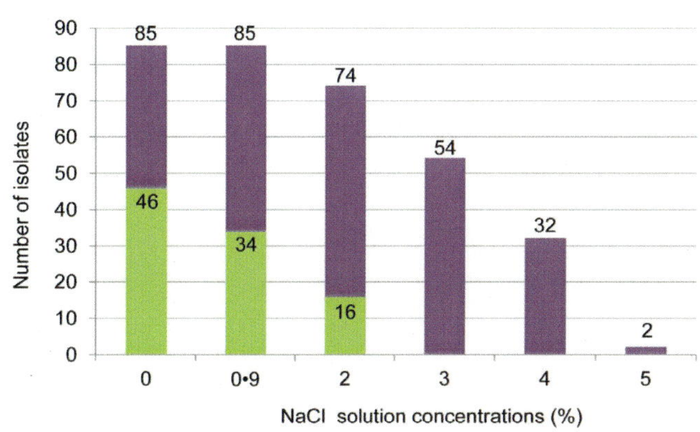

Figure 6. Rate of motile isolates according to NaCl concentration. Green bars show the number of motile isolates among isolates with non-inhibited growth (full bars).

when NaCl is used at 13% to 35% and could be used for treatment of root canal infection [28] or for locking tunneled hemodialysis catheters [29]. Considering the lower NaCl concentrations used in this study, the antimicrobial effect was probably not related to a direct hyperosmotic lysis. We presented arguments for an antimicrobial activity linked to an active biological process: i) NaCl was efficient mainly on bacteria in logarithmic phase of growth independently of the temperature and to a lesser extent on bacteria in stationary phase of growth at 37°C, ii) in stationary phase of growth at 4°C, which could be considered as metabolic standby conditions, HTS produced slight antimicrobial effects on *P. aeruginosa*, iii) variable response to HTS was observed among the population, and iv) loss of motility occurred from 2% NaCl solution. In summary, because the response to NaCl depended on the bacterial physiological status and varied among the population of *P. aeruginosa*, we assumed that NaCl bactericidal effect could be due to complex regulated mechanisms rather than to a mere hyperosmotic effect.

Several bioclinical answers remain to be addressed. Particularly, longitudinal studies are needed to monitor the evolution of NaCl MICs and MBCs of *P. aeruginosa* isolates recovered from the respiratory tract in patients under HTS treatment. In this study, only one patient was under HTS treatment for 4 years and isolates displayed high MBC and low MIC values. For this purpose, methods first proposed in this study for NaCl antimicrobial activity evaluation appeared suitable because of their good reproducibility. In addition, evaluating the NaCl action on several other CF pathogens including viruses, yeast, and fungi would be of interest because recent studies suggested NaCl-altered growth beyond NaCl concentration used in therapeutics for some viruses and yeasts not involved in CF [30,31]. The effect of HTS on polymicrobial community of the CF respiratory tract should be investigated not only because halotolerant bacteria may be favored by such a treatment but also because any modification of the relative composition of this complex microbiota will impact intercellular interactions and communication involved in this polymicrobial disease with unknown consequences [2,32]. Finally, the antimicrobial mechanism of action of NaCl warrants further investigation because it is still not fully elucidated, particularly the hypothesis of the possible induction of lytic activity of *P. aeruginosa* bacteriophages by NaCl has to be explored. Indeed, several environmental factors such as temperature or pH but also salinity could influence the transition from lysogenic to lytic phage [33,34].

Over the last decade, treatment strategies have shifted from controlling chronic infection to attempting to eradicate *P. aeruginosa* in the early stages of infection. Whatever the strategy, the antibiotic resistance makes the need for alternative approaches obvious and non-antibiotic treatments may expand the therapeutic repertoire. NaCl, as a simple and basic compound, may become a pivotal resource in CF care and in fighting *P. aeruginosa*. Beside polyvalent effects on the CF respiratory tract, we gave insights into antimicrobial activities of NaCl. NaCl kills *P. aeruginosa* but also acts on a range of its core eco-physiological functions such as biofilm formation and motility. Future studies should go further toward evaluating the role of NaCl in bacteriophage predation. Taken together, results and hypotheses on NaCl effects open research paths to treat CF as an eco-pathology of the respiratory tract. More widely, the efficacy of NaCl alone or in association with current available therapeutics should be more deeply investigated in infectious diseases.

Author Contributions

Conceived and designed the experiments: ALM HM EJB. Performed the experiments: ALM. Analyzed the data: ALM HM EJB BL. Wrote the paper: ALM. Acquisition of data: ALM RC. Performed statistical analyses: ALM BL. Critically revised the manuscript: HM RC BL EJB.

References

1. Clunes MT, Boucher RC (2007) Cystic Fibrosis: the mechanisms of pathogenesis of an inherited lung disorder. Drug Discov Today Dis Mech 4: 63–72.
2. Sibley CD, Rabin H, Surette MG (2006) Cystic fibrosis: a polymicrobial infectious disease. Future Microbiol 1: 53–61.
3. Emerson J, Rosenfeld M, McNamara S, Ramsey B, Gibson RL (2002) *Pseudomonas aeruginosa* and other predictors of mortality and morbidity in young children with cystic fibrosis. Pediatr Pulmonol 34: 91–100.
4. Boucher RC (2007) Evidence for airway surface dehydration as the initiating event in CF airway disease. J Intern Med 261: 5–16.
5. Reeves EP, Molloy K, Pohl K, McElvaney NG (2012) Hypertonic saline in treatment of pulmonary disease in cystic fibrosis. Scientific World Journal 465230.
6. Elkins MR, Robinson M, Rose BR, Harbour C, Moriarty CP, et al. (2006) A controlled trial of long-term inhaled hypertonic saline in patients with cystic fibrosis. N Engl J Med 354: 229–240.
7. Dmello D, Nayak RP, Matuschak GM (2011) Stratified assessment of the role of inhaled hypertonic saline in reducing cystic fibrosis pulmonary exacerbations: a retrospective analysis. BMJ Open 1:e000019.
8. Eng PA, Morton J, Douglass JA, Riedler J, Wilson J, et al. (1996) Short-term efficacy of ultrasonically nebulized hypertonic saline in cystic fibrosis. Pediatr Pulmonol 21: 77–83.
9. Ballmann M, Von der Hardt H (2002) Hypertonic saline and recombinant human DNase: a randomised cross-over pilot study in patients with cystic fibrosis. J Cyst Fibros 1: 35–37.
10. Wark P, McDonald V (2009) Nebulised hypertonic saline for cystic fibrosis. Cochrane Database Syst Rev CD001506.
11. Donaldson SH, Bennett WD, Zeman KL, Knowles MR, Tarran R, et al. (2006) Mucus clearance and lung function in cystic fibrosis with hypertonic saline. N Engl J Med 354: 241–250.
12. Cystic Fibrosis Consensus Conference May 17–18, 1994. Microbiology and infectious disease in cystic fibrosis. Bethesda, MD, Cystic Fibrosis Foundation, 1994; Vol. 5, Section 1, pp. 1–26.
13. Patel JB, Tenover FC, Turnidge JD, Jorgensen JH (2011) Susceptibility test methods: dilution and disk diffusion methods. In: Versalovic J, Carroll KC, Funke G, Jorgensen JH, Landry ML, Warnock DW, editors. Manual of Clinical Microbiology, 10th edn. Washington, DC: American Society for Microbiology press, pp 1122–1143.
14. Courvalin P, Leclercq R, Rice L (2009) Antibiogram, 3rd edn. Washington, DC: American Society for Microbiology press.
15. Stepanovic S, Vukovic D, Dakic I, Savic B, Svabic-Vlahovic M (2000) A modified microtiter-plate test for quantification of staphylococcal biofilm formation. J Microbiol Methods 40: 175–179.
16. Deligianni E, Pattison S, Berrar D, Ternan NG, Haylock RW, et al. (2010) *Pseudomonas aeruginosa* Cystic Fibrosis isolates of similar RAPD genotype exhibit diversity in biofilm forming ability *in vitro*. BMC Microbiol 10: 38.
17. Pompilio A, Crocetta V, Scocchi M, Pomponio S, Di Vincenzo V, et al. (2012) Potential novel therapeutic strategies in cystic fibrosis: antimicrobial and anti-biofilm activity of natural and designed α-helical peptides against *Staphylococcus aureus*, *Pseudomonas aeruginosa*, and *Stenotrophomonas maltophilia*. BMC Microbiol 12: 145.
18. Bye PT, Elkins MR (2007) Other mucoactive agents for cystic fibrosis. Paediatr Respir Rev 8:30–39.
19. Havasi V, Hurst CO, Briles TC, Yang F, Bains DG, et al. (2008) Inhibitory effects of hypertonic saline on *P. aeruginosa* motility. J Cyst Fibros 7: 267–269.
20. O'Toole GA, Kolter R (1998) Flagellar and twitching motility are necessary for *Pseudomonas aeruginosa* biofilm development. Mol Microbiol 30: 295–304.
21. Behrends V, Ryall B, Wang X, Bundy JG, Williams HD (2010) Metabolic profiling of *Pseudomonas aeruginosa* demonstrates that the anti-sigma factor MucA modulates osmotic stress tolerance. Mol Biosyst 6: 562–569.
22. Williams HD, Behrends V, Bundy JG, Ryall B, Zlosnik JE (2010) Hypertonic saline therapy in cystic fibrosis: do population shifts caused by the osmotic sensitivity of infecting bacteria explain the effectiveness of this treatment? Front Microbiol 1: 120.

23. Abdelraouf K, Kabbara S, Ledesma KR, Poole K, Tam VH (2011) Effect of multidrug resistance-conferring mutations on the fitness and virulence of *Pseudomonas aeruginosa*. J Antimicrob Chemother 66: 1311–1317.
24. Bergsson G, Reeves EP, McNally P, Chotirmall SH, Greene CM, et al. (2009) LL-37 complexation with glycosaminoglycans in cystic fibrosis lungs inhibits antimicrobial activity, which can be restored by hypertonic saline. J Immunol 183: 543–551.
25. O'Connell OJ, O'Farrell C, Harrison MJ, Eustace JA, Henry MT, et al. (2011) Nebulized hypertonic saline via positive expiratory pressure versus via jet nebulizer in patients with severe cystic fibrosis. Respir Care 56: 771–775.
26. Robinson M, Hemming AL, Regnis JA, Wong AG, Bailey DL, et al. (1997) Effect of increasing doses of hypertonic saline on mucociliary clearance in patients with cystic fibrosis. Thorax 52: 900–903.
27. Tarran R, Grubb BR, Parsons D, Picher M, Hirsh AJ, et al. (2001) The CF salt controversy: *in vivo* observations and therapeutic approaches. Mol Cell 8: 149–158.
28. Van der Waal SV, Van der Sluis LWM, Özok AR, Exterkate RA, van Marle J, et al. (2011) The effects of hyperosmosis or high pH on a dual-species biofilm of *Enterococcus faecalis* and *Pseudomonas aeruginosa*: an in vitro study. Int Endod J 44: 1110–1117.
29. Oguzhan N, Pala C, Sipahioglu MH, Cilan H, Durmaz S, et al. (2012) Locking tunneled hemodialysis catheters with hypertonic saline (26% NaCl) and heparin to prevent catheter-related bloodstream infections and thrombosis: a randomized, prospective trial. Ren Fail 34: 181–188.
30. Parmar JH, Bhartiya S, Venkatesh KV (2011) Characterization of the adaptive response and growth upon hyperosmotic shock in *Saccharomyces cerevisiae*. Mol Biosyst 7: 1138–1148.
31. Seo K, Lee JE, Lim MY, Ko G (2012) Effect of temperature, pH, and NaCl on the inactivation kinetics of murine norovirus. J Food Prot 75: 533–540.
32. Peters BM, Jabra-Rizk MA, O'May GA, Costerton JW, Shirtliff ME (2012) Polymicrobial interactions: impact on pathogenesis and human disease. Clin Microbiol Rev 25: 193–213.
33. Williamson SJ, Paul JH (2006) Environmental factors that influence the transition from lysogenic to lytic existence in the phiHSIC/Listonella pelagia marine phage-host system. Microb Ecol 52: 217–225.
34. Shkilnyj P, Koudelka GB (2007) Effect of salt shock on stability of lambdaimm434 lysogens. J Bacteriol 189: 3115–3123.

Correcting the Cystic Fibrosis Disease Mutant, A455E CFTR

Liudmila Cebotaru[1,2], Daniele Rapino[1,2], Valeriu Cebotaru[3], William B. Guggino[2]*

1 Department of Ophthalmology, School of Medicine, The Johns Hopkins University, Baltimore, Maryland, United States of America, **2** Department of Physiology, School of Medicine, The Johns Hopkins University, Baltimore, Maryland, United States of America, **3** Department of Medicine, School of Medicine, The Johns Hopkins University, Baltimore, Maryland, United States of America

Abstract

Cystic fibrosis is caused by more than 1000 mutations, the most common being the ΔF508 mutation. These mutations have been divided into five classes [1], with ΔF508 CFTR in class II. Here we have studied the class V mutation A455E. We report that the mature and immature bands of A455E are rapidly degraded primarily by proteasomes; the short protein half-life of this mutant therefore resembles that of ΔF508 CFTR. A455E could be rescued by treatment of the cells with proteasome inhibitors. Furthermore, co-transfection of A455E with the truncation mutant Δ264 CFTR also rescued the mature C band, indicating that A455E can be rescued by transcomplementation. We found that Δ264 CFTR bound to A455E, forming a bimolecular complex. Treatment with the compound correctors C3 and C4 also rescued A455E. These results are significant because they show that although ΔF508 belongs to a different class than A455E, it can be rescued by the same strategies, offering therapeutic promise to patients with Class V mutations.

Editor: Effie C. Tsilibary, National Center for Scientific Research Demokritos, Greece

Funding: This work was supported in part by a CFTR Folding Consortium Grant from the Cystic Fibrosis Foundation. The funders had no role in study design, data collection and analysis, decision to publish, or preparation of the manuscript.

Competing Interests: The authors have declared that no competing interests exist.

* E-mail: wguggino@jhmi.edu

Introduction

Cystic fibrosis (CF) is caused by mutations in the cystic fibrosis transmembrane conductance regulator (CFTR) [2]. Symptoms of CF include higher-than-normal sweat chloride, thick airway mucus, persistent lung infections, pancreatic enzyme insufficiency, intestinal blockage, and infertility in males [3]. These classic symptoms of CF can range in severity from mild to severe. Extensive effort has been made to understand the genotype of CF patients, with over 1000 gene mutations identified thus far [4]. These mutations in the CF gene have been divided into five different classes: Class I mutations result in defective protein production. Class II mutations result in a protein whose processing is blocked in the ER. The most common CFTR mutation, △F508 CFTR [2], is a class II mutation. Like other class II mutations, △F508 CFTR is retained in the ER, incompletely glycosylated, and rapidly degraded in proteasomes [5]. Class III mutations produce a protein that has defective regulation; the most common is the G551D mutation, which reaches the cell surface but does not conduct chloride [6,7]. Class IV mutations cause defects in channel conductance. Finally, class V mutations affect protein synthesis or splicing, causing less protein to be made. One of these class V mutations is A455E.

The A455E mutation is located in NBD1. It was originally found in French Canadian patients and is associated with a mild phenotype, with borderline high sweat, moderate lung disease, and sufficient pancreatic function [8,9]. Unlike other mild missense mutations such as R117H that have altered channel conductance [10] and are considered class IV mutations, the single-channel characteristics of A445E resemble those of wild-type CFTR [11,12] . Thus, because the mild disease resulting from A455E is thought to arise from reduced protein expression, it is considered a class V mutation. Thus, an effective pharmacological approach to treating this mutation should involve increasing the protein levels of A455E.

Our group has been interested in transcomplementation [13,14] using △264 CFTR, which is a truncated version of CFTR missing the first four transmembrane domains. When monkey lungs are infected with an adeno-associated viral vector rAAV-△264 CFTR, the △264 CFTR produced can increase the levels of endogenous wild-type CFTR protein [15]. We have also shown in cotransfection studies that △264 CFTR increases wild-type CFTR protein levels and increases the degree of maturation of the immature band B to the mature C band of △F508 CFTR. The purpose of the current study was to determine whether analogous transcomplementation can be used to enhance the protein processing of A455E.

Experimental Procedures

Cell culture

African green monkey kidney cells (Cos7) were maintained in Dulbecco's modified Eagle's medium-high glucose 1x (DMEM), penicillin (100 U/ml), streptomycin (100 μg/ml), and 10% fetal bovine serum as described previously [14]).

Plasmids and constructs

The construct pEGFP A455E was a gift from Dr. Gary Cutting at Johns Hopkins U. The plasmids were transfected into Cos 7 cells using Lipofectamine 2000 (Invitrogen) as we have previously described. After 48 h of transfection, the cells were harvested and used for immunoprecipitation and immunoblotting.

Immunoblotting and immunoprecipitation

Cells were harvested and processed as described previously [16] using the (C-terminus) antibody (1:1500; R&D Systems, Inc.). Glyceraldehyde 3-phosphate dehydrogenase (GAPDH), used as a loading control, was detected with monoclonal anti-GAPDH antibody (1:10,000; US Biological).

For immunoprecipitation, cells were harvested and processed as described previously. For pull-down experiments, 10 µl of anti-GFP antibody (Roche) were added to the lysate and allowed to incubate for 30 min. with 50 µl of A/G-agarose beads (Santa Cruz Biotechnology, Inc.). CFTR was detected as described above.

Statistics

Western blots were evaluated by one-way ANOVA followed by LSD post hoc tests. Statistical significance was set at $P<0.05$, and data are presented as mean±2SEM. All experiments were normalized for the control. SPSS (version 17.0 SPSS, Inc, Chicago, III) was used for data analysis

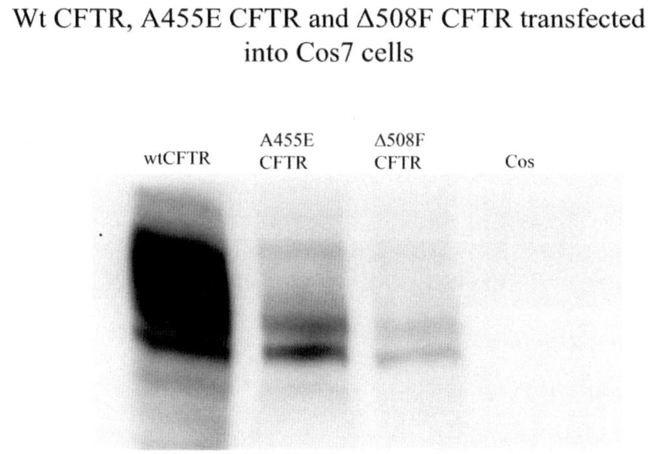

Figure 1. A455E has reduced expression of mature CFTR. Cos7 cells were transfected with 2 µg of wild-type, A455E, or ΔF508 CFTR constructs. After 48 h, the cells were lysed, and the total lysate was analyzed by western blotting with anti-human CFTR antibodies. Note that there is much less mature C band in the A455E sample than in the wild-type sample. In this and subsequent blots, some mature C band was detected with A455E (n = 8).

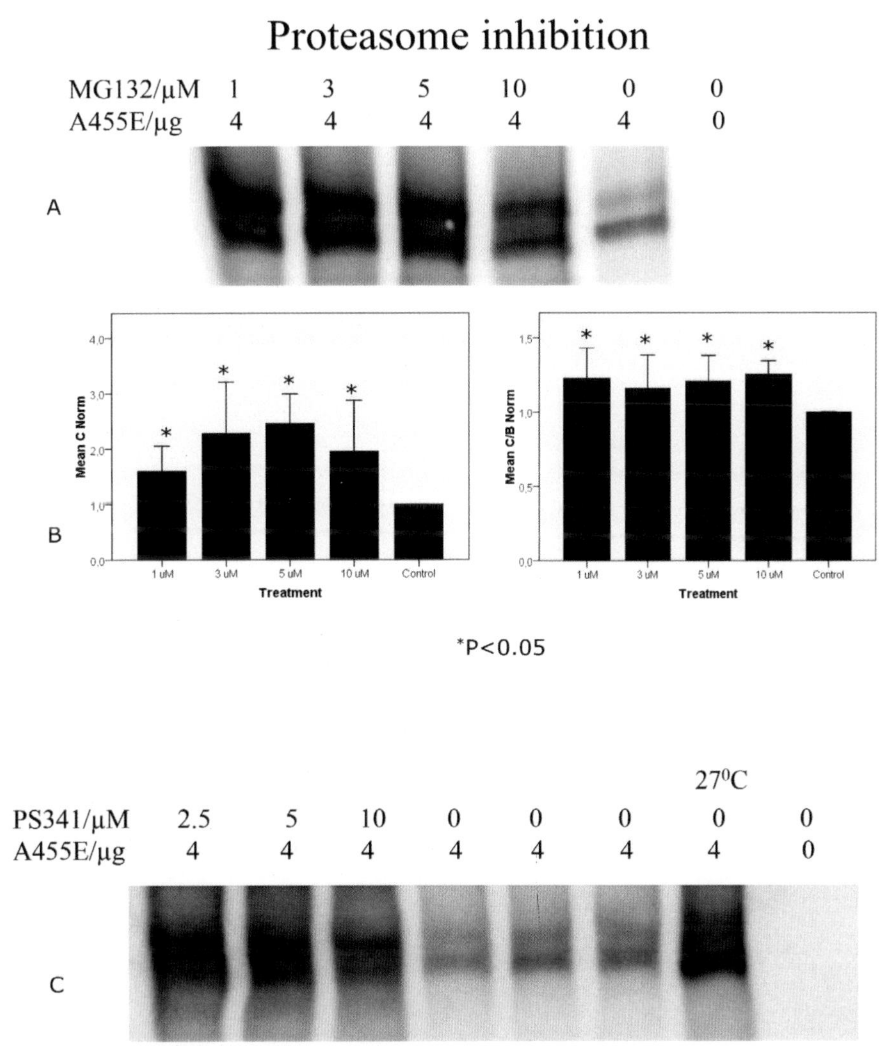

Figure 2. Proteasome inhibition. Cells transfected with A455E cDNA were treated either with MG132, a more general inhibitor (n = 6) (**A, B**), or the more specific inhibitor of proteasomes, PS341 (n = 2) (**C**). Note that in both cases, proteasome inhibition caused an increase in both the immature B and mature C bands of A455E.

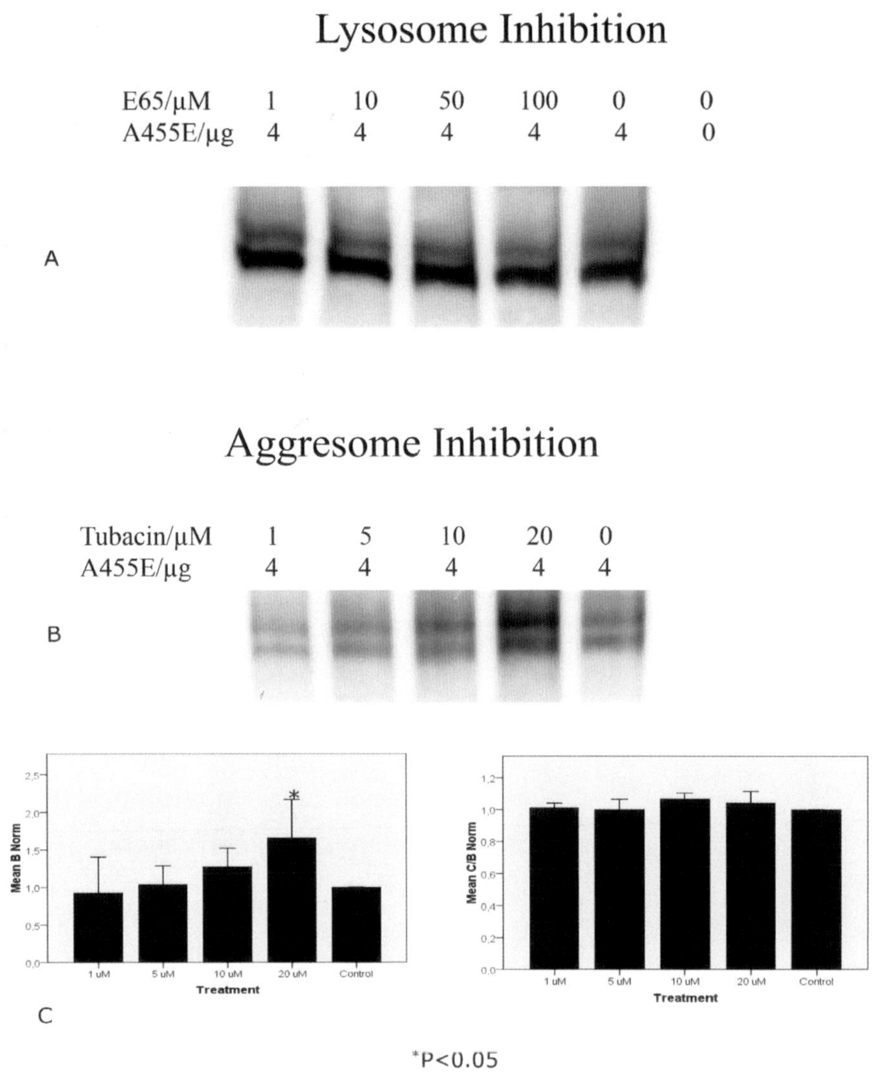

Figure 3. Lysosome/aggresome inhibition. Cos7 cells were transfected with A455E CFTR cDNA and treated for 16 h with the lysosome inhibitor E64 (n = 4) (**A**) There was very little change in band density in any of the treated groups or in the presence of the inhibitors when compared to the control or the HDAC6 inhibitor tubacin to inhibit aggresomes (n = 3) (**B, C**). Note that there is a significant increase with the highest concentration used.

Results

Expression of A455E

When we compared the expression of the A455E mutant to that of both wild-type and △F508 CFTR (Fig. 1) by western blotting, we found that the amount of CFTR protein was greatly reduced in the Cos7 cells transfected with the A455E mutant. To evaluate the degradation of A455E CFTR, we treated the cells with MG132, a non-specific inhibitor of proteasomal degradation. Fig. 2 shows that in the presence of MG132, the protein expression of both the B and C bands of A455E CFTR increased dramatically. A similar effect was seen when we used the more specific proteasome inhibitor, PS341. PS341 also caused an increase in both the B and C bands of A455E. Furthermore, we noted that A455E could be rescued by growing the cells at a reduced temperature, as had previously been observed for ΔF508 [13]. In sharp contrast, there was no increase in the protein expression of A455E CFTR when the cells were treated with the aggresome inhibitor tubacin or the lysosomal inhibitor E64 (Fig. 3). These data suggest that A455E is degraded primarily in proteasomes.

To evaluate how rapidly the A455E CFTR protein is degraded, we treated the transfected cells with cycloheximide for between 1 and 7 hours (Fig 4). Surprisingly, both the B and C bands of A455E CFTR rapidly disappeared in the cells treated with cycloheximide (Fig. 4), suggesting that it is rapidly degraded, as is ΔF508 CFTR (see [13]).

△264 CFTR increases the processing of band B to band C of A455E CFTR

We then tested whether the truncation mutant, △264 CFTR, was capable of transcomplementation with A455E (Fig. 5). In order to determine whether Δ264 CFTR affects the maturation of A455E CFTR, we cotransfected Δ264 CFTR and A455E CFTR into Cos7 cells and found that the mature C band from A455E CFTR was increased in cells cotransfected with Δ264 CFTR, as compared to cells transfected with A455E cDNA alone (Fig. 5).

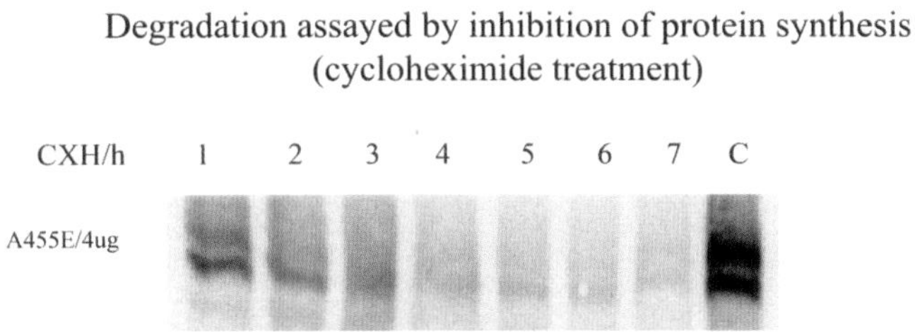

Figure 4. Effect of protein synthesis inhibition on the degradation of A455E. Cos7 cells were transfected with A455E cDNA and treated with cycloheximide (25 μg/ml) for the indicated times. Note the rapid decay of both the mature C and immature B bands of A455E. (n = 4).

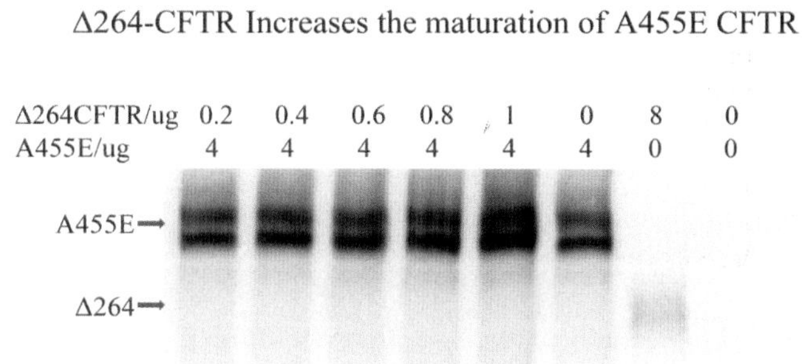

Figure. 5. Transcomplementation of A455E by Δ27-264 CFTR. Both the C and B bands of A455E CFTR were increased when cells were cotransfected with Δ27-264 CFTR, showing that A455E could be rescued by transcomplementation. (n = 11).

△264 CFTR binds to A455E CFTR, forming a biomolecular complex

We and others have shown that transcomplementation can occur via direct binding of truncated forms of CFTR to ΔF508-CFTR and via chaperone displacement [17]. In order to assess these possibilities in A455E CFTR, we conducted co-immunprecipitation experiments. Fig. 6 shows that Δ264-CFTR did indeed bind to A455E, in both the absence and presence of the proteasome inhibitor MG123.

Correctors 4A (C4) and VX325 (C3) increase the processing of band B to band C of A455E CFTR

We next asked whether small-molecule correctors might be effective in rescuing A455E CFTR (Fig. 7). We chose two well-known correctors, 4A (C4) [18] and VX325 (C3) [19]. We found that corrector C4 does have a robust effect on A455E CFTR; in contrast, C3 had only a minimal effect on A455E (Fig. 7).

Discussion

Transcomplementation of △F508-CFTR by fragments of CFTR has been observed [13,14,17,20,20]. These fragments are themselves extremely efficiently degraded; they bind to ΔF508 CFTR and improve the maturation from the immature band B to mature band C. Although transcomplementation has been observed by at least three different groups, it has never been demonstrated with other mutations. Here we show that A455E can also be rescued by transcomplementation. This finding is significant because it provides a new way to treat mutations other than ΔF508 CFTR and also provides insight into the mechanism of transcomplementation.

ΔF508 CFTR is associated with a least two major problems, an unstable NBD1 and defective interactions with intracellular loops (ICL), especially ICL4 [21–23]. These two defects disrupt both trafficking and channel activity. The A455E mutation, on the other hand, is located within the F1-type ATP-binding core subdomain near to the ABC protein signature, the Walker A domain [24]. Given the proximity to the Walker A domain, one might expect that A455E would have alterations in gating. However, electrophysiological studies have shown that its single-channel properties are similar to those of wild-type CFTR [11]. A455E also functions well as a regulator of other channels [25]. Thus, its ability to act as a conductance regulator is intact. What appears to be causing the disease, then, is a drastic reduction in the processing of the mature protein. At least two studies have failed to detect mature band C from A455E [11,26], although the results of their electrophysiological studies suggested that some mature band C must have been present at the plasma membrane in order to generate chloride currents [11]. In our study, we do detect some mature band C at the plasma membrane, but when the cells are treated with cycloheximide to evaluate protein degradation, it is clear that the mature band C of A455E is rapidly degraded along with the immature B band. This situation is similar to that in ΔF508 CFTR, in which both the immature mature bands of temperature-rescued ΔF508 CFTR are rapidly degraded. Van Oene et al. 2000.] have shown that A455E has a pattern of degradation that is clearly different from that of ΔF508 CFTR. A455E appears to be proteolytically cleaved within the NBD1-R domain to form C-terminal aggregates. This cleavage does not appear to occur via the 26S proteasome, but perhaps within the cystosol [26]. Clearly, these results show that the A455E mutant is distinctly different from ΔF508 CFTR.

Nevertheless, A455E shows some similarity to ΔF508 CFTR. Although A455E is uniquely cleaved in the cytoplasm, our results show that it is still degraded in the proteasome, because treatment with two types of proteasome inhibitors led to significant increases in steady-state protein levels. In fact, we saw a rather large increase in the mature band of A455E after proteasome inhibition. This result is in contrast to the response of A455E to lysosomal inhibitors, which were without effect. Inhibiting the aggresome

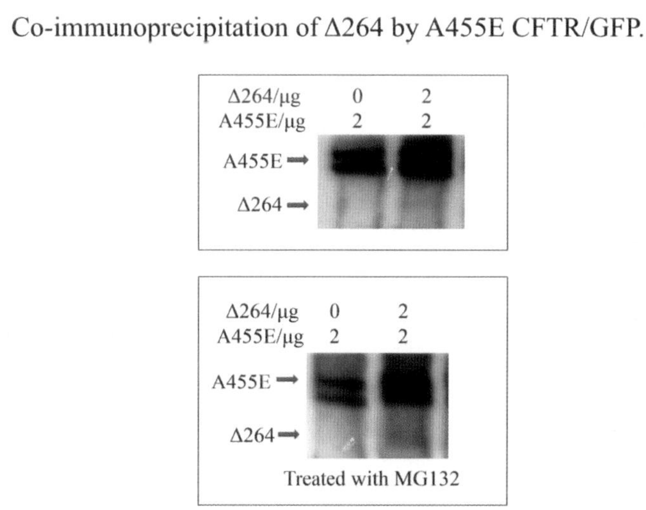

Figure 6. A455E binds to △27-264 CFTR. Cos7 cells were transfected with both Δ27-264 CFTR and an A455E CFTR construct bearing a GFP tag. Anti-GFP antibodies were used to pull down A455E, and the gels were blotted with anti-CFTR antibody. (n = 3).

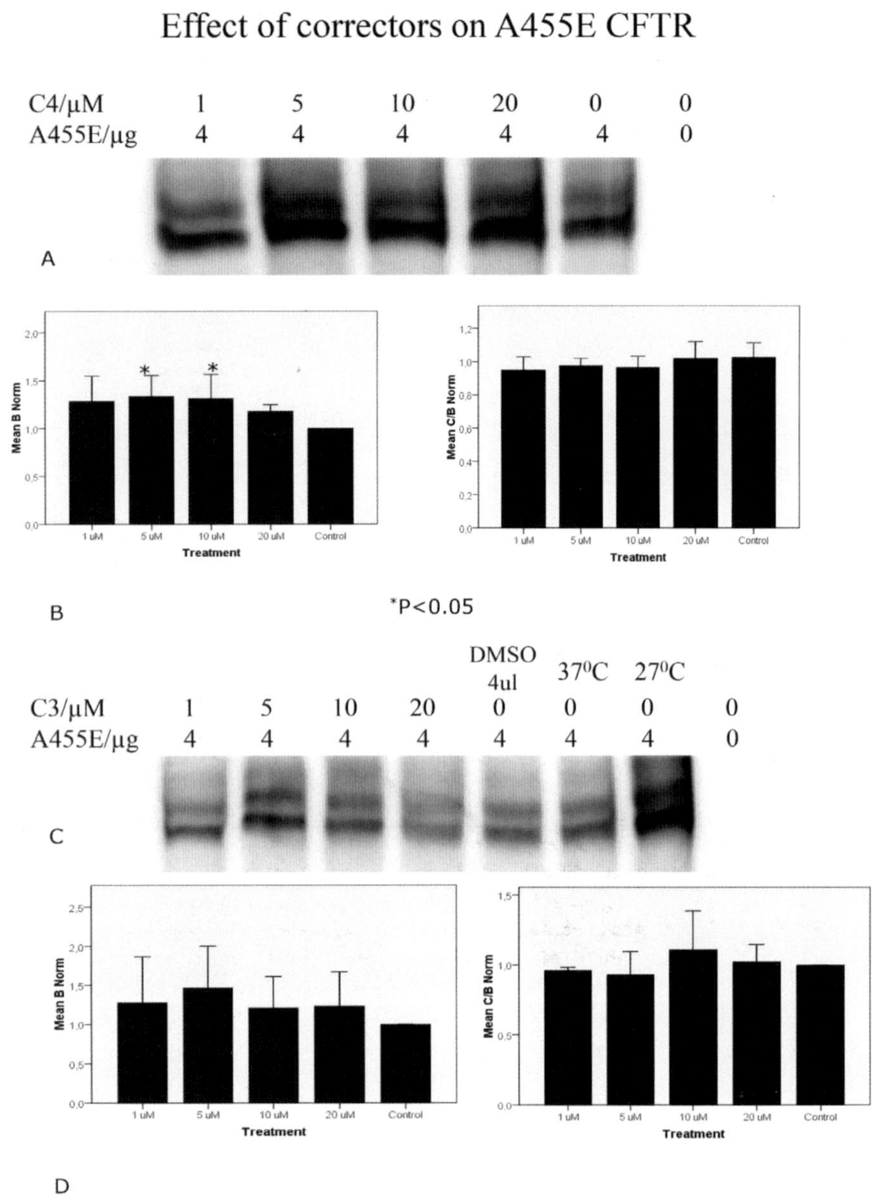

Figure 7. Correctors can rescue A455E. Cos7 cells were transfected with A455E and treated with the correctors C3 or C4 for 16 h at the specified concentrations. Note that C4 had a profound effect on the immature B band of A455E as well as causing an increase in the mature C band (**A, B**). C3 did not have a significant effect (**C, D**). (n = 3).

was also without effect. Taken together, our data suggest that A455E, like ΔF508 CFTR, is processed by proteasomes.

Δ264 CFTR rescues A455E and forms a molecular complex between the two molecules. It has been shown that CFTR forms an intramolecular dimer through an interaction between the Walker sites in the two NBDs that involves ATP. Indeed, Lewis et al. [27] have shown that the crystal structure indicates that two isolated NBD1s of CFTR readily form a head-to-tail dimer when both the regulatory insert and extension are removed. It is possible that a similar interaction occurs between Δ264 and A455E. Two other groups have shown that small fragments of CFTR can rescue ΔF508 CFTR, through either a bimolecular interaction [20] or chaperone displacement [17]. One group used a truncation that included TMD1 and NBD1 [20], and the other NBD1 plus the R domain [17]. What these truncations have in common with ours is that each contains NBD1. Thus, it is plausible to suggest that the transcomplementation most likely occurs by an interaction between the NBD1 moieties of the truncated and the mutant proteins. The observation that A455E is readily rescued by Δ264 CFTR suggests that transcomplementation may be influencing NBD1 in the region of the Walker sites. One then may ask why the interaction with the normal NBD2 of A455E does not rescue its own NBD1. One reason may be that NBD2 is translated much later than NBD1 [28]. By the time NBD2 is translated, the mutant NBD1 may already doom the molecule to be degraded by endoplasmic reticulum-associated degradation (ERAD). One might envision that the truncated and mutant CFTRs immediately form a complex during cotranslation of the NBD1s from the two molecules. Thus, the truncated NBD1 could act as a molecular chaperone to rescue the other molecule.

Therapeutic transcomplementation to rescue A455E would require gene transfer via a virus or non-viral particle. Several gene therapy approaches are currently being developed for both purposes [29].

Another way to rescue mutant CFTR is with corrector compounds that either bind to mutant CFTR or alter some component of the ERAD pathway. Several groups utilizing high-throughput methods to screen large compound libraries have identified correctors that rescue ΔF508 CFTR. For example, the C4 corrector utilized here was identified in an academic laboratory [30], whereas C3 was developed commercially [19]. Although many compounds have been identified, only VX 809 has reached clinical trials [31]. Although it has shown promise in laboratory experiments in clinical trials involving patients bearing the ΔF508 mutation, VX-809 [31] had a small effect on sweat chloride and no effect on pulmonary function or rescue of ΔF508 CFTR in rectal biopsies. Our demonstration that both C3 and C4 can rescue A455E suggests that A455E CFTR may be a better candidate for correction with either compound correctors or transcomplementation than is ΔF508 CFTR.

Acknowledgments

The authors thank Dr. Deborah McClellan for editorial assistance and Rahul Grover and Miqueias Lopes-Pacheco for help with experimental setups.

Author Contributions

Conceived and designed the experiments: LC WBG. Performed the experiments: VC. Analyzed the data: LC WBG DR. Contributed reagents/materials/analysis tools: VC. Wrote the paper: WBG.

References

1. Welsh MJ, Smith AE (1993) Molecular mechanisms of CFTR chloride channel dysfunction in cystic fibrosis. Cell 73: 1251–1254.
2. Rommens JM, Iannuzzi MC, Kerem B-S, Drumm ML, Melmer G, et al. (1989) Identification of the cystic fibrosis gene: Chromosome walking and jumping. Science 245: 1059–1065.
3. Rosenstein BJ, Cutting GR (1998) The diagnosis of cystic fibrosis: a consensus statement. Cystic Fibrosis Foundation Consensus Panel. J Pediatr 132: 589–595.
4. Cutting GR (1993) Spectrum of mutations in cystic fibrosis. J Bioenerg Biomembr 25: 7–10.
5. Cheng SH, Gregory RJ, Marshall J, Paul S, Souza DW, et al. (1990) Defective intracellular transport and processing of CFTR is the molecular basis of most of cystic fibrosis. Cell 63: 827–834.
6. Mickle JE, Cutting GR (2000) Genotype-phenotype relationships in cystic fibrosis. Med Clin North Am 84: 597–607.
7. Van GF, Hadida S, Grootenhuis PD, Burton B, Cao D, et al. (2009) Rescue of CF airway epithelial cell function in vitro by a CFTR potentiator, VX-770. Proc Natl Acad Sci U S A 106: 18825–18830. 0904709106 [pii];10.1073/pnas.0904709106 [doi].
8. Stansberg PM, Noreau D, McGlynn-Steele L, Koultchitski G, Ray PN (1997) PCR-based test for two cystic fibrosis mutations (A455E, 711+1G-->T) common among French Canadians. Clin Chem 43: 1083–1084.
9. De BM, Allard C, Leblanc JP, Simard F, Aubin G (1997) Genotype-phenotype correlation in cystic fibrosis patients compound heterozygous for the A455E mutation. Hum Genet 101: 208–211.
10. Sheppard DN, Rich DP, Ostedgaard LS, Gregory RJ, Smith AE, et al. (1993) Mutations in CFTR associated with mild-disease-form Cl- channels with altered pore properties. Nature 362: 160–164. 10.1038/362160a0 [doi].
11. Sheppard DN, Ostedgaard LS, Winter MC, Welsh MJ (1995) Mechanism of dysfunction of two nucleotide binding domain mutations in cystic fibrosis transmembrane conductance regulator that are associated with pancreatic sufficiency. EMBO J 14: 876–883.
12. Fulmer SB, Schwiebert EM, Morales MM, Guggino WB, Cutting GR (1995) Two cystic fibrosis transmembrane conductance regulator mutations have different effects on both pulmonary phenotype and regulation of outwardly rectified chloride currents. Proc Natl Acad Sci U S A 92: 6832–6836.
13. Cebotaru L, Woodward O, Cebotaru V, Guggino WB (2013) Transcomplementation by a truncation mutant of CFTR enhances {triangleup}F508 processing through a biomolecualr interaction. J Biol Chem . M112.420489 [pii];10.1074/jbc.M112.420489 [doi].
14. Cebotaru L, Vij N, Ciobanu I, Wright J, Flotte T, Guggino WB (2008) Cystic fibrosis transmembrane regulator missing the first four transmembrane segments increases wild type and DeltaF508 processing. J Biol Chem 283: 21926–21933.
15. Fischer AC, Smith CI, Cebotaru L, Zhang X, Askin FB, et al. (2007) Expression of a truncated cystic fibrosis transmembrane conductance regulator with an AAV5-pseudotyped vector in primates. Mol Ther 15: 756–763.
16. Cheng J, Moyer BD, Milewski M, Loffing J, Ikeda M, et al. (2002) A Golgi-associated PDZ domain protein modulates cystic fibrosis transmembrane regulator plasma membrane expression. J Biol Chem 277: 3520–3529.
17. Sun F, Mi Z, Condliffe SB, Bertrand CA, Gong X, Lu X, et al. (2008) Chaperone displacement from mutant cystic fibrosis transmembrane conductance regulator restores its function in human airway epithelia. FASEB J .
18. Pedemonte N, Lukacs GL, Du K, Caci E, Zegarra-Moran O, et al. (2005) Small-molecule correctors of defective DeltaF508-CFTR cellular processing identified by high-throughput screening. J Clin Invest 115: 2564–2571.
19. Van GF, Straley KS, Cao D, Gonzalez J, Hadida S, et al. (2006) Rescue of DeltaF508-CFTR trafficking and gating in human cystic fibrosis airway primary cultures by small molecules. Am J Physiol Lung Cell Mol Physiol 290: L1117–L1130. 00169.2005 [pii];10.1152/ajplung.00169.2005 [doi].
20. Cormet-Boyaka E, Jablonsky M, Naren AP, Jackson PL, Muccio DD, et al. (2004) Rescuing cystic fibrosis transmembrane conductance regulator (CFTR)-processing mutants by transcomplementation. Proc Natl Acad Sci U S A 101: 8221–8226.
21. Mendoza JL, Schmidt A, Li Q, Nuvaga E, Barrett T, et al. (2012) Requirements for efficient correction of DeltaF508 CFTR revealed by analyses of evolved sequences. Cell 148: 164–174. S0092-8674(11)01367-5 [pii];10.1016/j.cell.2011.11.023 [doi].
22. Du K, Sharma M, Lukacs GL (2005) The DeltaF508 cystic fibrosis mutation impairs domain-domain interactions and arrests post-translational folding of CFTR. Nat Struct Mol Biol 12: 17–25.
23. He L, Aleksandrov LA, Cui L, Jensen TJ, Nesbitt KL, et al. (2010) Restoration of domain folding and interdomain assembly by second-site suppressors of the DeltaF508 mutation in CFTR. FASEB J 24: 3103–3112. fj.09-141788 [pii];10.1096/fj.09-141788 [doi].
24. Lewis HA, Buchanan SG, Burley SK, Conners K, Dickey et al. (2004) Structure of nucleotide-binding domain 1 of the cystic fibrosis transmembrane conductance regulator. EMBO J 23: 282–293.
25. Schwiebert EM, Benos DJ, Egan ME, Stutts MJ, Guggino WB (1999) CFTR is a conductance regulator as well as a chloride channel. Physiol Rev 79: S145–S166.
26. Van Oene M, Lukacs GL, Rommens JM (2000) Cystic fibrosis mutations lead to carboxyl-terminal fragments that highlight an early biogenesis step of the cystic fibrosis transmembrane conductance regulator. Journal of Biological Chemistry 275: 19577–19584.
27. Atwell S, Brouillette CG, Conners K, Emtage S, Gheyi T, et al. (2010) Structures of a minimal human CFTR first nucleotide-binding domain as a monomer, head-to-tail homodimer, and pathogenic mutant. Protein Eng Des Sel 23: 375–384. gzq004 [pii];10.1093/protein/gzq004 [doi].
28. Kim SJ, Skach WR (2012) Mechanisms of CFTR Folding at the Endoplasmic Reticulum. Front Pharmacol 3: 201. 10.3389/fphar.2012.00201 [doi].
29. Boucher RC (1996) Current status of CF gene therapy. Trends Genet 12: 81–84.
30. Pedemonte N, Sonawane ND, Taddei A, Hu J, Zegarra-Moran O, et al. (2005) Phenylglycine and sulfonamide correctors of defective delta F508 and G551D cystic fibrosis transmembrane conductance regulator chloride-channel gating. Mol Pharmacol 67: 1797–1807.
31. Clancy JP, Rowe SM, Accurso FJ, Aitken ML, Amin RS, et al. (2012) Results of a phase IIa study of VX-809, an investigational CFTR corrector compound, in subjects with cystic fibrosis homozygous for the F508del-CFTR mutation. Thorax 67: 12–18. thoraxjnl-2011-200393 [pii];10.1136/thoraxjnl-2011-200393 [doi].

Voice Disorder in Cystic Fibrosis Patients

Bruna Mendes Lourenço[1,2], Kauê Machado Costa[1¤a¤b], Manoel da Silva Filho[1]*

1 Institute of Biological Sciences, Federal University of Pará, Belém, Pará, Brazil, 2 João de Barros Barreto University Hospital, Federal University of Pará, Belém, Pará, Brazil

Abstract

Cystic fibrosis is a common autosomal recessive disorder with drastic respiratory symptoms, including shortness of breath and chronic cough. While most of cystic fibrosis treatment is dedicated to mitigating the effects of respiratory dysfunction, the potential effects of this disease on vocal parameters have not been systematically studied. We hypothesized that cystic fibrosis patients, given their characteristic respiratory disorders, would also present dysphonic symptoms. Given that voice disorders can severely impair quality of life, the identification of a potential cystic fibrosis-related dysphonia could be of great value for the clinical evaluation and treatment of this disease. We tested our hypothesis by measuring vocal parameters, using both objective physical measures and the GRBAS subjective evaluation method, in male and female cystic fibrosis patients undergoing conventional treatment and compared them to age and sex matched controls. We found that cystic fibrosis patients had a significantly lower vocal intensity and harmonic to noise ratio, as well as increased levels of jitter and shimmer. In addition, cystic fibrosis patients also showed higher scores of roughness, breathiness and asthenia, as well as a significantly altered general grade of dysphonia. When we segregated the results according to sex, we observed that, as a group, only female cystic fibrosis patients had significantly lower values of harmonic to noise ratio and an abnormal general grade of dysphonia in relation to matched controls, suggesting that cystic fibrosis exerts a more pronounced effect on vocal parameters of women in relation to men. Overall, the dysphonic characteristics of CF patients can be explained by dysfunctions in vocal fold movement and partial upper airway obstruction, potentially caused by the accumulation of mucus and chronic cough characteristic of CF symptomatology. Our results show that CF patients exhibit significant dysphonia and suggest they may potentially benefit from voice therapy as a parallel treatment strategy.

Editor: Donald A. Robin, University of Texas Health Science Center at San Antonio, Research Imaging Institute, United States of America

Funding: This study was supported by the Federal University of Pará and the João de Barros Barreto University Hospital. MSF is a research fellow of the National Council for Research and Development (CNPQ). The funders had no role in study design, data collection and analysis, decision to publish, or preparation of the manuscript. Funder's websites: http://www.ufpa.br/, http://www.barrosbarreto.ufpa.br/, http://www.cnpq.br/.

Competing Interests: The authors have declared that no competing interests exist.

* E-mail: manoel@ufpa.br

¤a Current address: International Max Planck Research School for Neural Circuits, Max Planck Institute for Brain Research, Frankfurt am Main, Germany
¤b Current address: Institute for Neurophysiology, Johann Wolfgang Goethe University Frankfurt, Frankfurt am Main, Germany

Introduction

Voice disorders, or dysphonias, can be caused by neurological, structural or functional problems affecting breathing, phonation, articulation, resonance and prosody or the production of sounds at the level of the larynx [1]. A variety of respiratory tract disorders, including chronic cough and laryngeal tension, can lead to reduced voice quality [2]. Dysphonias can cause severe drawbacks in communication and significantly impair quality of life [3,4]. Given the importance of vocal communication to human interaction, subjects with abnormal voice patterns are at high risk for anxiety disorders and depression [5]. Patients with voice disorders score significantly lower on all health status subscales, as measured by the SF-36 form, a highly validated questionnaire assessing quality of life [4].

Cystic fibrosis (CF) is a common autosomal recessive disorder, with a prevalence of approximately 1:2500 live births in people of European descent [6]. This disease is caused by mutations in the cystic fibrosis transmembrane regulator gene, which encodes an epithelial chloride channel. Dysfunctions in this ion channel lead to abnormal transport of chloride and sodium across epithelial membranes and result in the production of thick, viscous secretions in various organs, including the respiratory tract [6,7]. Respiratory dysfunctions, such as shortness of breath and chronic cough, are a hallmark of CF and a major cause of morbidity in CF patients. Therefore, in current medical practice a large part of CF treatment is dedicated to mitigating the effects of respiratory dysfunction [7,8]. However, the potential effects of CF respiratory complications on the vocal capacity of CF patients have not been studied in detail.

We hypothesized that CF patients, given their characteristic respiratory disorders, would also present intrinsic voice alterations. If this is true, CF patients could potentially benefit from voice therapy as a way to improve their quality of life. We tested our hypothesis by measuring vocal parameters, using both objective and subjective clinical evaluation methods, in male and female CF patients undergoing conventional treatment and compared them to age and sex matched controls.

Methods

Subject selection and Ethics Statement

Subjects aged between 10 and 30 years were divided into four groups: a male control group ($n = 25$), a female control group ($n = 16$), male patients with CF ($n = 15$) and female patients with CF ($n = 8$). For some analyses, CF patients ($n = 23$) and control subjects ($n = 41$) were pooled independently of their sex. CF patients were diagnosed based on the standard sweat test, family

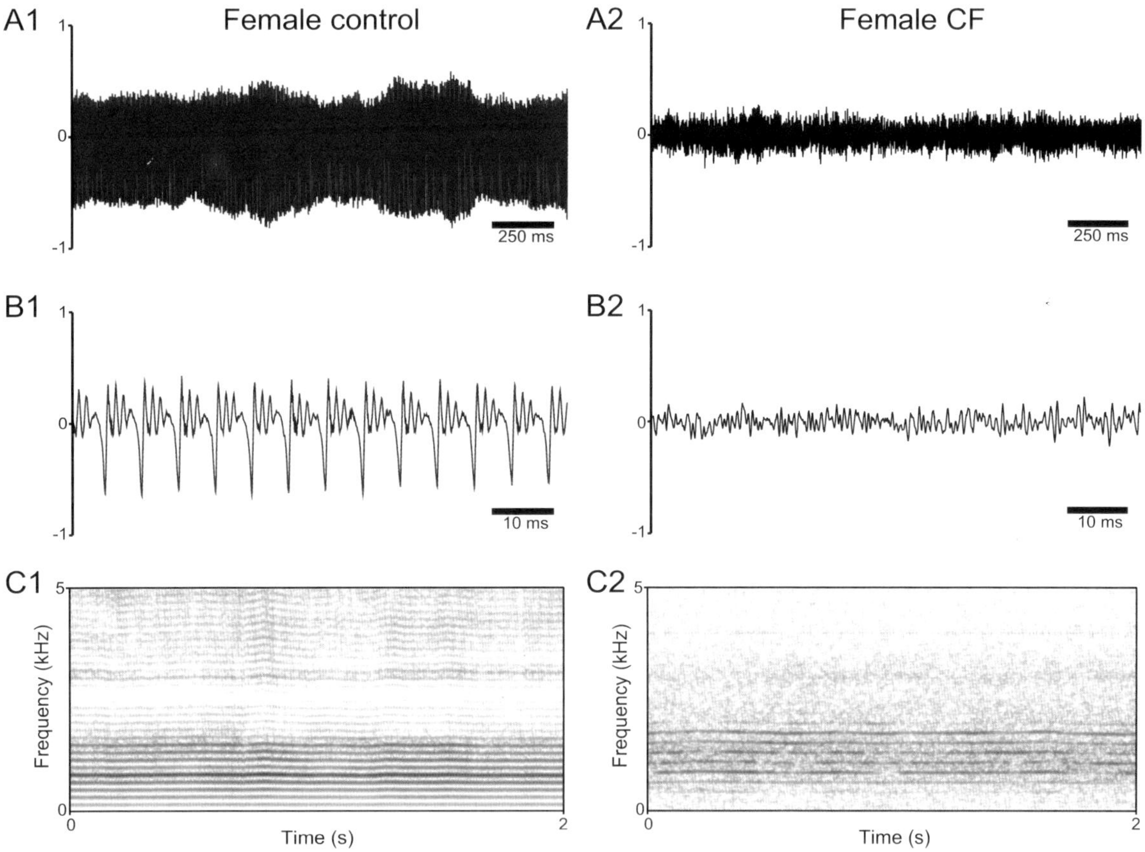

Figure 1. Representative voice recordings and spectrograms of female patients with CF (red) and healthy controls (blue). A: Sound recordings of/a/vowel phonations from a female control subject (A1) and a female patient with CF (A2); note the markedly reduced amplitude range of the signal from the CF patient in relation to the control. B: Amplified views of the recordings presented in A1 and A2; note the irregularity of the voice signal from the CF patient in relation to the control. C: Spectrogram (frequency domain) representations of the recordings presented in A1 and A2; note the higher level of background noise and low formant segregation in the CF patient in relation to the healthy control.

history and the presence of chronic pulmonary disease and pancreatic insufficiency. Previous laryngoscopic examination (conducted prophylactically as part of the patients' clinical monitoring) confirmed that the selected CF patients had no drastic vocal cord dysfunctions or laryngeal diseases, such as vocal cord polyps, laryngeal carcinoma or laryngeal paralysis. CF patients and control subjects had never received voice therapy.

Patients with CF were receiving, individually, regular treatment accompanied by physician, dietician, physiotherapist and psychologist. At the time of the study, none of the CF patients had signs of infection and were not being medicated with inhalatory antibiotics or hypertonic saline. Further information on the clinical status of the subjects can be found in Tables S1–S4, including body mass index (BMI) and FEV1 (a common measure of lung function defined as the volume of air that is exhaled in the first second of forced expiration and normalized by the mean values for the population). The low number of CF patients of each sex is a limitation of this study and was due to the limited pool of willing CF patients which fitted the necessary criteria. This study was approved by the research ethics committee of the João de Barros Barreto University Hospital (#112/09) and all subjects or their legal caretakers signed an informed consent form.

Vocal recordings

Subjects were asked to produce a sustained/a/vowel phonation in their usual intensity for a maximum voicing time. Voice recordings were conducted using a hand-held microphone (PG42-LC, Shure) always positioned six centimeters from the subject's mouth and at a 45° angle to ensure comparable intensity measurements. The initial second of the recording was always excluded from the analysis and parameters were measured over the three second time window that followed this period. Signals were recorded with a sampling rate of 44.1 kHz and analyzed with the Praat 5.1.36 software.

Objective vocal analysis

We measured the following quantitative vocal parameters: fundamental frequency (F_0), intensity, jitter (index of F_0 variability), shimmer (index of intensity variability) and the harmonics to noise ratio (HNR; index of glottal turbulence noise and hoarseness). These parameters have been extensively validated as quantitative, objective measures of vocal quality and are routinely used by voice care professionals as diagnostic tools [9]. Low values of vocal intensity and HNR, high values of jitter and shimmer and altered F_0 are all potential signs of dysphonia.

Subjective vocal analysis

In addition to these objective acoustic variables, we also conducted a perceptual assessment of voice quality in CF and control subjects using the GRBAS (Grade, Roughness, Breathiness, Asthenia, Strain) scale [10]. This vocal assessment method evaluates a patient's general grade of dysphonia (represented by

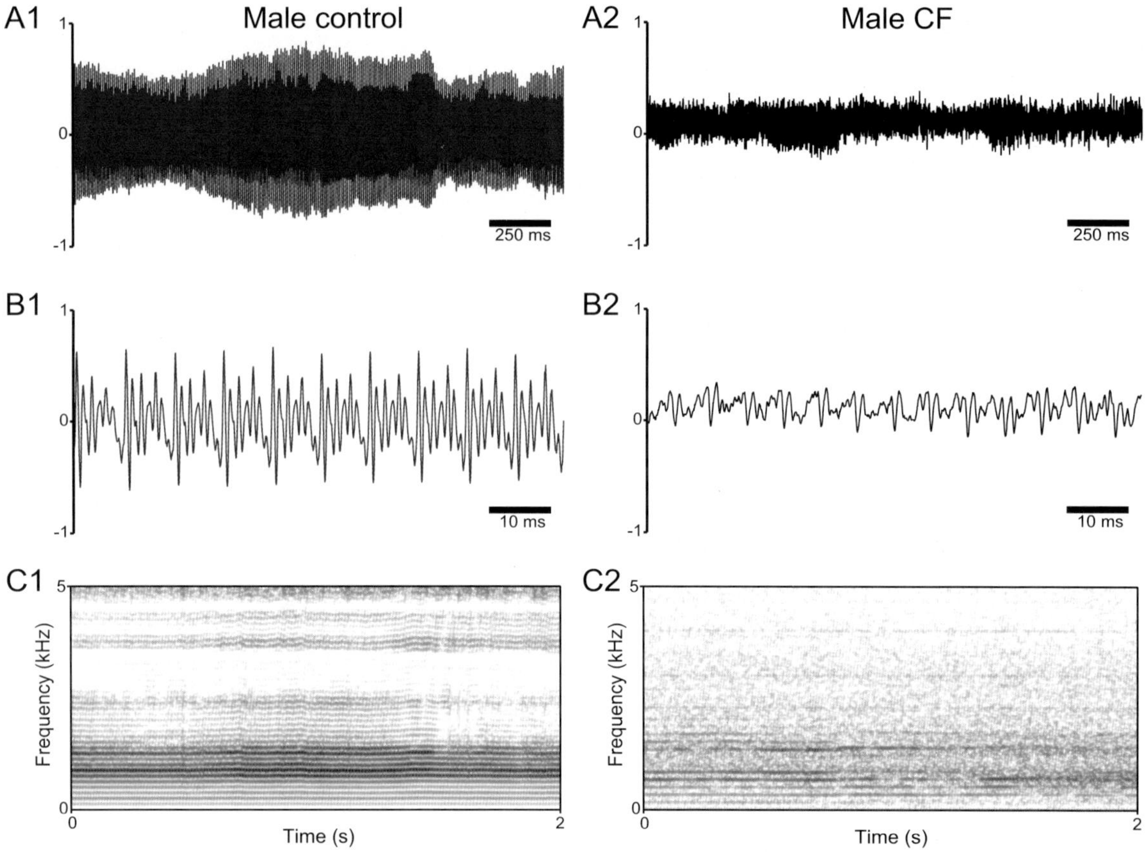

Figure 2. Representative voice recordings and spectrograms of male patients with CF (red) and healthy controls (blue). A: Sound recordings of/a/vowel phonations from a male control subject (A1) and a male patient with CF (A2); note the markedly reduced amplitude range of the signal from the CF patient in relation to the control. B: Amplified views of the recordings presented in A1 and A2; note the irregularity of the voice signal from the CF patient in relation to the control. C: Spectrogram (frequency domain) representations of the recordings presented in A1 and A2; note the higher level of background noise and low formant segregation in the CF patient in relation to the healthy control.

the letter G) through four subjective parameters: roughness (R), breathiness (B), asthenia (A), and strain (S). These variables are determined by a voice care professional, who quantifies his perception of the patients voice as zero (normal), one (mild alteration), two (moderate alteration) or three (severe alteration) on each of the abovementioned factors. The reliability of this method has been extensively validated [10–13]. In order to avoid any confirmation bias in our analyses, we asked an independent practicing clinical voice therapist, with no ties to the research project, to perform the GRBAS evaluation of all our recordings. The evaluator received the recordings in a pseudo-randomized order and was completely blind to the structure of the experimental protocol, the project's objective and the identification and diagnosis of each subject. The evaluator had 9 years of professional experience in voice therapy and GRBAS analysis methods and was instructed to analyze our recordings exactly as it would be performed in clinical practice.

Data analysis and statistics

Differences in objective and subjective vocal parameters were evaluated with the Mann-Whitney test. Data distribution was non-Gaussian for many variables, as defined by the Shapiro-Wilk normality test (Table S5), and therefore data are represented as median values or median and interquartile range (IQR). Statistical significance level was initially set at $P<0.05$; to account for multiple comparisons within the objective and subjective categories of vocal parameters, the Bonferroni correction method was applied. This procedure adjusted the significance level to $P<0.01$ for all analyses.

Results

Representative recordings

Voice signal recordings and spectrograms of representative individuals from all studied groups are shown in Figures 1 and 2. In the control group, recordings show clear features of a euphonic voice [14], such as high periodicity and wide amplitude ranges (Figures 1-B1 and 2-B1). In contrast, signals from subjects in the CF group showed remarkable aperiodicity and reduced amplitude (Figures 1-B2 and 2-B2). The spectrograms of CF patients also showed high noise levels and the loss of high frequency harmonics in relation to the controls (Figures 1-C2 and 2-C2).

CF-related changes in vocal parameters

Analysis of objective voice parameters revealed that CF patients presented a significant decrease in intensity (Figure 3-B; $P<0.0001$), an increase in jitter (Figure 3-C: $P<0.0001$) and shimmer (Figure 3-D; $P<0.0001$) and a much lower HNR (Figure 3-E; $P<0.0001$) in relation to controls. No differences were observed in F_0 (Figure 3-A; $P>0.01$) between the two groups.

The perceptual assessment of voice quality on the GRBAS scale also revealed clear signs of dysphonia in CF patients. In relation to

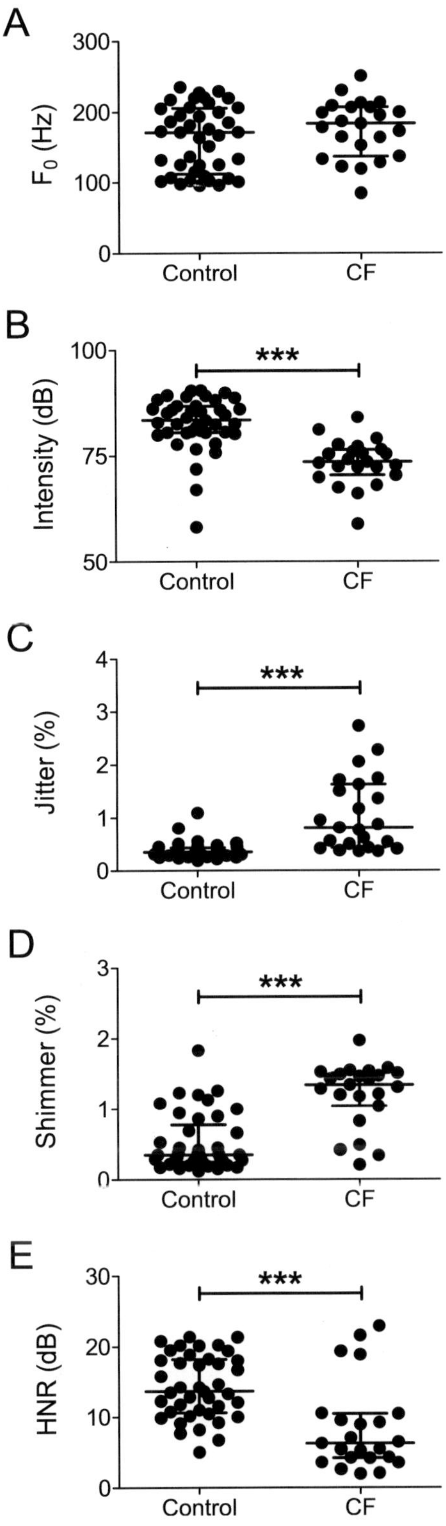

Figure 3. Objective measurements of vocal parameters of control subjects and CF patients. Horizontal lines and error bars represent median±IQR for all variables. Subjects were pooled independently of their sex. **A:** Values of F_0 for each group. **B:** Values of intensity for each group; note the significant reduction in intensity in the CF group. **C:** Values of jitter for each group; note the significant increase in jitter in the CF group. **D:** Values of shimmer for each group; note the significant increase in shimmer in the CF group. **E:** Values of HNR for each group; note the significant reduction in this variable in the CF group. *** $= P < 0.0001$.

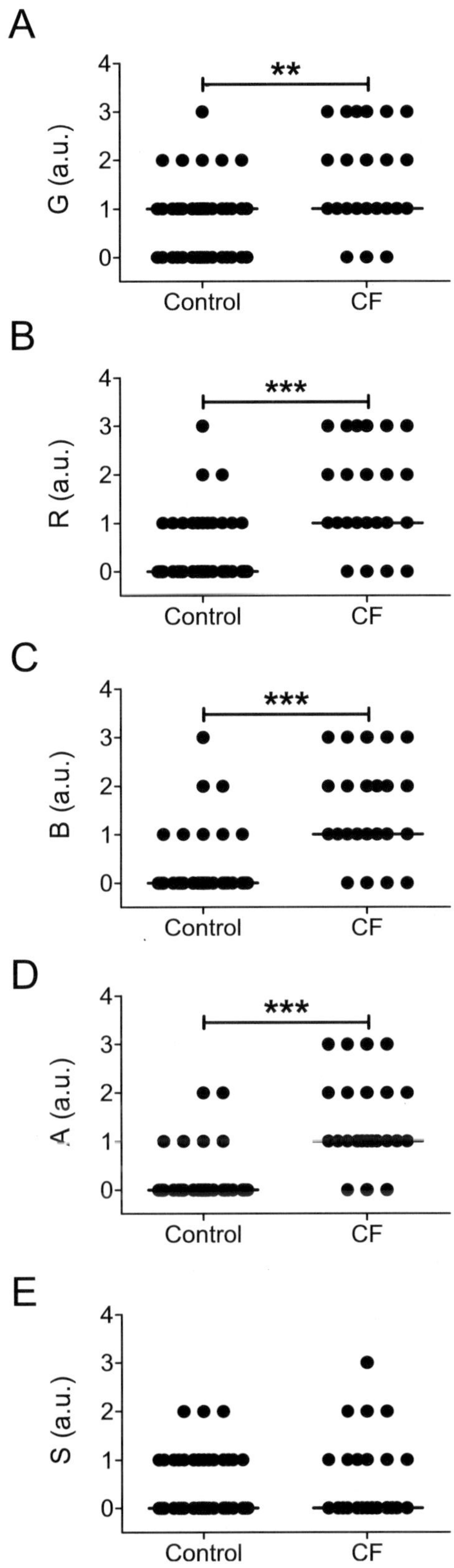

Figure 4. Subjective measurements of vocal parameters of male and female control subjects and CF patients. Horizontal lines and error bars represent the median value of each group. Subjects were pooled independently of their sex. **A:** Values of G for each group; note the significant increase in G in the CF group. **B:** Values of R for each group; note the significant increase in R in the CF group. **C:** Values

of B for each group; note the significant increase in B in the CF group. **D:** Values of A for each group; note the significant increase in A in the CF group. **E:** Values of S for each group. ** $=P<0.001$; *** $=P<0.0001$.

the control group, patients with CF presented an overall increase in R (Figure 4-B; $P<0.0001$), B (Figure 4-C; $P<0.0001$) and A (Figure 4-D; $P<0.0001$). In addition, CF patients showed an increase in G in relation to controls (Figure 4-A; $P=0.0012$). Interestingly, no difference was observed in the S score between CF patients and healthy controls (Figure 4-E; $P>0.01$). All median values and IQRs for the studied variables and statistical comparisons between groups are summarized in Table S6.

It is important to note that it is highly unlikely that the CF-related changes in vocal parameters are related to the age or lung function of the subjects, as none of the objective variables that were affected in CF patients had any significant correlation with age or FEV1 (Figures S1 and S2; $r2<0.2$ and $P<0.01$ for correlations of age or FEV1 with intensity, jitter, shimmer and HNR).

Influence of sex in CF-related dysphonia

We also analyzed our data segregating the control and CF groups according to sex, in order to reveal any possible influence of sex in CF-related dysphonia. These analyses revealed that both male and female CF patients, in relation to their matched controls, presented a significant decrease in intensity (Figure 5-B1 and 5-B2; $P<0.0001$ for both males and females) and an increase in jitter (Figure 5-C1 and 5-C2; for males: $P=0.001$ for females and $P<0.0001$ for males) and shimmer (Figure 5-D1 and 5-D2; $P=0.0001$ for females and $P=0.0038$ for males). Interestingly, while female CF patients showed drastically lower values of HNR (Figure 5-E1; $P=0.0002$) in relation to the control group, this feature was not observed in male CF patients (Figure 5-E2; $P>0.01$) compared to their respective controls. No differences between CF patients and control subjects were observed in F_0 for both sexes (Figure 5-A1 and 5-A2; $P>0.01$ for both comparisons).

In relation to the subjective vocal parameters analyzed on the GRBAS scale, both male and female patients with CF presented an overall increase in R (Figure 6-B1 and 6-B2; $P=0.0019$ for females and $P=0.0025$ for males), B (Figure 6-C1 and 6-C2; $P=0.0003$ for females and $P=0.0004$ for males) and A (Figure 6-D1 and 6-D2; $P=0.0003$ for females and $P<0.0001$ for males) compared to matched controls. However, only female CF patients showed an increase in G in relation to controls (Figure 6-A1; $P=0.0081$), which was not observed in male subjects (Figure 6-A2; $P=0.0293$). No difference was observed in the S score between CF patients and healthy controls of both sexes (Figure 6-E1 and 6-E2; $P>0.01$ for both comparisons). All median values and IQRs for the studied variables and statistical comparisons between CF patients and control subjects segregated by sex are summarized in Table S7.

Discussion

Our results show that subjects with CF present significantly altered vocal parameters, both objectively and subjectively. To our knowledge, this is the first systematic investigation of voice dysfunction in CF. Our findings suggest that dysphonia is a relevant manifestation of CF pathology.

Objective vocal parameters affected by CF were intensity, jitter, shimmer and HNR. Changes in vocal intensity can be observed in cases of vocal microtrauma, neurological dysfunction and obstructive respiratory diseases [15]. Vocal intensity depends fundamentally of subglottal air pressure, upper airway airflow and glottal resistance [16]. The observed decrease in intensity in CF patients could thus be explained by the inefficient lung function and partial upper airway obstruction characteristic of CF physiopathology [6,8]. Chronic cough, a major symptom of CF, could also contribute to this effect [2,6,7,15].

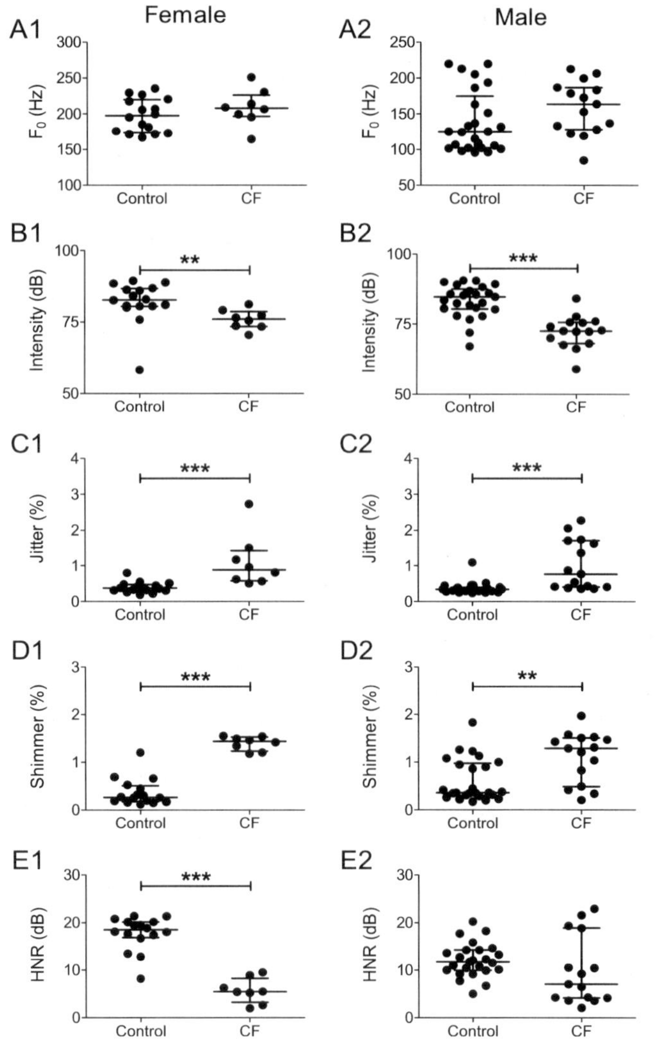

Figure 5. Objective measurements of vocal parameters of male and female control subjects and CF patients. Horizontal lines and error bars represent median±IQR for all variables. **A:** Values of F_0 for female (A1) and male (A2) subject groups. **B:** Values of intensity for female (A1) and male (A2) subject groups. **C:** Values of jitter for female (A1) and male (A2) subject groups. **D:** Values of shimmer for female (A1) and male (A2) subject groups. **E:** Values of HNR for female (A1) and male (A2) subject groups; note that only female CF patients have a lower HNR in relation to the matched controls. ** $=P<0.001$; *** $=P<0.0001$.

Changes in jitter and shimmer are typically related to irregularities in vocal fold vibration, and are also usually related to vocal harshness and the presence of noise in the vocal signal [9,17,18]. The differences in these variables observed in our dataset can be due to the presence of thick mucous secretions in the vocal folds of CF patients, which can potentially interfere in the oscillatory motion of the vocal folds [19,20]. In addition, chronic cough is also known to cause dysfunction of vocal fold movement [2].

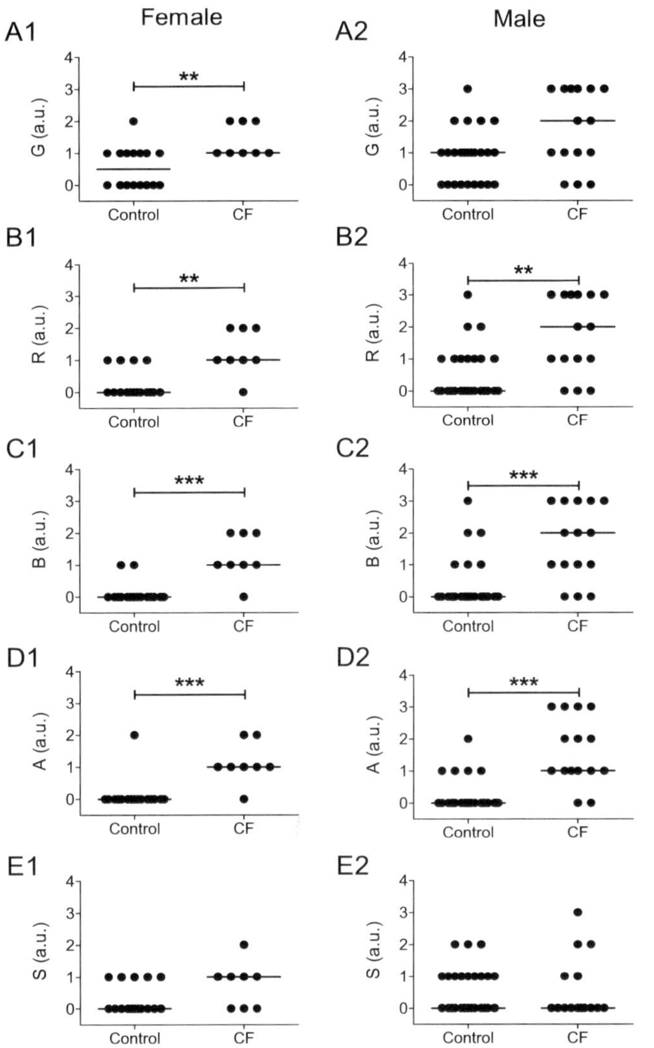

Figure 6. Subjective measurements of vocal parameters of male and female control subjects and CF patients. Horizontal lines and error bars represent the median value of each group. **A:** Values of G for female (A1) and male (A2) subject groups; note that only female patients have a significant change in G in relation to the matched controls. **B:** Values of R for female (A1) and male (A2) subject groups. **C:** Values of B for female (A1) and male (A2) subject groups. **D:** Values of A for female (A1) and male (A2) subject groups. **E:** Values of S for female (A1) and male (A2) subject groups. ** $=P<0.001$; *** $=P<0.0001$.

Decreases in HNR are caused by increases in the variation of vocal amplitude and frequency and in upper airway turbulence. This produces distortions in the vocal signal, emphasizing the subharmonic components and vocal breaks and, consequently, reducing the relative contribution of harmonic components to the overall vocal signal [21]. More importantly, it has been reported that high vocal noise (low HNR) is the most characteristic sign of dysphonia [13]. CF patients showed drastically low HNR values, which can be considered pathologically hoarse and highly detrimental to a normal voice production [15,22]. This decrease in HNR could have the same physiological underpinning as the changes in jitter and shimmer, namely the accumulation of mucus and chronic cough.

The changes in objective vocal parameters in CF patients were confirmed in the subjective evaluation of vocal quality using the GRBAS scale. CF patients showed significant differences in most perceptual vocal parameters, with the exception of S [23]. Previous studies have shown that increases in R and B are strongly related with increases in shimmer [23], which is in agreement with our finding that all three variables are higher in CF patients in relation to the controls. Increases in A are caused by decreases in airflow rate in the upper airways, a common feature of many respiratory diseases [24]. In these cases, subglottal pressure does not rise to the appropriate levels during voice production, causing asthenia and hoarseness. In our dataset of CF patients, this feature can be related to the observed decrease in intensity.

Differences in G represent the general degree of vocal disorder, i.e. a subjective summation of all other perceptual parameters [11,12]. This makes G the most important index within the GRBAS scale [10]. The significantly higher values of G in CF patients indicated that the individual changes in R, B and A combine to produce a noticeable condition of dysphonia.

A notable finding of our study is that female CF patients appear to have more vocal alterations in relation to the controls than male CF patients. When data from each sex was analyzed separately, only female CF patients presented significant lower values of HNR, and higher values of G compared to matched controls. This difference between sexes may be due to the intrinsic differences in the structure of the vocal apparatus observed between men and women. On average, men have thicker vocal folds, larger glottal area and airflow, and lower laryngeal airway resistance than women [25–28]. Our data show that CF vocal pathology is probably due to disorders in vocal fold oscillation and obstruction of the upper airways, and these dysfunctions can be exacerbated when associated to thinner vocal folds and higher airway resistance, respectively. Taken together, these gender-related structural differences are likely to be a major factor in making female patients more susceptible to CF-related dysphonia.

In addition, several other studies have reported that healthy males have voices with significantly lower HNR than healthy females across different languages and age ranges [29–32]. This is also the case in our dataset, as recordings from male control subjects had significantly lower HNRs than female control subjects (Figure 5-E1 and 5-E2; $P=0.0001$ between female and male controls). This intrinsic difference might be explained both by the already mentioned gender related differences in the structure of the vocal apparatus and by social influences, as some authors speculate that women have better vocal training than men, as they use their voices more frequently [29]. Because the perception of what is a normal or appropriate voice depends on what is expected from a person's gender, age and social group, deviations in vocal parameters must be compared with matched controls. Indeed, because healthy women might be expected to have higher HNRs than men, it is fair to predict that the significantly larger decrease in HNR observed in female CF patients might have a highly deleterious impact in their quality of life.

Our data suggests that, as a group, only female patients have their voices affected by the pathophysiology of CF to a degree in which the general perception of their voice, and presumably its communication function, is significantly affected. Nevertheless, it is important to point out that 6 out of 15 subjects in the male CF patient group also presented very low values of HNR (under 5dB), even though the median values of the group were not significantly different from the control. In addition, 6 male CF subjects also presented levels of G above 2, while no such values were observed in the male control group. This would mean that, even though female CF patients might be more susceptible to the deleterious effects of CF on vocal capacity (and thus present more dysphonic symptoms than males), some individual male CF patients might also develop significant changes in HNR and G.

Our results open the possibility that CF patients may benefit from voice therapy as a clinical intervention strategy to reduce dysphonia and increase life quality. Voice therapy consists of a series of techniques applied to the mitigation of voice disorders, which include enhancing the patient's awareness of his or her dysphonia, application of vocal health guidelines, hearing training, muscle relaxation and psychodynamic vocal training [33,34]. This form of therapy has been shown to be an effective treatment in reducing dysphonic symptoms in several diseases, including respiratory disorders, and is capable of at least partially restoring quality of life to affected patients [35–37].

The dysphonic characteristics observed in CF patients can be potentially attributed to dysfunctions in vocal fold movement and partial upper airway obstruction, both of which can be caused by the accumulation of mucus and chronic cough, which are standard symptoms of CF respiratory pathology. While there is no available data on which therapy would be adequate for CF patients, therapy for vocal disorders with hyperfunctional origins have been shown to be effective in patients with chronic cough [2]. Given that chronic cough is a major manifestation of CF pathology, this strategy could potentially be applied to CF patients. This type of intervention is usually based on voice education and vocal hygiene as strategies for cough suppression and also applies exercises that improve dysfunctional vocal fold vibration [2], which according to our data are probably the major features of CF-related dysphonia. Of course, further studies must be conducted to confirm the efficacy of this form of treatment, as well as any other form of voice therapy, for patients with CF.

Conclusion

We showed that patients with CF exhibit symptoms of dysphonia, with changes in both objective and subjective vocal parameters. This may be a relevant feature of CF pathology and morbidity. Voice alterations were more pronounced in female patients, which exhibited a marked reduction in both HNR and overall subjective voice quality. Our results suggest that CF patients might potentially benefit from voice therapy.

Supporting Information

Figure S1 Linear correlation analyses between age and objective vocal parameters for the control and CF groups. *P* values indicate if the slope of the linear regression line is significantly different from zero. **A:** Linear correlation between age and F_0 for each group; note that there is a relatively high inverse correlation (r^2 around 0.2) between these two variables in both the control and CF groups. **B:** Linear correlation between age and intensity for each group. **C:** Linear correlation between age and jitter for each group. **D:** Linear correlation between age and shimmer for each group. **E:** Linear correlation between age and HNR for each group. ** = $P<0.001$.

Figure S2 Linear correlation analyses between FEV1 and objective vocal parameters in the CF group. FEV1 is a common measure of lung function, defined as the volume of air that is exhaled in the first second of forced expiration and normalized to the mean values for the population. *P* values indicate if the slope of the linear regression line is significantly different from zero. Note that only very small correlations were found between FEV1 and each objective vocal parameter. **A:** Linear correlation between FEV1 and F_0 for each group. **B:** Linear correlation between FEV1 and intensity. **C:** Linear correlation between FEV1 and jitter. **D:** Linear correlation between FEV1 and shimmer. **E:** Linear correlation between FEV1 and HNR.

Table S1 Age and body mass index (BMI) for all subjects of the female control group.

Table S2 Age and body mass index (BMI) for all subjects of the male control group.

Table S3 Age, body mass index (BMI), FEV1 and medical status of the female cystic fibrosis group.

Table S4 Age, body mass index (BMI), FEV1 and medical status of the male cystic fibrosis group.

Table S5 Summary of mean ± standard error values and normality test results for all studied groups.

Table S6 Summary of median and IQR values for pooled data of CF and control subjects, with statistical comparison including values for the Mann-Whitney U (U), Z-score (Z), effect size (r) and P.

Table S7 Summary of median and IQR values for data of CF and control subjects segregated according to sex, with statistical comparison including values for the Mann-Whitney U (U), Z-score (Z), effect size (r) and P.

Acknowledgments

We thank Dr. Francisco Palheta Neto for his assistance in diagnosing and selecting the subjects. We also thank Milena Freitas for performing the blind GRBAS evaluation of our acoustic data. We are grateful to Ivaylo Borislavov Iotchev and Dr. Felipe Camargo Munhoz for critically reviewing the manuscript and providing important suggestions.

Author Contributions

Conceived and designed the experiments: BML MSF. Performed the experiments: BML. Analyzed the data: BML KMC. Contributed reagents/materials/analysis tools: BML KMC MSF. Wrote the paper: KMC BML MSF.

References

1. Cohen SM, Elackattu A, Noordzij JP, Walsh MJ, Langmore SE (2009) Palliative Treatment of Dysphonia and Dysarthria. Otolaryngol Clin North Am 42: 107–121. doi:10.1016/j.otc.2008.09.010.
2. Gibson PG, Vertigan AE (2009) Speech pathology for chronic cough: a new approach. Pulm Pharmacol Ther 22: 159–162. doi:10.1016/j.pupt.2008.11.005.
3. Murry T, Medrado R, Hogikyan ND, Aviv JE (2004) The relationship between ratings of voice quality and quality of life measures. J Voice 18: 183–192. doi:10.1016/j.jvoice.2003.11.003.
4. Wilson JA, Deary IJ, Millar A, Mackenzie K (2002) The quality of life impact of dysphonia. Clin Otolaryngol Allied Sci 27: 179–182.
5. Deary IJ, Scott S, Wilson IM, White A, MacKenzie K, et al. (1997) Personality and psychological distress in dysphonia. Br J Health Psychol 2: 333–341. doi:10.1111/j.2044-8287.1997.tb00547.x.
6. Ratjen F, Döring G (2003) Cystic fibrosis. The Lancet 361: 681–689. doi:10.1016/S0140-6736(03)12567-6.

7. Yankaskas JR, Marshall BC, Sufian B, Simon RH, Rodman D (2004) Cystic fibrosis adult care: consensus conference report. Chest 125: 1S–39S.
8. Zemanick ET, Harris JK, Conway S, Konstan MW, Marshall B, et al. (2010) Measuring and improving respiratory outcomes in cystic fibrosis lung disease: opportunities and challenges to therapy. J Cyst Fibros Off J Eur Cyst Fibros Soc 9: 1–16. doi:10.1016/j.jcf.2009.09.003.
9. Baken RJ, Orlikoff RF (2000) Clinical Measurement of Speech and Voice. Cengage Learning. 628 p.
10. Hirano M (1981) Clinical examination of voice. Springer London, Limited. 124 p.
11. Nemr K, Simões-Zenari M, Cordeiro GF, Tsuji D, Ogawa AI, et al. (2012) GRBAS and Cape-V scales: high reliability and consensus when applied at different times. J Voice 26: 812.e17–22. doi:10.1016/j.jvoice.2012.03.005.
12. De Bodt MS, Wuyts FL, Van de Heyning PH, Croux C (1997) Test-retest study of the GRBAS scale: Influence of experience and professional background on perceptual rating of voice quality. J Voice 11: 74–80. doi:10.1016/S0892-1997(97)80026-4.
13. Bhuta T, Patrick L, Garnett JD (2004) Perceptual evaluation of voice quality and its correlation with acoustic measurements. J Voice Off J Voice Found 18: 299–304. doi:10.1016/j.jvoice.2003.12.004.
14. Kosztyła-Hojna B, Andrzejewska A, Moskal D, Rogowski M, Falkowski D, et al. (2011) Morphological aspects of the euphonic voice. Folia Histochem Cytobiol Pol Acad Sci Pol Histochem Cytochem Soc 49: 72–79.
15. Pontes PAL, Vieira VP, Gonçalves MIR, Pontes AAL (2002) Characteristics of hoarse, rough and normal voices: acoustic spectrographic comparative analysis. Rev Bras Otorrinolaringol 68: 182–188. doi:10.1590/S0034-72992002000200005.
16. Hodge FS, Colton RH, Kelley RT (2001) Vocal intensity characteristics in normal and elderly speakers. J Voice 15: 503–511. doi:10.1016/S0892-1997(01)00050-9.
17. Yelken K, Gultekin E, Guven M, Eyibilen A, Aladag I (2010) Impairment of voice quality in paradoxical vocal fold motion dysfunction. J Voice 24: 724–727. doi:10.1016/j.jvoice.2009.05.004.
18. Maryn Y, Corthals P, De Bodt M, Van Cauwenberge P, Deliyski D (2009) Perturbation measures of voice: a comparative study between Multi-Dimensional Voice Program and Praat. Folia Phoniatr Logop Off Organ Int Assoc Logop Phoniatr IALP 61: 217–226. doi:10.1159/000227999.
19. Grini-Grandval MN, Bingenheimer S, Maunsell R, Ouaknine M, Giovanni A (2002) Phonatory threshold pressure in a healthy population before and after aerosol treatment, a preliminary study. Rev Laryngol – Otol – Rhinol 123: 311–314.
20. Verdonck-de Leeuw IM, Festen JM, Mahieu HF (2001) Deviant vocal fold vibration as observed during videokymography: the effect on voice quality. J Voice Off J Voice Found 15: 313–322. doi:10.1016/S0892-1997(01)00033-9.
21. Franca MC (2012) Acoustic comparison of vowel sounds among adult females. J Voice 26: 671.e9–17. doi:10.1016/j.jvoice.2011.11.010.
22. Yumoto E, Gould WJ, Baer T (1982) Harmonics-to-noise ratio as an index of the degree of hoarseness. J Acoust Soc Am 71: 1544–1549.
23. Lopes LW, Barbosa Lima IL, Alves Almeida LN, Cavalcante DP, de Almeida AAF (2012) Severity of voice disorders in children: correlations between perceptual and acoustic data. J Voice 26: 819.e7–12. doi:10.1016/j.jvoice.2012.05.008.
24. Omori K (2011) Diagnosis of Voice Disorders. JMAJ 54: 248–253.
25. Hollien H (1962) Vocal fold thickness and fundamental frequency of phonation. J Speech Hear Res 5: 237–243.
26. Holmes LC, Leeper HA, Nicholson IR (1994) Laryngeal Airway Resistance of Older Men and Women as a Function of Vocal Sound Pressure Level. J Speech Hear Res 37: 789–799.
27. Lucero JC, Koenig LL (2005) Simulations of temporal patterns of oral airflow in men and women using a two-mass model of the vocal folds under dynamic control. J Acoust Soc Am 117: 1362–1372. doi:10.1121/1.1853235.
28. Holmberg EB, Hillman RE, Perkell JS (1988) Glottal airflow and transglottal air pressure measurements for male and female speakers in soft, normal, and loud voice. J Acoust Soc Am 84: 511–529. doi:10.1121/1.396829.
29. Dehqan A, Ansari H, Bakhtiar M (2010) Objective voice analysis of Iranian speakers with normal voices. J Voice Off J Voice Found 24: 161–167. doi:10.1016/j.jvoice.2008.07.005.
30. Naufel de Felippe AC, Grillo MHMM, Grechi TH (2006) Standardization of acoustic measures for normal voice patterns. Braz J Otorhinolaryngol 72: 659–664.
31. Ferrand CT (2000) Harmonics-to-noise ratios in normally speaking prepubescent girls and boys. J Voice Off J Voice Found 14: 17–21.
32. Toran KC, Lal BK (2009) Objective analysis of voice in normal young adults. Kathmandu Univ Med J KUMJ 7: 374–377.
33. Holmberg EB, Hillman RE, Hammarberg B, Södersten M, Doyle P (2001) Efficacy of a behaviorally based voice therapy protocol for vocal nodules. J Voice 15: 395–412. doi:10.1016/S0892-1997(01)00041-8.
34. Schindler A, Mozzanica F, Maruzzi P, Atac M, De Cristofaro V, et al. (2013) Multidimensional assessment of vocal changes in benign vocal fold lesions after voice therapy. Auris Nasus Larynx 40: 291–297. doi:10.1016/j.anl.2012.08.003.
35. Gartner-Schmidt JL, Roth DF, Zullo TG, Rosen CA (2013) Quantifying Component Parts of Indirect and Direct Voice Therapy Related to Different Voice Disorders. J Voice 27: 210–216. doi:10.1016/j.jvoice.2012.11.007.
36. Speyer R (2008) Effects of Voice Therapy: A Systematic Review. J Voice 22: 565–580. doi:10.1016/j.jvoice.2006.10.005.
37. Mueller PB, Larson GW (1992) Voice therapy practices and techniques: A survey of voice clinicians. J Commun Disord 25: 251–260. doi:10.1016/0021-9924(92)90019-S.

Reduced Mucosal Associated Invariant T-Cells Are Associated with Increased Disease Severity and *Pseudomonas aeruginosa* Infection in Cystic Fibrosis

Daniel J. Smith[1,2,4]*, Geoffrey R. Hill[3], Scott C. Bell[1,2,5], David W. Reid[1,2,4]

1 Department of Thoracic Medicine, The Prince Charles Hospital, Brisbane, Queensland, Australia, **2** School of Medicine, University of Queensland, Brisbane, Queensland, Australia, **3** Bone Marrow Transplant Laboratory, QIMR Berghofer Medical Research Institute, Brisbane, Queensland, Australia, **4** Infection and Inflammation Laboratory, QIMR Berghofer Medical Research Institute, Brisbane, Queensland, Australia, **5** Queensland Children's Medical Research Institute, Royal Children's Hospital, Brisbane, Queensland, Australia

Abstract

Background: Primary defects in host immune responses have been hypothesised to contribute towards an inability of subjects with cystic fibrosis (CF) to effectively clear pulmonary infections. Innate T-lymphocytes provide rapid pathogen-specific responses prior to the development of classical MHC class I and II restricted T-cell responses and are essential to the initial control of pulmonary infection. We aimed to examine the relationship between peripheral blood lymphocyte phenotype and clinical outcomes in adults with CF.

Methods: We studied 41 subjects with CF and 22, age matched, non-smoking healthy control subjects. Lymphocytes were extracted from peripheral blood samples and phenotyped by flow-cytometry. Lymphocyte phenotype was correlated with sputum microbiology and clinical parameters.

Results: In comparison to healthy control subjects, mucosal associated invariant T (MAIT)-lymphocytes were significantly reduced in the peripheral blood of subjects with CF (1.1% versus 2.0% of T-lymphocytes, $P = 0.002$). MAIT cell concentration was lowest in CF subjects infected with *P. aeruginosa* and in subjects receiving treatment for a pulmonary exacerbation. Furthermore a reduced MAIT cell concentration correlated with severity of lung disease.

Conclusion: Reduced numbers of MAIT cells in subjects with CF were associated with *P. aeruginosa* pulmonary infection, pulmonary exacerbations and more severe lung disease. These findings provide the impetus for future studies examining the utility of MAIT cells in immunotherapies and vaccine development. Longitudinal studies of MAIT cells as biomarkers of CF pulmonary infection are awaited.

Editor: Johan K. Sandberg, Karolinska Institutet, Sweden

Funding: Internal funding was received from QIMR Berghofer Medical Research Institute. The institute had no role in decision to publish the manuscript.

Competing Interests: The authors have declared that no competing interests exist.

* Email: daniel.smith@health.qld.gov.au

Introduction

Cystic fibrosis (CF) pulmonary disease is typified by a vicious cycle of bacterial infection and exuberant, but ineffective host immune response [1]. The inability of the intense inflammatory response to clear infection has led to speculation that intrinsic immune defects may contribute to the persistence of pathogens in CF [2]. At the level of the airway lumen, the cellular immune response is dominated by activated neutrophils. However, in contrast, airway epithelial biopsies demonstrate a profound T lymphocyte (T-cell) infiltrate, supporting an important role for adaptive immune responses in the orchestration of a sustained inflammatory response [3].

To date, studies of peripheral, adaptive immune responses in CF have largely focused on the classic dichotomy of T-helper (Th)-1 and Th-2 responses [4]. These early studies suggested a skew towards a Th2 in most CF subjects with *P. aeruginosa* infection, which resulted in increased pulmonary inflammation and disease progression [4–6]. The activation of the "classical" adaptive immune response involves antigen recognition, followed by T-cell recruitment and clonal expansion at the site of infection. Consequently, there is a time lag between the host's recognition of the presence of a pathogen and the development of an effective, adaptive immune response. In recent times, an increasing number of unconventional "innate" T-cell populations have been described (including γ/δ, semi-invariant natural killer (iNKT) and M3-restricted T-cells), which are capable of mounting a more immediate response to pathogens than was previously thought possible. Mucosal associated invariant T (MAIT) cells are a recently described sub-class of innate T-cells, which can be differentiated from other T-cells by the presence of an evolutionary conserved T-cell receptor (TCR)

(Vα7.2–Jα33). MAIT cells recognise bacterial and fungal metabolites presented on the major histocompatibility complex (MHC) related protein-1 (MR1) (including the common CF pathogens *Pseudomonas aeruginosa* and *Staphylococcus aureus*), but not viruses [7,8]. These "innate" T-cell populations provide rapid pathogen-specific responses prior to the development of classical MHC class I and II restricted T-cell responses and importantly may also provide a sustained cytokine response in chronic infection [9,10].

To date, there is limited knowledge of how changes in circulating lymphocyte populations may relate to pulmonary infection in CF [11]. In this study we performed extensive phenotyping of peripheral blood mononuclear cell populations (PBMCs) obtained from subjects with CF and compared these profiles to those in healthy, age matched, controls. Our particular focus was on the correlation of γ/δ and MAIT innate T-cell values with clinical and microbiological parameters.

Methods

Participants and sample collection

Forty-one subjects with CF attending the Adult CF Centre, The Prince Charles Hospital, Queensland, Australia and 22 age-matched, non-smoking, healthy control subjects each supplied a single venous blood sample.

In subjects with CF, total white cell count (WCC), C-reactive protein (CRP) and clinical demographics including, age, CF genotype, lung function, body mass index, pulmonary exacerbation frequency and pulmonary pathogens (based on standard sputum microbiological testing) were recorded. Longitudinal rate of decline in forced expiratory volume in one second (FEV_1) was determined in CF subjects by means of linear regression analysis (limited to subjects with at least five FEV_1 measurements recorded over a minimum surveillance period of 2 years).

To explore the effect of pulmonary exacerbations on lymphocyte concentrations a sub-set of 13 "stable" CF subjects (stable respiratory symptoms and a CRP <5 mg L^{-1} at time of blood collection) were compared to eight CF subjects in whom blood was collected within 72 hours of admission to hospital for the intravenous antibiotic treatment of a "pulmonary exacerbation", defined as increased respiratory symptoms (cough, sputum volume or purulence, dyspnoea) (Figure S1 in File S1).

Ethics approval was obtained from The Prince Charles Hospital, Queensland, Australia, Human Research and Ethics Committee (HREC/11/QPCH/36 and HREC2008:2885) and all subjects provided written, informed consent.

Separation and storage of peripheral blood mononuclear cells (PBMCs)

Twelve millilitres of venous blood was collected into lithium heparinised tubes and separated into plasma and cellular components. The cellular component was re-suspended in RPMI (Gibco)+2% heat inactivated Foetal Calf Serum (HiFCS) and PBMCs separated by means of Histopaque 1.077 (Sigma-Aldrich) density gradient separation, as per the manufacturer's protocol.

Table 1. Subject demographics.

	Healthy Controls	Cystic Fibrosis	P value
Sex (Female:Male)	11:11	17:24	0.5
Age (years)	26 (25–32)	28 (22–32)	0.9
BMI (kg/metre^2)	24.6 (21.4–28.3)	23.5 (20.5–25.8)	0.3
FEV_1 (Litres)	4.1 (3.5–4.7)	2.2 (1.4–2.5)	<0.001
FEV_1% Predicted (%)	110 (101–120)	58 (37–75)	<0.001
FVC (Litres)	4.9 (4.4–5.7)	3.1 (2.6–4.1)	<0.001
FVC % Predicted (%)	107 (95–112)	76 (58–84)	<0.001
CFTR Genotype			
F508del Homozygotes		20	
F508del Heterozygotes		18	
Other mutations		3	
Sputum Microbiology*			
Pseudomonas aeruginosa		36	
Staphylococcus aureus		12	
Aspergillus fumigatus		5	
Haemophilus influenzae		4	
Stenotrophomonas maltophilia		3	
Chryseobacterium indologenes		2	
Scedosporium apiospermum		2	
Mycobacterium intracellulare		1	
Burkholderia gladioli		1	
Achromobacter xylosoxidans		1	
Methicillin resistant *S. aureus*		1	

Data presented as median (interquartile range).
*Summary data, subjects may have had more than one pathogen isolated in sputum, individual microbiological data available in Table S1 in File S2.

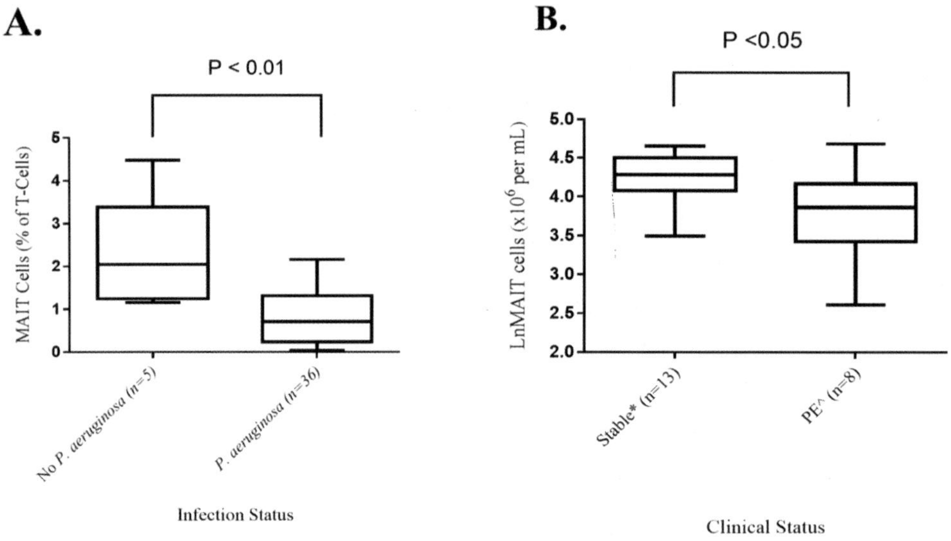

Figure 1. MAIT Cell percentage in CF subjects based on A. Presence of *P. aeruginosa* in sputum cultures, B. Clinical status. PE: pulmonary exacerbations, *two and ^one not infected with *P. aeruginosa*, between group differences determined by Mann-Whitney U test.

Following separation, PBMCs were washed twice, re-suspended in RPMI and 15% dimethyl sulfoxide (DMSO), gradually frozen to −80°C and transferred to storage in liquid nitrogen for later batch analysis (concentration 5–20×10^6 cells/ml).

Flow Cytometry

PBMCs were rewarmed and re-suspended by drop-wise addition of 10 ml of RPMI+2%HiFCS, washed twice and re-suspended in phosphate buffered saline (PBS) with 1% HiFCS (FACS buffer). A cell count was performed and the volume adjusted to obtain a cell concentration of 10×10^6 cells/ml.

One hundred micro-litre aliquots of cells were incubated with each of two antibody staining panels as follows:

Panel 1 [adapted from [12]]: FITC anti-human CD16, Pacific Blue anti-human CD14, APC anti-human CD1c, Alexa Fluor700 anti-human CD3, APC/Cy7 anti-human HLA-DR, PE/Cy7 anti-human CD56, PE/Cy7 anti-human CD20, Anti-CD8 antibody – PE Texas (Abcam) and V500 anti-CD4 (BD biosciences) were added to 100 µL of cells and incubated in the dark for 15 minutes. Cells were washed twice in 1 ml of FACS buffer and fixation was performed by incubation with 500 µl of Cytofix (BD biosciences) for 10 minutes. Finally, samples were washed and suspended in 300 µl of FACS buffer.

Table 2. Comparison of lymphocyte sub-sets between CF and healthy control subjects.

Lymphocyte Population (size gated, CD14−)	CF (n = 41)	Non-CF (n = 22)	P-Value
T-Cells (CD3+CD16−)	**72.6 (68.1–79.6)**	**74.9 (67.9–79.0)**	0.6
CD4+CD8−	65.2 (56.1–70.5)	65.1 (59.9–71.4)	0.6
CD8+CD4−	25.7 (21.1–32.5)	27.4 (22.7–32.8)	0.6
MAIT Cells (CD161+, TCR Va7.2+)	1.1 (0.4–1.9)	2.0 (1.4–3.1)	**0.002**
γ/δ T-cells (TCR γ/δ+)	10.4 (6.5–13.4)	6.4 (4.6–9.4)	**0.012**
CD4+CD8+	0.3 (0.2–1.0)	0.4 (0.3–1.7)	0.1
CD4−CD8−*	2.1 (0.9–3.3)	1.6 (1.1–2.3)	0.3
B-Cells (CD3−CD16−CD20+HLA-DR+)	**9.5 (4.9–14.3)**	**4.8 (3.9–8.7)**	0.1
Non-Resting (CD1c−)	64.6 (57.0–74.4)	71.6 (60.5–75.1)	0.5
Resting (CD1c+)	35.0 (24.8–43.	28.1 (25.0–38.3)	0.4
NK-Cells (CD3−)	**9.5 (6.9–12.2)**	**13.1 (8.0–18.0)**	**0.013**
CD16+CD56dim HLA-DR−	75.1 (61.0–86.7)	88.0 (84.7–92.6)	**0.001**
CD16−CD56+HLA-DR−	8.9 (6.1–13.2)	6.1 (4.5–9.1)	**0.016**
CD16−CD56+HLA-DR+	14.4 (5.1–24.1)	4.3 (2.7–9.2)	**0.005**
CD3+CD16+	**2.2 (1.1–3.8)**	**1.8 (1.1–3.6)**	0.7
Contaminants/Undefined	**3.7 (3.0–5.2)**	**2.4 (1.9–3.9)**	0.013

*After exclusion of MAIT and γ/δ T-cells. Values expressed as percentage of parent population, Median (interquartile range). Significance of between group differences determined by Mann-Whitney U test.

A.

	LnMAIT Cell Concentration (cells per mL)	γ/δ T-Cell Concentration (cells per mL)
FEV_1% predicted	r = 0.47 p = 0.003	r = 0.35 p = 0.030
FEV_1% predicted decline per year	r = 0.28 p = 0.10	r = 0.31 p = 0.06
FVC% predicted	r = 0.43 p = 0.006	r = 0.33 p = 0.042
Body Mass Index (kg/m²)	r = 0.12 P = 0.48	r = -0.03 P = 0.86
C-reactive protein (mg/L)	r = -0.39 p = 0.021	r = -0.44 p = 0.008

B.

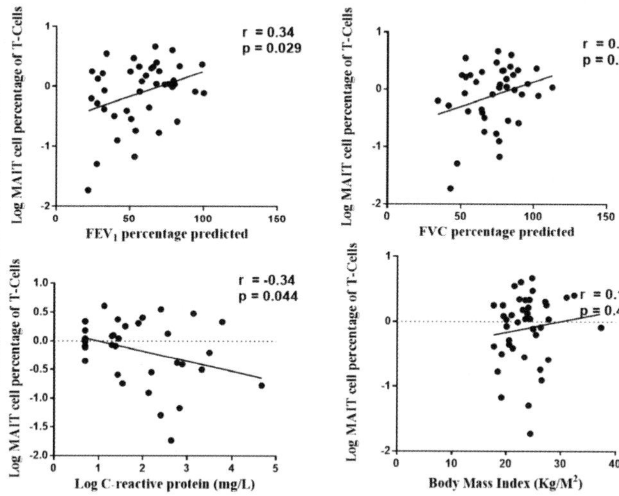

Figure 2. Relationship between MAIT and γ/δ T-cell counts and percentages with lung function. A. Pearson's Correlation co-efficient (r) and significance value (p) of MAIT and γ/δ T-cells and B. Correlation plots for MAIT Cell expressed as percentage of T-cell population, with FEV_1 and FVC % predicted, C-reactive protein and body mass index. MAIT: Mucosal invariant T-Lymphocytes, γ/δ T-Cell: Gamma-Delta T-lymphocytes, FEV_1: Forced expiratory volume in one second, FVC: Forced vital capacity.

Table 3. Lymphocyte sub-set phenotypes in CF subjects based on the presence of *P. aeruginosa* infection compared to healthy control subjects.

	CF, No *P. aeruginosa* (n = 5)	**CF, *P. aeruginosa* infection (n = 36)**	**P-Value^**	**Non-CF (n = 22)**	**P-Value$**
Sex (Female:Male)	3:2	14:22	0.4	11:11	1.0
Age (years)	23.3 (18.4–41.7)	28 (24.5–32.6)	0.8	26 (25–32)	0.5
BMI (kg/metre²)	24.7 (19.9–31.7)	23.4 (20.5–25.3)	0.5	24.6 (21.4–28.3)	0.8
FEV_1% Predicted (%)	72.4 (59.1–88.8)	63.6 (43.4–80.1)	0.3	110 (101–120)	**0.001**
FVC % Predicted (%)	83.9 (68.1–95.9)	79.3 (71.1–88.7)	0.5	107 (95–112)	**0.012**
Lymphocyte Population (size gated, CD14−)					
T-Cells (CD3+CD16−)	**68.2 (63.4–76.8)**	**72.9 (68.3–81.3)**	0.1	**71.9 (67.9 79.0)**	0.3
CD4+CD8−	64.4 (49.6–70.0)	65.2 (56.9–70.5)	0.6	65.1 (59.9–71.4)	0.5
CD8+CD4−	26.2 (22.8–38.8)	25.1 (20.5–33.1)	0.6	27.4 (22.7–32.8)	0.9
MAIT Cells (CD161+, TCR Va7.2+)	2.4 (1.4–3.6)	1.0 (0.3–1.8)	**0.023**	2.0 (1.4–3.1)	1.0
γ/δ T-cells (TCR γ/δ+)	8.0 (6.0–16.0)	10.5 (6.6–13.4)	0.7	6.4 (4.6–9.4)	0.2
CD4+CD8+	0.2 (0.2–0.2)	0.3 (0.2–1.1)	**0.014**	0.4 (0.3–1.7)	**0.004**
CD4−CD8−*	3.1 (1.6–4.1)	2.1 (0.7–2.8)	0.2	1.6 (1.1–2.3)	0.1
B-Cells (CD3−CD16−CD20+HLA-DR+)	**17.2 (14.0–20.9)**	**8.5 (3.6–13.0)**	**0.002**	**4.8 (3.9–8.7)**	**0.003**
Non-Resting (CD1c−)	74.5 (69.1–79.0)	64.1 (55.5–73.7)	0.1	71.6 (60.5–75.1)	0.1
Resting (CD1c+)	24.9 (20.3–30.5)	35.9 (25.3–43.9)	0.1	28.1 (25.0–38.3)	0.1
NK-Cells (CD3−)	**9.6 (4.6–10.9)**	**9.5 (7.8–12.5)**	**0.5**	**13.1 (8.0–18.0)**	**0.039**
CD16+CD56dim HLA-DR−	69.2 (48.5–80.9)	76.1 (63.8–88.1)	0.2	88.0 (84.7–92.6)	**0.006**
CD16−CD56+HLA-DR−	10.9 (7.1–14.5)	8.5 (6.1–13.3)	0.5	6.1 (4.5–9.1)	**0.1**
CD16−CD56+HLA-DR+	21.4 (10.8–37.4)	14.2 (4.5–23.8)	0.2	4.3 (2.7–9.2)	**0.006**
CD3+CD16+	**2.0 (0.9–2.6)**	**2.5 (1.0–4.2)**	0.4	**1.8 (1.1–3.6)**	0.9
Contaminants/Undefined	**1.8 (1.6–3.5)**	**3.7 (3.1–5.4)**	0.017	**2.4 (1.9–3.9)**	**0.4**

^CF No *P. aeruginosa versus* CF *P. aeruginosa* infection. $CF No *P. aeruginosa versus* Non-CF. *After exclusion of MAIT and γ/δ T-cells. Values expressed as percentage of parent population, Median (interquartile range). Significance of between group differences determined by Mann-Whitney U test.

Table 4. Lymphocyte sub-sets in CF subjects based on clinical stability and compared to healthy control subjects.

	CF, Pulmonary exacerbation (n = 8)	CF, Stable (n = 13)	P-Value^	Non-CF (n = 22)	P-Value$
Sex (Female:Male)	1:7	8:5	**0.027**	11:11	0.5
Age (years)	32.2 (30.1–39.1)	22.7 (20.5–26.9)	**0.001**	26 (25–32)	**0.010**
BMI (kg/metre^2)	24.6 (23.5–26.0)	23.0 (21.5–27.0)	0.4	24.6 (21.4–28.3)	0.7
FEV_1% Predicted (%)	49.7 (40.3–68.5)	83.2 (74.1–88.8)	**0.001**	110 (101–120)	**<0.001**
FVC % Predicted (%)	74.6 (71.2–79.3)	90.0 (85.9–96.4)	**0.001**	107 (95–112)	**0.001**
Lymphocyte Population (size gated, CD14−)					
T-Cells (CD3+CD16−)	**71.6 (68.1–82.3)**	**71.3 (67.1–77.1)**	0.6	**74.9 (67.9–79.0)**	0.3
CD4+CD8−	65.9 (52.2–76.2)	58.3 (55.3–68.9)	0.5	65.1 (59.9–71.4)	0.1
CD8+CD4−	23.8 (16.4–37.8)	29.2 (23.6–35.3)	0.3	27.4 (22.7–32.8)	0.7
MAIT Cells (CD161+, TCR Va7.2+)	1.1 (0.3–2.1)	1.1 (0.9–1.9)	0.7	2.0 (1.4–3.1)	**0.018**
γ/δ T-cells (TCR γ/δ+)	11.1 (7.1–16.5)	10.5 (6.4–13.6)	0.8	6.4 (4.6–9.4)	**0.017**
CD4+CD8+	0.2 (0.2–1.0)	0.2 (0.2–0.3)	0.5	0.4 (0.3–1.7)	**0.010**
CD4−CD8−*	2.6 (1.4–3.5)	2.2 (1.3–3.4)	0.6	1.6 (1.1–2.3)	0.1
B-Cells (CD3−CD16−CD20+HLA-DR+)	**9.6 (2.5–14.0)**	**13.1 (8.5–16.7)**	0.3	**4.8 (3.9–8.7)**	**0.001**
Non-Resting (CD1c−)	73.4. (65.5–79.9)	70.4 (59.9–79.9)	0.8	71.6 (60.5–75.1)	0.7
Resting (CD1c+)	25.6 (19.9–34.1)	29.3 (18.1–40.1)	0.8	28.1 (25.0–38.3)	0.7
NK-Cells (CD3−)	**10.1 (5.9–12.6)**	**9.6 (5.4–11.8)**	0.7	**13.1 (8.0–18.0)**	**0.020**
CD16+CD56dim HLA-DR−	70.7 (52.9–83.7)	69.2 (55.3–80.5)	0.9	88.0 (84.7–92.6)	**<0.001**
CD16−CD56+HLA-DR−	9.9 (8.6–12.6)	8.0 (6.7–13.3)	0.6	6.1 (4.5–9.1)	**0.026**
CD16−CD56+HLA-DR+	19.4 (5.8–37.2)	21.4 (13.2–30.6)	0.8	4.3 (2.7–9.2)	**<0.001**
CD3+CD16+	**2.0 (1.2–4.0)**	**2.5 (1.1–4.2)**	1.0	**1.8 (1.1–3.6)**	0.7
Contaminants/Undefined	**3.6 (3.1–4.2)**	**3.5 (2.5–4.1)**	0.6	**2.4 (1.9–3.9)**	**0.4**

^CF pulmonary exacerbation *versus* CF stable, $CF stable *versus* Non-CF. *After exclusion of MAIT and γ/δ T-cells. Values expressed as percentage of parent population, Median (interquartile range). Significance of between group differences determined by Mann-Whitney U test.

Panel 2: Surface staining was performed by incubation with V500 anti-CD4, FITC anti-TCR Va7.2, PerCP/Cy5.5 anti-CD161, APC/Cy7 anti-CD3, PE anti-TCR γ/δ, PE Texas red Anti-CD8 for 15 minutes at room temperature in the dark. Cells were washed twice in 1 ml of FACS buffer, fixed and resuspended in 300 µl of buffer solution.

Unless stated otherwise, antibodies were obtained for Biolegend, San Diego. Antibody titration was performed to optimise antibody-cell concentration prior to testing.

Sample analysis was performed on a Fortessa IV flow cytometer (BD Biosciences). A lymphocyte gate was set based on forward and side scatter properties and a minimum of 50,000 gated events were capture for each sample.

MAIT cells were defined as $CD3^+/CD4^-/CD8^+$or$-$/$CD161^+$/TCR $Va7.2^+$ [13].

For subjects with CF, automated haemocytometer, absolute lymphocyte counts were obtained and T-cell sub-types were considered as both, absolute numbers of cells per mL of blood and percentage of the whole T-cell population.

Data analysis was performed using Flowjo version 7.6 (Treestar), representative gating plots are available in Figure S2 in File S1.

Statistical Analysis

Statistical analysis was performed using PASW, version 18 (SPSS Inc. Chicago IL, USA) and Graph-pad Prism, version 6. Between group differences in PBMC populations were examined using student's t-test or Mann-Whitney U test. Shapiro-Wilk test and q-q plots were used to determine normal distribution of continuous variables. Non-normally distributed continuous variables (WCC, CRP, MAIT cell absolute count and percentage, B-cell count, NKT-cell and NK-cell percentage) were natural logarithm transformed and Pearson's correlation used to determine relationships between variables. A p-value<0.05 was considered to represent statistical significance.

Results

The characteristics of subjects with CF and healthy controls are provided in Table 1. Thirty-six of the 41 subjects with CF had chronic pulmonary infection with *P. aeruginosa* (either in isolation or in combination with another CF respiratory pathogen) on routine microbiological cultures. The remaining five subjects did not have *P. aeruginosa* infection on current, or previous sputum cultures (Table S1 in File S1 for complete sputum microbiological data).

A greater number of subjects in the pulmonary exacerbation group were male, these subjects were also older, with more severe lung disease, when compared to the stable subjects.

Comparison of lymphocyte sub-sets between groups, demonstrated a reduction in the percentage of MAIT cells in subjects with CF, compared to healthy controls (median 1.1% versus 2.0%, $p = 0.002$), with an accompanying increase in the percentage of γ/δ T-cells (median 10.4% versus 6.4%, $p = 0.012$). CF subjects also displayed reduced percentages of NK-cells (median 9.5% versus

13.1%, $p = 0.013$). The percentage of cells in all of the other major lymphocyte sub-sets was similar between groups (Table 2).

Relationship between MAIT cells, microbiological and clinical parameters in subjects with CF

Absolute MAIT cell concentrations and the proportion of T-cells that were MAIT cells (MAIT cell percentage), in the five subjects without *P. aeruginosa* infection were significantly higher than in patients with chronic *P. aeruginosa* infection (Table 3 and Figure 1A). MAIT cell percentages in subjects not infected with *P. aeruginosa* were similar to healthy controls subjects. No difference was seen in the MAIT cell percentage of subjects with a *P. aeruginosa* infection, based on their co-pathogen (Figure S3 in File S1).

Absolute blood MAIT cell counts in the sub-group of stable CF subjects were higher, when compared to subjects sampled early in the course of treatment for a pulmonary exacerbation (Figure 1B). However, the MAIT cell percentage was similar between stable and pulmonary exacerbation subjects (Table 4).

Absolute MAIT cell count and MAIT cell percentage correlated positively with FEV_1 and FVC percentage predicted. A weak relationship was seen between increased rate of FEV_1 decline and MAIT cells counts, but this did not reach statistical significance (Figure 2).

MAIT cell percentage and absolute MAIT cell concentrations were inversely correlated with CRP ($r = -0.34$, $p = 0.044$ and $r = -0.39$, $p = 0.021$, respectively), however, there was no relationship between MAIT cells and total WCC.

Relationship between γ/δ T-cells, microbiological and clinical parameters in subjects with CF

Absolute γ/δ T-cell counts correlated with FEV_1 and FVC percentage predicted values. A trend toward more rapid rate of lung function decline in FEV_1 was seen in subjects with lower γ/δ T-cells numbers (Figure 2A). No relationship between γ/δ T-cells when expressed as a percentage of total T-cells and lung function parameters was observed (Figure 2B).

γ/δ T-cell percentage and absolute cell number were inversely correlated with CRP ($r = -0.44$, $p = 0.008$) and absolute γ/δ T-cell number was higher in stable CF subjects compared to subjects experiencing a pulmonary exacerbation (Figure S4 in File S1).

There was no relationship between γ/δ T-cell counts or percentages and absolute WCC or profile of infection with *P. aeruginosa* (Table 3).

Relationship between other lymphocyte sub-subset and clinical parameter

Absolute blood lymphocyte count was positively correlated with FEV_1 and FVC (litres and percentage predicted), however, no relationship was seen between absolute WCC and the percentage of the major lymphocyte sub-sets (T-cells, B-cells, NK-cells, CD3+/CD16+ cells) or lung function (Table S2 in File S1).

Total lymphocyte count was decreased in CF subjects being treated for a pulmonary exacerbation.

B-cell percentage was higher in subjects not infected with *P. aeruginosa*, compared to CF subjects with chronic *P. aeruginosa* infection and healthy controls. There was a trend towards lower B-cell percentages in CF subjects during a pulmonary exacerbation compared to stable CF patients (Figure S5A and B in File S1).

Discussion

In this study we demonstrate for the first time that the peripheral blood of subjects with CF is characterized by a relative lymphopenia and major reductions in circulating MAIT cells and to a lesser extent an increase in γ/δ T-cells compared to normal healthy controls, consistent with both quantitative and qualitative differences in innate T-cell immunity in CF. Importantly, lung disease severity, systemic inflammation, clinical status and the presence or absence of chronic *P. aeruginosa* infection were all significantly related to the number of circulating MAIT cells in peripheral blood.

The reduction in absolute lymphocyte counts as lung disease severity increases in the current study is consistent with a single previous study of peripheral blood lymphocytes in children with CF [11]. Similar to this earlier study, a reduction in the percentage of NK-cells was also seen in subjects with CF, however, in contrast, no difference in the percentage of CD4+ T cells was seen and the percentages of other major lymphocyte subsets were similar between CF subjects and healthy control subjects [11]. NK-cells represent an innate, cytotoxic subset of lymphocyte which primarily respond to viral infections and tumour cells [14]. In addition, NK cells provide critical support to the eradication of bacterial pulmonary infection (including *P. aeruginosa*), principally through the generation of Th2 cytokines and IFN-γ [15,16].

A higher percentage of B-cells was seen in CF subjects not infected with *P. aeruginosa* and a trend towards lower concentrations in subjects who were undergoing treatment for an acute pulmonary exacerbation. B-cells are critical for pulmonary protection against encapsulated bacteria and B-cells cultured *in vitro* respond to the mucoid exopolysaccharide of *P. aeruginosa* [17]. Further longitudinal studies are required to delineate the role of B-cells during acute pulmonary exacerbations and to determine whether changes in circulating numbers can be attributed to peripheral destruction, tissue sequestration or transformation to plasma cells.

The association between MAIT cells counts and *P. aeruginosa* infection, severe lung function impairment, increased systemic inflammation and acute pulmonary exacerbations in subjects with CF may suggest that MAIT cell deficiency is associated with susceptibility to pulmonary infection in CF. However, the sub-group of CF subjects undergoing a pulmonary exacerbation may have been biased towards a lower MAIT cell concentration, as more subjects in this sub-group were male and in general they had poorer baseline lung function [18]. Furthermore, these data are cross-sectional and do not inform on whether low MAIT cell numbers contribute to *P. aeruginosa* colonisation and disease progression, or whether low numbers simply reflect depletion of MAIT cells in the circulation, because of recruitment to the airway mucosa.

MAIT cells provide a pivotal link between the innate and adaptive immune responses. The semi-invariant T-cell receptor on MAIT cells recognises metabolite derivatives of pathogens (e.g. vitamin B (riboflavin and folic acid)) presented combined to MR-1 [19]. Activated MAIT cells produce high concentrations of pro-inflammatory interleukin (IL)-17 [20], which invokes a potent cascade of cytokines and chemokines (e.g. IL-8 and G-CSF) that promote neutrophil migration into the airways. Interleukin-17 is involved in neutrophil recruitment in CF and high concentrations have been described in sputum and bronchoalveolar lavage fluid of subjects with CF infected with *P. aeruginosa* and also in those patients with severe disease [21–23].

Mouse models demonstrate MAIT cell recruitment into the lungs at a very early stage of bacterial infection and sustained

MAIT cell responsiveness during the late stages of infection contributes towards an ongoing cytokine response [10]. In mice with selective MAIT cell deficiency the immune response was ineffective in controlling pulmonary infection [10].

Whilst we provide the first description of circulating MAIT cells in CF, understanding of the role of MAIT cells in human disease is limited. A reduction in the proportion of circulating MAIT cells has been reported in subjects with human immunodeficiency virus (HIV), *Mycobacterium tuberculosis* (MTB) and other severe pulmonary infections, and sepsis [7,8,24–26]. In HIV infection, blood MAIT cells concentrations decrease progressively from time of infection, however, MAIT cell density remains relatively preserved in rectal mucosa, suggesting possible preferential recruitment and thus loss from the circulating pool [27,28]. Similarly, MTB reactive MAIT cells are enriched in lung lymph of healthy people when compared to matched blood samples [29]. Collectively, the results of these earlier studies and our current work suggest that although blood MAIT cell counts may not reflect tissue concentrations, they may still prove to be a useful, surrogate biomarker of the immune response within the lung [30]. We demonstrate a strong, inverse relationship between MAIT cell counts and CRP and the specificity of MAIT cell responsiveness to bacterial and fungal infections, offers the potential for improved specificity compared to CRP, which will respond to both viruses and non-infective sources of systemic inflammation [31]. Further mechanistic studies of MAIT cells in CF, including assessment in the actual airway will provide novel insights into their role in innate and adaptive immunity in the CF lung, including whether effective vaccines can be developed that boost MAIT cell function to allow eradication of key bacterial pathogens.

γ/δ T-cells represent a minor population of circulating T-cells, which has the capacity to expand rapidly in response to bacterial infection [32]. γ/δ T-and MAIT cells share many similarities; they both produce IL-17 and preferentially migrate to mucosal surfaces from the circulation [33]. In murine pulmonary infection models, γ/δ T-cells rapidly accumulate in the lung, in response to a range bacterial pathogens, where they facilitate the influx of neutrophils and subsequent bacterial clearance [32]. The small increase in the proportion of γ/δ T-cells in the blood of CF subjects in the current study is consistent with findings of a single previous study in CF [34]. However, the relationship between γ/δ T-cells and clinical parameters in CF subjects were only significant when absolute γ/δ T-cell concentrations were considered and these relationships may simply reflect changes in the absolute numbers of T-cells, rather than any implying any specific role for γ/δ T-cell in pathology.

Our current study has several limitations. Firstly, cross-sectional data collection, does not inform whether a causal relationships exists between lymphocytes subsets and clinical parameters. Furthermore, the limited number of patients included in the analysis of stable disease *versus* pulmonary exacerbation, and inclusion of only five patients not infected with *P. aeruginosa* means type I statistical errors are possible. Longitudinal studies which collect blood samples from the same subject before and after the acquisition of *P. aeruginosa,* or during a pulmonary exacerbation and again during a period of stable disease are required. Finally, blood lymphocyte population may not reflect airway populations and studies which correlate lymphocyte concentrations in airway biopsies to those in the blood are anticipated.

Conclusion

In summary, we describe important differences in the proportions of circulating MAIT and γ/δ T-cell in adult patients with CF, compared to healthy control subjects. Reduced numbers of MAIT cells were associated with *P. aeruginosa* pulmonary infection and more severe lung disease. Our findings provide the impetus for future studies examining the utility of MAIT cells in immunotherapies and vaccine development, and longitudinal studies of MAIT cells as biomarkers of CF pulmonary infection.

Supporting Information

File S1 Tables S1, S2, and Figures S1–S5. Table S1 in File S1. Sputum microbiology of CF subjects. Table S2 in File S1. Relationship between White cell count and lymphocyte subsets, and C-reactive protein, body mass index and lung function. Figure S1 in File S1 Flow diagram of subjects include in sub-group analysis. Figure S2 in File S1 Representative flow-cytometry gating plots. Figure S3 in File S1. MAIT cell percentage in CF subjects with *Pseudomonas aeruginosa* and a co-pathogen in sputum culture. Figure S4 in File S1. Comparison of γ/δ T-cell counts in stable subjects and subjects undergoing antibiotic treatment for a pulmonary exacerbation. Figure S5 in File S1. Comparison of lymphocyte counts and percentage of lymphocyte sub-sets between A. Stable and pulmonary exacerbations B. *P. aeruginosa* infected and non-infected CF subjects.

File S2 Individual Subject Raw Data.

Author Contributions

Conceived and designed the experiments: DS DR GH SB. Performed the experiments: DS. Analyzed the data: DS. Contributed reagents/materials/analysis tools: DS DR GH. Contributed to the writing of the manuscript: DS DR GH SB.

References

1. Elizur A, Cannon CL, Ferkol TW (2008) Airway inflammation in cystic fibrosis. Chest 133: 489–495.
2. Ratner D, Mueller C (2012) Immune responses in Cystic Fibrosis; are they intrinsically defective? Am J Respir Cell Mol Biol.
3. Regamey N, Tsartsali L, Hilliard TN, Fuchs O, Tan HL, et al. (2012) Distinct patterns of inflammation in the airway lumen and bronchial mucosa of children with cystic fibrosis. Thorax 67: 164–170.
4. Moser C, Jensen PO (2011) Adaptive Immune Responses and Biofilm Infections. Biofilm Infections: 201–214.
5. Hartl D, Griese M, Kappler M, Zissel G, Reinhardt D, et al. (2006) Pulmonary T(H)2 response in Pseudomonas aeruginosa-infected patients with cystic fibrosis. J Allergy Clin Immunol 117: 204–211.
6. Moser C, Kjaergaard S, Pressler T, Kharazmi A, Koch C, et al. (2000) The immune response to chronic Pseudomonas aeruginosa lung infection in cystic fibrosis patients is predominantly of the Th2 type. APMIS 108: 329–335.
7. Gold MC, Lewinsohn DM (2013) Co-dependents: MR1-restricted MAIT cells and their antimicrobial function. Nat Rev Microbiol 11: 14–19.
8. Le Bourhis L, Martin E, Peguillet I, Guihot A, Froux N, et al. (2010) Antimicrobial activity of mucosal-associated invariant T cells. Nat Immunol 11: 701–708.
9. Lanier LL (2013) Shades of grey–the blurring view of innate and adaptive immunity. Nat Rev Immunol 13: 73–74.
10. Meierovics A, Yankelevich WJ, Cowley SC (2013) MAIT cells are critical for optimal mucosal immune responses during in vivo pulmonary bacterial infection. Proc Natl Acad Sci U S A 110: E3119–3128.
11. Hausler M, Schweizer K, Biesterfel S, Opladen T, Heimann G (2002) Peripheral decrease and pulmonary homing of CD4+CD45RO+ helper memory T cells in cystic fibrosis. Respir Med 96: 87–94.
12. Autissier P, Soulas C, Burdo TH, Williams KC (2010) Evaluation of a 12-color flow cytometry panel to study lymphocyte, monocyte, and dendritic cell subsets in humans. Cytometry A 77: 410–419.
13. Martin E, Treiner E, Duban L, Guerri L, Laude H, et al. (2009) Stepwise development of MAIT cells in mouse and human. PLoS Biol 7: e54.
14. Hamerman JA, Ogasawara K, Lanier LL (2005) NK cells in innate immunity. Curr Opin Immunol 17: 29–35.

15. Culley FJ (2009) Natural killer cells in infection and inflammation of the lung. Immunology 128: 151–163.
16. Wesselkamper SC, Eppert BL, Motz GT, Lau GW, Hassett DJ, et al. (2008) NKG2D is critical for NK cell activation in host defense against Pseudomonas aeruginosa respiratory infection. J Immunol 181: 5481–5489.
17. Daley L, Pier GB, Liporace JD, Eardley DD (1985) Polyclonal B cell stimulation and interleukin 1 induction by the mucoid exopolysaccharide of Pseudomonas aeruginosa associated with cystic fibrosis. J Immunol 134: 3089–3093.
18. Novak J, Dobrovolny J, Novakova L, Kozak T (2014) The decrease in number and change in phenotype of mucosal-associated invariant T cells in the elderly and differences in males and females of reproductive age. Scand J Immunol.
19. Lopez-Sagaseta J, Dulberger CL, McFedries A, Cushman M, Saghatelian A, et al. (2013) MAIT recognition of a stimulatory bacterial antigen bound to MR1. J Immunol 191: 5268–5277.
20. Dusseaux M, Martin E, Serriari N, Peguillet I, Premel V, et al. (2011) Human MAIT cells are xenobiotic-resistant, tissue-targeted, CD161hi IL-17-secreting T cells. Blood 117: 1250–1259.
21. McAllister F, Henry A, Kreindler JL, Dubin PJ, Ulrich L, et al. (2005) Role of IL-17A, IL-17F, and the IL-17 receptor in regulating growth-related oncogene-alpha and granulocyte colony-stimulating factor in bronchial epithelium: implications for airway inflammation in cystic fibrosis. J Immunol 175: 404–412.
22. Tan HL, Regamey N, Brown S, Bush A, Lloyd CM, et al. (2011) The Th17 pathway in cystic fibrosis lung disease. Am J Respir Crit Care Med 184: 252–258.
23. Tiringer K, Treis A, Fucik P, Gona M, Gruber S, et al. (2013) A Th17- and Th2-skewed cytokine profile in cystic fibrosis lungs represents a potential risk factor for Pseudomonas aeruginosa infection. Am J Respir Crit Care Med 187: 621–629.
24. Grimaldi D, Le Bourhis L, Sauneuf B, Dechartres A, Rousseau C, et al. (2014) Specific MAIT cell behaviour among innate-like T lymphocytes in critically ill patients with severe infections. Intensive Care Med 40: 192–201.
25. Wong EB, Akilimali NA, Govender P, Sullivan ZA, Cosgrove C, et al. (2013) Low levels of peripheral CD161++CD8+ mucosal associated invariant T (MAIT) cells are found in HIV and HIV/TB co-infection. PLoS One 8: e83474.
26. Jiang J, Wang X, An H, Yang B, Cao Z, et al. (2014) Mucosal-associated Invariant T-Cell Function Is Modulated by Programmed Death-1 Signaling in Patients with Active Tuberculosis. Am J Respir Crit Care Med 190: 329–339.
27. Cosgrove C, Ussher JE, Rauch A, Gartner K, Kurioka A, et al. (2013) Early and nonreversible decrease of CD161++/MAIT cells in HIV infection. Blood 121: 951–961.
28. Leeansyah E, Ganesh A, Quigley MF, Sonnerborg A, Andersson J, et al. (2013) Activation, exhaustion, and persistent decline of the antimicrobial MR1-restricted MAIT-cell population in chronic HIV-1 infection. Blood 121: 1124–1135.
29. Gold MC, Cerri S, Smyk-Pearson S, Cansler ME, Vogt TM, et al. (2010) Human mucosal associated invariant T cells detect bacterially infected cells. PLoS Biol 8: e1000407.
30. Shoki AH, Mayer-Hamblett N, Wilcox PG, Sin DD, Quon BS (2013) Systematic review of blood biomarkers in cystic fibrosis pulmonary exacerbations. Chest 144: 1659–1670.
31. Levy H, Kalish LA, Huntington I, Weller N, Gerard C, et al. (2007) Inflammatory markers of lung disease in adult patients with cystic fibrosis. Pediatr Pulmonol 42: 256–262.
32. Ito M, Kojiro N, Ikeda T, Ito T, Funada J, et al. (1992) Increased proportions of peripheral blood gamma delta T cells in patients with pulmonary tuberculosis. Chest 102: 195–197.
33. Sutton CE, Mielke LA, Mills KH (2012) IL-17-producing gammadelta T cells and innate lymphoid cells. Eur J Immunol 42: 2221–2231.
34. Raga S, Julia MR, Crespi C, Figuerola J, Martinez N, et al. (2003) Gammadelta T lymphocytes from cystic fibrosis patients and healthy donors are high TNF-alpha and IFN-gamma-producers in response to Pseudomonas aeruginosa. Respir Res 4: 9.

Swimming Motility in a Longitudinal Collection of Clinical Isolates of *Burkholderia cepacia* Complex Bacteria from People with Cystic Fibrosis

James E. A. Zlosnik*, Paul Y. Mori, Derek To, James Leung, Trevor J. Hird, David P. Speert

Centre for Understanding and Preventing Infection in Children, Department of Pediatrics, Faculty of Medicine, University of British Columbia, Vancouver, British Columbia, Canada

Abstract

Chronic bacterial lung infections in cystic fibrosis (CF) are the leading cause of morbidity and mortality. While a range of bacteria are known to be capable of establishing residence in the CF lung, only a small number have a clearly established link to deteriorating clinical status. The two bacteria with the clearest roles in CF lung disease are *Pseudomonas aeruginosa* and bacteria belonging to the *Burkholderia cepacia* complex (BCC). A number of common adaptations by *P. aeruginosa* strains to chronic lung infection in CF have been well described. Typically, initial isolates of *P. aeruginosa* are nonmucoid and display a range of putative virulence determinants. Upon establishment of chronic infection, subsequent isolates ultimately show a reduction in putative virulence determinants, including swimming motility, along with an acquisition of the mucoid phenotype and increased levels of antimicrobial resistance. Infections by BCC are marked by an unpredictable, but typically worse, clinical outcome. However, in contrast to *P. aeruginosa* infections in CF, studies describing adaptive changes in BCC bacterial phenotype during chronic lung infections are far more limited. To further enhance our understanding of chronic lung infections by BCC bacteria in CF, we assessed the swimming motility phenotype in 551 isolates of BCC bacteria from cystic fibrosis (CF) lung infections between 1981 and 2007. These data suggest that swimming motility is not typically lost by BCC during chronic infection, unlike as seen in *P. aeruginosa* infections. Furthermore, while we observed a statistically significant link between mucoidy and motility, we did not detect any link between motility phenotype and clinical outcome. These studies highlight the need for further work to understand the adaptive changes of BCC bacteria during chronic infection in the CF lung.

Editor: Tom Coenye, Ghent University, Belgium

Funding: This work was supported by a Cystic Fibrosis Canada (www.cysticfibrosis.ca) operating grant to DPS (20R32976) and a fellowship to JZ. The funders had no role in study design, data collection and analysis, decision to publish, or preparation of the manuscript.

Competing Interests: The authors have declared that no competing interests exits.

* Email: jzlosnik@cfri.ubc.ca

Introduction

People with cystic fibrosis (CF) experience chronic lung infections, lasting years and sometimes decades. These lung infections are the main cause of morbidity and mortality in CF, leading to either lung transplantation or death through cumulative damage to the lungs. A number of bacterial species are associated with chronic infection in the CF endobronchial space [1,2]. Bacteria belonging to the *Burkholderia cepacia* complex (BCC) are particularly concerning to the CF community due to their well-documented capacity for inter-patient transmission and an association with an unpredictable but typically worse outcome [1,3,4]. The BCC comprises at least 18 distinct species of bacteria and all, except for *B. ubonensis*, have been isolated from the lungs of people with CF [5,6]. Historically, *B. cenocepacia* has been the most common and problematic species in many CF centres. However, the epidemiology of BCC bacteria in CF appears to be changing, with *B. multivorans* becoming the most common cause of new BCC infection in CF in number of studies [1,7]

The most common pathogen in CF is *Pseudomonas aeruginosa* [1]. Numerous studies have described a range of common adaptations to chronic infection by *P. aeruginosa*. The current paradigm for *P. aeruginosa* infections in CF involves infection with a virulent nonmucoid strain, which, upon establishment of chronic infection, ultimately converts to the mucoid phenotype through the production of exopolysaccharide alginate [8]. In addition, a range of other adaptations have been described, which presumably enhance the capacity for survival in the CF lung [9,10]. These often include the loss of a range of putative virulence determinants such as a quorum sensing and swimming motility as well as acquisition of other traits such as increased antibiotic resistance, serum sensitivity through loss of LPS O-polysaccharide and hypermutability [10–15].

Currently published data suggest that the pathogenic mechanisms employed by BCC bacteria in chronic CF lung infections may in fact be distinct from those observed in *P. aeruginosa*. For instance, a recent survey of sequential clinical isolates from a number of CF patients attending the Vancouver CF clinics who had been chronically infected with BCC indicated that, unlike *P.*

aeruginosa, BCC maintain quorum sensing systems during chronic infection in the CF lung [16]. Recent transcriptomic and proteomic studies on isolates of *B. cenocepacia* from a single chronic infection have also suggested that virulence may be increased in isolates taken from later in chronic infection [17,18]. In addition to these experimental data, the apparent aggressiveness of BCC bacteria in CF is also consistent with BCC bacteria deploying differential pathogenic mechanisms during chronic infections. Most notable is the well described capacity for BCC to cause a typically fatal invasive necrotizing pneumonia known as 'cepacia syndrome', which has commonly been associated with *B. cenocepacia* but is also known to occur in other species including *B. multivorans* and *B. dolosa* [19–21]. Invasive disease is rarely, if ever, seen in *P. aeruginosa* infections in CF.

In contrast to *P. aeruginosa*, studies on adaptation to chronic lung infections in CF by BCC are very limited. We have previously shown that, unlike *P. aeruginosa*, the nonmucoid phenotype is associated with a worse outcome in terms of lung function decline and survival, while mucoid to nonmucoid transitions are common in adaptation to chronic infection [22,23]. Other studies have also documented BCC phenotypic colonial morphology variation in the context of chronic CF lung infections [24]. Variation in some other phenotypic traits has been described in clinical isolates of BCC bacteria, most notably, in antimicrobial susceptibility profiles, in the context of chronic CF infections [25,26]. Recently, whole genome sequencing of sequential isolates from multiple patients in an outbreak of *B. dolosa* in the United States also revealed a number of candidate pathogenicity genes that appear to be commonly mutated during chronic infection and may confer elevated virulence on this species [27].

We have previously described an association between colonial morphology and motility, whereby increased flagellin protein production and swimming motility were detected in a shiny colony clonal variant that was obtained from an infection model where the infection had been established with an isolate that demonstrated a matte colony morphology [28,29]. The swimming motility phenotype is also of interest, due to the well described capacity for bacterial flagella to stimulate inflammation through the TLR5 pathogen recognition receptor as well as its involvement in epithelial invasion by BCC bacteria [30–34]. In this study we examine the clinical significance of motility in BCC bacteria. We report the largest assessment to date of swimming motility from a longitudinal collection of over 550 BCC isolates, collected at least annually from 100 CF patients attending the Vancouver clinics during the period June 1981–June 2007.

Materials and Methods

Bacterial isolates

Bacteria were collected from CF patients at least annually between June 1981 and June 2007 from the Vancouver CF clinics as described previously [23]. Briefly we examined 551 isolates from 100 patients. For patients culturing BCC this collection typically contains at least one isolate per year. Bacteria were routinely stored by freezing confluent growth, taken from a purity plate, at $-80°C$ in Mueller Hinton broth (Oxoid) plus 8% dimethyl sulfoxide. For experiments, bacteria were revived on a Columbia Blood Agar plate, and a fresh culture was established the day prior to the experiment on a Luria Bertani (LB) agar plate (10 g l^{-1} tryptone, 5 g l^{-1} yeast extract, 10 g l^{-1} sodium chloride) containing 1.5% agar. All plates were incubated overnight at 35°C.

Swimming motility

Swimming motility for each isolate was individually assessed on LB supplemented with 0.3% agar plates as previously described [11]. Briefly, plates were poured on the bench with no drying time and then used the same day. Growth from the confluent area of a freshly cultured plate was inoculated into the center of the swimming motility agar plates using a sterilized wooden stick. Motility plates were then incubated for 48 hours at 35°C in stacks 4 plates high, the plates were kept upright and not inverted. At 48 hours the diameter of the colonial growth was measured. Isolates with less than or equal to 10 mm growth at 48 hours were classified as nonmotile, while those with >10 mm growth were classified as motile. Motile and nonmotile controls, *P. aeruginosa* PAK and *P. aeruginosa* PAK *ΔfliC* [35], were run in all experiments.

Western blotting

Whole protein extractions from BCC bacteria were prepared as described previously [11]. Briefly, bacterial growth was scraped from the confluent area of a freshly grown agar plate using a sterile wooden stick and resuspended in 1 ml of 1.5 mM Tris.Cl pH 7.5. The bacteria were then added to an equal volume of 0.1 mm diameter glass beads in a 2 ml screw cap centrifuge tube (Lysing Matrix B, MP Biomedicals). Bacterial cells were then broken with 3 rounds of beating in a FastPrep ribolyzer (ThermoSavant) set to speed 6.5 for 45 seconds. Cellular debris was pelleted by centrifugation at 18,400 x *g* in a Hettich Mikro 200 microcentrifuge. 250 µl of supernatant was then removed to harvest the extracted protein. Protein concentration was determined using the Micro BCA protein assay kit (Pierce). 15 or 25 µg of protein was separated on a 12% acrylamide gel, proteins were transferred to a PVDF membrane by electroblotting and then probed using a 1 in 10,000 dilution of an anti-*Burkholderia pseudomallei* flagellin antibody [36] as described previously [37]. Blots were visualized either using chemiluminensce (Amersham ECL detection kit, GE Healthcare) with a 1 in 10,000 dilution of an anti-rabbit HRP linked secondary antibody (Cell Signalling) or green fluorescence using a 1 in 10,000 dilution of a goat anti-rabbit IRDye 800CW secondary antibody (Licor) on an Odyssey (Licor) infrared imaging system. Blots were performed in at least triplicate for all isolates examined.

TLR5 stimulatory assays

TLR5 activation was assessed using a TLR5-NF-κB luciferase reporter system as described previously [32]. Briefly, bacterial cells were grown overnight in 3 mls of LB broth at 37°C on an orbital rotator. Bacterial cells were harvested by centrifugation (2,340 x *g* for 5 minutes) and washed twice in phosphate buffered saline and adjusted to 2.5×10^6 CFU ml^{-1}. Heat killed bacteria (30 mins at 65°C) were then added to 5×10^4 freshly cultured CHO-K1 cells containing the TLR5-NF-κB luciferase reporter, representing an MOI of 50:1, and incubated for 4 hrs in 96-well plates. CHO-K1 cells were routinely cultured both before and during experiments in F-12 K media (Gibco). Activation of the TLR5-NF-κB luciferase reporter was then assessed using a luciferase assay (Promega) and a Tecan Infinite M200 plate reader. Luminescence was measured by injecting 50 µl of substrate into each well, with an injection speed of 200 µl sec^{-1}, and luminescence was measured over an integration time of 5 seconds. All values are expressed relative to an unstimulated control containing only the reporter cell line and no bacteria. TLR5 activation assays were performed on five separate occasions for each isolate and in triplicate on each occasion.

Clinical data

Clinical data were previously collected for all patients included in the study [22]. We employed the same inclusion/exclusion criteria in this study. The clinical data included in this manuscript was obtained following approval the Providence Healthcare Research Ethics Board - part of the UBC Research Ethics Boards (H07-01396). Informed consent was not required as the data was analysed in aggregate and de-linked from any patient identifiers.

Statistical analysis

All motility data were collected and stored in a Microsoft Access 2010 database. For analysis, data were exported initially to Microsoft Excel 2010 and then transferred to GraphPad Prism V.4. Data were graphed using either Microsoft Excel 2010 directly or exported to GraphPad Prism V.4. All statistical analyses were performed with appropriate statistical tests using GraphPad Prism V.4.

Results

Prevalence of the motile phenotype in clinical isolates of BCC in the Vancouver CF population 1981–2007

Isolates from people with CF infected with BCC are routinely collected and stored in our laboratory at least annually. We have previously reported data from this collection, describing the prevalence of the mucoid phenotype in Vancouver isolates of BCC from CF infections between June 1981 and June 2007 [23]. Given the well-described loss of swimming motility in *P. aeruginosa* during chronic CF lung infections, we assessed our isolate collection for swimming motility in order to understand the significance of swimming motility during chronic BCC infections in CF. An examination of the full isolate collection revealed that both motile and nonmotile isolates of all species were present, with the exception of *B. cepacia* for which there were only four isolates that were all motile and *B. metallica* for which the sole isolate was motile (Table 1). In total we examined 551 isolates from 100 patients. *B. cenocepacia* is traditionally considered the most virulent of the BCC species, so it is notable that a larger percentage - 38% - of *B. cenocepacia* isolates examined were nonmotile as opposed to 14% of *B. multivorans* (Table 1). We also assessed the extent of motility displayed by these isolates, in terms of the diameter of the resultant colony when *B. cenocepacia* and *B. multivorans* were grown on swimming motility agar. These data show that, consistent with this trend, *B. cenocepacia* isolates on average exhibit considerably smaller diameter of colonial growth than *B. multivorans* on swim plates (Fig 1). In fact only 1% of *B. cenocepacia* isolates in our collection possessed the capacity to swim across the entire plate, whereas 16% of *B. multivorans* isolates possessed this capacity (Fig 1).

Motility and the mucoid phenotype

Previous studies of clonal variants in *B. cenocepacia* taken from a CF lung infection have found that nonmucoid variants demonstrated loss of swimming motility capacity [24,38]. Unlike *P. aeruginosa*, the mucoid phenotype is not visually detectable on LB-agar motility plates [23]. Therefore any differences observed in the diameter of growth on swimming motility plates used in this study is due to the swimming motility phenotype, rather than excess elaboration of exopolysaccharide in mucoid isolates. Even though the mucoid phenotype does not manifest itself visually on LB agar plates it is conceivable there still could be a link between EPS production capacity and swimming motility. As we have previously assessed the mucoid phenotype in these isolates [23], we examined the swimming motility phenotype in relation to the mucoid phenotype. These data support previous observations, showing a general, but not absolute, correlation between the extent of mucoidy, scored from – to +++ and capacity for swimming motility as measured by the diameter of bacterial growth after 48 hours at 35°C (Fig 2). This trend was statistically significant (Kruskal-Wallis $p<0.0001$). Breaking down these data into species, the same trend was observable for both *B. multivorans* and *B. cenocepacia* (Fig 2), which was statistically significant for both species (data not shown).

The motility phenotype in relation to clinical outcome in BCC lung infections in people with cystic fibrosis

Given that initial colonizing isolates of *P. aeruginosa* infection in CF are typically motile, while phenotype switches to nonmotility are commonly seen in later isolates, we were interested in assessing the clinical significance of the BCC swimming motility phenotype. In the context of the 89 clinical infections where there was infection by a single clone, 51/89 infections only ever had motile BCC isolated while 19/89 were only ever nonmotile, indicating that nonmotile isolates of BCC may be competent to initiate and maintain infection (Fig. 3A). We also examined the dataset to look at infections where there was clear evidence of chronic infection (defined as the presence in our collection of at least three different isolates of the same strain type over the period of at least a year, $n = 48$). Swimming motility phenotype switches were detected during chronic infection, but only in a minority of cases (11/48). Like *P. aeruginosa*, these switches were always motile to nonmotile, although they were often accompanied by subsequent isolation of motile variants (data not shown). Previous RAPD typing of these isolates [23] indicated that all cases of swimming motility phenotype switching took place in sequential clonal isolates and therefore were not replacement infections (data not shown). In total these data represent over 214 patient years of BCC infection data and an average of 8.5 isolates per patient for chronic infections.

We also sought to assess the clinical impact of the different phenotypes (Fig 3B). Patient data were previously collected and this study was approved by the UBC research ethics boards [22]. For cases for which we have suitable follow up clinical data ($n = 52$), as defined by our previous criteria [22], we assessed the post infection decline in lung function, using Forced Expiratory Volume in one second (FEV1), % predicted. The mean annual post-infection lung function decline was 4.0% FEV1 % predicted for those infected with motile BCC bacteria ($n = 32$), while those only infected with nonmotile BCC bacteria ($n = 5$) had a mean annual decline of 8.2% FEV1% predicted. Patients who were colonized with either mixed motile phenotypes ($n = 5$) or those where there was clear evidence of a motile to nonmotile phenotype switch ($n = 10$) had annual post-infection FEV1% predicted declines of 4.4% and 3.0% respectively. Among all groups, these data demonstrated no significant differences between patients infected with motile or nonmotile BCC, irrespective of whether we examined all cases (Kruskal-Wallis $p = 0.273$, Fig. 3B) or just those for whom chronic infection (defined as the presence in our collection of 3 or more isolates over a period of a year or more) was documented ($n = 34$, Kruskal-Wallis $p = 0.174$, data not shown).

The effects of loss of motility on the biological properties of BCC bacteria during chronic infection

To assess the biological consequence of the motile to nonmotile switches, we investigated the production of flagellum protein by Western blot using a polyclonal antibody [36] raised against *B.*

Table 1. Prevalence of swimming motility in isolates of *B. cepacia complex* from cystic fibrosis infections in Vancouver from 1981–2008.

	Total number of isolates tested, *n*	Nonmotile, *n* (%)	Motile, *n* (%)
B. cepacia	4	0 (0)	4 (100)
B. multivorans	207	29 (14)	178 (86)
B. cenocepacia	294	111 (38)	183 (62)
B. stabilis	10	3 (30)	7 (70)
B. vietnamiensis	35	23 (66)	12 (34)
B. metallica	1	0 (0)	1 (100)

pseudomallei flagellin, as described previously [37]. We examined isolates from 5 patients in whom there was a switch from motility to nonmotility in later isolates. These cases were selected to represent *B. multivorans* as well as most of the major epidemic lineages of *B. cenocepacia* (RAPD types 01, 04 and 06). In addition, we also examined a well-described isolate of the RAPD02/ET-12 lineage, K56-2. In most cases, lack of motility was associated with a loss of detectable flagellin protein, however flagellin protein was detected in 2 nonmotile isolates (C9343 and VC8402) from two patients in which there had been a phenotype switch from motile to nonmotile (Table 1). Given the role flagella play in activating inflammation through the pattern recognition receptor TLR5, we also assessed TLR5 activation in these isolates using a TLR5-NF-κB luciferase reporter assay system as described previously [32]. Motile isolates demonstrated significantly increased TLR5 activation compared to nonmotile isolates (2.88 vs 2.10 fold compared to unstimulated controls, unpaired one tailed *t*-test $p = 0.0092$).

Discussion

Chronic bacterial infections in CF are particularly difficult to model *ex-vivo*, in part due to the length of time that bacteria are resident in the CF lung, making it hard to mimic conditions of the CF lung using either *in vitro* or animal/plant model systems. The inability to effectively model CF lung infections in the laboratory makes it challenging to understand the contribution any given bacterial trait may have towards disease severity or to understand the adaptive mechanisms bacteria use to facilitate chronic residence in the CF lung. There are a large range of putative virulénce determinants now described for BCC bacteria, for a recent review see [39], however, for the most part, the clinical significance of these determinants is unclear. In addition, there is a growing range of *ex-vivo* models for BCC infection, however there is little consistency among these models in terms of conserved virulence determinants and in any case none of the models truly mimics CF infection [40].

Swimming motility is well described as an adaptive trait in *P. aeruginosa* infections in CF whereby initial infection is typically by

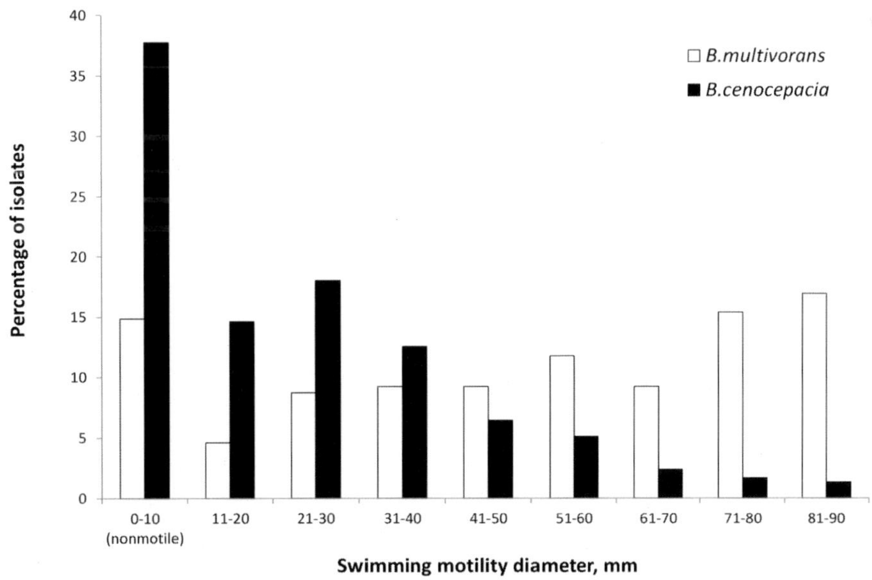

Figure 1. Analysis of swimming motility capacity of *B. multivorans* (white bars) and *B. cenocepacia* (black bars) isolates from cystic fibrosis lung infections in Vancouver between 1981 and 2008. Motility was assessed by inoculating bacteria into the center of a motility agar plate and incubating for 48 hrs, after which the diameter was measured. Isolates were classified as motile if colonial diameter was >10 mm and nonmotile if the diameter was less than or equal to 10 mm.

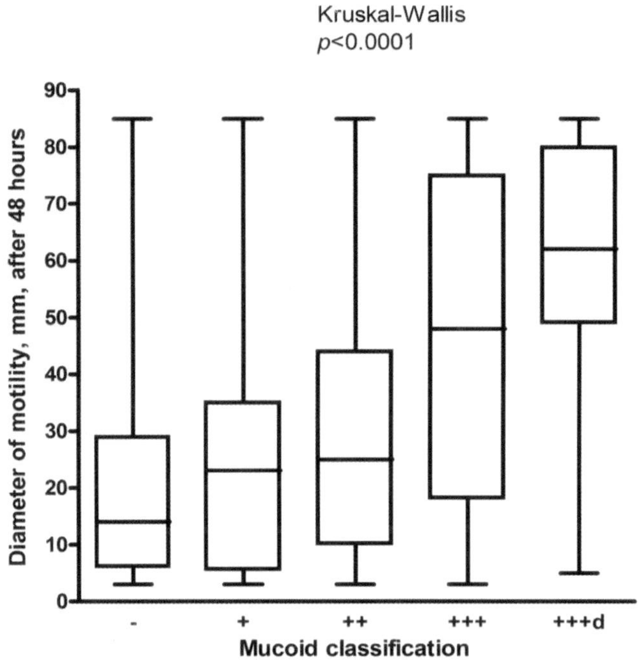

All BCC isolates, median (IQR)	**14 (6-29)**	**23 (5.5-35)**	**25 (10-44)**	**48 (18-75)**	**62 (49-80)**
B. cenocepacia, median (IQR)	14 (5-28.5)	25.5 (10.5-37)	25 (9-38)	24 (7.5-51)	49 (27.5-62.5)
B. multivorans, median (IQR)	29 (13-52)	38 (6-56)	38.5 (14.5-65.5)	64.5 (7.5-51)	70 (53.5-84)
BCC other species, median (IQR)	11.5 (6.5-19.5)	4 (3.5-10.5)	9 (5-13)	8 (-)	85 (-)

Figure 2. Motility and the mucoid phenotype in BCC. Box and Whisker plot of motility phenotype compared to the mucoid phenotype (as previously assessed: [23]) in all isolates of *B. cepacia* complex assessed for which we had corresponding mucoid scores ($n = 541$). Statistical significance was assessed by the non parametic Kruskal-Wallis one-way analysis of variance in GraphPad Prism v.4. Data were also analyzed separately for *B. cenocepacia* ($n = 288$) and *B. multivorans* ($n = 203$) as well as all the remaining species examined ($n = 50$) and the medians and inter-quartile range (IQR) are provided in the box below the figure. IQRs could not be calculated for BCC other species scored +++ and +++d because there were only 3 and 1 isolates in those categories respectively.

a motile isolate which can convert to a nonmotile phenotype later in chronic infection [11,14]. The swimming motility phenotype is also well described in BCC bacteria and is mediated by a single polar flagellum [41–43]. *In-vitro* experiments have shown that the BCC flagellum facilitates invasion into epithelial cells *in-vitro* and promotion of inflammatory markers [34,44]. The clinical significance of motility in chronic BCC lung infections in CF, however, is not clear.

In order to describe the significance of motility in clinical isolates of BCC we examined our collection of BCC taken on a regular basis from people with CF. Aside from the longitudinal nature of our BCC collection, a strength of this study is that our collection contains large numbers of the two most commonly isolated species from the BCC: *B. cenocepacia* and *B. multivorans*. Our data reveal that both motile and nonmotile isolates can be recovered from CF lung infections for all species examined, except for *B. cepacia* for which we only had 4 isolates from a single infection and *B. metallica* for which we had only one isolate (Table 1). Stratifying infections into 'motility phenotypes' revealed that isolates from the majority of chronic infections most commonly display the motile phenotype throughout the infection and do not normally switch to nonmotile (Fig 3A). We identified a limited number of infections where nonmotile isolates were the only phenotype ever isolated, suggesting that nonmotile BCC bacteria are also competent to initiate infection. However, these data must be understood in the context that although they were the first recovered isolates, the duration of colonization prior to the first positive culture cannot be determined. Additionally, although there was minimal passage of the bacteria between the lung and storage, it is still conceivable that phenotype switching may have already taken place as a consequence of adaptation to growth either in the lung or in the lab. Nonetheless, by examining archived bacterial isolates, the approach we have taken in this study is identical to that used by us to describe the evolution of *P. aeruginosa* motility in the CF lung [11].

A number of studies have examined adaptation of BCC bacteria to various *in-vitro* growth environments [45–49]. However, there are currently little data on adaptive strategies of BCC bacteria to chronic pulmonary infection in CF. This study adds to other evidence [16,22] which suggest that at least some of the mechanisms of pathogenesis in BCC bacterial lung disease are distinct from those described for *P. aeruginosa*. Our data indicate

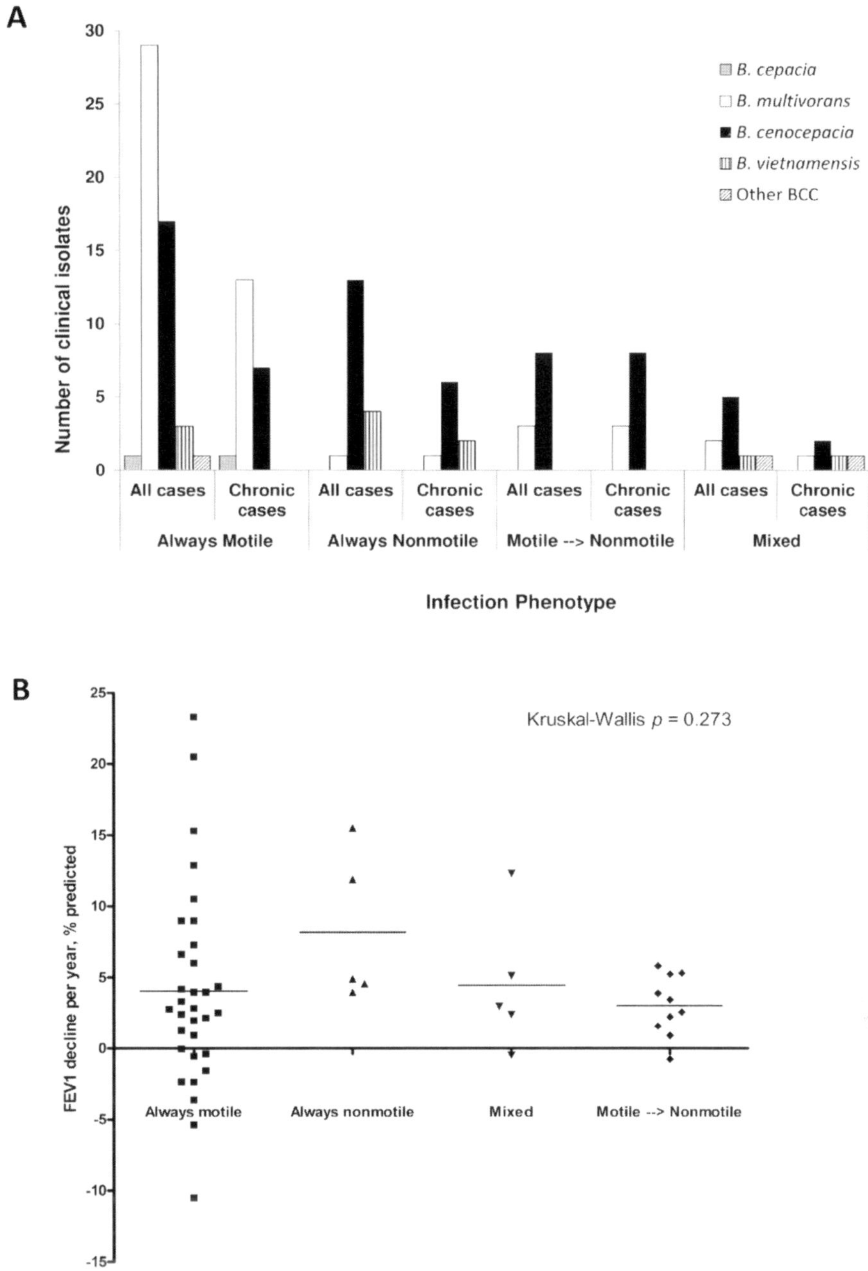

Figure 3. Assessment of clinical significance of swimming motility in BCC bacteria. A) CF lung infections categorized by species and motility phenotype. Data are displayed for all cases ($n = 89$) and for cases where chronic infection ($n = 48$) was clearly established (defined as the presence in our collection of at least 2 or more isolates of the same strain type that were collected at least a year apart). Grey bars = *B. cepacia*, white bars = *B. multivorans*, black bars = *B. cenocepacia*; vertical striped bars = *B. vietnamiensis* and diagonal striped bars = other BCC species. Infections were categorized as: isolates were always motile; always nonmotile; motile to nonmotile phenotype switches detected during infection (as defined by an initial isolation of at least 2 separate motile isolates on separate months followed by a nonmotile isolate at any point thereafter) or mixed (there was no clear established initial swimming motility phenotype as the first two isolates stored for patients on separate months demonstrated both motile and nonmotile phenotypes). One case was also classified as mixed (FEV1% predicted decline −0.5%) as most isolates were nonmotile, however several marginally motile (diameter 11 and 12 mm) isolates were detected during the course of the patients' infection. B) Assessment of the impact of motility phenotype on FEV1 decline following initial infection with BCC. FEV1 data were collected from the patient charts as described previously. Criteria for inclusion were established previously [22]. Data were analyzed in GraphPad Prism v.4 and the non-parametric Kruskal-Wallis test calculated to assess difference.

that loss of motility is not a common adaptive feature in BCC bacteria to chronic lung infection, as opposed to *P. aeruginosa* (Fig 3A). Examination of the biological properties of sequential clonal isolates from infections where there was switch from motile to nonmotile phenotypes (Table 2), revealed that loss of motility is often, but not always, associated with a loss of detectable flagellin protein by Western blot. Consistent with published data [33], we also show that conversion to the nonmotile phenotype was associated with a reduction in TLR-5 stimulator capacity (Table 2).

Table 2. Biological characteristics of motile and nonmotile CF clinical isolates of *Burkholderia cepacia* complex bacteria.

Patient	Isolate	Species	Date of isolation	Strain type (RAPD)	Motility	Flagella Western blot	TLR5 activity
A	C3921	BC	Oct 1990	001	+	+	1.95 (0.44)
	C8963	BC	Jan 2000	001	–	–	2.00 (0.27)
	C9343	BC	Oct 2000	001	–	+	2.99 (0.56)
B	VC3868	BC	Aug 1990	004	+	+	3.35 (0.69)
	VC9670	BC	Jun 1999	004	–	–	1.82 (0.26)
	VC13450	BC	Jul 2006	004	–	–	1.99 (0.29)
C	VC6432	BC	Jul 1994	006	+	+	3.38 (0.78)
	VC8402	BC	Sep 1997	006	–	+	2.47 (0.59)
D	VC2307	BC	Apr 1987	006	+	+	3.71 (1.00)
	VC6905	BC	Mar 1995	006	–	–	1.82 (1.00)
E	VC12201	BC	Jan 2004	009	+	+	3.10 (0.58)
	VC13307	BC	Mar 2006	009	–	–	1.87 (0.25)
F	VC12539	BM	Sep 2004	BM-044	+	+	1.86 (0.25)
	VC13732	BM	Mar 2007	BM-044	–	–	1.85 (0.32)
n/a	K56-2	BC	–	002	+	+	3.03 (0.41)

Date of isolation = month/year. Species: BC = *B. cenocepacia*, BM = *B. multivorans*. Strain types were determined previously for these isolates by RAPD [23,50]. Western blotting was performed on whole cell extracts using a polyclonal anti-*B. pseudomallei* flagella antibody [36] as we have described previously [37]. Results are representative of three independent experiments and are positive or negative for the presence of a band at either 45 kDa or 55 kDa – the variants of flagella known to be produced by BCC bacteria [41]. TLR5 activation values are the mean of assays performed in triplicate on five separate occasions, with standard error of the mean in brackets.

These data further support the contention that the adaptive strategies used by BCC in chronic CF lung infections are distinct from those described for *P. aeruginosa* and therefore BCC merits separate consideration. While phenotype conversion, from motile to nonmotile, did occur during chronic infection, it was not common and was often accompanied by the subsequent isolation of motile isolates from the same infection (Figure 3A). Other data from this isolate collection also supports this suggestion. One study has shown that BCC maintain functional quorum sensing signaling systems during chronic infection, whereas isolation of quorum sensing mutants during chronic *P. aeruginosa* infections in CF is common [16,22]. Meanwhile we have also shown that conversion to the nonmucoid phenotype in BCC infections is common, while the extent of mucoidy is inversely related to survival and outcome, also in contrast to *P. aeruginosa* [22,23].

Our data are supportive of a link between motility and the mucoid phenotype as has previously been described by others [24,38]. This correlation was seen both when all isolates were examined and in both *B. multivorans* and *B. cenocepacia* isolates when examined separately (Figure 2). Nonetheless, it is notable that there is considerable variation in all mucoid classes in their capacity for swimming motility and we identified both nonmotile and motile nonmucoid isolates (considered as mucoid scores – and +) as well as nonmotile and motile mucoid isolates (considered as mucoid scores ++/+++/+++d) (Fig 2). Therefore our data indicate that, while there is a significant trend, the connection between swimming motility and the mucoid colonial morphology phenotype is not absolute. Given our previously described link between mucoidy and outcome [22,23], the link described here between mucoidy and motility might suggest that there would be a link with patient outcome in terms of lung function decline. However, we did not observe a link between motility and clinical outcome (Fig 3B). Conclusions from these data are limited by the small numbers of cases in the nonmotile group in particular ($n = 5$) and therefore this question requires further investigation in another population containing larger numbers of nonmotile infections.

We believe this study is the most comprehensive analysis to date of the swimming motility phenotype in clinical isolates of BCC bacteria. Based on these data, it appears that differences in the motility phenotype do not contribute significantly to the severity of BCC lung disease in CF. We suggest, however, that these data and others indicate that the pathogenic mechanisms of BCC bacteria in CF lung disease need to be considered separately from those that have been observed for *P. aeruginosa*. The assertion is supported by the clinical picture, where BCC have a well-established elevated risk of mortality/lung transplantation and can result in an invasive necrotizing pneumonia known as 'cepacia syndrome' rarely if ever seen in *P. aeruginosa* infections [3,20]. As a consequence further studies on adaptation to the CF lung, using clinical isolates with matched clinical data from patients are merited.

Acknowledgments

We would like to thank Don Woods for the generous provision of the anti-*Burkholderia pseudomallei* flagellum antibody. We would also like to thank Stuart Turvey for the provision of reagents and the TLR-5 reporter cell line. This work was supported by a Cystic Fibrosis Canada operating grant to DPS (20R32976) and a Cystic Fibrosis Canada Postdoctoral Fellowship to JEAZ.

Author Contributions

Conceived and designed the experiments: JZ DS. Performed the experiments: JZ PM DT JL TH. Analyzed the data: JZ. Contributed to the writing of the manuscript: JZ DS.

References

1. Lipuma JJ (2010) The changing microbial epidemiology in cystic fibrosis. Clin Microbiol Rev 23: 299–323. doi:10.1128/CMR.00068-09.
2. Hauser AR, Jain M, Bar-Meir M, McColley SA (2011) Clinical Significance of Microbial Infection and Adaptation in Cystic Fibrosis. Clin Microbiol Rev 24: 29–70. doi:10.1128/CMR.00036-10.
3. Corey M, Farewell V (1996) Determinants of mortality from cystic fibrosis in Canada, 1970–1989. Am J Epidemiol 143: 1007–1017.
4. LiPuma JJ, Dasen SE, Nielson DW, Stern RC, Stull TL (1990) Person-to-person transmission of Pseudomonas cepacia between patients with cystic fibrosis. Lancet 336: 1094–1096.
5. Vandamme P, Dawyndt P (2011) Classification and identification of the Burkholderia cepacia complex: Past, present and future. Syst Appl Microbiol 34: 87–95. doi: 10.1016/j.syapm.2010.10.002.
6. Peeters C, Zlosnik JEA, Spilker T, Hird TJ, Lipuma JJ, et al. (2013) Burkholderia pseudomultivorans sp. nov., a novel Burkholderia cepacia complex species from human respiratory samples and the rhizosphere. Syst Appl Microbiol 36: 48–489. doi: 10.1016/j.syapm.2013.06.003.
7. Govan JR, Brown AR, Jones AM (2007) Evolving epidemiology of Pseudomonas aeruginosa and the Burkholderia cepacia complex in cystic fibrosis lung infection. Futur Microbiol 2: 153–164. doi: 10.2217/17460913.2.2.153.
8. Martin DW, Schurr MJ, Mudd MH, Govan JR, Holloway BW, et al. (1993) Mechanism of conversion to mucoidy in Pseudomonas aeruginosa infecting cystic fibrosis patients. Proc Natl Acad Sci U S A 90: 8377–8381.
9. Ciofu O, Mandsberg L, Hengzhuag W, Hoiby N (2012) Phenotypes selected during chronic lung infection in cystic fibrosis patients: implications for the treatment of Pseudomonas aeruginosa biofilm infections. FEMS Immunol 65: 215–225. doi:10.1111/j.1574-695X.2012.00983.x.
10. Folkesson A, Jelsbak L, Yang L, Johansen HK, Ciofu O, et al. (2012) Adaptation of Pseudomonas aeruginosa to the cystic fibrosis airway: an evolutionary perspective. Nat Rev Microbiol 10: 841–851. doi:10.1038/nrmicro2907.
11. Mahenthiralingam E, Campbell ME, Speert DP (1994) Nonmotility and phagocytic resistance of Pseudomonas aeruginosa isolates from chronically colonized patients with cystic fibrosis. Infect Immun 62: 596–605.
12. Huse HK, Kwon T, Zlosnik JEA, Speert DP, Marcotte E, et al. (2013) Pseudomonas aeruginosa Enhances Production of a Non-alginate Exopolysaccharide During Long-term Colonization of the Cystic Fibrosis Lung. PLoS One 8: e82621. doi:10.1371/journal.pone.0082621.
13. Rau MH, Hansen SK, Johansen HK, Thomsen LE, Workman CT, et al. (2010) Early adaptive developments of Pseudomonas aeruginosa after the transition from life in the environment to persistent colonization in the airways of human cystic fibrosis hosts. Environ Microbiol 12: 1643–1658. doi:10.1111/j.1462-2920.2010.02211.x.
14. Smith EE, Buckley DG, Wu Z, Saenphimmachak C, Hoffman LR, et al. (2006) Genetic adaptation by Pseudomonas aeruginosa to the airways of cystic fibrosis patients. Proc Natl Acad Sci U S A 103: 8487–8492. doi: 10.1073/pnas.0602138103.
15. Ciofu O, Riis B, Pressler T, Enghusen H, Høiby N, et al. (2005) Occurrence of Hypermutable Pseudomonas aeruginosa in Cystic Fibrosis Patients Is Associated with the Oxidative Stress Caused by Chronic Lung Inflammation Occurrence of Hypermutable Pseudomonas aeruginosa in Cystic Fibrosis Patients Is Associated with the. Antimicrob Agents Chemother 49: 2276–2282. doi:10.1128/AAC.49.6.2276.
16. McKeon SA, Nguyen DT, Viteri DF, Zlosnik JEA, Sokol PA (2011) Functional quorum sensing systems are maintained during chronic Burkholderia cepacia complex infections in patients with cystic fibrosis. J Infect Dis 203: 383–392. doi:10.1093/infdis/jiq054.
17. Mira NP, Madeira A, Moreira AS, Coutinho CP, Sá-Correia I (2011) Genomic Expression Analysis Reveals Strategies of Burkholderia cenocepacia to Adapt to Cystic Fibrosis Patients' Airways and Antimicrobial Therapy. PLoS One 6: e28831. doi:10.1371/journal.pone.0028831.
18. Madeira A, Dos Santos SC, Santos PM, Coutinho CP, Tyrrell J, et al. (2013) Proteomic Profiling of Burkholderia cenocepacia Clonal Isolates with Different Virulence Potential Retrieved from a Cystic Fibrosis Patient during Chronic Lung Infection. PLoS One 8: e83065. doi:10.1371/journal.pone.0083065.
19. Nash EF, Thomas A, Whitmill R, Rashid R, Barker B, et al. (2011) "Cepacia syndrome" associated with Burkholderia cepacia (genomovar I) infection in an adolescent with cystic fibrosis. Pediatr Pulmonol 46: 512–514. doi: 10.1002/ppul.21404.
20. Isles A, Maclusky I, Corey M, Gold R, Prober C, et al. (1984) Pseudomonas cepacia infection in cystic fibrosis: an emerging problem. J Pediatr 104: 206–210.
21. Kalish LA, Waltz DA, Dovey M, Potter-Bynoe G, McAdam AJ, et al. (2006) Impact of Burkholderia dolosa on lung function and survival in cystic fibrosis. Am J Respir Crit Care Med 173: 421–425. doi: 10.1164/rccm.200503-344OC.

22. Zlosnik JEA, Costa PS, Brant R, Mori PYB, Hird TJ, et al. (2011) Mucoid and Nonmucoid Burkholderia cepacia Complex Bacteria in Cystic Fibrosis Infections. Am J Respir Crit Care Med 183: 67–72. doi:10.1164/rccm.201002-0203OC.
23. Zlosnik JEA, Hird TJ, Fraenkel MC, Moreira LM, Henry DA, et al. (2008) Differential mucoid exopolysaccharide production by members of the Burkholderia cepacia complex. J Clin Microbiol 46: 1470–1473. doi:10.1128/JCM.02273-07.
24. Coutinho CP, de Carvalho CCCR, Madeira A, Pinto-de-Oliveira A, Sá-Correia I (2011) Burkholderia cenocepacia phenotypic clonal variation during a 3.5-year colonization in the lungs of a cystic fibrosis patient. Infect Immun 79: 2950–2960. doi:10.1128/IAI.01366-10.
25. Larsen GY, Stull TL, Burns JL (1993) Marked phenotypic variability in Pseudomonas cepacia isolated from a patient with cystic fibrosis. J Clin Microbiol 31: 788–792.
26. Leitão JH, Sousa S A, Cunha MV, Salgado MJ, Melo-Cristino J, et al. (2008) Variation of the antimicrobial susceptibility profiles of Burkholderia cepacia complex clonal isolates obtained from chronically infected cystic fibrosis patients: a five-year survey in the major Portuguese treatment center. Eur J Clin Microbiol Infect Dis 27: 1101–1111. doi:10.1007/s10096-008-0552-0.
27. Lieberman TD, Michel J-B, Aingaran M, Potter-Bynoe G, Roux D, et al. (2011) Parallel bacterial evolution within multiple patients identifies candidate pathogenicity genes. Nat Genet 43: 1275–1280. doi:10.1038/ng.997.
28. Chung JW, Altman E, Beveridge TJ, Speert DP (2003) Colonial morphology of Burkholderia cepacia complex genomovar III: implications in exopolysaccharide production, pilus expression, and persistence in the mouse. Infect Immun 71: 904–909.
29. Chung JW, Speert DP (2007) Proteomic identification and characterization of bacterial factors associated with Burkholderia cenocepacia survival in a murine host. Microbiology 153: 206–214. doi: 10.1099/mic.0.2006/000455-0.
30. Smith KD, Andersen-Nissen E, Hayashi F, Strobe K, Bergman MA, et al. (2003) Toll-like receptor 5 recognizes a conserved site on flagellin required for protofilament formation and bacterial motility. Nat Immunol 4: 1247–1253. doi:10.1038/ni1011.
31. de C Ventura GM, Le Goffic R, Balloy V, Plotkowski MC, Chignard M, et al. (2008) TLR 5, but neither TLR2 nor TLR4, is involved in lung epithelial cell response to Burkholderia cenocepacia. FEMS Immunol Med Microbiol 54: 37–44. doi: 10.1111/j.1574-695X.2008.00453.x.
32. Blohmke CJ, Victor RE, Aaron F, Elias IM, Hancock DG, et al. (2008) Innate immunity mediated by TLR5 as a novel antiinflammatory target for cystic fibrosis lung disease. J Immunol 180: 7764–7773.
33. Urban TATAA, Griffith A, Torok AMAM, Mark E, Burns JL, et al. (2004) Contribution of Burkholderia cenocepacia flagella to infectivity and inflammation. Infect Immun 72: 5126–5134. doi:10.1128/IAI.72.9.5126.
34. Tomich M, Herfst CA, Golden JW, Mohr CD (2002) Role of flagella in host cell invasion by Burkholderia cepacia. Infect Immun 70: 1799–1806. doi: 10.1128/IAI.70.4.1799-1806.2002.
35. Simpson DA, Ramphal R, Lory S (1992) Genetic analysis of Pseudomonas aeruginosa adherence: distinct genetic loci control attachment to epithelial cells and mucins. Infect Immun 60: 3771–3779.
36. Brett PJ, Mah DCW, Woods DE (1994) Isolation and Characterization of Pseudomonas pseudomallei Flagellin Proteins. Infect Immun 62: 1914–1919.
37. Zlosnik JEA, Speert DP (2010) The Role of Mucoidy in Virulence of Bacteria from the Burkholderia cepacia Complex: A Systematic Proteomic and Transcriptomic Analysis. J Infect Dis 202: 770–781. doi:10.1086/655663.
38. Silva IN, Ferreira AS, Becker JD, Zlosnik JEA, Speert DP, et al. (2011) Mucoid morphotype variation of Burkholderia multivorans during chronic cystic fibrosis lung infection is correlated with changes in metabolism, motility, biofilm formation and virulence. Microbiology: 3124–3137. doi:10.1099/mic.0.050989-0.
39. Loutet SA, Valvano MA (2010) A decade of Burkholderia cenocepacia virulence determinant research. Infect Immun 78: 4088–4100. doi:10.1128/IAI.00212-10.
40. Uehlinger S, Schwager S, Bernier SP, Riedel K, Nguyen DT, et al. (2009) Identification of specific and universal virulence factors in Burkholderia cenocepacia strains by using multiple infection hosts. Infect Immun 77: 4102–4110. doi:10.1128/IAI.00398-09.
41. Hales BA, Morgan JAW, Hart CA (1998) Variation in Flagellin Genes and Proteins of Burkholderia cepacia Variation in Flagellin Genes and Proteins of Burkholderia cepacia. J Bacteriol 180: 1110–1118.
42. Montie T, Stover G (1983) Isolation and characterization of flagellar preparations from Pseudomonas species. J Clin Microbiol 18: 452–456.
43. Mahenthiralingam E, Urban TA, Goldberg JB (2005) The multifarious, multireplicon Burkholderia cepacia complex. Nat Rev Microbiol 3: 144–156. doi: 10.1038/nrmicro1085.
44. Urban TA, Goldberg JB, Forstner JF, Sajjan US (2005) Cable pili and the 22-kilodalton adhesin are required for Burkholderia cenocepacia binding to and transmigration across the squamous epithelium. Infect Immun 73: 5426–5437. doi: 10.1128/IAI.73.9.5426-5437.2005.
45. Traverse CC, Mayo-smith LM, Poltak SR, Cooper VS (2012) Tangled bank of experimentally evolved Burkholderia biofilms reflects selection during chronic infections. 110. doi: 10.1073/pnas.1207025110.
46. Ellis CN, Cooper VS (2010) Experimental adaptation of Burkholderia cenocepacia to onion medium reduces host range. Appl Environ Microbiol 76: 2387–2396. doi:10.1128/AEM.01930-09.
47. O'Grady EP, Sokol PA (2011) Burkholderia cenocepacia differential gene expression during host-pathogen interactions and adaptation to the host environment. Front Cell Infect Microbiol 1: 15. doi:10.3389/fcimb.2011.00015.
48. Pessi G, Braunwalder R, Grunau A, Omasits U, Ahrens CH, et al. (2013) Response of Burkholderia cenocepacia H111 to Micro-Oxia. PLoS One 8: e72939. doi:10.1371/journal.pone.0072939.
49. Drevinek P, Holden MTG, Ge Z, Jones AM, Ketchell I, et al. (2008) Gene expression changes linked to antimicrobial resistance, oxidative stress, iron depletion and retained motility are observed when Burkholderia cenocepacia grows in cystic fibrosis sputum. BMC Infect Dis 8: 121. doi:10.1186/1471-2334-8-121.
50. Mahenthiralingam E, Campbell ME, Henry DA, Speert DP (1996) Epidemiology of Burkholderia cepacia infection in patients with cystic fibrosis: analysis by randomly amplified polymorphic DNA fingerprinting. J Clin Microbiol 34: 2914–2920.

20

Effect of Different Breathing Aids on Ventilation Distribution in Adults with Cystic Fibrosis

Markus Wettstein[1], Lorenz Radlinger[2], Thomas Riedel[3]*

1 Physiotherapy Institute, Inselspital, Bern University Hospital and University of Bern, Bern, Switzerland, **2** Bern University of Applied Sciences, Health, Bern, Switzerland, **3** Paediatric and Neonatal Intensive Care Medicine, Department of Paediatrics, Inselspital, Bern University Children's Hospital and University of Bern, Bern, Switzerland

Abstract

Background and objectives: We investigated the effect of different breathing aids on ventilation distribution in healthy adults and subjects with cystic fibrosis (CF).

Methods: In 11 healthy adults and 9 adults with CF electrical impedance tomography measurements were performed during spontaneous breathing, continuous positive airway pressure (CPAP) and positive expiratory pressure (PEP) therapy randomly applied in upright and lateral position. Spatial and temporal ventilation distribution was assessed.

Results: The proportion of ventilation directed to the dependent lung significantly increased in lateral position compared to upright in healthy and CF. This effect was enhanced with CPAP but neutralised with PEP, whereas the effect of PEP was larger in the healthy group. Temporal ventilation distribution showed exactly the opposite with homogenisation during CPAP and increased inhomogeneity with PEP.

Conclusions: PEP shows distinct differences to CPAP with respect to its impact on ventilation distribution in healthy adults and CF subjects EIT might be used to individualise respiratory physiotherapy.

Editor: Dominik Hartl, University of Tübingen, Germany

Funding: The authors have no support or funding to report.

Competing Interests: The authors have declared that no competing interests exist.

* Email: thomas.riedel@insel.ch

Introduction

Respiratory Physiotherapy (RPT) is often used for the promotion of lung expansion, minimisation of atelectasis and the airway clearing. RPT contains breathing manoeuvres, positioning, mobilisation/ambulation, exercise therapy and different airway clearance techniques (ACTs) using different devices.

Improved mucus clearance is considered essential in optimising respiratory performance (airway obstruction, atelectasis, ventilation inhomogeneity, increased work of breathing) and might reduce the progression of lung disease in Cystic Fibrosis (CF). [1] Some ACTs have been shown to lead to significantly greater sputum expectoration compared to breathing manoeuvres alone [2].

Probably the most frequently used airway clearance devices are the positive expiratory pressure (PEP) devices. [1] They provide a constant backpressure to the airways during expiration. It has been hypothesised that PEP increases gas pressure behind the mucus via collateral ventilation and maintains airway patency by stabilising the airways during expiration, thereby improving mucus clearance. [3,4] A recent study showed superiority of PEP over high frequency chest wall oscillation as the primary form of airway clearance in CF patients. [5] Ventilation distribution is mainly influenced by factors like gravity (posture), ventilation patterns (tidal volume, flow rate) or breathing manoeuvres (type of respiratory aid) and the quality (age, body weight, genetics) and/or pathology of the lung. [6–11] Hence, to increase their efficacy, ACT's are often combined with positioning and breathing aids such as continuous positive airway pressure (CPAP) or positive expiratory pressure (PEP), in order to benefit from postural drainage effects or changes in ventilation distribution [12,13].

In healthy lungs, most of the tidal volume is directed to the dependent parts of the lung. [11,14] In certain lung diseases and in elderly, children or obese patients these findings may be different, due to early airway closure and lung collapse in the dependent lung during expiration. [15–17] These gravitational effects have been shown to be enhanced with CPAP. [14] PEP devices may homogenise the ventilation distribution and may counteract the early airway closure [3].

To achieve the optimal combination of position and device for each individual patient, it is essential to be aware of the effects of different breathing aids on ventilation distribution in different body positions.

Conventional techniques to assess ventilation distribution such as multiple breath washout (MBW), radio nuclear lung scans or ventilation MRI are either nearly impossible to perform during RPT or give only an overall measure of ventilation distribution without being able to show regional differences. Electrical impedance tomography (EIT) is a imaging technique for bedside monitoring of ventilation distribution. [18] EIT accurately measures tidal volumes and changes in end-expiratory level and describes regional ventilation distribution by measurement of local impedance change and has the advantage of a high temporal resolution [14,19–22].

With the present work, we aimed to compare the effect of different breathing aids on gravity-dependent ventilation distribution in subjects with CF and healthy adults. We hypothesised that the different devices have variable impact on gravity-dependent ventilation distribution in both groups.

Materials and Methods

Ethics Statement

This study was designed as a randomised cross-over study and approved by the ethics committee of the region of Bern, Switzerland. Written informed consent from all subjects was obtained at enrolment.

Subjects

We investigated 11 healthy physiotherapists (5 female), median (range) age 33 (23–45) years and 9 subjects with advanced CF lung disease (2 female), age 31 (19–48) years. All of them were familiar with the use of breathing aids and RPT. Subjects with CF were recruited from outpatient chest clinics at Bern University Hospital, Switzerland. CF subjects showed a forced expiratory volume in the first second (FEV_1) of median (range) 41 (16–63)% predicted, whereas forced vital capacity (FVC) was 48 (20–70)% predicted. FEV_1 and FVC in healthy subjects was 108 (95–118)% predicted and 111 (98–121)% predicted, respectively. In healthy as well as in CF there were no smokers.

Measurements

For each subject, three repetitive recordings of EIT were performed during spontaneous breathing, CPAP (VPAPIII, Resmed AG, Basel, Switzerland) and PEP (PARI-PEP, PARI GmbH, Starnberg, Germany) in upright and right lateral position with the respective commonly used breathing pattern. CPAP pressure were set to 15 mbar in healthy (similar to PEP pressure) and to 10 mbar for CF (according to the hospital guidelines). CPAP was applied by full face mask, PEP was applied by using a mouthpiece and expiratory time was limited to 7 seconds. Body position and the different devices within each body position were applied in a random order. Randomisation was achieved by using sealed envelopes. In between the measurements was a break of at least one minute to check electrodes. Measurements with the new device/position were started after a stabilisation phase of one minute. Based on our own experience this time has shown to lead to stable conditions.

Data acquisition and processing

A Goettingen GoeMF II EIT tomograph (CareFusion, Houten, The Netherlands) was used with a frame rate of 13 Hz and a recording time of 45 seconds in combination with self-adhesive ECG electrodes (Blue Sensor T, Synmedic, Switzerland). EIT scans were generated from the collected potential differences and the known excitation currents with weighted back-projection in a 32×32 pixel matrix using the software provided with the EIT device. The EIT signal was low-pass filtered below the cardiac frequency and a cut-off mask of 20% of the maximum standard deviation of the mean impedance change (912 pixels) was used. [19,23] The proportion of ventilation distributed into the right and left parts of the lung (spatial distribution), relative change in end-expiratory level (EEL), relative change in tidal volume and local filling characteristics (temporal distribution) were calculated adapted to previously-published methods in Matlab R2013a (The MathWorks Inc., Nattick, MA, USA). [14] For the calculation of the temporal distribution the time course of the impedance signal of the region of interest was plotted against the global impedance signal breath by breath. The resulting curve was fitted to the equation $I(g) = a * g^{FI} + c$, where the filling index (FI) describes the shape of the curve. The region of interest is filling faster than the rest of the lung if $FI < 1$ and slower if $FI > 1$ [24].

Statistics

For spatial distribution EIT results are expressed as the percentage of ventilation directed to the right parts of the lung. For filling characteristics FI-values of the right parts of the lung are reported. Changes in EEL from spontaneous breathing within the same body position were normalised for the impedance change during spontaneous tidal breathing in upright position. Changes in EIT tidal volumes are expressed as percentage change from average EIT tidal volume during spontaneous breathing in the corresponding body position. All data were tested for normal distribution with the Shapiro-Wilk test. The mean value of the three measurements was used for analysis. Descriptive data are presented as means and standard deviation.

Comparison of breathing aids and body positions

Differences in terms of spatial and temporal distribution and change in EEL between spontaneous breathing, CPAP and PEP and between the different body positions within groups were assessed with paired t-tests or two way analysis of variance test with Tukey correction for multiple comparisons where applicable. Comparisons between groups (CF and healthy) were assessed with unpaired t-tests.

A p-value <0.05 was considered significant. All statistics were performed using StatsDirect, version 2.7.9 (StatsDirect Ltd., GB).

Results

Ventilation distribution

In upright position we found no difference in either spatial or temporal ventilation distribution between the right and left lung irrespective of the breathing aid in CF as well as in healthy. In right lateral position there was a significant shift of spatial distribution towards the right lung during spontaneous breathing in CF and healthy. This effect was enhanced by the use of CPAP and neutralised with PEP in both groups. (Figure 1) Temporal distribution showed a lag of the right lung in right lateral position (CF and healthy). This effect was reduced with CPAP and increased with PEP in healthy but no significant difference was noted in CF (Table 1).

Additional results: End-expiratory Level (EEL) and tidal volumes

Compared to spontaneous breathing we found an increase in EEL with CPAP and a decrease in EEL with PEP. This effect was only statistically significant in the healthy group. (Table 2) Tidal volumes during PEP compared to spontaneous breathing increased significantly in upright and right lateral position in both groups. No significant differences in tidal volumes were found between spontaneous breathing and CPAP. Between CPAP and PEP differences were only significant in upright position (Table 3).

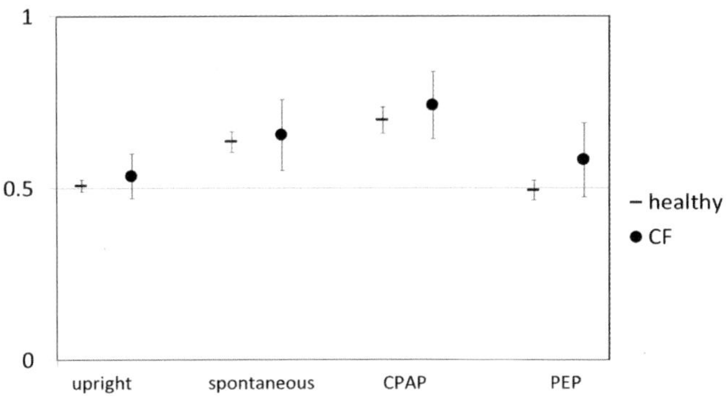

Figure 1. Spatial ventilation distribution with different breathing aids. Mean (95% CI) of the percentage of ventilation directed to the right lung in right lateral position for healthy and CF. For comparison spontaneous breathing in upright position is shown. Values >0.5 indicate more ventilation of the right lung, values <0.5 more ventilation of the left lung.

Discussion

Summary

In healthy adults and subjects with CF gravitational effects on spatial ventilation distribution in both right and left lateral position are enhanced by CPAP but neutralised by PEP. Spatial ventilation inhomogeneity is inversely related to temporal inhomogeneity.

Differences between breathing aids

It is well known that ventilation is increased in the dependent lung during spontaneous breathing and CPAP has been shown previously to enhance gravitational effects in healthy adults, but to our knowledge this is the first study investigating ventilation distribution during PEP therapy. [14] So far the differences between breathing aids have mainly been studied with respect to their clinical effects such as mucus clearance, improvement of gas exchange or improvement of spirometry [25–28].

In our study we compared two devices commonly used during RPT. It has been hypothesised that their effect on mucus clearance is caused by stabilising the airways and by enhancing gravitational effects on ventilation distribution [1,6,29] If it is accepted by the patient and if there are no unwanted side effects, gravity assisted positioning (without any device) as a possibility to enhance mucus clearance is recommended in patients with cystic fibrosis or non-cystic fibrosis-related bronchiectasis [30].

We demonstrated that the investigated devices had a different influence on ventilation distribution in the lateral position, with CPAP enhancing the effect of gravity on spatial distribution whereas PEP appeared to counteract it. Temporal distribution showed the opposite.

We can only speculate on the underlying mechanisms leading to the presented differences between CPAP and the PEP devices. In healthy lungs, the gravity-dependent strain on the independent parts of the lung will lead to a decrease in compliance, corresponding to a shift towards the right, flatter part of the pressure-volume curve. This decrease in compliance will tend to reduce ventilation in these parts of the lung. The application of continuous pressure during inspiration as well as expiration (CPAP) will lead to a further decrease in compliance of the independent parts of the lung and thus decreased local tidal volume. This effect has been described before. [14] As expected from the different breathing patterns used during these therapies end-expiratory level compared to spontaneous breathing was increased with CPAP and decreased with PEP, leading to different lung volumes at the beginning of inspiration. This will influence both spatial and temporal ventilation distribution as shown in healthy adults by Schnidrig et al. [11] With the combination of slightly reduced EEL (healthy −0.38; CF −0.31) and the significantly higher tidal volume (1.8 times normal in both groups) with PEP compared to spontaneous breathing we would expect a shift of ventilation to the right lung in right lateral position. This is not the case in both groups so our results cannot be explained by the change in breathing pattern during PEP therapy alone. PEP is only active during expiration, possibly leading to a homogenisation of the compliance of the lungs at the end of expiration. Similar compliance of the lungs during inspiration will minimise

Table 1. Temporal ventilation distribution: Filling index of the right lung in different body positions.

	spontaneous	CPAP	PEP
upright healthy	0.97 (0.06)	0.96 (0.04)	0.95 (0.06)
		n.s.#	n.s.#
upright CF	0.96 (0.05)	0.95 (0.06)	0.96 (0.04)
		n.s.#	n.s.#
right lateral healthy	1.08 (0.03)	1.01 (0.01)	1.21 (0.11)
	p = 0.006*	p = 0.02*	p<0.001*
	[0.11 (0.07–0.15)]‡	[0.05 (0.03–0.07)]‡	[0.26 (0.19–0.33)]‡
		p = 0.008#	p<0.001#
right lateral CF	1.10 (0.17)	1.05 (0.10)	1.13 (0.24)
	p = 0.021*	p = 0.035*	p = 0.042*
	[0.14 (0.09–0.19)]‡	[0.10 (0.03–0.17)]‡	[0.17 (0.02–0.32)]‡
		n.s.#	n.s.#

Results are given as mean (standard deviation). An index >1 indicating a lag (slower filling than the rest of the lung) and an index <1 a lead (faster filling than the rest of the lung). Mean difference (95% confidence interval) to spontaneous breathing is noted in square brackets‡.
p-values provided for comparison with the upright position* and for comparison with spontaneous breathing within the respective body position#.
n.s. not significant; CF cystic fibrosis; CPAP continuous positive airway pressure; PEP positive end-expiratory pressure.

Table 2. Change in end-expiratory level (EEL) to spontaneous breathing in the corresponding body position expressed as percentage of the average tidal volume during spontaneous breathing in upright position.

	CPAP	PEP
upright healthy	+53 (38–68)%*	−59 (−40–−78)%*
upright CF	+66 (26–106)%	−43 (−10–−76)%
right lateral healthy	+41 (23–59)%*	−38 (−20–−56)%*
right lateral CF	+2 (−16–20)%	−0.31 (−67–5)%

Results are given as mean (95% confidence interval).
All RPT devices showed significant differences in EEL compared to spontaneous breathing in both body positions in healthy (*p<0.001) but not CF.
CF cystic fibrosis; CPAP continuous positive airway pressure; PEP positive end-expiratory pressure.

differences of tidal volumes directed to the dependent and independent parts of the lungs.

The much higher inter-subject variability in CF compared to healthy most likely reflects the differences in disease severity. The effect of different devices cannot be predicted by the diagnosis of CF and conventional lung function tests and EIT might help to further individualise RPT in CF.

Strength and weaknesses of the study

To our knowledge this is the first study assessing the influence of different breathing aids on gravity-dependent ventilation distribution in healthy adults and subjects with CF. All participants were familiar with the use of the different devices. EIT itself does not influence the breathing pattern unlike other lung function techniques which use special breathing manoeuvres. With the random order of application of devices/body positions and the consistency of the measured effects we can rule out long lasting effects of one specific device, body position or a potential effect of cardiac oscillations.

Nevertheless, our study has some limitations. First, as the duration of EIT measurements was fixed at 45 seconds for all subjects, the number of breaths analysed was variable. Given the statistical analysis used (intra-subject comparison) and the highly significant differences shown in all subjects this is unlikely to be of any importance. Multiple studies have been performed to evaluate the value of EIT in assessing regional differences of ventilation in animals, infants and adults. EIT has been validated against computer tomography, ventilation scintigraphy and positron emission tomography and a variety of EIT derived indices showed a very good reproducibility. [31–33] In our study we compared ventilation of the right and left lung, which might have led to a certain loss of spatial information. Nevertheless, we were able to show clear differences between breathing aids.

We only investigated young adults. Thus, any conclusions drawn from this study may not apply for elderly people or very young children. This needs to be investigated in different clearly specified disease groups especially since the devices are applied on sick and usually not on healthy lungs.

Pressures for CPAP and PEP were different in CF (10 mbar) and healthy (15 mbar) which might at least partly explain the slightly lower effect of PEP in CF. Nevertheless the distinct differences between devices remain visible even with lower pressures.

Finally, in the present study we did not directly measure tidal volume, which possibly may influence ventilation distribution. We estimated tidal volume using the EIT signal normalised for tidal volume during spontaneous breathing. In right lateral position where we found the biggest differences in spatial and temporal

Table 3. Change in tidal volume expressed as percentage of the average tidal volume during spontaneous breathing in the respective body position.

	CPAP	PEP
upright healthy	11 (−1–43)%	103 (50–156)%
	n.s.*	p<0.001*
		p = 0.004#
upright CF	15 (−2–32)%	97 (51–143)%
	n.s.*	p<0.001*
		p = 0.007#
right lateral healthy	37 (23–51)%	75 (25–125)%
	n.s.*	p = 0.025
		n.s.#
right lateral CF	28 (−1–57)%	77 (19–135)%
	n.s.*	p = 0.029*
		n.s.#

Results are given as mean difference (95% confidence interval).
p-values provided for comparison with spontaneous breathing* and for comparison of CPAP and PEP# in the respective body position.

ventilation distribution tidal volumes were only significantly different between spontaneous breathing and PEP.

Clinical relevance

Given the importance of physiotherapy in different pulmonary diseases and the frequent use of breathing aids, it is important to understand the mechanisms of this therapy. We have demonstrated that breathing aids have different effects on ventilation distribution with a very effect size, but the therapeutic effect remains unclear. Whether PEP or CPAP is better for individual subjects needs to be evaluated in an interventional study assessing clinically relevant endpoints. Based on our results one could speculate that for CF PEP combined with lateral position might be superior for mucus clearance and CPAP combined with lateral position might be superior to overcome atelectasis. Nevertheless, EIT might help to find the optimal breathing aid for each patient and to apply individualised, patient-tailored therapy.

Conclusion

Breathing aids show distinct differences in their effects on gravity-dependent ventilation distribution in healthy adults and CF. EIT might be used for individualised RPT in CF. In future studies individualised techniques need to be combined with measures of efficiency such as gas exchange, mucus clearance or other functional outcomes.

Author Contributions

Conceived and designed the experiments: MW LR TR. Performed the experiments: MW. Analyzed the data: MW LR TR. Contributed reagents/materials/analysis tools: TR. Contributed to the writing of the manuscript: MW LR TR.

References

1. Elkins MR, Jones A, van der Schans C (2006) Positive expiratory pressure physiotherapy for airway clearance in people with cystic fibrosis. Cochrane Database Syst Rev: CD003147.
2. Thomas J, Cook DJ, Brooks D (1995) Chest physical therapy management of patients with cystic fibrosis. A meta-analysis. Am J Respir Crit Care Med 151: 846–850.
3. Groth S, Stafanger G, Dirksen H, Andersen JB, Falk M, et al. (1985) Positive expiratory pressure (PEP-mask) physiotherapy improves ventilation and reduces volume of trapped gas in cystic fibrosis. Bull Eur Physiopathol Respir 21: 339–343.
4. Oberwaldner B, Evans JC, Zach MS (1986) Forced expirations against a variable resistance: a new chest physiotherapy method in cystic fibrosis. Pediatr Pulmonol 2: 358–367.
5. McIlwaine MP, Alarie N, Davidson GF, Lands LC, Ratjen F, et al. (2013) Long-term multicentre randomised controlled study of high frequency chest wall oscillation versus positive expiratory pressure mask in cystic fibrosis. Thorax 68: 746–751.
6. Reid WD, Chung F (2004) Clinical Management Notes and Case Histories in Cardiopulmonary Physical Therapy. Thorofare, NJ, USA: SLACK incorporated.
7. Frerichs I, Dudykevych T, Hinz J, Bodenstein M, Hahn G, et al. (2001) Gravity effects on regional lung ventilation determined by functional EIT during parabolic flights. J Appl Physiol 91: 39–50.
8. Tucker B, Jenkins S (1996) The effect of breathing exercises with body positioning on regional lung ventilation. Aust J Physiother 42: 219–227.
9. Tucker B, Jenkins S, Cheong D, Robinson P (1999) Effect of unilateral breathing exercises on regional lung ventilation. Nucl Med Commun 20: 815–821.
10. Crawford AB, Makowska M, Engel LA (1986) Effect of tidal volume on ventilation maldistribution. Respir Physiol 66: 11–25.
11. Schnidrig S, Casaulta C, Schibler A, Riedel T (2013) Influence of end-expiratory level and tidal volume on gravitational ventilation distribution during tidal breathing in healthy adults. Eur J Appl Physiol 113: 591–598.
12. Holland AE, Denehy L, Ntoumenopoulos G, Naughton MT, Wilson JW (2003) Non-invasive ventilation assists chest physiotherapy in adults with acute exacerbations of cystic fibrosis. Thorax 58: 880–884.
13. Placidi G, Cornacchia M, Polese G, Zanolla L, Assael BM, et al. (2006) Chest physiotherapy with positive airway pressure: a pilot study of short-term effects on sputum clearance in patients with cystic fibrosis and severe airway obstruction. Respir Care 51: 1145–1153.
14. Riedel T, Richards T, Schibler A (2005) The value of electrical impedance tomography in assessing the effect of body position and positive airway pressures on regional lung ventilation in spontaneously breathing subjects. Intensive Care Med 31: 1522–1528.
15. Frerichs I, Braun P, Dudykevych T, Hahn G, Genee D, et al. (2004) Distribution of ventilation in young and elderly adults determined by electrical impedance tomography. Respir Physiol Neurobiol 143: 63–75.
16. Davies H, Helms P, Gordon I (1992) Effect of posture on regional ventilation in children. Pediatr Pulmonol 12: 227–232.
17. Hurewitz AN, Susskind H, Harold WH (1985) Obesity alters regional ventilation in lateral decubitus position. J Appl Physiol 59: 774–783.
18. Frerichs I (2000) Electrical impedance tomography (EIT) in applications related to lung and ventilation: a review of experimental and clinical activities. Physiol Meas 21: R1–21.
19. Dunlop S, Hough J, Riedel T, Fraser JF, Dunster K, et al. (2006) Electrical impedance tomography in extremely prematurely born infants and during high frequency oscillatory ventilation analyzed in the frequency domain. Physiol Meas 27: 1151–1165.
20. Frerichs I, Dargaville PA, Dudykevych T, Rimensberger PC (2003) Electrical impedance tomography: a method for monitoring regional lung aeration and tidal volume distribution? Intensive Care Med 29: 2312–2316.
21. Riedel T, Kyburz M, Latzin P, Thamrin C, Frey U (2009) Regional and overall ventilation inhomogeneities in preterm and term-born infants. Intensive Care Med 35: 144–151.
22. Frerichs I, Hahn G, Schiffmann H, Berger C, Hellige G (1999) Monitoring regional lung ventilation by functional electrical impedance tomography during assisted ventilation. Ann N Y Acad Sci 873: 493–505.
23. Pulletz S, van Genderingen HR, Schmitz G, Zick G, Schadler D, et al. (2006) Comparison of different methods to define regions of interest for evaluation of regional lung ventilation by EIT. Physiol Meas 27: S115–127.
24. Grant CA, Fraser JF, Dunster KR, Schibler A (2009) The assessment of regional lung mechanics with electrical impedance tomography: a pilot study during recruitment manoeuvres. Intensive Care Med 35: 166–170.
25. App EM, Kieselmann R, Reinhardt D, Lindemann H, Dasgupta B, et al. (1998) Sputum rheology changes in cystic fibrosis lung disease following two different types of physiotherapy: flutter vs autogenic drainage. Chest 114: 171–177.
26. Gondor M, Nixon PA, Mutich R, Rebovich P, Orenstein DM (1999) Comparison of Flutter device and chest physical therapy in the treatment of cystic fibrosis pulmonary exacerbation. Pediatr Pulmonol 28: 255–260.
27. Bellone A, Lascioli R, Raschi S, Guzzi L, Adone R (2000) Chest physical therapy in patients with acute exacerbation of chronic bronchitis: effectiveness of three methods. Arch Phys Med Rehabil 81: 558–560.
28. Thompson CS, Harrison S, Ashley J, Day K, Smith DL (2002) Randomised crossover study of the Flutter device and the active cycle of breathing technique in non-cystic fibrosis bronchiectasis. Thorax 57: 446–448.
29. Main E, Prasad A, Schans C (2005) Conventional chest physiotherapy compared to other airway clearance techniques for cystic fibrosis. Cochrane Database Syst Rev: CD002011.
30. Bott J, Blumenthal S, Buxton M, Ellum S, Falconer C, et al. (2009) Guidelines for the physiotherapy management of the adult, medical, spontaneously breathing patient. Thorax 64 Suppl 1: i1–51.
31. Victorino JA, Borges JB, Okamoto VN, Matos GF, Tucci MR, et al. (2004) Imbalances in regional lung ventilation: a validation study on electrical impedance tomography. Am J Respir Crit Care Med 169: 791–800.
32. Hinz J, Neumann P, Dudykevych T, Andersson LG, Wrigge H, et al. (2003) Regional ventilation by electrical impedance tomography: a comparison with ventilation scintigraphy in pigs. Chest 124: 314–322.
33. Richard JC, Pouzot C, Gros A, Tourevieille C, Lebars D, et al. (2009) Electrical impedance tomography compared to positron emission tomography for the measurement of regional lung ventilation: an experimental study. Crit Care 13: R82.

21

Proteomic Analysis of Nasal Epithelial Cells from Cystic Fibrosis Patients

Ludovic Jeanson[1,2]¶, Ida Chiara Guerrera[2,3]¶, Jean-François Papon[4,5], Cerina Chhuon[2,3], Patricia Zadigue[4], Virginie Prulière-Escabasse[5], Serge Amselem[1], Estelle Escudier[1], André Coste[4,5], Aleksander Edelman[2,3]*

1 Service de Génétique et Embryologie Médicales, Unité Mixte de Recherche_Scientifique 933, Institut National de la Santé et de la Recherche Médicale, Université Pierre et Marie Curie – Paris 6, and Assistance Publique – Hôpitaux de Paris, Hôpital Armand Trousseau, Paris, France, **2** Unité_1151, Institut National de la Santé et de la Recherche Médicale, Université Paris Descartes, Paris, France, **3** Plateau Proteome Necker, Structure Fédérative de Recherche de Necker, Université Paris Descartes, Paris, France, **4** Unité Mixte de Recherche_Scientifique 855, Institut National de la Santé et de la Recherche Médicale, Université Paris 12, Faculté de Médecine, Créteil, France, **5** Service d'Otorhinolaryngologie et de chirurgie cervico-faciale, Assistance Publique – Hôpitaux de Paris, Hôpital inter-communal et Groupe Hospitalier Henri Mondor-Albert Chenevier, Créteil, France

Abstract

The pathophysiology of cystic fibrosis (CF) lung disease remains incompletely understood. New explanations for the pathogenesis of CF lung disease may be discovered by studying the patterns of protein expression in cultured human nasal epithelial cells (HNEC). To that aim, we compared the level of protein expressions in primary cultures of HNEC from nasal polyps secondary to CF (CFNP, n = 4), primary nasal polyps (NP, n = 8) and control mucosa (CTRL, n = 4) using isobaric tag for relative and absolute quantification (iTRAQ) labeling coupled with liquid chromatography (LC)-MS-MS. The analysis of the data revealed 42 deregulated protein expressions in CFNP compared to NP and CTRL, suggesting that these alterations are related to CF. Overall, AmiGo analysis highlighted six major pathways important for cell functions that seem to be impaired: metabolism, G protein process, inflammation and oxidative stress response, protein folding, proteolysis and structural proteins. Among them, glucose and fatty acid metabolic pathways could be impaired in CF with nine deregulated proteins. Our proteomic study provides a reproducible set of differentially expressed proteins in airway epithelial cells from CF patients and reveals many novel deregulated proteins that could lead to further studies aiming to clarify the involvement of such proteins in CF pathophysiology.

Editor: Andy T. Y. Lau, Shantou University Medical College, China

Funding: Funding was provided by Agence Nationale pour la Recherche -05-MRAR-02201; European Community: Life Sciences and Health Grant (LSHG-CT-2005-512044) NEUPROCF; French Foundation for Cystic Fibrosis: "Vaincre la Mucoviscidose"; Legs Poix from Chancellerie des Universités. The funders had no role in study design, data collection and analysis, decision to publish, or preparation of the manuscript.

Competing Interests: The authors have declared that no competing interests exist.

* Email: aleksander.edelman@inserm.fr

¶ These authors contributed equally to this work.

Introduction

Chronic inflammation, which represents one of the most serious causes of morbidity/mortality in the world, is a severe complication common to both frequent and rare disorders. Among chronic inflammatory disorders, cystic fibrosis (CF) is the most common recessively inherited disease in the Western world. CF is caused by mutations in the gene encoding the cystic fibrosis transmembrane conductance regulator (CFTR) protein [1], which is expressed in airway epithelial cells and acts as a chloride channel activated by cyclic AMP. The most frequent mutation of CF alleles is F508del, a deletion of phenylalanine in the intra-cytosolic nucleotide binding domain 1 of CFTR.

Primary nasal polyposis, a common disorder of the upper airways [2] which affects almost 4% of the population, is an inflammatory disease of unknown etiology. Interestingly, CF is often associated with nasal polyps [3] that constitute an accessible model to study CF pathophysiology.

Global approaches may be useful to unmask abnormal cellular pathways in complex chronic inflammatory diseases. A few proteomic studies have been performed in CF with different sample sources: sputum [4,5], bronchio-alveolar lavage fluid [6] or serum [7]. Only three global proteomic studies have been performed in airway epithelial cells which are one of the main targets in CF: two in lung epithelial cell lines IB3-1 (i.e. immortalized bronchial epithelial cell line isolated from a patient homozygous for the F508del mutation) and C38 (i.e. IB3-1 "corrected" by transfection with wild type *CFTR*) [8,9] and the last one in cells obtained by nasal brushing (including blood, inflammatory and epithelial cells) from CF patients [10]. To our knowledge, no proteomic studies have been done on primary cultures of pure airway epithelial cells from CF patients (i.e. not contaminated with blood and/or inflammatory cells). This culture system allows epithelial cell differentiation at the air/liquid interface and is useful to study chronic inflammation in airways [11].

The effects of F508del CFTR are complex at the cellular level and are known to alter many different functions [11–13]. Among them, metabolism, G protein process, inflammation, oxidative stress response, protein folding, proteolysis and structural proteins are known to be abnormal but the proteins implicated in those malfunctions are largely unknown.

The aim of the present study was to compare the levels of protein expressions in primary cultures of human nasal epithelial cells (HNEC) from control mucosa (CTRL), primary nasal polyps (NP) and NP secondary to CF (CFNP). We chose differential quantitative global proteomic analysis based on isobaric tag for relative and absolute quantification (iTRAQ) labeling coupled with liquid chromatography (LC)-MS-MS that permitted reproducible protein quantification in the different patients evaluated in this study. The iTRAQ method is based on the covalent labeling of the amines from proteins with isobaric tags containing a different distribution of heavy isotopes. The fragmentation of the attached tag generates a low molecular mass reporter ion that can be used to relatively quantify the peptides and the proteins from which they originated.

The results provided new insights into the comprehension of abnormal airway epithelial cell functions that might exist in CF pathogenesis.

Materials and Methods

Subjects

In order to evaluate the differential protein expression related to CF four patients with CFNP were randomly matched to four non-CF patients affected by NP (CFNP *vs.* NP), and four other non-CF patients with NP were matched to four CTRL patients without nasal polyposis (NP *vs.* CTRL) (Figure 1).

All NP samples were collected from patients requiring surgery for their nasal polyposis. Patients were requested to stop all treatments at least one month before surgery except for CF patients who were prepared for surgery by systemic antibiotics adapted to nasal bacteriology. Four control mucosa from the inferior turbinate were obtained from individuals who underwent turbinectomy for snoring. All the patients did not mention any allergic background and were negatively tested with skin prick tests. All non-CF patients with NP presented typical primary nasal polyposis and did not suffer from recurrent airway infections. In order to avoid, as much as possible, heterozygous carriers of the F508del mutation, nasal polyps occurring in a context of purulent chronic sinusitis were not included [14]. All four CF patients were homozygous for the F508del mutation. The CTRL and NP patients were not genotyped for CF mutations. Characteristics of the patients are given in Table 1. This protocol was approved by the ethics committee of our institution (Comité de Protection des Personnes-Ile-de-France IX CHU Henri Mondor). The participants provided their verbal consent to participate in the study and their non opposistion to the use of their data. Parental consent was obtained for minor subjects. The nasal mucosa collected for the experiments were either nasal polyps or turbinates obtained during ethmoidectomy or turbinectomy, respectively. All these samples were surgical waste, usually discarded during surgery. Our procedure is based on French law n°2004-800 of 6 August 2004 on Bioethics ("loi relative à la bioéthique") which was codified in the French Public Health Code (L. 1235-2 and L. 1245-2). The surgeon recorded in the patient's file the non-opposition for using the discarded nasal mucosa.

Material

Reagents for mass spectrometry and protein biochemistry experiments. dithiothreitol (DTT), pronase, ethylenediamine tetra-acetic acid (EDTA), collagen IV, urea, thio-urea, orthovanadate, glycerol, TRIS, iodoacetamide, NaCl, detergents (CHAPS, sodium deoxychotate, Triton X100), NH4CO3 and the Glu-fibrinopeptide were from Sigma-Aldrich (Saint-Quentin Fallavier, France). Anti-proteases were from Roche (Neuilly sur Seine, France). Bromophenol blue, SDS, acrylamide, silver staining kit were from Biorad (Marnes la Coquette, France). Trypsin for mass spectrometry was of highest grade purchased from Promega (Charbonnieres-les-bains, France). Acetonitril (ACN) and Tri-fluoro-acetic acid (TFA) were from Carlo Erba (Val de Reuil, France), Alpha-Cyano-4-Hydroxycinnamic Acid

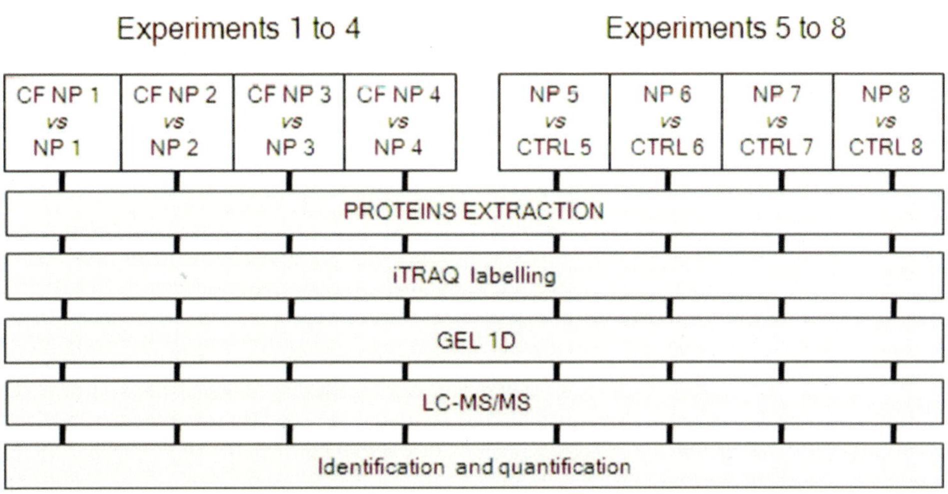

Figure 1. Workflow for the study. Two series of independent experiments were compared: (i) experiments 1 to 4 for proteins derived from HNEC cultures obtained from 4 CF NP patients *vs.* 4 NP patients (non CF); (ii) experiments 5 to 8 for proteins derived from HNEC cultures obtained from 4 NP patients (non CF) *vs.* 4 controls patients. Each couple of samples was matched randomly. For quantification of proteins, iTRAQ labeling coupled to LC-MS/MS was performed (see methods for details).

Table 1. Description of patients.

Patient	Sex	Age (years)	Associated disease	Cigarette smoke
CTRL				
CTRL 5	M	32	None	No
CTRL 6	F	24	None	No
CTRL 7	M	28	None	No
CTRL 8	M	20	None	Yes
CFNP*				
CFNP 1	M	21	None	No
CFNP 2	F	15	None	No
CFNP 3	M	22	None	No
CFNP 4	F	25	None	No
CFNP 5	F	19	None	No
CFNP 6	M	21	None	No
CFNP 7	M	17	None	No
NP				
NP 1	M	25	Samster's disease	No
NP 2	F	29	Aspirin intolerance	Yes
NP 3	M	35	Asthma	No
NP 4	F	34	Asthma	No
NP 5	M	33	Samster's disease	No
NP 6	F	23	Asthma	No
NP 7	M	37	Asthma	No
NP 8	F	41	Samster's disease	No

*All CFNP patients are homozygous for the F508del *CFTR* mutation.

(HCCA) from Laser Biolabs (Sophia-Antipolis, France). iTRAQ reagents were from Applied Biosystems (Courtaboeuf, France)

Columns. C18 trap column (C18 pepmap100, 5 µm particles, 100 Å pores, 300 µm i.d., 5 mm length), and C18 analytical column (C18 pepmap100, 3 µm particles, 15 cm length, 75 µm inner diameter., 100 Å pores) were from Acclaim (Vandoeuvre, France). The Ultimate3000 series HPLC and the Probot fraction collector were purchased from Dionex (Voisins le Bretonneux, France).

Primary cultures of HNEC

Nasal samples were transported to the laboratory in order to perform primary cultures of HNEC as previously described [11]. Mucosa samples were rinsed in phosphate-buffered saline (PBS) with dithiothreitol (DTT, 5 mM) and antibiotics (100 U/ml of penicillin, 100 mg/ml of streptomycin, 2.5 µg/ml of amphotericin B and 100 mg/ml of gentamicin) and then placed overnight at 4°C in a PBS-antibiotics solution containing 0.1% pronase. The samples were incubated in DMEM/F12 with 5% fetal calf serum (FCS) before centrifugation (800 g, 7 min). Cell pellets were then suspended in 0.25% trypsin-EDTA solution for 3 min and incubated in DMEM/F12-antibiotics with 10% FCS. Finally, HNEC were plated on permeable polycarbonate supports at 1×10^6 cells/cm^2. All inserts had a diameter of 12-mm and were coated with type IV collagen. HNEC were incubated at 37°C in 5% CO_2. For the first 24 h, HNEC were incubated with 1 ml of DMEM/F12-antibiotics with 2% Ultroser G outside the insert and DMEM/F12-antibiotics with 10% FCS inside the insert. After 24 h, medium was removed inside the inserts in order to place the cells at an air-liquid interface, and medium outside the inserts was then changed daily. Transepithelial resistance and potential difference were measured every three days using a microvoltmeter (World Precision Instruments, Astonbury, UK). The primary culture of HNEC, differentiated at the air-liquid interface, provides functional cells closely resembling normal airway epithelium within one week that maintain their differentiation for at least four weeks [15]. We previously controlled that all cultured cells are epithelial cells, with viability around 95% during the first four weeks. For all experiments the cells were studied at day 7 after seeding, corresponding to the establishment of cell differentiation.

Protein preparation for proteomic experiments

Experiments for protein quantification were performed in primary cultures of HNEC from CFNP, NP and CTRL. Cells in Transwell filters were washed, scraped off the filters in ice-cold PBS, and centrifuged (800 g, 10 min, 4°C). The pellet was suspended in 100 µl/culture plate of lysis buffer, constituted of 0.5% w/v SDS, 50 mM Tris-HCl pH 7, before incubation at 95°C for 5 min. The total cellular proteins obtained were supplemented by 250 µl/culture plate of dissolution buffer, constituted of 8 M urea, 2.5 M thio-urea, 4% w/v CHAPS, 50 mM DTT, anti-protease 1X, 1 mM orthovanadate, and mixed one h at room temperature. Labeling of proteins with iTRAQ reagents, protein fractionation and digestion were performed according to previously described protocols [16].

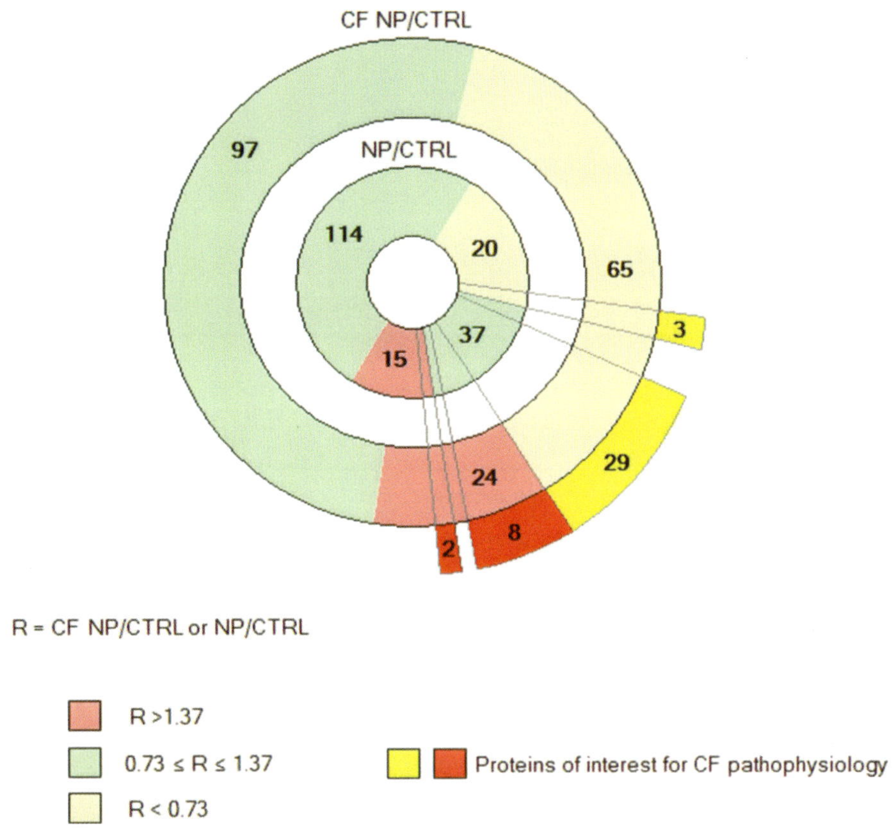

Figure 2. Distribution of the 186 common quantified proteins in CFNP (outer donut) and NP (inner donut) *vs* CTRL. Downregulated proteins are highlighted in yellow, upregulated proteins are highlighted in red and stable proteins are highlighted in green according to the ratio thresholds (R = CF NP/CTRL or NP/CTRL). 15 proteins are upregulated in NP compared to CTRL (inner donut) and 21 proteins are upregulated in CFNP compared to CTRL (outer donut). Among them, 11 proteins are upregulated in both CFNP and NP. 20 proteins are downregulated in NP compared to CTRL (inner donut) and 48 proteins are downregulated in CFNP compared to CTRL (outer donut). Among them, 16 proteins are downregulated in both CFNP and NP. Finally, among the proteins deregulated in common between CFNP and NP, two are more regulated in CFNP and three are more downregulated in CFNP. The 42 proteins of interest for CF pathophysiology are represented in intense red and intense yellow outside the outer donut.

iTRAQ labeling

After protein preparation, 25 µg of each sample were precipitated overnight at −20°C using 100% acetone and dissolved in 20 µl of denaturing buffer containing 1 µl denaturant and 2 µl reducing reagent (TCEP) as provided in the iTRAQ kit, followed by vortexing and incubation at 60°C for 1 h. One µl of cysteine blocking solution (iodoacetamide) was then added to each sample, followed by incubation at room temperature for 30 min. iTRAQ labeling was carried out by adding iTRAQ reagents 114, 115, 116 or 117 to either the NP, CF NP or CTRL samples followed by incubation at room temperature for 2 h. For the NP/CFNP experiments, iTRAQ reagent 114 was used for NP and the 116 was used for CFNP. For the NP/CTRL experiments: iTRAQ reagent 115 was used for NP and the 117 was used for CTRL. Subsequently, two samples/experiment (NP/CF NP or NP/CTRL) were mixed by vortexing, pooled together and dried in a Speedvac evaporator (Thermo Fisher Scientific, Courtaboeuf, France).

Trypsin digestion

Samples were digested according to Bensalem et al [17] with minor modifications. Briefly, prior to mass spectrometry analysis, the dry iTRAQ sample pellet was dissolved in Laemmli buffer, constituted of 10% glycerol, 0.05 M Tris-HCl (pH 6.8), 0.1% SDS, 50 mM DTT, and 0.01% (w/v) bromophenol blue, then supplemented by 1/5 H_2O dilution. Dissolved proteins were separated by electrophoresis (SDS-PAGE). Briefly, protein samples were loaded onto 10% w/v polyacrylamide gels and run at 25 mA for 2 to 3 h at room temperature. After electrophoresis, protein visualization was carried out by silver staining compatible with MS/MS analysis.

12 protein bands were excised from the SDS-PAGE gel and prepared as follows: each gel piece was destained for 5 min with 200 µl of destaining buffer (silver staining kit). Before drying the gel pieces in a Speedvac evaporator, they were washed with deionised water (Millipore, Guyancourt, France) and shrunk in the presence of Acetonitril for 15 min. The gel pieces were dried at room temperature for 20 min and followed by digestion with 0.8 µg (4 U) of trypsin in 8 µl of 25 mM NH_4/CO_3, overnight at 37°C. The peptide mixture was extracted from the gel plug with 10 µl of a 50% ACN, 0.1% tri-fluoro-acetic acid solution and dried in a Speedvac evaporator.

Nano-LC-MALDI-TOF-TOF

Nanochromatography protocol. Digested peptides were suspended in water with 0.1% TFA and 10% acetonitrile, separated with an Ultimate3000 series HPLC. Briefly: 10 µL of eluate were injected and trapped using solvent A (0.1%

SPECIFICALLY REGULATED in CFNP

	CFNP/CTRL	NP/CTRL
GRP78	3.60	3.13
ENPL	2.98	2.45
CATB	2.16	1.09
DPP2	1.95	1.16
K2C2A	1.74	0.92
LAMP1	1.73	0.98
K1C14	1.61	0.85
K1C17	1.57	0.77
SPB3	1.56	1.16
K2C5	1.44	0.92
ODPA	0.71	0.80
TERA	0.69	0.87
GDIR1	0.69	0.94
KPYM	0.68	0.93
MVP	0.68	0.85
1433B	0.67	0.92
SET	0.67	0.89
SYNC	0.66	0.89
STIP1	0.64	0.84
G6PD	0.63	0.88
ODO1	0.63	0.77

	CFNP/CTRL	NP/CTRL
ILEU	0.63	0.92
TBA1A	0.61	0.95
G6PI	0.61	0.92
ANXA1	0.61	0.83
HSP7C	0.60	0.89
ASSY	0.60	0.83
EZRI	0.59	0.90
TBA4A	0.59	0.86
1433S	0.56	0.87
HS90A	0.56	0.81
PGAM1	0.49	0.82
TKT	0.56	0.80
TALDO	0.65	0.80
ACADM	0.53	0.80
HSPB1	0.51	0.88
FAS	0.50	0.91
LOX15	0.41	0.75
GLNA	0.34	0.79
PRDX6	0.33	0.44
PRSX1	0.30	0.44
PRDX2	0.30	0.46

REGULATED in NP and CFNP

	CFNP/CTRL	NP/CTRL
PDIA3	3.05	2.84
PDIA4	3.03	2.79
FLNA	2.83	2.38
PDIA1	2.39	2.38
VIME	2.18	1.55
HSP71	2.07	2.20
MYH14	1.90	1.81
MYH9	1.56	2.34
G3P	1.56	2.81
HNRL2	1.42	1.43
CPNS1	1.43	1.75
K1C19	0.72	0.63
LG3BP	0.70	0.59
K1C13	0.69	0.69
VAPA	0.67	0.70
KCRU	0.66	0.65
DHE3	0.65	0.71
BAP31	0.63	0.57
HYEP	0.62	0.56
HNRPC	0.62	0.71
K2C1	0.60	0.56

	CFNP/CTRL	NP/CTRL
AT1A1	0.58	0.68
K1C18	0.55	0.60
RS17	0.53	0.65
AT1B1	0.43	0.48
RS18	0.40	0.71
K2C4	0.19	0.25

Legend: R>1.8; 1.5≤R≤1.8; 1.37≤R≤1.5; 0.73≤R≤1.37; 0.6≤R≤0.73; 0.5≤R≤0.6; R<0.5

Figure 3. Comparison of differentially expressed proteins in CFNP compared to NP and CTRL. On the left, we report the ratios of 42 proteins significantly modulated in CFNP/CTRL *vs* NP/CTRL patients. On the right, we report proteins that are modulated in both CFNP/CTRL and NP/CTRL patients. To obtain the CFNP/CTRL ratios, relative protein expressions ratios from CF NP/NP were normalized to the average of the ratios obtained in NP *vs* CTRL (CF NP/CTRL = CFNP/NP × NP/CTRL).

Trifuoroacetic acid, 2% ACN) at a 30 µl/min loading flow for 3 min in a C18 trap column. The microvalve then oriented the elution to back flow (300 nl/min) the peptides toward the analytical column with a gradient rising from 7% solvent B (80% acetonitrile, 20% solvent A) at microvalve switch to 16% in 7 min, from 16% to 32% in 20 min and from 32% to 50% in 7 min. Fractions were spotted on-line on a MALDI target using a Probot fraction collector. Spotted fractions were mixed 1:4 with 2 mg/ml of HCCA in 70% ACN 0.1% TFA and Glu fibrinopeptide at 30 fmoles/spot. 96 fractions were collected and analysed using a 4800 MALDI TOF/TOF analyser (ABI, Lyon - Rhône-Alpes, France).

MS mode. Spectra acquisition and processing were performed using the 4000 series explorer software (ABI) version 3.5.28193 build 1011 in positive reflectron mode at fixed LASER fluency with low mass gate and delayed extraction. External plate calibration was performed using 4 calibration points spotted throughout the plate, additional internal calibration was performed using the Glu-fibrinopeptide (M/Z = 1570.677) allowing a mass accuracy of few ppm. For each fraction, steps of 50 spectra in the range of 700 to 4000 Da were acquired at a 200 Hz LASER shot frequency. 500 spectra per sample were summed and processed to obtain monoisotopic values from isotopes clusters with a raw spectra s/n ratio of 20.

MS/MS mode. In each MS spectrum, the 8 most abundant peaks were selected for fragmentation starting with the least abundant. A cut off was applied at a minimum s/n of 20. Neighboring precursors within resolution of 200 were excluded. 1000 MS/MS spectra per precursor were summed by increments of 50. Processing included baseline subtraction and Stavitsky Golay smoothing with 15 points across peak and a polynomial order of 4. Peaklists reflect monoisotopic values from isotope clusters with a s/n ratio of minimum 22.

Peak list and quantification analysis. Generated MS/MS peaklists were subsequently submitted to an in-house Mascot version 2.2 search engine (Matrix science). The Swiss-Prot 55.5 release Swiss-Prot 20080610 (389046 sequences; 139778124 residues) release database was used with the Homo sapiens species. Parent and fragment mass tolerances were respectively set to 50 ppm and 0.3 Da. Variable modification, oxidation (M), iTRAQ 4plex (Y) and fixed modification, iTRAQ 4plex (N-term), iTRAQ 4plex (K), carbamidomethylation (C) were allowed. Trypsin digestion and possibility of one missed cleavage were selected. A filter was applied to the search in order to reduce false positives and matching redundancies of the same peptide in several hits. All matches above 1% risks of random matching were eliminated ($p<0.01$). The probability score calculated by the software was used as a primary criterion for correct identification. For Mascot scores slightly above the threshold of p value, measurement errors were carefully watched to detect possible false positives that usually give random mass measurement errors, while relevant identifications give constant measurement errors. Molecular weights from experimental and Mascot results were also compared. Whenever the result was ambiguous, the spectra either in MS or MS/MS were manually checked for proper matching and the result was accordingly rejected or accepted.

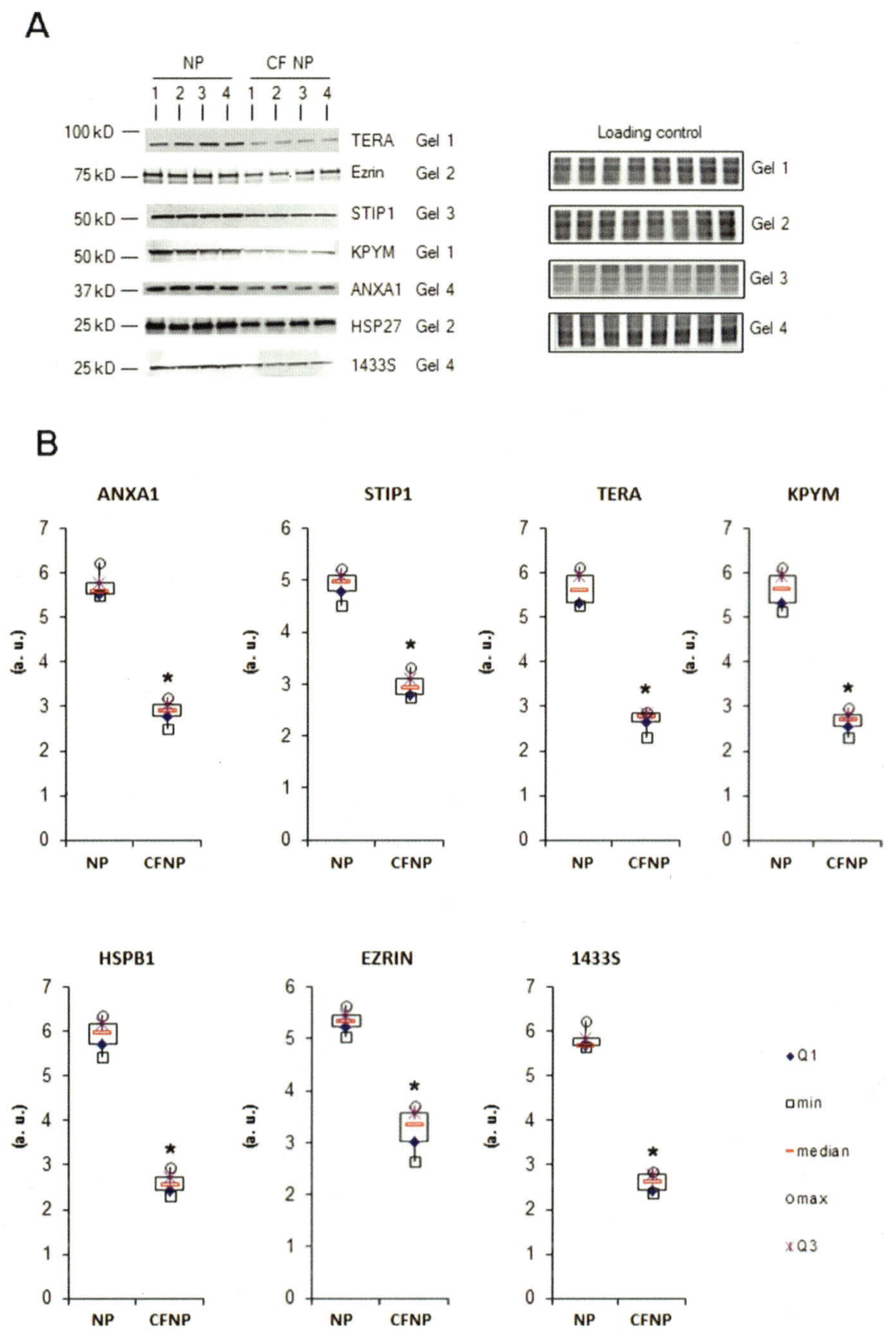

Figure 4. Western blot analysis of seven differentially expressed proteins. The Western blots from the 4 NP patients and the 4 CFNP patients used for proteomic experiments are shown with their respective loading controls. **A**: Each protein is analyzed in three technical replicates. For normalization, the acrylamide gels were stained with Coomassie blue (total migrated protein detection) just after electro-transfer and scanned using the Odyssey LI-COR. Using the Odyssey software, protein intensity values were normalized with their corresponding loading control intensity values. **B**: Box plots of the intensity calculated with the Odyssey software, *$p<0.01$, Mann and Whitney test. (a.u.: arbitrary units). We report Maximum (max), minimum (min), first quartile (Q1), third quartile (Q3).

Statistical analysis for proteomic experiments

For the quantification, the protein ratio type was the 'weighted' geometric mean, only 'bold face ratios' were considered (significantly different from 1 at a 95% confidence level), outlier removal was 'automatic' (Dixon's method and Rosner's method), the minimum number of peptides was two and at least two peptides were required to be the top ranking peptide matches ('bold and red type faces'). Selective criteria were adopted to obtain a consistently quantified set of proteins: (i) the intensity ratio must be calculated with at least two unique quantified peptides and (ii) the protein must be quantified in at least 3/4 experiments. Differences between expression of proteins in CFNP vs NP were evaluated by Mann-Whitney test p-value<0.05 (mostly confirmed by Student test with Aspin-Welch correction, p-value<0.05) (Table S1). Proteins were therefore considered up/down-regulated if the average of the ratio of the protein expression were >1.37 and $<$

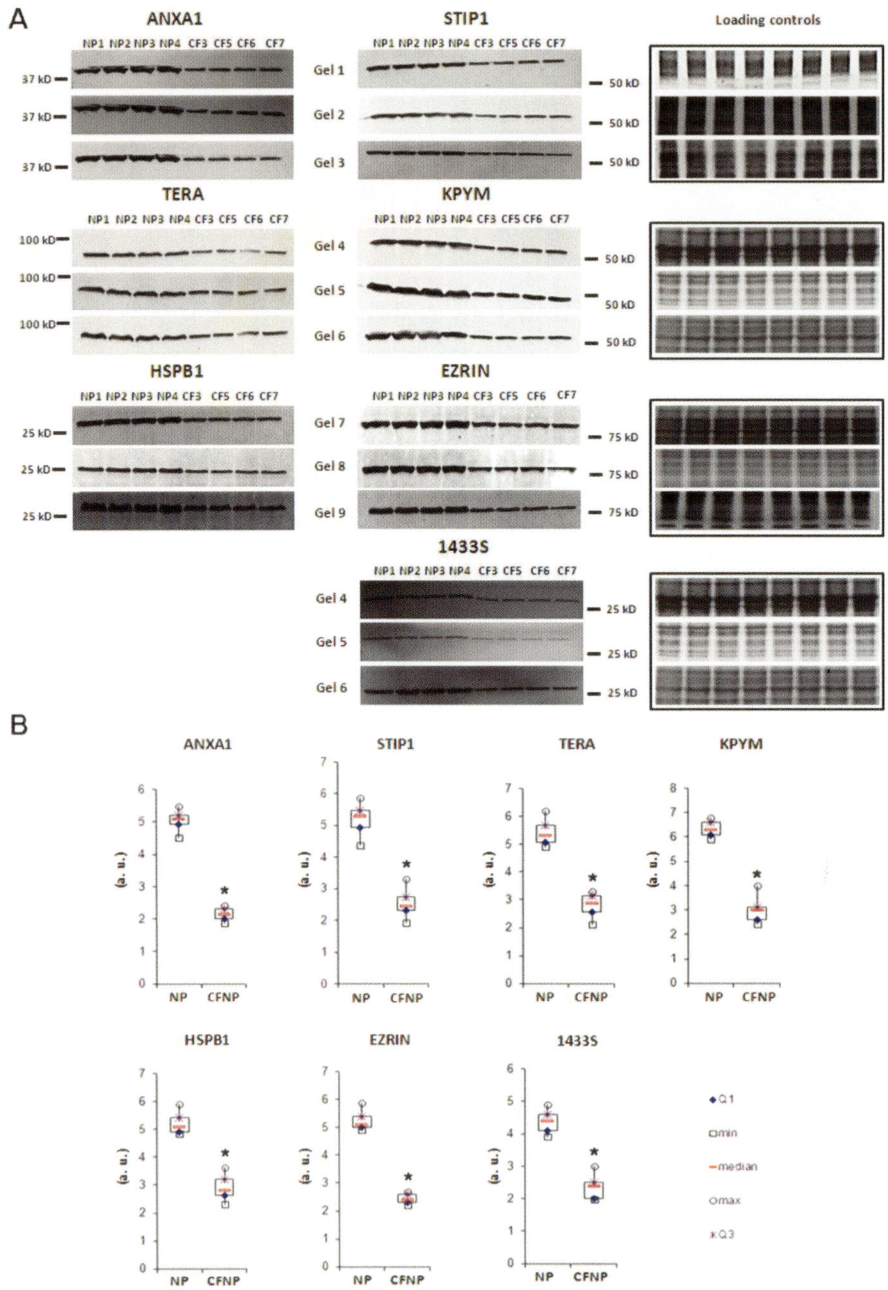

Figure 5. Western blot analysis of ANXA1, STIP1, TERA, KPYM, HSPB1, EZRIN and 1433S in primary cultures of human nasal epithelial cells (HNEC) from NP (n = 4) and CFNP (n = 4). A: Each protein was analyzed in three technical replicates. For normalization, the acrylamide gels were stained with Coomassie blue (total migrated protein detection) just after electro-transfer and scanned using the Odyssey LI-COR. Using the Odyssey software, protein intensity values were normalized with their corresponding loading control intensity values. **B**: Box plots of the intensity calculated with the Odyssey software, *$p < 0.01$, Mann and Whitney test. (a.u.: arbitrary units). We report Maximum (max), minimum (min), first quartile (Q1), third quartile (Q3).

0.73. To determine this threshold, we calculated the standard deviations of the protein ratios for each experiment, we normalized the Gaussian distributions and we calculated the average threshold to select the proteins upregulated (last 20% on the right of the Gaussian) and the more downregulated under-expressed (first 20% on the left of the Gaussian). These thresholds are in agreement with other studies using iTRAQ labeling [18]. Finally, the reliably quantified protein data set for both series of experiments were analysed using the AmiGO toolbox kit (http://amigo.geneontology.org/cgi-bin/amigo/term_enrichment and Cytoscape software).

SDS PAGE and Western blot

All Western blot analyses were performed according to previously described protocols [11]. Analysis of protein expression in HNEC was performed using antibodies directed against human STIP1, TERA, EZRI, ANXA1, 1433S, KPYM and HSPB1. All the used primary and secondary antibodies are listed in the

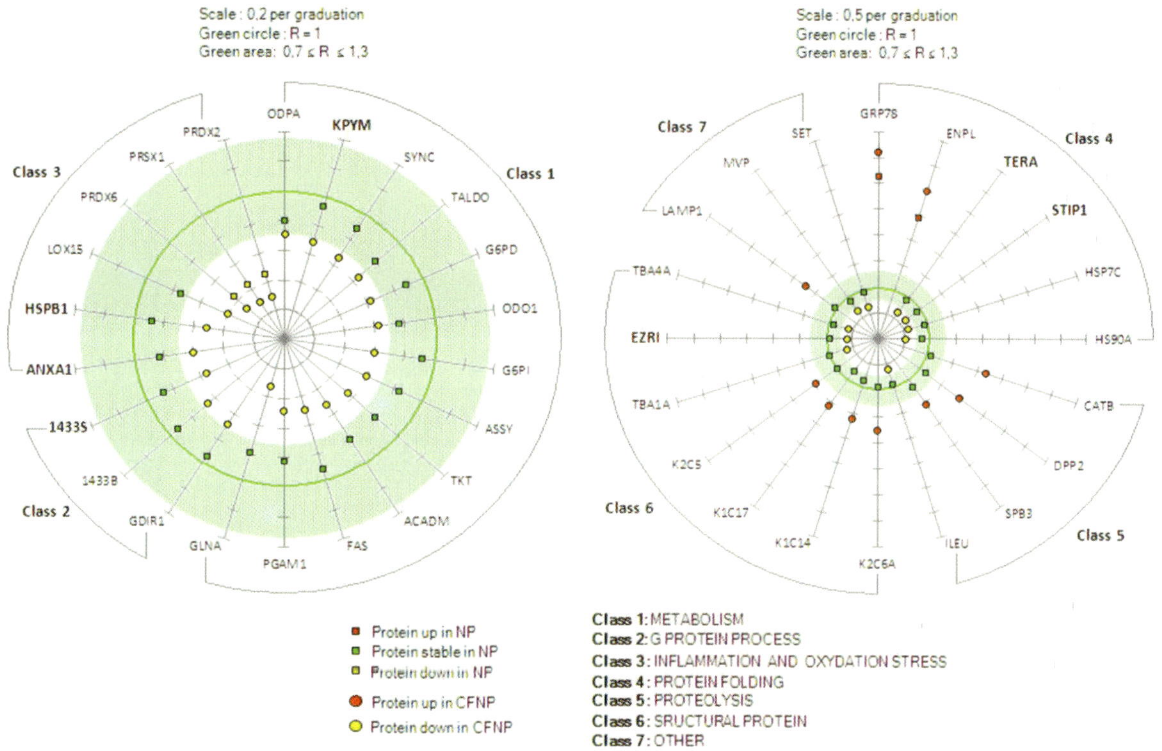

Figure 6. Expression pattern of the 42 differential proteins of interest in CF. The 42 differential proteins are displayed in seven different classes related to their functions (according to the AmiGO toolbox kit). Left graph: metabolism (class 1), G protein process (class 2), inflammation and oxidative stress (class 3); right graph): protein folding (class 4), proteolysis (class 5), structural protein (class 6), other (class 7). The green circle represent the absolute stable ratio value (R = 1) and the green area represent the ratio thresholds (0.73≤R≤1.37) (R = CFNP/CTRL or NP/CTRL). Scale graduations for R are 0.2 and 0.5 for left and right graph, respectively. The CFNP/CTRL ratio values of the differential proteins are represented by yellow dots (downregulated in CFNP) and red dots (upregulated in CFNP); the NP/CTRL ratio values are represented by yellow squares (downregulated in NP), red squares (upregulated in NP), and green squares (stable in NP). For the proteins in bold, the modulation was confirmed by Western blot. Protein names are from Swissprot, ratio values and p values are available in supplemental material (Table S1).

supplemental data with all the details including stock concentrations, used dilutions, manufacturer details and specificity (Table S2). For Western blots realized from NP 1, 2, 3, 4 and CFNP 3, 5, 6, 7, experiments were performed on four patients per category and in triplicate. Mann and Whitney test was used for comparison of data series and P values≤0.01 were considered statistically significant. Data are expressed with Box plots including median, maximum and minimum values and first and third quartiles.

SDS PAGE. Proteins were prepared as follows: first, HNEC from CF NP, NP and CTRL in Transwell filters were washed twice, scraped off the filters in ice-cold PBS, and centrifuged at 800 g for 10 min at 4°C. Second, the pellet was re-suspended in 500 µl of RIPA lysis buffer constituted of 150 mM NaCl, 50 mM Tris-HCl (pH 7.6), 1% v/v Triton X-100, 0.1% w/v SDS, 1% w/v sodium deoxychotate and antiprotease 1X, and kept on ice for 30 min under agitation. Third, the cell lysates were then centrifuged (20 000 g, 15 min) at 4°C. Finally, samples of the supernatants (20 µg protein in 1 volume Laemmli buffer containing 10% glycerol, 0.05 M Tris-HCl (pH 6.8), 0.1% SDS, 50 mM DTT, and 0.01% (w/v) bromophenol blue) were loaded onto 10% w/v polyacrylamide gels and run at 25 mA for 2 to 3 h at room temperature and electrically transferred at 200 mA for 90 min to nitrocellulose membranes.

Western blot analysis. The proteins of interest were detected using appropriate first and secondary antibodies all used at 1:15000 dilution. The infra-red signal was obtained by scanning with the Odyssey LI-COR (Techsciences, Cergy Saint Christophe, France). Quantification of protein levels was obtained using the Odyssey LI-COR software. For normalization, the acrylamide gels were stained with Coomassie blue (total migrated protein detection) just after electro-transfer [19] and scanned using the Odyssey LI-COR.

Results

Comparison of protein expression patterns in CFNP, NP and CTRL

186 proteins were quantified across eight patients in both sets of experiments (CFNP *vs.* NP and NP *vs.* CTRL). The distribution of modulated proteins was different in CF and NP: CFNP presented a higher proportion of deregulated proteins (24 upregulated and 65 downregulated) than NP patients (15 upregulated and 20 downregulated). In order to identify the proteins that were specifically deregulated in CFNP patients, we selected proteins that are significantly modulated in CFNP patients compared to NP patients. 8 proteins were upregulated in CFNP, but stable in NP patients, 29 were downregulated in CFNP but stable in NP, 3 proteins were significantly more downregulated and 2 proteins more upregulated in CFNP than in NP (Figure 2). In addition, 11 proteins were equally upregulated and 16 proteins were equally downregulated in both CFNP and NP. The expression ratios of the modulated proteins are presented in Figure 3 (Table S1 for full details). Seven of these 42 differential proteins (TERA, EZRIN, STIP1, KPYM, ANXA1, HSP27 and 1433S) were analyzed by

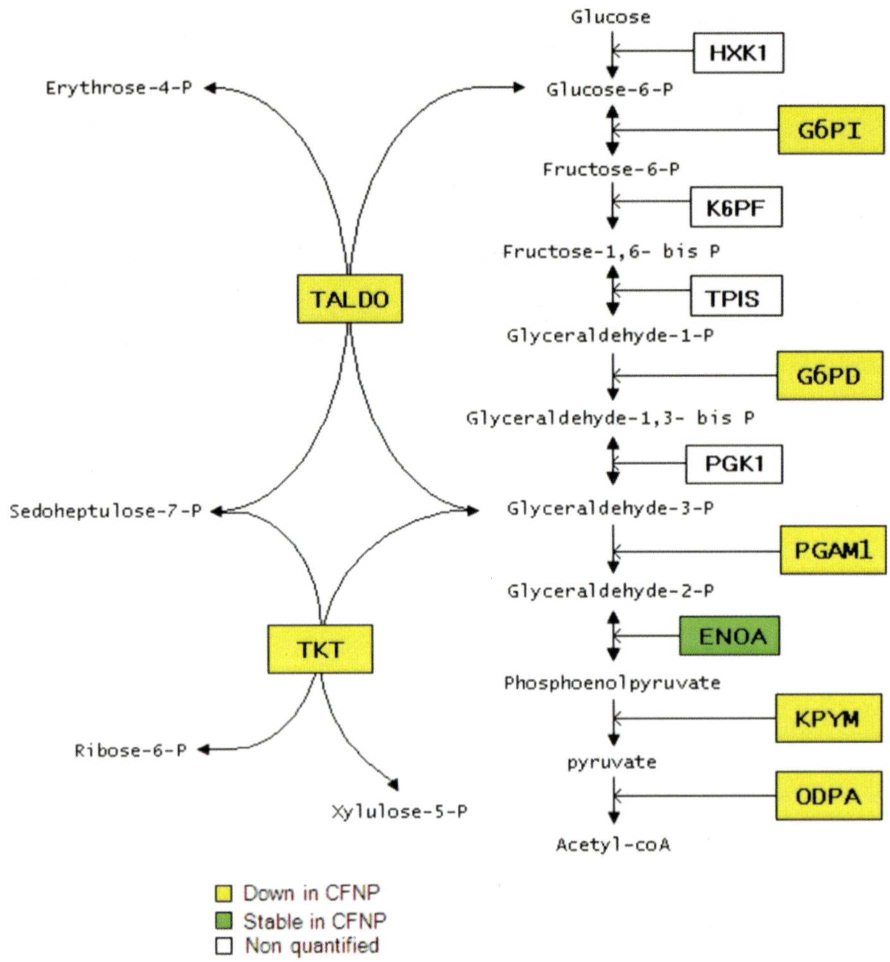

Figure 7. Diagram of the glycolysis/pentose pathway indicating the 7 downregulated proteins in CFNP.

Western blot on patients CFNP1, 2, 3, 4 and NP1, 2, 3, 4 (Figure 4). To extend our validation we repeated the Western blot analysis, on three new additional CFNP patients (CFNP5, 6, 7). Furthermore, technical reproducibility of Western blot analysis, was also assessed by performing three technical replicates for the seven above-mentioned proteins derived from NP1, 2, 3, 4 and CFNP3, 5, 6, 7 (Figure 5A). The statistical analysis of Western blot results confirmed fully the differential expressions observed in the proteomic quantification data (Figure 5B).

Functional distribution of the differential proteins in CFNP/CTRL

To further investigate the altered molecular mechanisms in CF epithelial cells, the differential proteins were analyzed using the AmiGO toolkit which allows highlighting the most represented classes of proteins in a given set. For the retained 42 proteins specifically modulated in CFNP, the AmiGO analysis revealed six major classes of proteins important for cell functions: metabolism, G protein process, inflammation and oxidative stress response, protein folding, proteolysis and structural proteins (Figure 6).

Metabolism (class 1). Thirteen proteins implicated in metabolism were downregulated specifically in CFNP. Among them, seven proteins implicated in glycolysis related metabolism (KPYM, G6PD, ODPA, G6PI, PGAM1, TALDO and TKT) were found downregulated in CFNP and stable in NP suggesting metabolism abnormalities related to CF. Four of these proteins are directly implicated in the canonical glycolytic pathway, pyruvate kinase (KPYM), glucose phosphate isomerase (G6PI), glucose phosphate dehydrogenase 1 (G6PD) and pyruvate dehydrogenase (ODPA). Three other proteins, phosphoglycerate mutase 1 (PGAM1), transketolase (TKT) and transaldolase (TALDO), are implicated in the interconnection between glycolysis and the pentose pathway (Figure 7). In addition, four proteins implicated in amino-acid metabolism, arginosuccinate synthase (ASSY), glutamine synthetase (GLNA), asparaginyl-tRNA synthetase (SYNC), oxoglutarate dehydrogenase (ODO1), and two proteins implicated in fatty acid metabolism, medium-chain specific acyl-CoA dehydrogenase (ACADM) and fatty acid synthase, (FAS) were also significantly downregulated in CFNP compared to NP and CTRL.

G protein process (class 2). Three proteins implicated in these pathways were significantly downregulated in CFNP compared to NP and CTRL, Rho GDP-dissociation inhibitor 1 (GDIR1), 14-3-3 proteins sigma and beta (1433S, 1433B), suggesting possible abnormalities in the ligand/receptor responsiveness in CF.

Inflammation and oxidative stress response (class 3). Six proteins implicated in enzymatic antioxidant response and inflammation were found to be downregulated in CFNP compared to NP and CTRL. Among them, three inflammation-related proteins, arachidonate 15-lipoxygenase (LOX15), annexin

A1 (ANXA1) and heat shock protein beta 1 (HSPB1) were stable in NP compared to control suggesting a CF specificity. Three proteins related to oxidative stress, the peroxiredoxins 1, 2 and 6, (PRDX1, 2 and 6), were downregulated in CFNP and NP compared to CTRL. However, these downregulations in CFNP were significantly lower compared to NP suggesting that these anomalies are present in both nasal polyposis but they are more severe in CF.

Protein folding (class 4). Four protein folding-related proteins were found significantly downregulated in CFNP whilst stable in NP. Interestingly, these proteins, heat shock protein 90-alpha and cognate 71 (HS90A, HSP7C), transitional endoplasmic reticulum ATPase (TERA), stress-induced-phosphoprotein 1 (STIP1), are known to participate in proper folding and degradation of CFTR [20–22]. In addition, two proteins related to protein folding in endoplasmic reticulum were upregulated in CFNP with significant differences with NP, glucose-regulated protein 78 (GRP78) and endoplasmin (ENPL). These proteins are known to be upregulated in the unfolded protein response (UPR) [23].

Proteolysis (class 5). Three proteins implicated in proteolysis were upregulated, serpin B3 (SPB3), cathepsin B (CATB) and dipeptidyl peptidase 2 (DPP2) and one downregulated, serpin B1 (ILEU), in CFNP and stable in NP suggesting proteolysis abnormalities related to CF.

Structural proteins (class 6). Focusing on the cytoskeleton, we observed four proteins upregulated, keratins 6A, 14, 17 and 5 (K2C6A, K1C14, K1C17, K2C5) and three downregulated, ezrin (EZRI), tubulins alpha 1A and 4A (TBA1A and TBA4A) in CFNP and stable in NP compared to CTRL suggesting a cytoskeleton reshuffle in CF.

Other (class 7). The HLA class II-associated protein I (SET) was downregulated in CF and is implicated in MAP kinase signaling since it regulates ERK1/2 phosphorylation [24]. We found an upregulation of the lysosome-associated membrane protein 1 (LAMP1), a well-known lysosomal membrane marker [25] suggesting an increased degradation activity in CF. Finally, the major vault protein (MVP) was downregulated in CF and is implicated in the bacterial resistance of lung epithelial cells [26].

Discussion

In this study we found 42 proteins significantly and specifically modulated in CFNP patients. For seven of these proteins the results were validated by Western blot in the eight patients analysed by proteomics and in three additional CF patients. Our data are also supported by previously published studies by us [11,13,27] and by others [9,10] showing deregulation of ANXA1 (in CFTR−/− mouse), of GRP78 for UPR activation (in both CFNP and NP), of PRDX6, PRDX2, CATB, HSPB1, PDIA3, ANXA1, VIME and EZRI (in CF cells). Importantly, we found many novel differentially expressed proteins in CF NP that could be of importance in CF pathophysiology.

Several proteins involved in CFTR synthesis/degradation were found to be dowregulated in CF (HSP7C, HS90A, STIP1, TERA and LAMP1), supporting previous observations of alteration of folding and degradation pathways in CF [20,21]. HSP7C, HS90A and STIP1 form a protein complex that assists correct CFTR protein folding and participates in the degradation of misfolded F508del CFTR by promoting ubiquitination [20,21,28]. In addition, TERA plays an essential role in endoplasmic reticulum-associated degradation [29] and is known to be involved in the ER-associated degradation of CFTR [22]. Of note, TERA, HSP7C and HS90A are present in the network of the CFTR physical interaction proteins (Figure 8). These downregulations observed in CF are surprising since F508del CFTR is mostly retained in ER for degradation and remain to be investigated. In addition, we observed an upregulation of a lysosomal membrane marker, LAMP1 [25], perhaps related to a raised turnover of the rescued F508del CFTR by the lysosomal pathway [30]. Altogether, these data may suggest a diminished folding-control/ER-degradation of F508del CFTR associated with a rise in lysosomal-mediated turnover, suggesting that F508del CFTR may be preferentially degraded by the lysosomal pathway in our model.

Several proteins involved in inflammation and oxidative stress were found to be deregulated in CF (PRDX1, 2 and 3, HSPB1, LOX15, ANXA1 and MVP), supporting previous studies [13,31,32]. PRDX1, 2 and 6 are implicated in enzymatic antioxidant defenses and we have previously shown a downregulation of PRDX6 under oxidative challenge in CFTR−/− mice lungs [13]. In another study, PRDX6 has also been found to be downregulated in HNEC of CF patients [10]. Another protein linked to oxidative stress, HSPB1 is able to raise intracellular glutathione levels [33] and activate ROS detoxification enzymes such as the peroxiredoxins mentioned above [34]. The decreased expression of these proteins in CFNP may result in lower protection against oxidative stress suggesting a susceptibility to oxidative damage in CF. LOX15 produces 15-hydroxyeicosatetraenoic acid (15-HPETE), an inhibitor of inflammatory mediators by promoting TNF mRNA decay [35]. ANXA1 is also known to have anti-inflammatory properties [36]. The downregulation of these two proteins participates in inflammation in CF by deregulating the eicosanoid-related pathway. Interestingly, MVP is known to participate in the resistance of airway cells to bacteria and may participate in the well-known lower resistance of CF patients to Pseudomonas aeruginosa infection [26].

Eight proteins belonging to the glucose and fatty acid metabolic pathways were found to be deregulated in CF (KPYM, G6PI, G6PD, ODPA, PGAM1, TALDO, TKT and ACADM). KPYM, G6PI, G6PD, ODPA, PGAM1, TALDO and TKT are directly implicated in the glycolysis/pentose pathway leading to NADPH and acyl-CoA production (Figure 7). Interestingly, a recent metabolomic study showed a diminished amount of glycolysis-related metabolites in CF cells (*i.e.* glucose, glucose-6-phosphate, fructose-6-phosphate) and concluded that glycolysis could be suppressed in CF [12]. However, a recent study showed upregulations of KPYM in IB3-1 cells compared to C38 cells, concluding that glycolysis could be increased in CF [8]. This discrepancy could be related to the differences between primary cells and transfected cellular lineages. ACADM is the medium chain of acyl-CoA dehydrogenase that is a key enzyme of fatty acid beta-oxidation leading to acyl-CoA production. The protein expression and activity of all these metabolic enzymes have never been directly investigated in CF. Altogether, our data show that the two major pathways leading to the production of NADPH and acetyl-CoA seem to be altered in CF and could further aggravate oxidative stress conditions.

Deregulation of proteases (SPB3 and CATB) and of a protease inhibitor (ILEU) may participate in lung fibrosis frequently observed in CF. SPB3, ILEU and CATB are important inflammation modulators. SPB3 and CATB (upregulated in this study) have been shown to promote lung, intestinal and liver fibrosis, respectively, in mouse models [37,38]. Furthermore, ILEU (downregulated in this study) is a leukocyte elastase inhibitor that prevents lung fibrosis in mice [39]. These anomalies, detected by us in upper airway epithelial cells, may represent at the cellular level the molecular anomalies that could lead to lung fibrosis. In addition, the upregulation of cytoplasmic structural proteins in CF

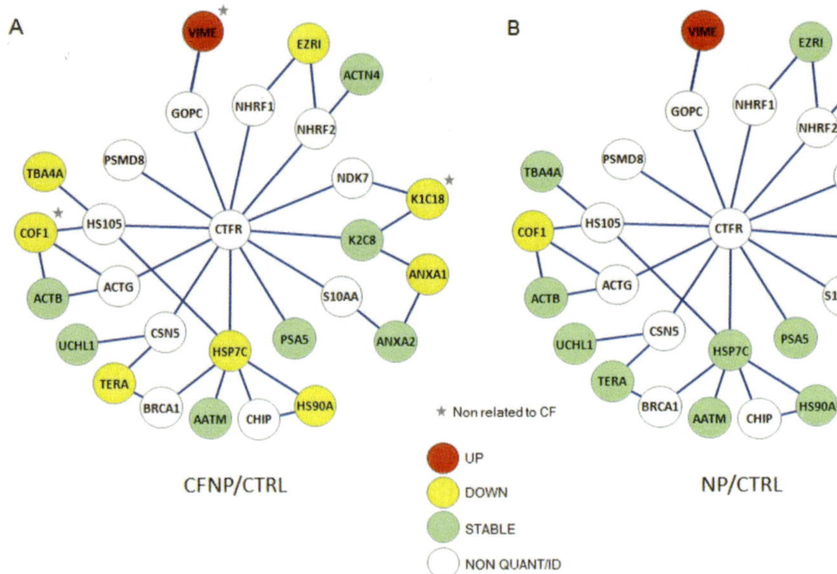

Figure 8. Quantified proteins present in the CFTR physical network. Proteomics quantitative analysis allowed us to reproducibly quantify 186 proteins. Of those, 16 could be mapped on a hand curated CFTR physical network based on the Biogrid interaction database (http://thebiogrid.org).This network is composed of 198 proteins selected according to experimental criteria for direct protein-protein interactions (surface plasmon resonance (SPR), pull-down and FRET experiments). To this bibliographic network, we have added proteins identified in our laboratory using SPR and DNA ligation assays. We built the CFTR protein interaction network by taking into account only proteins that directly interact with one another, at first and second degrees. In the graph, we represent the 16 proteins with a color code corresponding to their expression status in CF (**A**) and NP (**B**) compared to CTRL: upregulated (red), downregulated (yellow), stable (green). The network is completed by a minimal number of connecting proteins of the CFTR network (white) that could not be identified or quantified by MS/MS. Proteins that are up or downregulated in both CFNP and NP are marked by a grey star.

(K2C5, K1C14, K2C6A and K1C17) and the downregulation of TBA1A, TBA4A and EZRI, known to interact with CFTR by anchoring it to the tubulin cytoskeleton [40,41], suggest a possible intracellular remodeling of airway epithelial cells that could be related to trafficking and/or stabilization processes. All together, these results suggest a possible remodeling at the intra and extra cellular levels.

G protein related pathways were found to be altered in CF, suggesting numerous dysfunctions in CF cells. Three proteins related to G protein signaling (GDIR1, 1433B and 1433S) and one protein related to MAP kinase signaling (SET) (all downregulated) are multifunctional proteins that regulate most of the major cellular functions including proliferation, apoptosis, inflammatory response, epithelial cell polarization and secretory processes [42]. Those downregulations could be related to some or many alterations described above.

Finally, based on the Biogrid interaction database (http://thebiogrid.org), we built the CFTR protein interaction network by taking into account only proteins that directly interact with one another, at first and second degrees. This network is composed of 198 proteins selected according to experimental criteria for direct protein-protein interactions (surface plasmon resonance (SPR), pull-down and FRET experiments). To this bibliographic network we have added proteins identified in our laboratory using SPR and DNA ligation assays [43]. It is of interest to note that 16 of the 186 quantified proteins in the present study could be mapped on our handcurated CFTR physical network (Figure 8). Remarkably, 9 proteins out of these 16 were deregulated in CF patients (8 down and 1 up), while only 4 of the 16 proteins were downregulated (3) or upregulated (1) in NP patients (Figure 8). Those differentially expressed proteins are cytoskeleton or chaperon proteins that are all implicated in the folding, stability or degradation of CFTR. We suggest that some of the deregulated proteins in CF patients may be related to the perturbation of the CFTR/F508delCFTR physical network.

Overall, our proteomic study provides a reproducible set of differentially expressed proteins in airway epithelial cells from CF patients. While some of our findings correlate with previous studies, we have identified many novel differentially expressed proteins that have not been previously studied in CF pathophysiology.

Acknowledgments

We thank François Guillonneau and all the personnel of the 3P5 Proteomics facility, University Paris Descartes, Nicolas Cagnard of the Bioinformatic Platform University Paris Descartes and Dr. Charlotte Sumida for correcting the manuscript.

Author Contributions

Conceived and designed the experiments: AE EE LJ ICG. Performed the experiments: LJ ICG CC. Analyzed the data: ICG LJ. Contributed reagents/materials/analysis tools: AC JFP VPE PZ. Contributed to the writing of the manuscript: LJ ICG AE EE SA AC.

References

1. Rommens JM, Iannuzzi MC, Kerem B, Drumm ML, Melmer G, et al. (1989) Identification of the cystic fibrosis gene: chromosome walking and jumping. Science 245: 1059–1065.
2. Fokkens W, Lund V, Bachert C, Clement P, Helllings P, et al. (2005) EAACI position paper on rhinosinusitis and nasal polyps executive summary. Allergy 60: 583–601. doi:10.1111/j.1398-9995.2005.00830.x.
3. Beer H, Southern KW, Swift AC (2013) Topical nasal steroids for treating nasal polyposis in people with cystic fibrosis. Cochrane Database Syst Rev 4: CD008253. doi:10.1002/14651858.CD008253.pub3.
4. Sloane AJ, Lindner RA, Prasad SS, Sebastian LT, Pedersen SK, et al. (2005) Proteomic analysis of sputum from adults and children with cystic fibrosis and from control subjects. Am J Respir Crit Care Med 172: 1416–1426. doi:10.1164/rccm.200409-1215OC.
5. Pedersen SK, Sloane AJ, Prasad SS, Sebastian LT, Lindner RA, et al. (2005) An immunoproteomic approach for identification of clinical biomarkers for monitoring disease: application to cystic fibrosis. Mol Cell Proteomics MCP 4: 1052–1060. doi:10.1074/mcp.M400175-MCP200.
6. McMorran BJ, Patat SAO, Carlin JB, Grimwood K, Jones A, et al. (2007) Novel neutrophil-derived proteins in bronchoalveolar lavage fluid indicate an exaggerated inflammatory response in pediatric cystic fibrosis patients. Clin Chem 53: 1782–1791. doi:10.1373/clinchem.2007.087650.
7. Charro N, Hood BL, Faria D, Pacheco P, Azevedo P, et al. (2011) Serum proteomics signature of cystic fibrosis patients: a complementary 2-DE and LC-MS/MS approach. J Proteomics 74: 110–126. doi:10.1016/j.jprot.2010.10.001.
8. Ciavardelli D, D'Orazio M, Pieroni L, Consalvo A, Rossi C, et al. (2013) Proteomic and ionomic profiling reveals significant alterations of protein expression and calcium homeostasis in cystic fibrosis cells. Mol Biosyst 9: 1117–1126. doi:10.1039/c3mb25594h.
9. Pollard HB, Eidelman O, Jozwik C, Huang W, Srivastava M, et al. (2006) De novo biosynthetic profiling of high abundance proteins in cystic fibrosis lung epithelial cells. Mol Cell Proteomics MCP 5: 1628–1637. doi:10.1074/mcp.M600091-MCP200.
10. Roxo-Rosa M, da Costa G, Luider TM, Scholte BJ, Coelho AV, et al. (2006) Proteomic analysis of nasal cells from cystic fibrosis patients and non-cystic fibrosis control individuals: search for novel biomarkers of cystic fibrosis lung disease. Proteomics 6: 2314–2325. doi:10.1002/pmic.200500273.
11. Jeanson L, Kelly M, Coste A, Guerrera IC, Fritsch J, et al. (2012) Oxidative stress induces unfolding protein response and inflammation in nasal polyposis. Allergy 67: 403–412. doi:10.1111/j.1398-9995.2011.02769.x.
12. Wetmore DR, Joseloff E, Pilewski J, Lee DP, Lawton KA, et al. (2010) Metabolomic profiling reveals biochemical pathways and biomarkers associated with pathogenesis in cystic fibrosis cells. J Biol Chem 285: 30516–30522. doi:10.1074/jbc.M110.140806.
13. Trudel S, Kelly M, Fritsch J, Nguyen-Khoa T, Thérond P, et al. (2009) Peroxiredoxin 6 fails to limit phospholipid peroxidation in lung from Cftr-knockout mice subjected to oxidative challenge. PloS One 4: e6075. doi:10.1371/journal.pone.0006075.
14. Coste A, Girodon E, Louis S, Prulière-Escabasse V, Goossens M, et al. (2004) Atypical sinusitis in adults must lead to looking for cystic fibrosis and primary ciliary dyskinesia. The Laryngoscope 114: 839–843. doi:10.1097/00005537-200405000-00009.
15. Papon J-F, Coste A, Gendron M-C, Cordonnier C, Wingerstmann L, et al. (2002) HLA-DR and ICAM-1 expression and modulation in epithelial cells from nasal polyps. The Laryngoscope 112: 2067–2075. doi:10.1097/00005537-200211000-00030.
16. Guerrera IC, Quetier I, Fetouchi R, Moreau F, Vauloup-Fellous C, et al. (2014) Regulation of interleukin-6 in head and neck squamous cell carcinoma is related to papillomavirus infection. J Proteome Res 13: 1002–1011. doi:10.1021/pr401009f.
17. Bensalem N, Masscheleyn S, Mozo J, Vallée B, Brouillard F, et al. (2007) High sensitivity identification of membrane proteins by MALDI TOF-MASS spectrometry using polystyrene beads. J Proteome Res 6: 1595–1602. doi:10.1021/pr0606272.
18. Unwin RD, Griffiths JR, Whetton AD (2010) Simultaneous analysis of relative protein expression levels across multiple samples using iTRAQ isobaric tags with 2D nano LC-MS/MS. Nat Protoc 5: 1574–1582. doi:10.1038/nprot.2010.123.
19. Welinder C, Ekblad L (2011) Coomassie staining as loading control in Western blot analysis. J Proteome Res 10: 1416–1419. doi:10.1021/pr1011476.
20. Rubenstein RC, Zeitlin PL (2000) Sodium 4-phenylbutyrate downregulates Hsc70: implications for intracellular trafficking of DeltaF508-CFTR. Am J - Physiol Cell Physiol 278: C259–267.
21. Loo MA, Jensen TJ, Cui L, Hou Y, Chang XB, et al. (1998) Perturbation of Hsp90 interaction with nascent CFTR prevents its maturation and accelerates its degradation by the proteasome. EMBO J 17: 6879–6887. doi:10.1093/emboj/17.23.6879.
22. Boyault C, Gilquin B, Zhang Y, Rybin V, Garman E, et al. (2006) HDAC6-p97/VCP controlled polyubiquitin chain turnover. EMBO J 25: 3357–3366. doi:10.1038/sj.emboj.7601210.
23. Ma Y, Hendershot LM (2004) ER chaperone functions during normal and stress conditions. J Chem Neuroanat 28: 51–65. doi:10.1016/j.jchemneu.2003.08.007.
24. Yu L-G, Packman LC, Weldon M, Hamlett J, Rhodes JM (2004) Protein phosphatase 2A, a negative regulator of the ERK signaling pathway, is activated by tyrosine phosphorylation of putative HLA class II-associated protein I (PHAPI)/pp32 in response to the antiproliferative lectin, jacalin. J Biol Chem 279: 41377–41383. doi:10.1074/jbc.M400017200.
25. Sajjan US, Yang JH, Hershenson MB, LiPuma JJ (2006) Intracellular trafficking and replication of Burkholderia cenocepacia in human cystic fibrosis airway epithelial cells. Cell Microbiol 8: 1456–1466. doi:10.1111/j.1462-5822.2006.00724.x.
26. Kowalski MP, Dubouix-Bourandy A, Bajmoczi M, Golan DE, Zaidi T, et al. (2007) Host resistance to lung infection mediated by major vault protein in epithelial cells. Science 317: 130–132. doi:10.1126/science.1142311.
27. Bensalem N, Ventura AP, Vallée B, Lipecka J, Tondelier D, et al. (2005) Down-regulation of the anti-inflammatory protein annexin A1 in cystic fibrosis knock-out mice and patients. Mol Cell Proteomics MCP 4: 1591–1601. doi:10.1074/mcp.M500019-MCP200.
28. Onuoha SC, Coulstock ET, Grossmann JG, Jackson SE (2008) Structural studies on the co-chaperone Hop and its complexes with Hsp90. J Mol Biol 379: 732–744. doi:10.1016/j.jmb.2008.02.013.
29. Lim PJ, Danner R, Liang J, Doong H, Harman C, et al. (2009) Ubiquilin and p97/VCP bind erasin, forming a complex involved in ERAD. J Cell Biol 187: 201–217. doi:10.1083/jcb.200903024.
30. Cushing PR, Fellows A, Villone D, Boisguérin P, Madden DR (2008) The relative binding affinities of PDZ partners for CFTR: a biochemical basis for efficient endocytic recycling. Biochemistry (Mosc) 47: 10084–10098. doi:10.1021/bi8003928.
31. Kelly-Aubert M, Trudel S, Fritsch J, Nguyen-Khoa T, Baudouin-Legros M, et al. (2011) GSH monoethyl ester rescues mitochondrial defects in cystic fibrosis models. Hum Mol Genet 20: 2745–2759. doi:10.1093/hmg/ddr173.
32. Chen J, Kinter M, Shank S, Cotton C, Kelley TJ, et al. (2008) Dysfunction of Nrf-2 in CF epithelia leads to excess intracellular H_2O_2 and inflammatory cytokine production. PloS One 3: e3367. doi:10.1371/journal.pone.0003367.
33. Mehlen P, Kretz-Remy C, Préville X, Arrigo AP (1996) Human hsp27, Drosophila hsp27 and human alphaB-crystallin expression-mediated increase in glutathione is essential for the protective activity of these proteins against TNFalpha-induced cell death. EMBO J 15: 2695–2706.
34. Préville X, Salvemini F, Giraud S, Chaufour S, Paul C, et al. (1999) Mammalian small stress proteins protect against oxidative stress through their ability to increase glucose-6-phosphate dehydrogenase activity and by maintaining optimal cellular detoxifying machinery. Exp Cell Res 247: 61–78. doi:10.1006/excr.1998.4347.
35. Ferrante JV, Ferrante A (2005) Novel role of lipoxygenases in the inflammatory response: promotion of TNF mRNA decay by 15-hydroperoxyeicosatetraenoic acid in a monocytic cell line. J Immunol Baltim Md 1950 174: 3169–3172.
36. Jorge YC, Mataruco MM, Araújo LP, Rossi AFT, de Oliveira JG, et al. (2013) Expression of annexin-A1 and galectin-1 anti-inflammatory proteins and mRNA in chronic gastritis and gastric cancer. Mediators Inflamm 2013: 152860. doi:10.1155/2013/152860.
37. Lunardi F, Villano G, Perissinotto E, Agostini C, Rea F, et al. (2011) Overexpression of SERPIN B3 promotes epithelial proliferation and lung fibrosis in mice. Lab Investig J Tech Methods Pathol 91: 945–954. doi:10.1038/labinvest.2011.1.
38. Moles A, Tarrats N, Fernández-Checa JC, Marí M (2012) Cathepsin B overexpression due to acid sphingomyelinase ablation promotes liver fibrosis in Niemann-Pick disease. J Biol Chem 287: 1178–1188. doi:10.1074/jbc.M111.272393.
39. Takemasa A, Ishii Y, Fukuda T (2012) A neutrophil elastase inhibitor prevents bleomycin-induced pulmonary fibrosis in mice. Eur Respir J 40: 1475–1482. doi:10.1183/09031936.00127011.
40. Playford MP, Nurminen E, Pentikäinen OT, Milgram SL, Hartwig JH, et al. (2010) Cystic fibrosis transmembrane conductance regulator interacts with multiple immunoglobulin domains of filamin A. J Biol Chem 285: 17156–17165. doi:10.1074/jbc.M109.080523.
41. Castellani S, Guerra L, Favia M, Di Gioia S, Casavola V, et al. (2012) NHERF1 and CFTR restore tight junction organisation and function in cystic fibrosis airway epithelial cells: role of ezrin and the RhoA/ROCK pathway. Lab Investig J Tech Methods Pathol 92: 1527–1540. doi:10.1038/labinvest.2012.123.
42. Samanta AK, Chakraborty SN, Wang Y, Kantarjian H, Sun X, et al. (2009) Jak2 inhibition deactivates Lyn kinase through the SET-PP2A-SHP1 pathway, causing apoptosis in drug-resistant cells from chronic myelogenous leukemia patients. Oncogene 28: 1669–1681. doi:10.1038/onc.2009.7.
43. Colas J, Faure G, Saussereau E, Trudel S, Rabeh WM, et al. (2012) Disruption of cytokeratin-8 interaction with F508del-CFTR corrects its functional defect. Hum Mol Genet 21: 623–634. doi:10.1093/hmg/ddr496.

Testing Two Different Doses of Tiotropium Respimat in Cystic Fibrosis: Phase 2 Randomized Trial Results

Judy M. Bradley[1], Paul Koker[2], Qiqi Deng[2], Petra Moroni-Zentgraf[3], Felix Ratjen[4], David E. Geller[5], J. Stuart Elborn[6]* on behalf of the Tiotropium Cystic Fibrosis Study Group[¶]

1 Institute of Nursing and Health Research, University of Ulster, Ulster, Northern Ireland, **2** Boehringer Ingelheim Pharmaceuticals Inc, Ridgefield, Connecticut, United States of America, **3** Boehringer Ingelheim Pharma GmbH & Co KG, Ingelheim, Germany, **4** The Hospital for Sick Children, Toronto, Ontario, Canada, **5** Florida State University College of Medicine, Orlando, Florida, United States of America, **6** Centre for Infection and Immunity, Queen's University Belfast, Belfast, Northern Ireland

Abstract

Background: Tiotropium is a once-daily, long-acting anticholinergic bronchodilator with the potential to alleviate airway obstruction in cystic fibrosis. Our objective was to evaluate the efficacy and safety of 2.5 and 5 µg once-daily tiotropium delivered via the Respimat Soft Mist Inhaler vs. placebo in people with cystic fibrosis.

Methods: This phase 2, 12-week, randomized, double-blind, placebo-controlled parallel-group study of tiotropium Respimat as add-on to usual cystic fibrosis maintenance therapy included people with cystic fibrosis with pre-bronchodilator forced expiratory volume in 1 second (FEV_1) ≥25% predicted. Co-primary efficacy end points were change from baseline in percent-predicted FEV_1 area under the curve from 0 to 4 hours (FEV_1 AUC_{0-4h}), and trough FEV_1 at the end of week 12.

Findings: A total of 510 subjects with cystic fibrosis aged 5–69 years were randomized. Both doses of tiotropium resulted in significant improvement compared with placebo in the co-primary efficacy end points at the end of week 12 (change from baseline in percent-predicted FEV_1 AUC_{0-4h}: 2.5 µg: 2.94%, 95% confidence interval 1.19–4.70, p = 0.001; 5 µg: 3.39%, 95% confidence interval 1.67–5.12, p = 0.0001; in percent-predicted trough FEV_1:2.5 µg: 2.24%, p = 0.2; 5 µg: 2.22%, p = 0.02). There was a greater benefit with tiotropium 5 vs. 2.5 µg. No treatment-related adverse events or unexpected safety findings were observed in patients taking tiotropium.

Conclusions: Tiotropium significantly improved lung function in people with cystic fibrosis. The improvement was greater with the higher dose than the lower dose, with no difference in adverse events.

Editor: Leonardo M. Fabbri, University of Modena and Reggio Emilia, Italy

Funding: This study was funded by Boehringer Ingelheim. Boehringer Ingelheim was involved in the study design, data collection and analysis, decision to publish, and preparation of the manuscript.

Competing Interests: JSE acted as a consultant for Boehringer Ingelheim and was principal investigator for this study; JMB declares no conflicts; PK, QD, and PMZ are employees of Boehringer Ingelheim; FR acts as a consultant for Boehringer Ingelheim and is the principal investigator for the phase 3 study of tiotropium in CF; DEG declares no conflicts related to bronchodilators in CF.

* Email: s.elborn@qub.ac.uk

¶ Membership of the Tiotropium Cystic Fibrosis Study Group is provided in the Acknowledgments.

Introduction

Respiratory disease is the major cause of death in people with cystic fibrosis (CF), and new therapies addressing important pathophysiologic aspects of CF are urgently needed [1]. Treatments targeting airflow obstruction may provide clinical benefit to people with CF. Current standard therapy includes antibiotics, airway clearance techniques, dornase alfa, hypertonic saline, and inhaled bronchodilators [2]. Approximately 80% of people with CF use short- and/or long-acting bronchodilators, although their place as long-term therapy is not clearly defined and there are no bronchodilators with an approved indication for CF [3,4].

Bronchodilator agents improve pulmonary function and lessen wheezing in many people with CF [4]. The similar effectiveness of β_2 agonists and anticholinergics suggests that a significant proportion of airflow obstruction in CF is parasympathetically mediated [5]. Anticholinergic treatment may therefore prove a valuable add-on to current CF treatments.

A single dose of ipratropium bromide, a short-acting anticholinergic compound, has demonstrated lung function improvements in people with CF [6]. However, the long-term effects of maintenance therapy with ipratropium bromide have not been studied in CF. Tiotropium bromide (hereafter referred to as tiotropium), a long-acting anticholinergic compound delivered as an aqueous solution using the Respimat Soft Mist Inhaler, has consistently shown superior efficacy to ipratropium [7], and is well tolerated in the treatment of chronic obstructive pulmonary disease (COPD); these findings are consistent with those observed with the tiotropium 18 μg HandiHaler [8]. Tiotropium Respimat therefore has the potential to alleviate airflow obstruction in people with CF. Tiotropium Respimat was selected because the inhaler and formulation are suitable for populations of all ages. The inhaler is an active device that releases drug substance as an aerosol; hence, no minimal inspiratory flow is required by the patient. Suitability of the Respimat Soft Mist Inhaler was demonstrated in children aged <5 years using Respimat with a valved holding chamber and facemask [9,10]. Results from a phase 1 study *(manuscript in press)* showed that safety and tolerability of tiotropium are acceptable when compared with placebo in people with CF. Based on available data, tiotropium delivered by Respimat was tested at doses of 2.5 and 5 μg in this phase 2 study.

The primary objective was to evaluate the efficacy and safety of 12 weeks' treatment with tiotropium Respimat 2.5 or 5 μg once daily compared with placebo in people with CF. We hypothesized that treatment with tiotropium for 12 weeks is more effective in improving lung function compared with placebo, and that the higher dose of tiotropium (5 μg) is more effective than the 2.5 μg dose.

Methods

The protocol for this trial and supporting CONSORT checklist are available as supporting information; see Checklist S1 and Protocol S1.

Study Design

This was a double-blind, placebo-controlled, multicenter, multinational, parallel-group study to evaluate treatment with two doses of tiotropium (2.5 and 5 μg once daily, two inhalations at the same time of day) compared with placebo over 12 weeks (ClinicalTrials.gov identifier: NCT00737100). The trial period was from 23 September 2008 to 2 April 2010. The study was conducted at 94 centers in Australia, Europe, Canada, and the United States.

Ethical review was undertaken for each site/country by the local institutional review board/independent ethics committee and approval granted by the Competent Authority in each state.

Participants

Participants with documented CF had to be able to perform spirometric maneuvers according to American Thoracic Society (ATS) standards [11]. Patients of all ages were included, except in Russia, where patients aged <6 years were excluded. Subjects had to have a screening pre-bronchodilator forced expiratory volume in 1 second (FEV_1) ≥25% of predicted values [12,13] and inhale medication competently using the Respimat Soft Mist Inhaler. Patients were trained using a placebo Respimat device. They were to be clinically stable as defined by no evidence of acute respiratory tract infection or pulmonary exacerbation requiring use of antibiotics or oral corticosteroids within 4 weeks of screening. Pre-bronchodilator FEV_1 at week 0 or start of treatment had to be within 15% of FEV_1 at screening. All patients continued to receive their standard-of-care treatment during the study; tiotropium and placebo were considered add-on to usual therapy. If patients were diagnosed with a pulmonary exacerbation during the study period then this was recorded as an adverse event (AE) or serious AE, but there was no requirement to discontinue medication, and this decision was determined by the patient and physician. If taking long-term medication, participants had to agree to continue it throughout the study. Patients were allowed to continue using short-acting β-agonists (SABAs) and long-acting β-agonists (LABAs) if they were stabilized at least 4 weeks prior to randomization and throughout the study. Furthermore, patients taking SABAs and LABAs were required to have a 6-hour or 12-hour washout period, respectively, prior to all spirometry measurements.

Daily inhaled antibiotic use was allowed if stabilized for at least 6 weeks prior to and throughout the study period. Cyclic therapies (e.g., 4-week on/off tobramycin inhalation solution [TIS]) can impact treatment outcomes in short-term early phase trials. Cycled inhaled antibiotic use (e.g., TIS every other month) was allowed; however, the start of treatment had to be scheduled 2 weeks after the most recent TIS cycle and the last TIS cycle was to happen 2 weeks before the last treatment visit. This trial's 12-week design minimized the impact of cyclic medications by ensuring that baseline and final assessments were scheduled at a similar time point in the TIS cycle (i.e., both 2 weeks following completion of a TIS cycle). In order to comply with a 4-week on/off TIS regimen, the end-of-treatment visit may have been scheduled within 10–14 weeks after start of treatment to ensure baseline and end of study assessments occurred at mid-point of an off month in participants cycling TIS on alternate months. Physicians were advised to follow similar timing for other cycled medication use as for TIS, although this was not an official protocol procedure. Written informed consent was obtained from each patient or the patient's legal representative. Exclusion criteria (see Protocol S1 and File S1) included previous intolerance to tiotropium.

End Points

The co-primary end points for this trial were: i) the change from baseline (30 min prior to administration of first tiotropium dose at randomization; week 0) in percent-predicted FEV_1 area under the curve from time 0–4 hours (AUC_{0-4h}) at the end of week 12; and ii) the change from baseline (30 min prior to administration of first tiotropium dose at randomization; week 0) in percent-predicted trough FEV_1 at the end of week 12. The secondary outcomes in this study were changes from baseline in forced vital capacity (FVC), residual volume/total lung capacity (RV/TLC), forced expiratory flow (FEF) from 25% to 75% of vital capacity (FEF_{25-75}), Respiratory and Systemic Symptoms Questionnaire (RSSQ), and health-related quality of life (Cystic Fibrosis Questionnaire-Revised [CFQ-R]) at the end of week 12 [14]. AEs were also recorded. To measure exposure to the study drug, all patients were asked to return all dispensed Respimat inhalers.

Assessments

Pulmonary function tests (PFTs). The use of spirometers, including daily calibration, met ATS/European Respiratory Society criteria [15]. The qualifying PFTs (FEV_1 and FVC) were conducted at the screening visit. At weeks 0 and 12, PFTs were performed pre-dose (–10 minutes prior to study drug inhalation), at 30 minutes, and at 1, 2, 3, and 4 hours after inhalation of study drug. FEV_1 AUC_{0-4h} was calculated using the trapezoidal rule [16], divided by the duration (4 hours) reported in liters. Trough FEV_1 was defined as the FEV_1 value performed at –30 minutes prior to study drug inhalation. At weeks 4 and 8, PFTs were performed 30 minutes prior to drug administration. During the follow-up visit, after 30 days post-treatment (or at the time of premature study discontinuation), a single PFT was performed. Percent-predicted FEV_1 was calculated using the reference equations by Wang and colleagues [12] for pediatric/adolescents (aged 6–18 years) and by Knudson and colleagues [13] for adults (aged >18 years). RV/TLC measurements were performed as described in File S1.

Patient-reported outcomes. The proportion of patients with at least one pulmonary exacerbation during the double-blind period was analyzed using the RSSQ [17,18]. Health-related quality of life was assessed as the change from baseline in CFQ-R score [14]. Both methods are described in detail in File S1. For patients aged 6–13 years and depending on the patient's age and reading ability, the CFQ-R was administered to the patient directly, indirectly, or administered to their parent or caregiver. No patient under the age of 6 years completed the CFQ-R.

Safety. Medical history was recorded at screening. All patients were reviewed at screening and baseline entry into the study and at 2, 4, 8, and 12 weeks of therapy, and then at 30 days' post-treatment. Health status of patients who withdrew prematurely from the treatment period was followed up until their predicted study completion date. At each visit, all AEs and serious AEs, regardless of causality, were recorded.

Statistical Analyses

The primary analyses were performed in all randomized patients who received at least one dose of study drug and had both baseline and at least one post-dose PFT measurement at or before 12 weeks for either co-primary efficacy variable. Mean change from baseline in the co-primary efficacy variables (FEV_1 AUC_{0-4h} and trough FEV_1) was analyzed using a restricted maximum likelihood–based mixed-effect model with repeated measures (MMRM). To model the within-patient errors, an unstructured covariance matrix was used. Analyses were implemented using Statistical Analysis System software version 8.2 (SAS Institute Inc., Cary, NC, USA). The primary comparisons were between treatments after 12 weeks. The first co-primary end point, FEV_1 AUC_{0-4h}, was also stratified by age group. The age variable was dichotomized into patients aged 12 years and older and patients aged 11 years and younger, and was included in the model as a fixed effect. Other terms in the model were "treatment," "visit," "treatment-by-visit interaction," "baseline" and "baseline-by-visit interaction," and "random effect of center." Prespecified subgroup analyses for both primary end points included age group and baseline LABA use. The subgroup analyses were performed by adding subgroup, treatment-by subgroup, visit-by-subgroup, and treatment-by-visit-by subgroup interaction into the primary model.

All secondary end points on additional PFT parameters were analyzed as in the primary analysis, using the same MMRM model. For exacerbation analyses, Mantel-Haenszel test was adjusted for age group; treatment and age group were covariates for logistic regression analysis. The duration of pulmonary exacerbation was calculated based on the AE listings. Safety end points were summarized descriptively.

Data considered to be missing at random were not imputed, but handled in the analysis via the use of the MMRM model; only data that could be considered not missing at random were imputed. Randomly missing data with no subsequent non-missing values for that visit were imputed using the last observation carried forward technique (FEV_1, FVC, and FEF_{25-75} measurements).

In order to detect a difference of five units in the percentage change from baseline in FEV_1 values between tiotropium and placebo with 80% power at a two-sided significance level of 5%, a minimum of 465 patients in the full analysis set were required (155 in each treatment group). Based on a previous study [19], an approximate estimate of the expected standard deviation for FEV_1 percent-predicted value at screening was used (15.66). In this study, the ratio of adult to pediatric patients was approximately 2:1.

A detailed description of blinding and randomization and handling of missing data can be found in File S1.

Results

The study flow for this trial is summarized in Figure 1 [20].

Demographics and Other Baseline Characteristics

Of 620 recruited patients, a total of 510 patients (54% male) were randomized and treated (placebo, n = 168; tiotropium 2.5 µg, n = 166; tiotropium 5 µg, n = 176). Mean (SD) age was 20.9 (11.6) years (range, 5–69 years) and 27.1% were aged ≤11 years (range, 5–11 years). There were no clinically relevant differences between treatment groups (overall or by age group) in any demographic or baseline characteristic (Table 1).

Co-primary Efficacy End Points

For percent-predicted FEV_1 AUC_{0-4h} at the end of week 12, adjusted changes (improvements) from baseline were greater for both doses of tiotropium compared with placebo (tiotropium 2.5 µg: 1.20%; tiotropium 5 µg: 1.65%; placebo: –1.74%. Tiotropium 2.5 µg difference from placebo [95% CI]: 2.94% [1.19, 4.70], $p = 0.001$; tiotropium 5 µg difference from placebo [95% CI]: 3.39% [1.67, 5.12], $p = 0.0001$) (Fig. 2). The adjusted mean change was larger in the tiotropium 5 µg group than in the tiotropium 2.5 µg group (Fig. 2). The additional bronchodilator efficacy observed in the tiotropium 5 µg group was driven by the results obtained in patients younger than 12 years (Table 2). Both tiotropium dose groups had estimated mean changes (improvements), measured in liters at the end of week 12 (Table 2), that were statistically significantly greater than that of placebo.

Adjusted changes (improvements) from baseline in percent-predicted trough FEV_1 (at end of week 12) were greater for both doses of tiotropium compared with placebo (tiotropium 2.5 µg: 0.81%; tiotropium 5 µg: 0.78%; placebo: –1.44%. Tiotropium 2.5 µg difference from placebo [95% CI]: 2.24% [0.38, 4.11], $p = 0.02$; tiotropium 5 µg difference from placebo [95% CI]: 2.22% [0.38, 4.06], $p = 0.02$; Table 3). The mean adjusted change was similar between the tiotropium 2.5 µg and 5 µg groups and was not affected by age.

Other Lung Function Measures

Both the 2.5 and 5 µg doses of tiotropium had adjusted mean improvements from baseline in percent-predicted FVC AUC_{0-4h} response that were greater than placebo (tiotropium 2.5 µg: 0.53%; tiotropium 5 µg: 1.81%; placebo: –1.30%. Tiotropium 2.5 µg difference from placebo [95% CI]: 1.83% [–0.19, 3.86], $p = 0.08$; tiotropium 5 µg difference from placebo [95% CI]: 3.12% [1.12, 5.12], $p = 0.002$). The mean adjusted change was greater for tiotropium 5 than 2.5 µg and was only statistically significant for the tiotropium 5 µg group. The observed improvement for FVC AUC_{0-4h} in the tiotropium 5 µg group was largely driven by results in patients aged ≤11 years (described in detail in File S1).

Both doses of tiotropium had estimated adjusted mean improvements in percent-predicted trough FVC response that were greater than placebo, but not statistically significant (tiotropium 2.5 µg: 0.47%; tiotropium 5 µg: 0.81%; placebo: –0.39%. Tiotropium 2.5 µg difference from placebo [95% CI]: 0.85% [–1.08, 2.79], $p = 0.4$; tiotropium 5 µg difference from placebo [95% CI]: 1.19% [–0.72, 3.11], $p = 0.2$). FEF_{25-75} results were consistent with these results; static lung hyperinflation as measured by RV/TLC showed no difference between dose groups (described in detail in File S1).

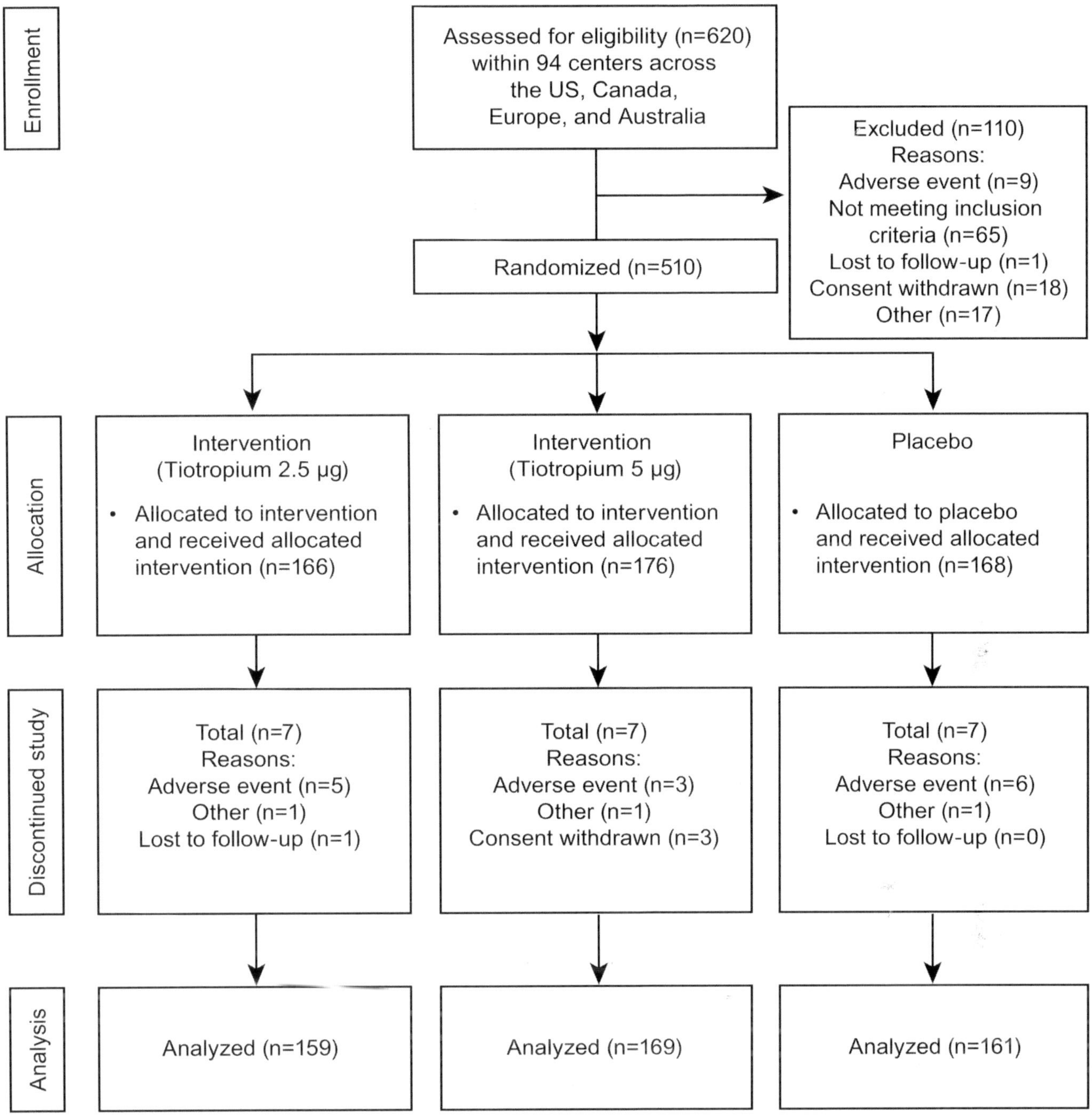

Figure 1. Flow diagram of participant recruitment and randomization [20].

Exposure

Overall exposure to study drug was acceptable, with a mean (SD) duration of treatment of 85.6 days (12.1); 87.5% of patients (446/510) took their study drug between >10 and ≤14 weeks. Approximately 9% of patients (47/510) took their study drug for ≥14 weeks.

Pulmonary Exacerbation as Assessed by RSSQ and Health-Related Quality of Life by CFQ-R

The proportions of patients who had at least one pulmonary exacerbation as determined by the RSSQ and intravenous antibiotic use were lower in the tiotropium 2.5 μg (7.8%) and 5 μg (6.9%) groups compared with the placebo group (9.6%; not statistically significant; $p = 0.9$ and $p = 0.6$ vs. placebo for tiotropium 2.5 μg and 5 μg respectively). Except for one pulmonary exacerbation in each treatment group, all events occurred in patients aged ≥12 years. The CFQ-R scores did not differ from baseline throughout the study period and no difference between the treatment groups was observed (additional results detailed in File S1).

Table 1. Patient demographics and characteristics of the study population at baseline.

	Placebo	Tiotropium 2.5 μg	Tiotropium 5 μg	Total
No. of patients	168	166	176	510
Male sex, n (%)	96 (57.1)	85 (51.2)	94 (53.4)	275 (53.9)
Age, years (mean, SD)	20.4 (11.6)	21.5 (12.0)	20.7 (11.3)	20.9 (11.6)
Age group, n (%)				
≤11 years	44 (26.2)	42 (25.3)	52 (29.5)	138 (27.1)
≥12 years	124 (73.8)	124 (74.7)	124 (70.5)	372 (72.9)
Percent-predicted FEV_1, (mean, SD)	76.6 (23.8)	75.4 (26.7)	75.9 (22.6)	76.0 (24.3)
≤11 years	94.9 (16.7)	98.8 (16.1)	90.3 (15.5)	94.3 (16.3)
≥12 years	70.1 (22.5)	67.5 (24.9)	69.9 (22.4)	69.2 (23.3)
BMI, kg/m^2 (mean, SD)	20.3 (4.4)	19.9 (4.0)	20.0 (4.1)	20.1 (4.2)
Baseline* concomitant pulmonary medications, n (%)	129 (76.8)	121 (72.9)	128 (72.7)	378 (74.1)
SABA	103 (61.3)	90 (54.2)	111 (63.1)	304 (59.6)
LABA	67 (39.9)	63 (38.0)	58 (33.0)	188 (36.9)

*Baseline includes all medications used on at least 1 day between informed consent and randomization (inclusive) and on at least 1 day between randomization and the first day of randomized drug intake (inclusive). BMI, body mass index; FEV_1, forced expiratory volume in 1 second; LABA, long-acting β-agonist; SABA, short-acting β-agonist; SD, standard deviation.

Subgroup Analysis

Differences in response to tiotropium by baseline LABA were explored by a prespecified subgroup analysis. In patients who used LABA at baseline, a larger difference compared with placebo (n = 64) was observed for the tiotropium 5 μg group (n = 56; 5.30% difference; 3.09% vs. −2.21%; 95% CI, 2.44–8.2; p = 0.0003) than for the tiotropium 2.5 μg (n = 60; 1.79% difference; −0.43% vs. −2.21%; 95% CI, −1.03 to −4.61; p = 0.2). In patients who did not use LABA at baseline, similar differences compared with placebo (n = 99) were observed for both tiotropium groups (tiotropium 2.5 μg: n = 98, 3.63% difference, 2.19% vs. −1.44%, 95% CI, 1.40–5.86, p = 0.002; tiotropium 5 μg: n = 113, 2.37% difference, 0.93% vs. −1.44%, 95% CI, 0.22–4.53, p = 0.03).

Adverse Events

The majority of patients (82.9%) reported one or more AE during the study. Most were mild to moderate in intensity and were primarily of respiratory nature; the most common AEs (defined as AE with an incidence >5% in any treatment group) were cough, exacerbation of CF, pyrexia, nasopharyngitis, and headache (Table 4). All deaths (two in the placebo group and one in the tiotropium 2.5 μg group) were due to exacerbation and/or complications of CF. An overall summary of AEs is provided in

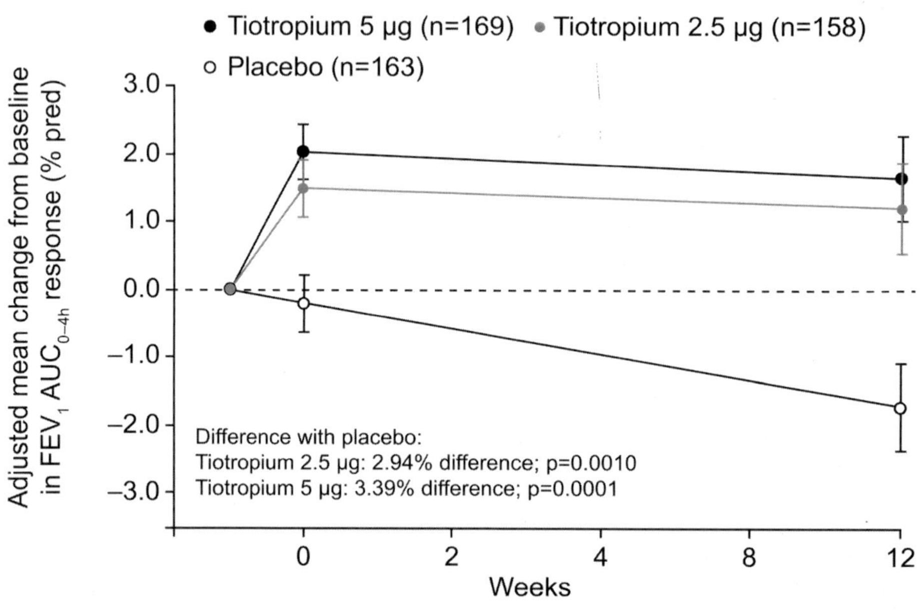

Figure 2. Adjusted mean FEV_1 AUC_{0-4h} (percent-predicted ± SE) change from baseline (full analysis set). AUC_{0-4h}, area under the curve from 0 to 4 hours; FEV_1, forced expiratory volume in 1 second.

Table 2. Adjusted mean (SE) changes from baseline in FEV_1 AUC_{0-4h} overall and in patients (aged ≤11 years and ≥12 years) treated with tiotropium (2.5 or 5 μg) or placebo after 12 weeks*.

Age group	Treatment	Difference from placebo		
Treatment	**Mean (SE)**	**Mean (SE)**	**p value**	**95% CI**
Overall, % predicted				
Placebo (n = 163)	−1.74 (0.65)			
Tiotropium 2.5 μg (n = 158)	1.20 (0.66)	2.94 (0.89)	0.0010	1.19–4.70
Tiotropium 5 μg (n = 169)	1.65 (0.63)	3.39 (0.88)	0.0001	1.67–5.12
Overall, L				
Placebo (n = 163)	−0.07 (0.02)			
Tiotropium 2.5 μg (n = 158)	0.02 (0.02)	0.09 (0.03)	0.0004	0.04–0.14
Tiotropium 5 μg (n = 169)	0.03 (0.02)	0.09 (0.02)	0.0002	0.05–0.14
≤11 years, % predicted				
Placebo (n = 43)	−0.32 (1.26)			
Tiotropium 2.5 μg (n = 42)	2.01 (1.29)	2.33 (1.74)	0.1801	−1.08 to 5.75
Tiotropium 5 μg (n = 50)	3.57 (1.16)	3.89 (1.67)	0.0199	0.62–7.17
≥12 years, % predicted				
Placebo (n = 120)	−2.55 (0.75)			
Tiotropium 2.5 μg (n = 116)	0.57 (0.76)	3.12 (1.04)	0.0028	1.08–5.17
Tiotropium 5 μg (n = 119)	0.55 (0.75)	3.11 (1.03)	0.0028	1.08–5.14

*Analysis of the full analysis set study group based on mixed-effect model with repeated measures model using unstructured covariance matrix.
AUC_{0-4h}, area under the curve from 0 to 4 hours; CI, confidence interval; FEV_1, forced expiratory volume in 1 second; SE, standard error.

Table 5 (and in File S1). Frequency of AEs was similar in all treatment arms and there was no evidence of a treatment relationship for any AE category; small differences between treatment groups were considered consequent to variability related to the overall small number of events.

Table 3. Adjusted mean (SE) changes from baseline in overall trough FEV_1 response and in patients (aged ≤11 years and ≥12 years) treated with tiotropium (2.5 or 5 μg) compared with placebo after 12 weeks*.

	Treatment	Difference from placebo		
Treatment	**Mean change (SE)**	**Mean change (SE)**	**p value**	**95% CI**
Overall, % predicted				
Placebo (n = 163)	−1.44 (0.71)			
Tiotropium 2.5 μg (n = 158)	0.81 (0.71)	2.24 (0.95)	0.0184	0.38–4.11
Tiotropium 5 μg (n = 169)	0.78 (0.69)	2.22 (0.93)	0.0179	0.38–4.06
Overall, L				
Placebo (n = 163)	−0.06 (0.02)			
Tiotropium 2.5 μg (n = 158)	−0.00 (0.02)	0.06 (0.03)	0.0330	0.00–0.11
Tiotropium 5 μg (n = 169)	−0.00 (0.02)	0.06 (0.03)	0.0281	0.01–0.11
≤11 years, % predicted				
Placebo (n = 43)	−0.83 (1.35)			
Tiotropium 2.5 μg (n = 42)	2.71 (1.38)	3.54 (1.86)	0.0577	−0.12 to 7.19
Tiotropium 5 μg (n = 50)	1.85 (1.24)	2.68 (1.78)	0.1322	−0.81 to 6.18
≥12 years, % predicted				
Placebo (n = 120)	−2.14 (0.80)			
Tiotropium 2.5 μg (n = 116)	−0.38 (0.81)	1.76 (1.11)	0.1128	−0.42 to 3.94
Tiotropium 5 μg (n = 119)	−0.11 (0.80)	2.03 (1.10)	0.0668	−0.14 to 4.20

*Analysis of the full analysis set study group based on mixed-effect model with repeated measures model using unstructured covariance matrix.
CI, confidence interval; FEV_1, forced expiratory volume in 1 second; SE, standard error.

Table 4. Summary of adverse events that occurred in >5% of patients in any treatment group (treated set).

	Placebo	Tiotropium 2.5 µg	Tiotropium 5 µg	Total
No. of patients, n	168	166	176	510
Cough, n (%)	34 (20.2)	35 (21.1)	46 (26.1)	115 (22.5)
Cystic fibrosis*, n (%)	17 (10.1)	23 (13.9)	25 (14.2)	65 (12.7)
Pyrexia, n (%)	17 (10.1)	9 (5.4)	18 (10.2)	44 (8.6)
Nasopharyngitis, n (%)	14 (8.3)	11 (6.6)	14 (8.0)	39 (7.6)
Headache, n (%)	18 (10.7)	7 (4.2)	14 (8.0)	39 (7.6)
Sputum increased	8 (4.8)	12 (7.2)	13 (7.4)	33 (6.5)
Abdominal pain	10 (6.0)	13 (7.8)	9 (5.1)	32 (6.3)
Hemoptysis	7 (4.2)	13 (7.8)	12 (6.8)	32 (6.3)
Oropharyngeal pain	13 (7.7)	5 (3.0)	11 (6.3)	29 (5.7)
Bronchitis	9 (5.4)	6 (3.6)	10 (5.7)	25 (4.9)
Upper respiratory tract infection	6 (3.6)	8 (4.8)	11 (6.3)	25 (4.9)
Rhinorrhea	9 (5.4)	6 (3.6)	9 (5.1)	24 (4.7)
Dyspnea	9 (5.4)	8 (4.8)	6 (3.4)	23 (4.5)
Nasal congestion	4 (2.4)	9 (5.4)	10 (5.7)	23 (4.5)
Sinusitis	6 (3.6)	3 (1.8)	9 (5.1)	18 (3.5)
Arthralgia	9 (5.4)	5 (3.0)	4 (2.3)	18 (3.5)

*The preferred adverse event term used for "CF exacerbation" was "cystic fibrosis."
A patient may have been counted in more than one preferred term. Percentages were calculated using the total number of patients per treatment as the denominator.
Medical Dictionary for Regulatory Activities (MedDRA) version used for reporting: 13.0.

Discussion

This is the first study to evaluate and provide evidence for the safety and efficacy of tiotropium in people with CF. Both doses of tiotropium resulted in statistically significant improvements compared with placebo in the co-primary efficacy end points of FEV_1 AUC_{0-4h} and trough FEV_1. Similarly, results for FEV_1 AUC_{0-4h} in liters and for FVC support the findings of the primary end points. Interestingly, a treatment benefit for respiratory symptoms (based on RSSQ) or health-related quality of life (based on CFQ-R) was not observed with either dose of tiotropium. Both doses of tiotropium were safe and well tolerated. The age subgroup analyses performed in our study demonstrate that tiotropium 5 µg is effective, with a favorable safety profile in children as well as in adults. The results from this study led to a phase 3 trial being performed using the 5 µg tiotropium dose [21].

Table 5. Overall summary of adverse events (treated set).

	Placebo	Tiotropium 2.5 µg	Tiotropium 5 µg	Total
No. of patients, n	168	166	176	510
Patients with any AE, n (%)	139 (82.7)	139 (83.7)	145 (82.4)	423 (82.9)
Patients with an SAE, n (%)	7 (4.2)	13 (7.8)	10 (5.7)	30 (5.9)
Patients with a study drug-related AE*, n (%)	14 (8.3)	15 (9.0)	18 (10.2)	47 (9.2)
Patients with other significant AE†, n (%)	3 (1.8)	2 (1.2)	3 (1.7)	8 (1.6)
Patients with AE leading to discontinuation of study drug, n (%)	6 (3.6)	6 (3.6)	3 (1.7)	15 (2.9)
Patients with SAEs, n (%)	21 (12.5)	28 (16.9)	21 (11·9)	70 (13.7)
Fatal, n	2	1	0	3
Immediately life-threatening, n	1	0	0	1
Disability/incapacity, n	0	0	1	1
Required hospitalization, n	21	28	21	70
Prolonged hospitalization, n	1	1	0	2
Congenital anomaly, n	0	0	0	0
Other, n	0	0	0	0

*As assessed by the study investigators. †As defined by International Conference on Harmonisation (ICH) E3 guidelines.
A patient may have been counted in more than one seriousness criterion. AE, adverse event; SAE, serious AE.

This study has a number of challenges in design, relating in particular to the use of cycled inhaled antibiotics. Study design was such that measurements were made on the off phase of inhaled antibiotic treatment for those on such treatment. The study was not sufficiently long to confidently determine the presence of any significant changes in symptoms or pulmonary exacerbations. The effects seen in the study should therefore be interpreted as demonstrating short- to medium-term effect of bronchodilator therapy by tiotropium. The study was, however, sufficiently powered to detect a meaningful change in FEV_1.

Despite widespread use, there is limited evidence supporting the use of bronchodilators in CF. A recent systematic review concluded that short-acting anticholinergics had no consistent effect on lung function tests in people with CF [22]. Efficacy of the LABA salmeterol in people with CF has only been investigated in several short-term (<1 week duration) clinical trials [23,24]. Results from one trial of longer-term use (24 weeks) showed improvement in FEV_1 in people with CF compared with treatment with salbutamol; however, no significant effect of salmeterol on other spirometric indices were detected in this trial, and therefore the clinical relevance of these results is debatable [25,22].

The highest tiotropium dose tested in this study, 5 µg daily, resulted in lung function improvement that was numerically above that observed for 2.5 µg. The study was not powered for differences between doses and no statistical comparison was performed; however, the effect of the 5 µg dose was about 15% greater than that of the 2.5 µg dose (percent-predicted FEV_1 AUC_{0-4h}) and the effect of the higher dose was more consistent across visits. Based on a numerically superior efficacy and a similar AE profile of both doses, 5 µg appeared to be the preferred dose for subsequent clinical development of tiotropium in people with CF. Longer term studies are required to evaluate the effect of tiotropium on symptoms.

Tiotropium Respimat 5 µg is also the approved dose for COPD patients, in whom evidence for improvements in lung function, exercise tolerance, and health-related quality of life, as well as reduction in the frequency of exacerbations, exists [26,27,28].

Effect sizes of lung function improvements for treatments used in CF patients vary widely [22] and it is difficult to compare the magnitude of improvement between different inhaled therapies such as mannitol [29,30], hypertonic saline [31], and TIS [32], as different variables are used (absolute change in FEV_1 from baseline vs. relative change). Currently, people with CF are recommended complex, time-intensive daily therapies that are often difficult to sustain over the long term, and the addition of new therapies usually increases that burden [33]. Drug delivery using the Respimat Soft Mist Inhaler is fast, easier than the more traditional metered-dose inhaler, and does not require a power source [34]. Furthermore, because it is effective over 24 hours, tiotropium only requires once-daily inhalation and therefore may ease the burden of the number of daily medications required in CF, contributing to improved compliance.

Conclusion

This study provides evidence of the efficacy and safety of inhaled tiotropium delivered by the Respimat Soft Mist Inhaler in people with CF and supports proceeding to further investigations in phase 3.

Acknowledgments

Writing and editorial assistance was provided by Sarah J Petit and Elena Garonna of PAREXEL. We also thank the Cystic Fibrosis Foundation Therapeutics - Therapeutic Development Network Coordinating Center and the European Cystic Fibrosis Society Clinical Trials Network for their support.

The principal investigators for the Tiotropium Cystic Fibrosis Study Group are (by country):

Australia: Barry Clements, Hugh Greville, Peter Middleton, David Serisier, Peter van Asperen;

Belgium: Lieven Dupont, Christiane Knoop, Anne Malfroot;

France: Chantal Belleguic, Raphael Chiron, Jocelyne Derelle, Stephane Dominique, Daniel Dusser, Jean-Louis Ginies, Marcel Guillot, Delphine Horeau-Langlard, Muriel Le Bourgeois, Sylvie Leroy, Christophe Marguet, Anne Munck, Jean-Claude Pautard, Philippe Reix, Marie-Laure Uffredi;

Germany: Manfred Ballmann, Joachim Bargon, Rainald Fischer, Felix Herth, Hans-Eberhard Heuer, Matthias Griese, Wolfgang Kamin, Martin Kohlhäufl, Lutz Nährlich, Joachim Riethmüller, Stephan Sorichter, Thomas Wagner;

United Kingdom: Lesley Bennett, Margaret Crawford, James Crossley, David Derry, Iolo Doull, J. Stuart Elborn, Mark Everard, Chris Groggins, Mary Johnson, Tim Lee, Rosemary Rayner, Alastair Reid, Alan Smyth, Kevin Southern, Douglas Thomas, Martin Walshaw, Joanna Whitehouse;

Italy: Cesare Braggion, Virginia De Rose, Rolando Gagliardini, Laura Minicucci;

Netherlands: M. Reijers, H.A.W.M. Tiddens;

New Zealand: Mark O'Carroll, Janice Wong;

Portugal: Celeste Barreto, Pilar Cardim, Mário Loureiro, Herculano Rocha, Maria Luisa Vaz;

Russia: Irina Asherova, Maria Chepurnaya, Alexander G. Chuchalin, Mikhail Ilkovich, Nikolay Kapranov, Alla Neretina; Alexander Orlov, Olga Simonova;

United States: Richard Ahrens, Ran Anbar, Julie Biller, Holly Carveth, Cori Daines, Stanley Fiel, Patrick Flume, Deborah Froh, James Harris III, Michelle Howenstine, Daniel Layish Susan Millard, Samya Nasr, H. Worth Parker, Mark Pian, James Royall, Carlos Sabogal, Matthias Salathe, Aruna Sannuti, David Schaeffer, Steven Strausbaugh, Debbie Toder, Santiago Reyes, Laurie Whittaker, Robert Zanni.

Author Contributions

Performed the experiments: JB PK QD PMZ FR DG JSE. Analyzed the data: JB PK QD PMZ FR DG JSE. Wrote the paper: JB PK QD PMZ FR DG JSE. Contributed to the planning and design of the trial: JB PK QD PMZ FR DG JSE.

References

1. Davis PB, Drumm M, Konstan MW (1996) Cystic fibrosis. Am J Respir Crit Care Med 154: 1229–1256.
2. Konstan MW, Butler SM, Schidlow DV, Morgan WJ, Julius JR, et al. (1999) Patterns of medical practice in cystic fibrosis: part II. Use of therapies. Investigators and Coordinators of the Epidemiologic Study of Cystic Fibrosis. Pediatr Pulmonol 28: 248–254.
3. Johnson C, Butler SM, Konstan MW, Morgan W, Wohl ME (2003) Factors influencing outcomes in cystic fibrosis: a center-based analysis. Chest 123: 20–27.

4. Colombo JL (2003) Long-acting bronchodilators in cystic fibrosis. Curr Opin Pulm Med 9: 504–508.
5. Cropp GJ (1996) Effectiveness of bronchodilators in cystic fibrosis. Am J Med 100: 19S–29S.
6. Avital A, Sanchez I, Chernick V (1992) Efficacy of salbutamol and ipratropium bromide in decreasing bronchial hyperreactivity in children with cystic fibrosis. Pediatr Pulmonol 13: 34–37.
7. Voshaar T, Lapidus R, Maleki-Yazdi R, Timmer W, Rubin E, et al. (2008) A randomized study of tiotropium Respimat Soft Mist inhaler vs. ipratropium pMDI in COPD. Respir Med 102: 32–41.
8. Bateman E, Singh D, Smith D, Disse B, Towse L, et al. (2010) Efficacy and safety of tiotropium Respimat SMI in COPD in two 1-year randomized studies. Int J Chron Obstruct Pulmon Dis 5: 197–208.
9. Kamin W, Bannemer-Schult K, Klemmer A, Schulze Schweinhorst P, Wachtel H, et al. (2010) Children below five years of age can handle Respimat Soft Mist inhaler [abstract]. Am J Respir Crit Care Med 181 A6254.
10. Kamin W, Bannemer-Schult K, Klemmer A, Schulze Schweinhorst P, Wachtel H, et al. (2011) Flow profile data indicate that Respimat with spacer is suitable for inhalation therapy of pre-school children. Presented at: International Society for Aerosols in Medicine Congress; 18–22 June 2011; Rotterdam, The Netherlands.
11. Farrell PM, Rosenstein BJ, White TB, Accurso FJ, Castellani C, et al. (2008) Guidelines for diagnosis of cystic fibrosis in newborns through older adults: Cystic Fibrosis Foundation consensus report. J Pediatr 153: S4–S14.
12. Wang X, Dockery DW, Wypij D, Gold DR, Speizer FE, et al. (1993) Pulmonary function growth velocity in children 6 to 18 years of age. Am Rev Respir Dis 148: 1502–1508.
13. Knudson RJ, Lebowitz MD, Holberg CJ, Burrows B (1983) Changes in the normal maximal expiratory flow-volume curve with growth and aging. Am Rev Respir Dis 127: 725–734.
14. Henry B, Aussage P, Grosskopf C, Goehrs JM (2003) Development of the Cystic Fibrosis Questionnaire (CFQ) for assessing quality of life in pediatric and adult patients. Qual Life Res 12: 63–76.
15. Miller MR, Hankinson J, Brusasco V, Burgos F, Casaburi R, et al. (2005) Standardisation of spirometry. Eur Respir J 26: 319–338.
16. Whittaker ET, Robinson G (1967) The trapezoidal and parabolic rules. The Calculus of Observations: an Introduction to Numerical Mathematics. 4th ed. Dover, New York, 156–158.
17. Goss CH, Burns JL (2007) Exacerbations in cystic fibrosis. 1: Epidemiology and pathogenesis. Thorax 62: 360–367.
18. Lymp J (2009) Pulmonary exacerbations in a phase 2 clinical trial of BIIL 284 BS in CF: development and implementation of a respiratory and systemic symptoms questionnaire (RSSQ) [abstract]. Pediatr Pulmonol S23 A221.
19. Koker P, Bhattacharya S, Staab A (2007) A randomized, double-blind, placebo controlled study to investigate the efficacy and safety of 24 weeks of oral treatment with BIIL 284 BS in adult (75 mg, 150 mg) and pediatric (75 mg) cystic fibrosis patients. Boeringher Ingelheim Report.
20. Moher D, Schulz KF, Altman DG (2001) The CONSORT statement: revised recommendations for improving the quality of reports of parallel group randomized trials. BMC Med Res Methodol 1: 2.
21. Ratjen F, Koker P, Geller D, Langellier-Cocteaux B, Maulf F Le, et al. (2013) Tiotropium Respimat in cystic fibrosis: efficacy and safety results of phase III randomized placebo-controlled trial [abstract]. J Cyst Fibros (Suppl 1): S64.
22. Halfhide C, Evans HJ, Couriel J (2005) Inhaled bronchodilators for cystic fibrosis. Cochrane Database Syst Rev: CD003428.
23. Hordvik NL, Sammut PH, Judy CG, Colombo JL (1999) Effects of standard and high doses of salmeterol on lung function of hospitalized patients with cystic fibrosis. Pediatr Pulmonol 27: 43–53.
24. Salvatore D, D'Andria M (2002) Effects of salmeterol on arterial oxyhemoglobin saturations in patients with cystic fibrosis. Pediatr Pulmonol 34: 11–15.
25. Hordvik NL, Sammut PH, Judy CG, Colombo JL (2002) Effectiveness and tolerability of high-dose salmeterol in cystic fibrosis. Pediatr Pulmonol 34: 287–296.
26. Ichinose M, Fujimoto T, Fukuchi Y (2010) Tiotropium 5 μg via Respimat and 18 μg via HandiHaler; efficacy and safety in Japanese COPD patients. Respir Med 104: 228–236.
27. van Noord JA, Cornelissen PJ, Aumann JL, Platz J, Mueller A, et al. (2009) The efficacy of tiotropium administered via Respimat Soft Mist Inhaler or HandiHaler in COPD patients. Respir Med 103: 22–29.
28. Spiriva RESPIMAT. Summary of Product Characteristics (2010) emc+ website. Available: http://www.medicines.org.uk/EMC/medicine/20134/SPC/Spiriva+Respimat+2.5+micrograms+solution+for+inhalation/. Accessed 9 June 2013.
29. Aitken ML, Bellon G, De BK, Flume PA, Fox HG, et al. (2012) Long-term inhaled dry powder mannitol in cystic fibrosis: an international randomized study. Am J Respir Crit Care Med 185: 645–652.
30. Bilton D, Bellon G, Charlton B, Cooper P, De BK, et al. (2013) Pooled analysis of two large randomised phase III inhaled mannitol studies in cystic fibrosis. J Cyst Fibros 12: 367–376.
31. Elkins MR, Robinson M, Rose BR, Harbour C, Moriarty CP, et al. (2006) A controlled trial of long-term inhaled hypertonic saline in patients with cystic fibrosis. N Engl J Med 354: 229–240.
32. Vandyke RD, McPhail GL, Huang B, Fenchel MC, Amin RS, et al. (2013) Inhaled tobramycin effectively reduces FEV1 decline in cystic fibrosis. An instrumental variables analysis. Ann Am Thorac Soc 10: 205–212.
33. Royce FH, Carl JC (2011) Health-related quality of life in cystic fibrosis. Curr Opin Pediatr 23: 535–540.
34. Kesser KC, Geller DE (2009) New aerosol delivery devices for cystic fibrosis. Respir Care 54: 754–767.

23

A Physiologically-Motivated Compartment-Based Model of the Effect of Inhaled Hypertonic Saline on Mucociliary Clearance and Liquid Transport in Cystic Fibrosis

Matthew R. Markovetz[1], Timothy E. Corcoran[1,2,6], Landon W. Locke[2], Michael M. Myerburg[2], Joseph M. Pilewski[2], Robert S. Parker[1,3,4,5]*

1 Department of Chemical and Petroleum Engineering, Swanson School of Engineering, University of Pittsburgh, Pittsburgh, PA, United States of America, **2** Pulmonary Allergy and Critical Care Medicine, University of Pittsburgh, Pittsburgh, PA, United States of America, **3** McGowan Institute of Regenerative Medicine, University of Pittsburgh, Pittsburgh, PA, United States of America, **4** Clinical Research, Investigation, and Systems Modeling of Acute Illness (CRISMA) Laboratories, University of Pittsburgh, Pittsburgh, PA, United States of America, **5** University of Pittsburgh Cancer Institute, University of Pittsburgh, Pittsburgh, PA, United States of America, **6** Department of Bioengineering, Swanson School of Engineering, University of Pittsburgh, Pittsburgh, PA, United States of America

Abstract

Background: Cystic Fibrosis (CF) lung disease is characterized by liquid hyperabsorption, airway surface dehydration, and impaired mucociliary clearance (MCC). Herein, we present a compartment-based mathematical model of the airway that extends the resolution of functional imaging data.

Methods: Using functional imaging data to inform our model, we developed a system of mechanism-motivated ordinary differential equations to describe the mucociliary clearance and absorption of aerosolized radiolabeled particle and small molecules probes from human subjects with and without CF. We also utilized a novel imaging metric *in vitro* to gauge the fraction of airway epithelial cells that have functional ciliary activity.

Results: This model, and its incorporated kinetic rate parameters, captures the MCC and liquid dynamics of the hyperabsorptive state in CF airways and the mitigation of that state by hypertonic saline treatment.

Conclusions: We postulate, based on the model structure and its ability to capture clinical patient data, that patients with CF have regions of airway with diminished MCC function that can be recruited with hypertonic saline treatment. In so doing, this model structure not only makes a case for durable osmotic agents used in lung-region specific treatments, but also may provide a possible clinical endpoint, the fraction of functional ciliated airway.

Editor: Nades Palaniyar, The Hospital for Sick Children and The University of Toronto, Canada

Funding: MRM is supported by a Graduate Assistantships in Areas of National Need (GAANN) fellowship (U.S. Department of Education (www.ed.gov), P200A120195). The functional imaging project in [6] and TEC were supported by National Institutes of Health (www.nih.gov) R01HL108929. RSP acknowledges support of the B.P. America Faculty Fellowship in the Swanson School of Engineering. MMM acknowledges support from National Institutes of Health (www.nih.gov) RO1HL112862. Work performed in HBE cell cultures was supported by the NIH (www.nih.gov) P30DK072506 and the Cystic Fibrosis Foundation (www.cff.org) Research Development Program. The content is solely the responsibility of the authors and does not necessarily represent the official views of the National Heart, Lung, and Blood Institute or the National Institutes of Health. The funders had no role in study design, data collection and analysis, decision to publish, or preparation of the manuscript.

* Email: rparker@pitt.edu

Introduction

Cystic Fibrosis (CF) is an autosomal recessive disease that arises from a defect in the Cystic Fibrosis Transmembrane Conductance Regulator (CFTR) gene. CF affects multiple organ systems, with the most detrimental effects occurring in the lungs [1]. CFTR encodes an anion channel on epithelial surfaces, that is dysfunctional or absent from the CF epithelium. The associated loss of Cl^- and HCO_3^- secretion along with a tendency to hyperabsorb Na^+ through the epithelial sodium channel (ENaC) results in osmotic gradients that favor rapid absorption of the airway surface liquid (ASL) layer, leading to dehydrated airway mucus secretions and impaired mucociliary clearance (MCC) [2], [3]. The inability to clear pathogens via MCC leads to chronic infection, inflammation, airway damage, and premature respiratory failure.

Inhaled agents that reverse osmotic gradients in the airways are used to treat the ASL dehydration defect associated with CF. Hypertonic saline (HS) is one such osmotic agent that has been shown to increase both MCC and lung function in patients with CF [4], [5]. More recently CFTR modulators have been developed that substantially improve lung function in individuals with specific CFTR mutations [6].

Outcome measures and biomarkers that quantify the basic pathophysiology of CF lung disease are needed to allow for the rapid screening of new therapeutics for CF. Ideally, these screening methods seek to quantify the basic pathophysiology of CF lung disease. Mucociliary clearance scans, which quantify the clearance of a radiolabeled particulate from the lungs, are one such functional imaging method for studying outcomes in CF. We have expanded this method to include measuring the clearance of a radiolabeled small-molecule that can be absorbed as well as cleared via MCC. Similar techniques have been used in the past to resolve the individual components of lung clearance [7], [8]. Our *in vivo* method utilizes Technetium 99m sulfur colloid (Tc-SC) as the non-absorbable particle probe and Indium 111-DTPA (DTPA) as the small molecule probe. The probes are delivered together in a liquid aerosol. Figure 1 presents a schematic for pharmaceutical clearance from the airway epithelium. We assume that MCC clears the probes at similar rates and that the difference in their clearance rates is therefore associated with the absorption of the small molecule. Previous *in vitro* studies have demonstrated a relationship between DTPA and airway surface liquid absorption rates [9]. DTPA absorption is increased both *in vivo* in CF airways and *in vitro* in CF airway cell cultures [9], [10]. Decreases in DTPA absorption after osmotic therapies have also been demonstrated *in vitro* and *in vivo* [9], [10]. Thus, multi-probe methods provide measurements of both MCC and ASL absorption rates [10]. Successful CF therapies should restore ASL volume by correcting defective airway epithelial ion transport [11], [12]. The restoration of airway hydration should be rapidly detectable through these multi-probe imaging methods as decreased liquid absorption rates are reflected through slower absorption of DTPA and improvements in MCC cause increased Tc-SC clearance.

Herein we present a compartment-based model of particle and small molecule clearance from the human respiratory tract that uses functional imaging data to inform model structure and quantitate parameter values. Our goal in developing this model is to better resolve the specific physiological mechanisms that contribute to the composite functional imaging result. We believe that these mechanism-specific measurements may provide more sensitive and specific evaluations of therapeutic efficacy than the currently used image-derived metrics. The challenge is to construct a mathematical representation of the physiology that can resolve the underlying mechanisms and their interactions.

There have been a number of compartment-based pharmacokinetic (PK) models for inhaled pharmaceuticals [13], [14], [15], [16], [17], but to our knowledge none have considered the PK behavior of the radiopharmaceuticals used for functional imaging from which our data originates, nor has anyone assessed absorption kinetics with the methodology we have employed. We hypothesize that by dividing the lung into a solely absorptive peripheral lung region and separate central lung region that has both absorptive and MCC capability, and by subdividing this central lung region into fractions with, and without, functional ciliated airway, we can reproduce the dynamics of simultaneous particle and small molecule probe clearance from the lung. We further hypothesize that (i) functional ciliated airway clears at the same rate in patients with CF and non-CF subjects; (ii) the fraction of functional ciliated airway (FFCA) is decreased in CF; and (iii) FFCA can be increased through inhalation of HS. Our models provide estimates of FFCA, MCC, and large airway and peripheral lung absorption, the latter of which we believe is related to liquid hyper-absorption in CF small airways. These measured parameters may substantially expand the utility of our functional imaging measurement by providing more mechanistic insight into lung physiology and response to therapeutic agents (a list of all abbreviations and their definition used in this work can be found in Table 1).

Results

Model Synthesis and Assumptions

Starting from the original model of Sakagami [15], we extend it structurally to account for the dynamics and kinetics observed in

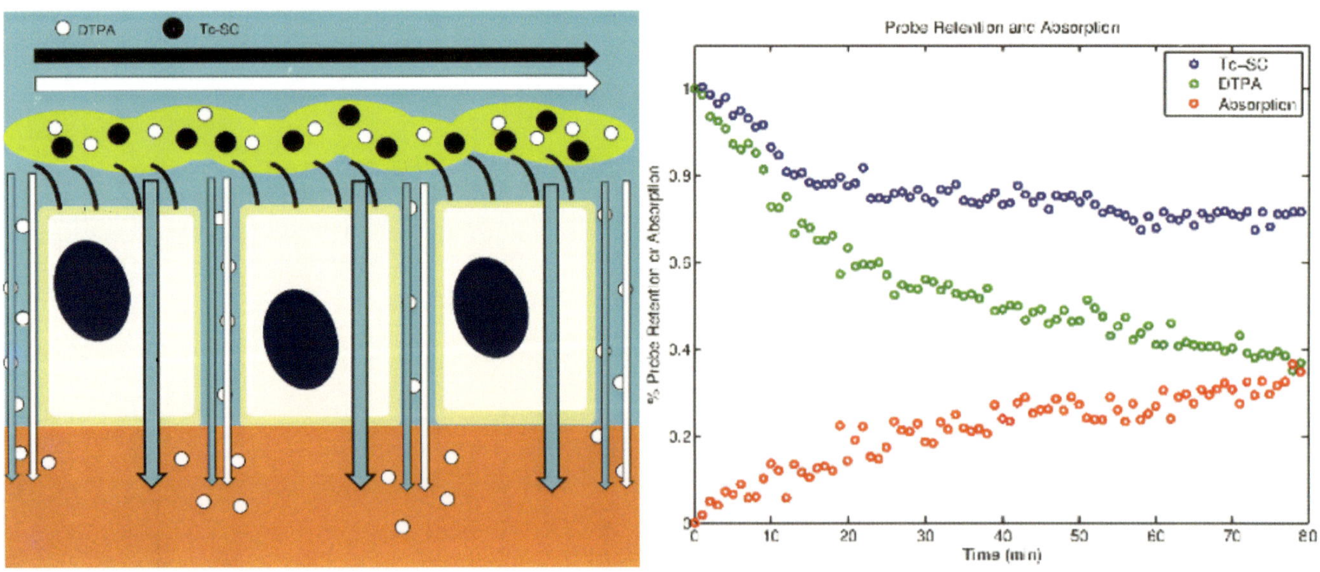

Figure 1. Left panel: schematic of transport routes in the airway epithelium. The black and white horizontal arrows represent mucociliary clearance of Tc-SC and DTPA, respectively. DTPA (downward white arrow) absorbs across the airway epithelium via the paracellular route. Water (downward blue arrow) also absorbs across the epithelium via the transcellular and paracellular route. Right panel: normalized Tc-SC (blue circles) and DTPA (green circles) retention curves with the difference between the respective datasets at each time point shown as absorption (red circles) in CF subject 8.

Table 1. Abbreviations and constants in the work presented herein.

Abbreviation	Description
AIC	Akaike Information Criterion; a Metric of Model Appropriateness
ASL	Airway Surface Liquid Layer
C	Imaging Region of Interest About the Central Lung; Analogous to L in Model
CF	Cystic Fibrosis
CFTR	Cystic Fibrosis Transmembrane Conductance Regulator
CI	Confidence Interval
DMEM	Dulbecco's Modified Eagle Medium
DTPA	Indium-111 Diethylene Triamine Pentaacetic Acid
ENaC	Epithelial Sodium Channel
FFCA	Fraction of Functional Ciliated Airway
HBE	Human Bronchial Epithelial (cell)
HS	Hypertonic Saline
IS	Isotonic Saline
k	Number of Free Parameters in Model
MCC	Mucociliary Clearance
N	Number of Data Points Analyzed for Model Fit
ODE	Ordinary Differential Equation
PK	Pharmacokinetic
Tc-SC	Technetium-99m Sulfur Colloid
W_i	Weighting Factor of the ith Element of the Dataset for AIC
y_i	i^{th} Value of Dataset
$\hat{y}_i$	i^{th} Value of Model Fit

the clinical data set. Founded on a basic understanding of lung anatomy and physiology, the lung structure can be lumped into two key dynamical structures as shown in Figure 2. Additional assumptions made in synthesizing this model are as follows:

- A fraction of the large airways (L), which are represented in the central (C) lung region of interest (ROI) [18], has functional MCC, with MCC in the remainder of L being non-functional. This allows the subdivision of L into two sub-compartments: L_F, which has functional MCC, and L_N, which has no functional MCC.
- The initial doses of the radiopharmaceuticals delivered to either the central (C_0) or peripheral (P_0) lung regions are described as the number of counts within C or in the area outside of C but within the whole lung ROI in the first image, respectively [10] (Figure S1 provides a visual representation of the C and P ROIs).
- 10% of inhaled radiopharmaceuticals were assumed to deposit in the trachea (T_0) [15]. However, neither counts in T nor the bloodstream (B) have a unique impact on the clearance of the Tc-SC and DTPA.
- MCC in the distal lung D, which contains small and intermediate-sized airways in addition to alveoli [18], is a slow process; given the 80-min timescale of our data this rate cannot be resolved with confidence. As a result, the MCC term from D to L, k_{DL}, is neglected.

The result of these assumptions is a three-compartment model for MCC in the lung wherein two compartments (D and L_N) are absorptive and one compartment (L_F) has MCC in addition to absorptive clearance, as shown in Figure 2.

Model Equations

Equations modeling the transport of both of the probes are outlined below. The model parameters k_{LT}, k_{DB}, k_{LB} and FFCA, the fraction of L with functional MCC, were determined by nonlinear least-squares regression as described in **Methods**. For Tc-SC clearance, k_{DB} and k_{LB} are set equal to 0. The mathematical description of this model, written as ODEs representing the change in counts in each model compartment, is as follows (see Table 2 for full list of model abbreviations):

$$\frac{dD}{dt} = -k_{DB}D \quad (1)$$

$$\frac{dL_N}{dt} = -k_{LB}L_N \quad (2)$$

$$\frac{dL_F}{dt} = -k_{LB}L_F - k_{LT}L_F \quad (3)$$

$$\frac{dT}{dt} = k_{LT}L_F \quad (4)$$

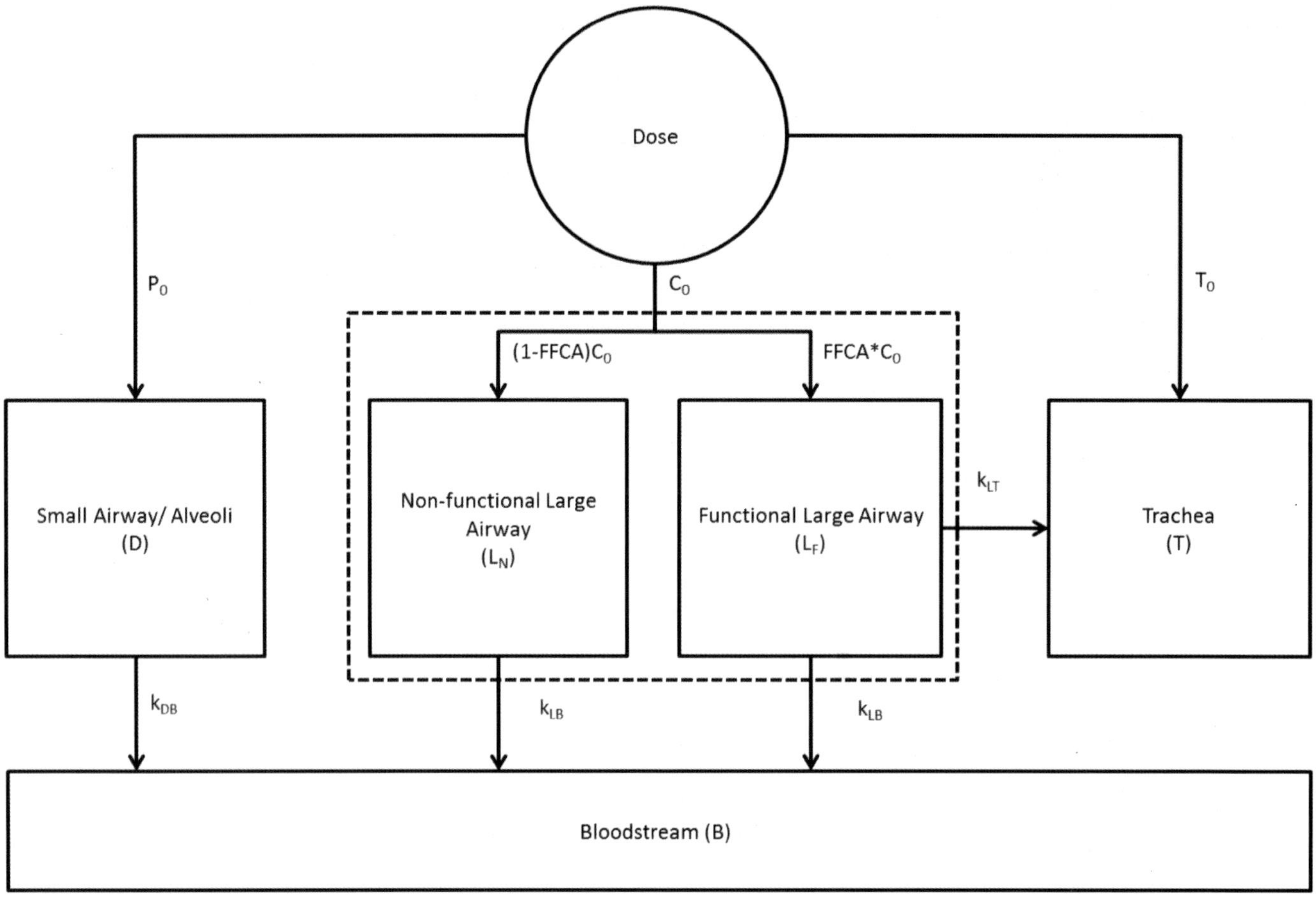

Figure 2. Schematic model structure describing the clearance of small molecule and particle probes from the lung. Initial depositions: T_0 = trachea, C_0 = central, P_0 = peripheral. See Table 1 for full list of model abbreviations.

$$\frac{dB}{dt} = k_{DB}D + k_{LB}(L_N + L_F) \quad (5)$$

Model Fit and Predictions

The ability of our model to reproduce therapeutic response after the inhalation of hypertonic saline was studied using imaging data from patients with CF who inhaled isotonic saline (IS) and hypertonic saline on alternating study days [10]. Retention of Tc-SC, which is a metric of MCC, is shown with model fit for each patient group in Figure 3 [3]. Data from pediatric patients with CF and healthy controls who inhaled isotonic saline is also shown. The model captured the dynamics of MCC in all patient groups. The previously described increases in MCC associated with HS inhalation are apparent in the image-derived data and the model fits. However, as previously reported, no statistical differences in baseline MCC were detected between the CF IS, pediatric CF, and control groups [10].

DTPA is assumed to deposit in the same regions and clear by MCC at the same rate as Tc-SC; DTPA absorption is then captured by regressing the parameters k_{DB} and k_{LB}. Additionally, our previous studies have shown that the absorption of DTPA indicates changes in the absorption of ASL [9]. As such, the effect of hypertonic saline on liquid absorption, using DTPA as an analog, is shown in Figure 4, along with the model fit for each group [10]. The model again captured the dynamics of absorption in all groups. Increased baseline rates of DTPA absorption are apparent in both adult and pediatric CF groups, as previously described [10].

Our model predicts that both Tc-SC retention and liquid absorption will follow trajectories within narrow envelopes based on the predicted upper and lower 95% confidence intervals (CIs) of the model parameters. These CI envelopes are derived using all possible combinations of the upper and lower 95% CIs and nominal values of the model parameters to generate the extreme values of model predictions. Figure 5 shows that predicted model trajectories lead to different final values of Tc-SC retention for all adult patient groups, with no overlap in trajectory envelopes of CF IS and non-CF groups for $t>18$ min and no overlap between non-CF and HS trajectories for $t>27$ min. In other words, the three adult patient subgroups have characteristically different total MCC behavior. Pediatric CF clearance trajectories closely resemble those of adult patients with CF, but are not shown for ease of interpretation. Patients with CF display less MCC than non-CF subjects, which appears to contradict our finding in [10]. However, the present work evaluates the entire time course of clearance, while the end of study value ($t = 80$ min) was used as the evaluation time point in [10]. By using the entire data sequence, particularly the dynamic response at short times, we are able to parametrically estimate and differentiate - with confidence - the MCC and absorption dynamics between patients with CF and

Table 2. Model parameters in the work presented herein.

Parameter	Description
B	Bloodstream Model Compartment (units counts)
C_0	Initial Counts in L (units counts)
D	Distal Lung Model Compartment (units counts)
FFCA	Free Parameter; Fraction of C_0 in L_F (units counts)
L	Large Airway Model Super-Compartment (units counts)
L_F	Sub-compartment of L with Functional MCC (units counts)
L_N	Sub-compartment of L without Functional MCC (units counts)
k_{DB}	Free Parameter; Rate Constant of Absorption in D (units min^{-1})
k_{DL}	Free Parameter (Unused in Final Model); Rate Constant of MCC from D to L (units min^{-1})
k_{LB}	Free Parameter; Rate Constant of Absorption in L (units min^{-1})
k_{LT}	Free Parameter; Rate Constant of MCC from L to T (units min^{-1})
P_0	Initial Counts in D (units counts)
T	Trachea Model Compartment (units counts)

non-CF subjects. These analyses also indicate that MCC function in patients with CF can be rescued by HS treatment, which caused total MCC to exceed that of non-CF subjects.

Figure 6 shows that the model-predicted trajectories for liquid absorption have no overlap for all $t>0$. Pediatric CF trajectories again resemble those of adult patients with CF, but are not shown. Patients with CF have higher absorption than non-CF subjects, which can be partially remediated by HS treatment. Combined, the results in Figures 5 and 6 indicate that HS has two distinct mechanisms of action, both rescuing MCC and ameliorating liquid hyperabsorption [4].

It has been proposed that the apparent increase of MCC following HS treatment occurs by increasing the rate at which MCC occurs [4], [19]. Our model suggests that the intrinsic rate of MCC is the same in all patient groups, and the rescue of MCC can be attributed to the recruitment of inactive portions of the airway. Figure 7A shows that the rate of MCC, k_{LT}, is not significantly different between all patient groups ($p>0.05$).

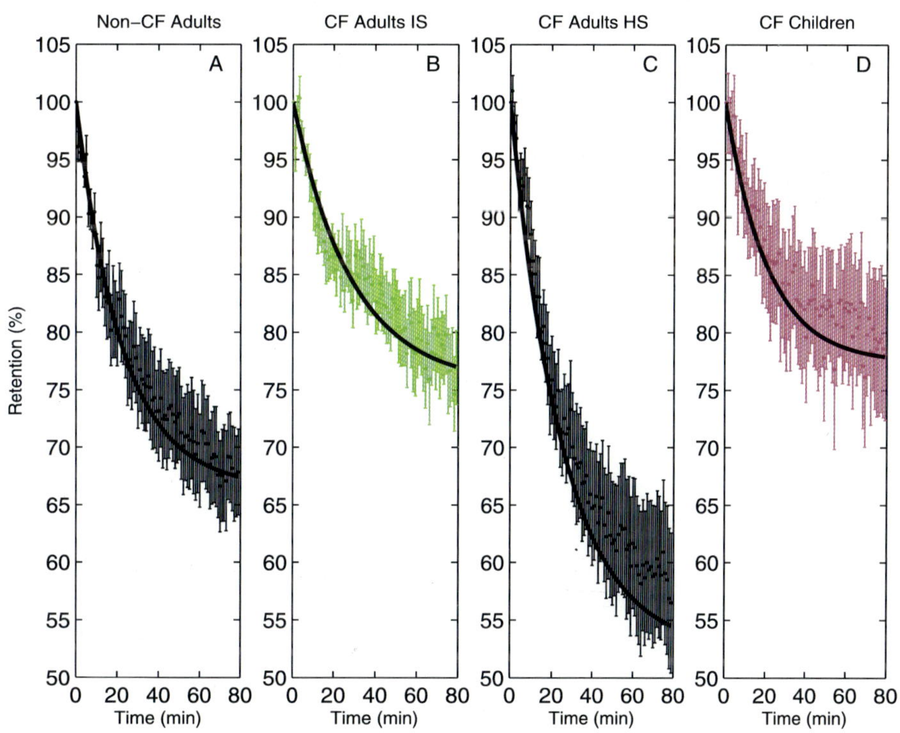

Figure 3. Tc-SC retention (mean ±SEM) vs. model fit (black line) for four patient subgroups. (A) Non-CF subjects (n = 9) (B) patients with CF (n = 12). (C) patients with CF after inhalation of hypertonic saline (n = 11). (D) Pediatric patients with CF. Data from [10].

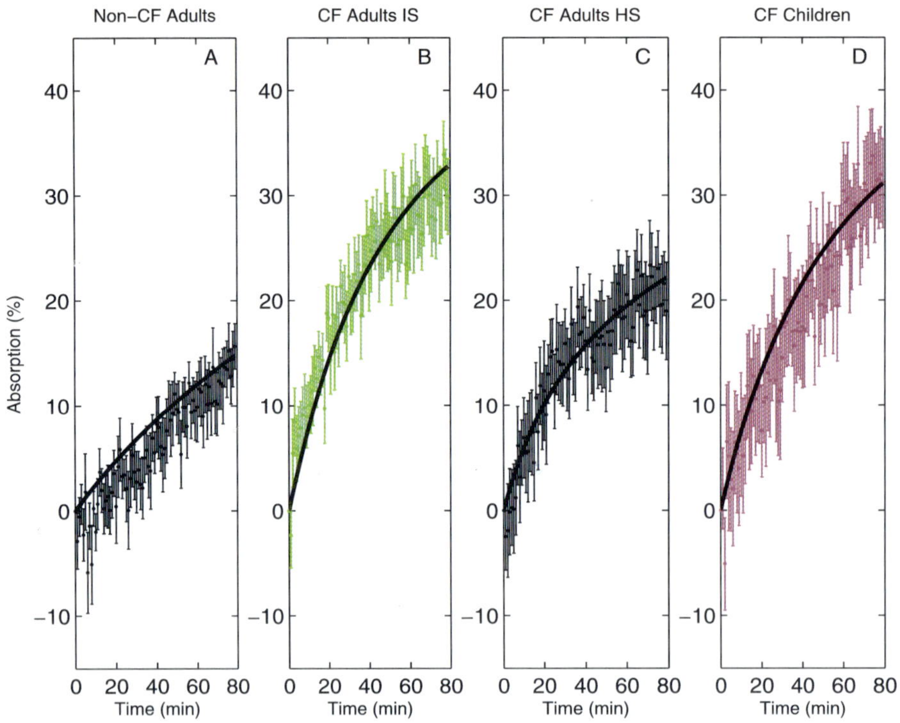

Figure 4. DTPA absorption (mean ±SEM) vs. model fit (line) for four patient subgroups. (A) Non-CF subjects (n = 9) (B) patients with CF (n = 12). (C) patients with CF after inhalation of hypertonic saline (n = 11). (D) Pediatric patients with CF. Data from [10].

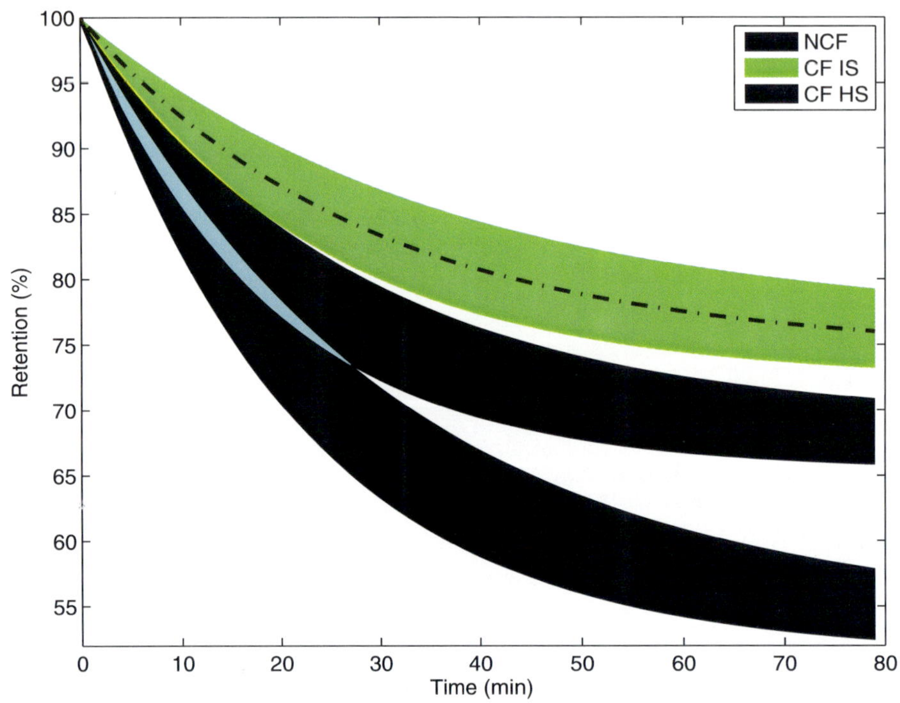

Figure 5. Estimated Tc-SC retention trajectories for three patient subgroups. Non-CF (red with dashed line), CF IS (green with dotted dashed line), CF HS (blue with line). Shaded envelope characterizes 95% confidence interval (CI) of retention prediction by the model. Pediatric CF subjects not shown due to overlap with adult CF.

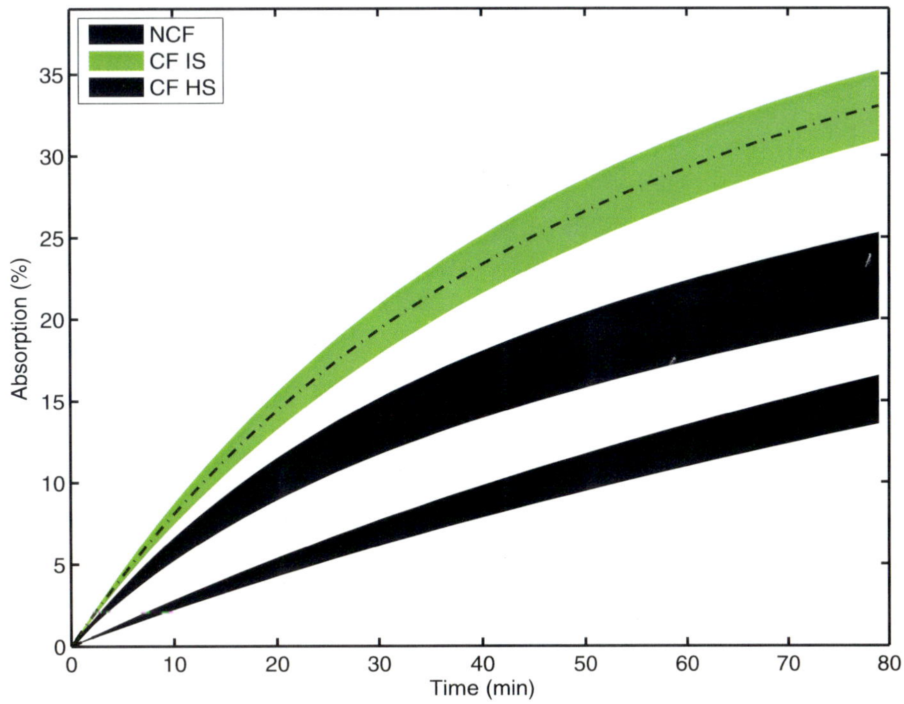

Figure 6. Estimated DTPA absorption trajectories for three groups. Non-CF (red with dashed line), CF IS (green with dotted dashed line), CF HS (blue with line). Shaded envelope characterizes 95% confidence interval (CI) of retention prediction by the model. Pediatric CF subjects not shown due to overlap with adult CF.

However, the parameter FFCA (Figure 7B), which describes the fractional area of large airways with functional MCC, is significantly lower in patients with CF versus non-CF subjects ($p<0.05$). Patients with CF given HS, however, show a significantly increased FFCA ($p<0.05$). This would support the concept of increased MCC, not through an intrinsic rate increase, but through an increase in the overall epithelial area contributing to MCC.

Our model also agrees with the previous reports that absorption, represented by k_{DB} and k_{LB} in our model, is increased in patients with CF vs. non-CF subjects ($p<0.001$ both parameters). The model demonstrates that HS inhalation decreases absorption in the peripheral lung (k_{DB}), which includes both small and intermediate sized airways and alveolar regions, more than IS inhalation ($p<0.001$). All model parameters are similar when comparing baseline measurements in the pediatric and adult CF IS groups (p = NS). Our parameters, as well as those of similar studies, are shown in Table 3.

In Vitro Evaluation of Model Prediction

In order to verify that hydration increases the fraction of functional ciliated area, we imaged CF HBE cultures (6 lines, n = 12) before and after addition of 10 μL of Dulbecco's Modified Eagle Media (DMEM) (Sigma-Aldrich, St. Louis, MO, USA), a liquid cell culture media, to the apical surface and again after a second addition of 10 μL of DMEM. We determined that hydration of HBE cells by addition of 10 μL significantly increases the fraction of functional ciliated area ($p<0.0005$) above baseline. No further increase in FFCA was observed following a second addition of 10 μL DMEM (p = NS), as shown in Figure 8A. CF HBE cells were imaged following apical addition of either 5 μL IS (n = 6) or HS (n = 6). A comparison of relative effect of IS and HS in CF HBE cells is shown in Figure 8B. Both IS and HS additions increase functional area ($p<0.05$ and $p<0.001$, respectively). However, HS increases functional area significantly more than IS ($p<0.01$).

Discussion

The failure of the CF airway epithelium to secrete Cl^- and absorb Na^+ in a normal manner results in a net osmotic gradient that favors rapid absorption of liquid from the ASL, resulting in diminished MCC and an accumulation of dehydrated mucus in the airways. Nuclear imaging methods have been previously developed to measure MCC and have been used as biomarkers of therapeutic efficacy. A novel method that measures both MCC and ASL absorption has been explored more recently [10]. This method involves the inhalation of radiolabeled particle and small molecule probes (Tc-SC and DTPA, respectively). The difference between total DTPA clearance and Tc-SC clearance can be used to estimate the absorption of DTPA, and previous studies have demonstrated: (i) a positive and significant correlation between DTPA and ASL absorption rates [9]; (ii) DTPA absorption response to the use of osmotic therapies both *in vivo* and *in vitro* [10], [9].

We have developed a model that considers the basic mechanisms governing small molecule and particle probe clearance from physiologically distinct compartments of the lung. The combination of these mechanisms is reflected in the imaging result. Compartment or mechanism specific results provide additional insight into CF lung pathophysiology and therapeutic mechanisms of action. They may also provide more sensitive and accurate predictions of therapeutic efficacy than analyses of the composite imaging data as the compartmental description incorporates the inherent time-correlation of mass transport within the model structure.

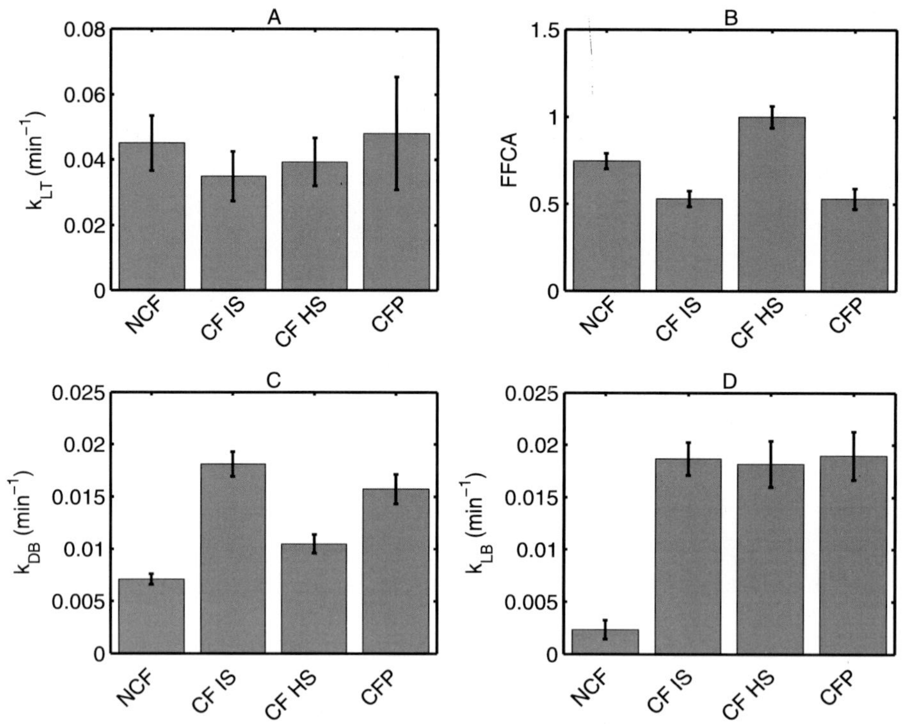

Figure 7. Least-squares solutions for model parameters are shown with 95% confidence intervals for four groups: Non-CF (NCF), CF HS, CF IS, and Pediatric CF (CFP). (A) MCC rate constant (k_{LT}) (min^{-1}). (B) Fraction (FFCA) of large airway with functional MCC. (C) Peripheral lung absorptive rate constant (k_{DB}) (min^{-1}). (D) Large airway absorptive rate constant (k_{LB}) (min^{-1}).

Model Structure Selection and Analysis

Our physically descriptive model includes central and peripheral lung compartments. The central zone includes large airways, intermediate and small airways, and alveoli while the peripheral zone includes only intermediate and small airways and alveoli [18], [20] (See Figure S1). The peripheral zone includes both smaller airways and alveoli in a single compartment. The model also includes compartments for the trachea and blood. As determined by Akaike Information Criterion (AIC) [21] analysis, a quantitative metric that weights the model accuracy (as measured by sum-squared error) against the cost of model complexity (quantified by the number of parameters in a model), the most appropriate model given the timeframe of our data assumed zero MCC from the peripheral compartment. Model rate constants describing MCC from the functional large airway compartment (k_{LT}), absorption from the small airway/alveolar compartment (k_{DB}), large airway absorption (k_{LB}), and FFCA were fit to the data. The fixed mathematical structure of the model is able to capture the dynamics of both MCC and the absorption of DTPA in the lungs of all patient groups.

An alternative, and more highly parameterized, model than that shown in Figure 2 would include parameter k_{DL} as an MCC rate constant from compartment D to compartment L, in addition to MCC rate constant k_{LT} and absorption rate constants k_{DB} and k_{LB}. All kinetics were assumed to be first order. Furthermore, the initial dosing of probes was included using a free dosing parameter (C/P), representing the ratio of radiopharmaceutical doses delivered to the large airways and peripheral lung. Under the assumption that Technetium 99m-labeled Sulfur Colloid (Tc-SC) is not absorbed in any lung region, the MCC curve was found to be bi-exponential, as suggested previously [15]. However, regression and analysis of the model parameters via the MATLAB

Table 3. Pharmacokinetic Lung Clearance Parameter Values.

Study	$k_{LT}(min^{-1})$	$k_{DB}(min^{-1})$
NCF	0.0450 ± 0.0085	0.0071 ± 0.0005
CF HS	0.0393 ± 0.0073	0.0105 ± 0.0009
CF IS	0.0349 ± 0.0076	0.0181 ± 0.0012
CF Pediatric	0.0481 ± 0.0173	0.0157 ± 0.0014
Sakagami* [14]	0.022 ± 0.002	0.048 ± 0.003

Values from this study are shown with ±95.
*PK model in isolated perfused rat lung. Three fluorescent markers used, but only the parameter values for sodium fluorescein (F-Na) are shown since $MW_{F-Na} = 376Da \approx MW_{DTPA}$.

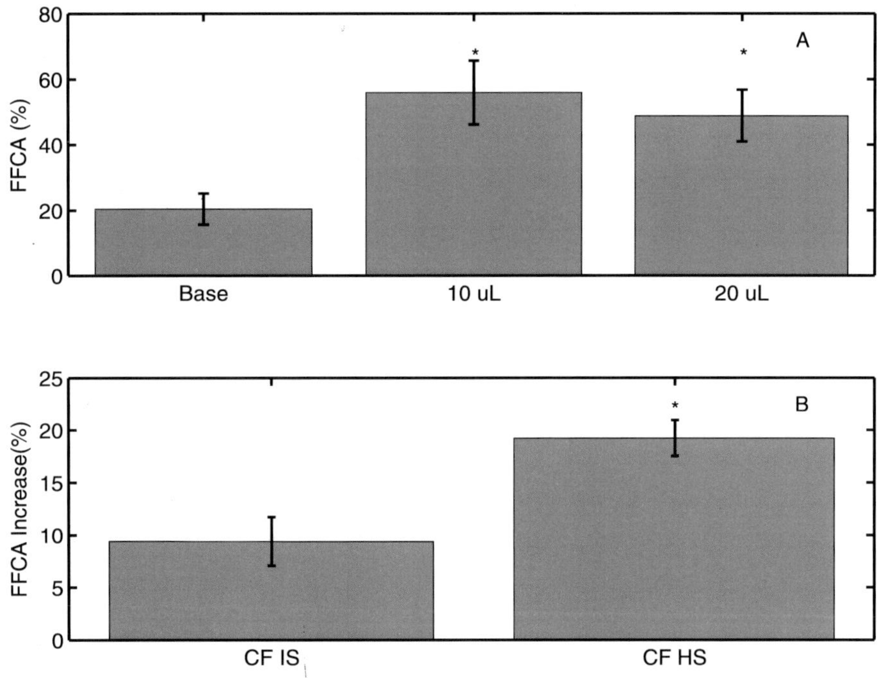

Figure 8. FFCA determined *in vitro* in CF HBE cells is shown ± SEM. (A) Activated area is significantly greater between 10 μL and baseline (* $p<0.0005$) and 2×10 μL and baseline (* $p<0.0005$). Activated area is not significantly greater between hydrated groups ($p>0.05$). (B) A two-tailed t-test with unequal variances assumed reveals that the increase in active area induced by HS in cells is significantly greater than that of IS (* $p<0.01$).

functions *lsqnonlin* (a nonlinear least-squares regression algorithm) and *nlparci* (an algorithm that computes confidence intervals on estimated parameters from the covariance matrix) yielded wide parameter confidence intervals, approximately ± 10 times the nominal parameter value. By eliminating k_{DL} the confidence intervals on parameter estimates are tightened dramatically (the worst case parameter CI from the model herein is k_{LB} in non-CF subjects which has CI's that are $\pm 39\%$ of the nominal value).

While a two-compartment model, like that proposed by Sakagami in [15], may be used to describe clearance, the parameters may not be able to be estimated with confidence if a physiological rate process captured by a parameter in the model is on the timescale of the experiment, or longer. The 80-minute functional imaging session inherently limits the confidence that can be derived for slower physiological processes. Therefore we hypothesized that the departure from monoexponential clearance seen in the retention curves could be explained by a non-zero steady state value for pharmaceutical retention. While this is aphysiologic over a period of days, an apparent non-zero baseline would manifest if a slow clearance process was occurring and data collection was short by comparison to the half-life of the clearance. This behavior can be realized in a number of ways in a kinetic model. In the present study, it is most easily incorporated by adding a new compartment that has no apparent MCC mechanism over the experimental timescale. Thus, while we believe that MCC in D can be observed on a longer timescale, we consider its mechanism to be practically unidentifiable (i.e. there is insufficient data to inform this parameter) over the timescale examined in the present work [22].

The model structure presented in Figure 2, and its grounding assumptions discussed in the **Results** section may fail to include mechanisms that could manifest on timescales longer than the 80 minute imaging period. To address the question of model appropriateness on the timescales of our data, we compared our model to the following alternative model structures with AIC as the basis for quantitative comparison:

Case 1. Exclude k_{LB}: DTPA absorption in L, represented by rate constant k_{LB}, is not appreciable over the 80-minute functional imaging timescale and should not be regressed to achieve model fit

Case 2. Include k_{DL}: MCC in D, represented by rate constant k_{DL}, is significant over the 80-minute functional imaging study timescale

The AIC values of each case above, in comparison to the model in Figure 2, are given in Table 4. These values demonstrate that the Figure 2 model displays the best combination of model fit and parsimony for the data set from [10]. Parsimony was especially important for model selection between the nominal case and Case 2, where the difference between AIC of the two cases was less than $\pm 1\%$. However, it is important to again note that there may in fact be clearance mechanisms from D, L_N, and L_F that are not accounted for in this model because of constraints on our ability to quantitatively resolve their effects with confidence over the timescale of imaging. This is illustrated graphically in Figure 9, where it is clear that we cannot confidently identify the parameter k_{DL} employed in Case 2 above.

Parametric Considerations

In non-CF subjects, FFCA is found to be <1. To our knowledge, the notion that not all of the surface of the conducting airways has functional cilia is a novel finding in humans. Hoegger *et al.* [23] recently report that even in the trachea, the most conductive airway, of newborn pigs without CF $\approx 70\%$ of particles clear in ten minutes and that those same particles are only actively moving $\approx 80\%$ of the time. While this timeframe is considerably shorter than the one in our study, it has been established that particles can be retained in the conducting airways of non-CF animals for a potentially significant amount of time. It would be reasonable to assume that particles deposited deeper in the

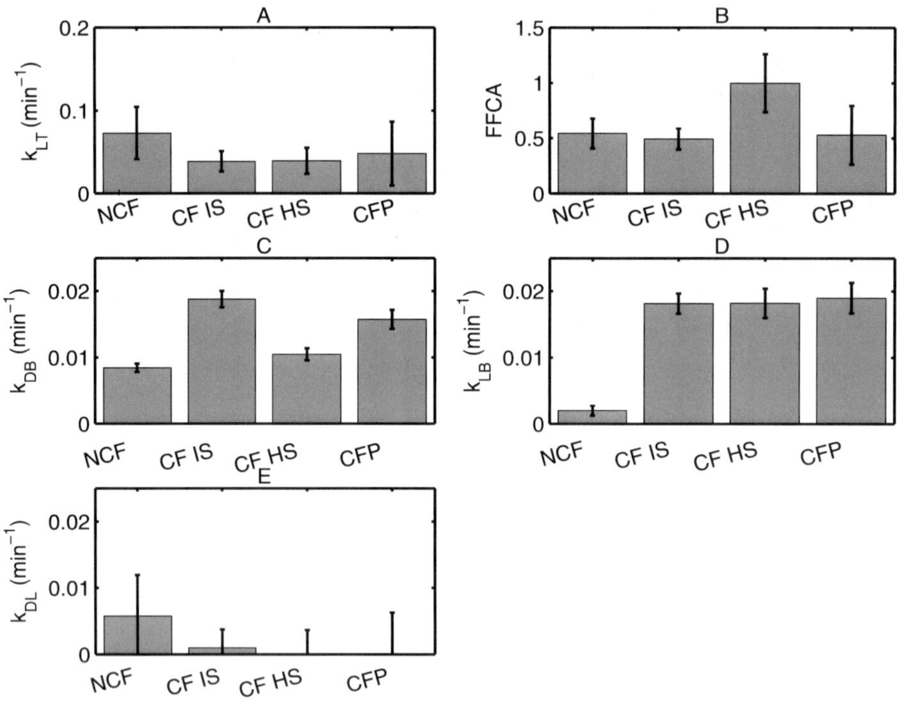

Figure 9. Least-squares solutions for model parameters in case 2 of Table 3 are shown for comparison to the selected model with 95% confidence intervals for four patient groups: Non-CF (NCF), CF HS, CF IS, and Pediatric CF (CP). (A) MCC rate constant (kLT) (min-1) reiterates that kLT is the same in all groups. (B) Fraction (FFCA) of large airway with functional MCC. (C) Peripheral lung absorptive rate constant (kDB) (min-1) and (D) large airway absorptive rate constant (kLB) are nearly identical to their analogs in the selected model. (E) MCC rate constant (kDL) (min-1) from D to L is clearly unidentifiable, and the nominal value is much smaller than kLT in each group. Confidence intervals are also widened in all parameters directly related to MCC.

airways, like those in our study, would be retained longer. Thus we have further reason to believe, in addition to the *in vitro* findings presented here, that our estimation of FFCA as a model parameter is grounded in realistic physiology.

Our model asserts that the rate of DTPA absorption (k_{DB}) is increased in the peripheral lung (small airway and alveoli) compartment of patients with CF as compared to non-CF subjects. Hypertonic saline slows this rate to nearly non-CF levels. Previous *in vitro* studies have related DTPA hyperabsorption to liquid hyperabsorption [9]. It is assumed that DTPA hyperabsorption occurs via a paracellular mechanism, driven by increased paracellular liquid absorption, as DTPA has no known transcellular route by which to absorb. Therefore, it is likely that our current result reflects the basic liquid absorption defect associated with CF. The aerosol delivery techniques utilized to deliver the radiopharmaceuticals targeted large and small airways through a specialized breathing pattern. Additionally, transient correction of the absorption defect would be expected after administration of an inhaled osmotic therapy based on most current hypotheses of airway disease in CF [24]. However, we cannot completely exclude the possibility of alveolar effects that may be related to yet undocumented physiological differences between the alveolar regions of CF and non-CF lungs.

The rate at which DTPA absorbs in the large airways (k_{LB}) is similar to k_{DB} in the CF IS, CF pediatric and non-CF groups. However, while hypertonic saline decreases the value of k_{DB} in patients with CF, it has no significant effect on k_{LB}. MCC is the dominant clearance mode in the large airways in both IS and HS cases. We have shown *in vitro* that HS modulates the FFCA of the airway epithelium and have shown *in vivo* that increased MCC can be attained by modulating FFCA without requiring change in MCC rate. The two rate constants in the central region (k_{LT} and k_{LB}) describe competing and correlated processes, whereas FFCA describes a more macroscopic phenomenon. Therefore, we would

Table 4. AIC Values for Various Model Structures.

	Model	Case 1	Case 2
NCF	−2546.28	−2535.65	−2543.38
CF HS	−2430.25	−2227.60	−2426.25
CF IS	−2775.62	−2287.07	−2775.57
CF Pediatric	−1858.37	−1597.47	−1854.37

The Akaike Information Criterion (AIC) is a metric for determining the most appropriate model for a system, where better fit is balanced against a penalty for overparameterization. Total AIC is shown as calculated from Equation 7 for all cases: 1) exclude k_{LB} from model structure; 2) include k_{PL} in model structure.

expect that a change in one rate constant in L would induce a corresponding change in the other. Between IS and HS days there is no change in k_{LT} (the dominant process), so we would not expect a change in k_{LB} either. However, due to the increase in FFCA, total MCC increases in the central lung after HS inhalation, which results in less DTPA being present and able to absorb in accordance with its unchanged rate constant. In effect, the underlying rate of DTPA absorption is unchanged, but an increase in total MCC as a result of increased FFCA leads to less DTPA being available for absorption and a smaller total quantity of DTPA absorbed in the CF HS case. In the case of D, however, we have assumed there is no competing, certainly no governing, MCC term in D. Thus, conditions affecting D must result changes in k_{DB}.

Study Limitations

A primary limitation of the functional imaging method utilized is its inability to uniquely discern airways and alveoli. Given the three dimensional nature of the lung architecture, small airways and alveoli are likely to be included in any zone analyzed via 2D imaging. The small sizes of these structures make them impossible to differentiate from each other through direct imaging, though other physiological measurements (such as 24 hr MCC) may help to differentiate their functional effects. The limited time scale of imaging (80 minutes) in the current study may have also limited assessment of small airway mucociliary clearance. Extended-duration imaging studies may yield additional data that can inform processes with slower rates and model parameters such as k_{DL}, which was excluded from the Figure 2 model on AIC grounds.

Physiological Implications

Our original study (see [10]) described significant differences in baseline whole lung DTPA absorption when comparing CF and healthy subjects. MCC was decreased in the CF groups, but not at statistically significant levels. In this study we find that MCC is decreased (in a statistically significant way) in the CF IS group for $t > 18$ minutes. The difference between these two findings arises from differences in the analysis tools used in this work versus the endpoint analysis performed in [10]. The confidence intervals presented here are around the parameters of the model, as opposed to being derived from statistical analysis of a final retention value, as in [10]. Our parameters govern the entire time-course of clearance, and thus are informed by the entire dynamic of the data given in [10]. The resulting confidence-interval-derived envelopes in Figures 5 and 6 capture the uncertainty of each physiologically descriptive parameter in the model. This is achieved by simulating the model at all possible combinations of upper and lower CIs for each parameter and determining the extreme values of model prediction at every time point. Hence, the CIs about our parameters are used to generate physiologically, as opposed to empirically, informed predictions of clearance behavior in each subject group population. The narrowness of our parameter CIs indicates confidence in the model parameter estimates (in that they are well informed from the dynamic data in [10]) and generates narrow prediction envelopes in each case, indicating a physiological difference in MCC dynamics between patients with CF and non-CF subjects that is not found via our previous endpoint-analysis methods.

Response to HS inhalation was apparent in terms of both decreased absorption and increased MCC as compared to IS inhalation. These trends are reflected in our modeled result. Our model suggests that the observed increase in MCC following HS inhalation is due to an increase in FFCA rather than an increase in MCC rate, and a detailed analysis of this hypothesis using the *in vivo* imaging data is ongoing. The model also predicts that FFCA is reduced in patients with CF as compared to the healthy population. We used this prediction as a hypothesis about inducing a functional change *in vivo* that can be tested *in vitro*. To further elucidate this phenomenon, and validate that such behavior is possible, we performed *in vitro* studies with HBE cell cultures. A quantitative visual assay of ciliary movement demonstrated that a larger fraction of the cell culture surface was activated after the addition of hypertonic saline vs. isotonic saline.

Clinical Relevance

Some previous imaging studies have shown significant differences in whole lung MCC between CF and non-CF subjects [25], [26] while others have not [4]. By ascribing a fixed mathematical structure to our model, we constrained the clearance curves to a single family of dynamical forms, which allows for more sensitive comparisons between the dynamical, and also endpoint, behavior present from one patient group to another. This ultimately increases our confidence in the model assertion that MCC is decreased in patients with CF and can be increased by hypertonic saline inhalation and, subsequently, that our model offers a better tool than statistical models for use in clinically gauging MCC.

Applications of this model may include the design of dosing regimens for agents targeting changes in MCC and/or absorption. For example, the timeline of the effects associated with an osmotic therapy (correction of liquid absorption defects) could be assessed independently of the resulting secondary effects (recruitment of functional ciliated airway, large and small airway clearance). Dosing timed in accordance with the duration of the counter-absorptive effect may provide more continuous clearance from the lungs and patient benefit, though outcome assessment is beyond the scope of the model at present. The model could also be used to resolve the pharmacodynamics of medications with subtle, complex, or multiple therapeutic effects, to the degree that these agents impact MCC and absorption.

Conclusions

Our physiologically motivated compartmental model is able to reproduce the clearance behavior of both large particle (Tc-SC) and small molecule (DTPA) radiolabeled probes as informed by functional imaging data. The model asserts that liquid absorption rate is increased in the peripheral lung of patients with CF as compared to non-CF subjects, and that hypertonic saline will decrease the rate of absorption in patients with CF to near non-CF levels. Our model also attributes increased MCC induced by hypertonic saline treatment to an increase in airway surface area with functional ciliary clearance, as opposed to an increased rate of clearance. The physiology inherent to the model structure and parameterization allow for increased sensitivity in gauging the effects of hypertonic saline *in vivo* in a real-time manner. This model should, therefore, be extendable to other treatments, both present and future, that target the liquid hyperabsorption and MCC deficiency present in cystic fibrosis.

Materials and Methods

Functional Imaging Methods

Data from previously reported clinical imaging studies were utilized [10]. These studies included both adult ($n = 12$) and pediatric ($n = 9$) patients with CF and healthy controls ($n = 9$). Raw imagining data from this study can be found in Table S1. An aerosol based functional imaging technique that measures the clearance of two different radiopharmaceutical probes from the lungs over 80 minutes was used. Indium-111-labeled diethylene triamine pentaacetic acid (DTPA) is a small molecule probe ($\approx$500 Da) that is cleared from the lung through both absorption and MCC while Technetium-99m-labeled sulfur colloid (Tc-SC) is a particle probe ($\approx$300nm) that is cleared only by MCC. DTPA absorption is calculated by subtracting the Tc-SC clearance rate (MCC) from the total In-DTPA clearance rate. Both probes were mixed and delivered together via nebulizer in the same liquid aerosol. All patient studies were approved by the University of Pittsburgh Institutional Review Board (clinicaltrial.gov numbers NCT01223183 and NCT01486199).

The aerosolized probes were delivered simultaneously by nebulizer using a technique that deposited aerosol primarily in the airways [10]. Their clearance (normalized decrease in radioactive counts over time) was then independently assessed over 80 minutes using dynamic planar scintigraphy. Whole, peripheral and central lung zones were considered, where the central zone was defined as a rectangle with $\frac{1}{2}$ the height and width of the whole lung region of interest postioned along the medial lung border and centered vertically. At t = 10 minutes (11th imaging frame) subjects inhaled nebulized saline treatments for 10 minutes. Adult patients with CF inhaled 7% hypertonic saline (HS, n = 11) on one testing day and isotonic saline (IS) on the other. Control and pediatric CF subjects performed a single testing day with isotonic saline. Previous *in vitro* studies have demonstrated a relationship between DTPA and ASL absorption. Since DTPA has no known route for intracellular transport this relationship is presumably due to the contribution of paracellular liquid flows. Changes in DTPA absorption in response to osmotic therapies have previously been demonstrated both *in vitro* [9] and *in vivo* [10]. Analysis of the Tc-SC and DTPA retention curves as well as DTPA absorption plotted with a logarithmic ordinate showed that the data did not follow a monoexponential profile, which guided selection of the model structure and kinetics necessary to accurately reproduce the data.

Initial Model Structure

Sakagami [15] proposed a robust modeling scaffold for inhaled pharmaceuticals that takes into account the regional pharmacokinetic differences between the large conducting airways (*L*) and the distal lung (*D*), consisting of smaller airways and alveoli. Analysis of the corresponding system of compartment-based ordinary differential equations (ODEs) yielded a bi-exponential retention curve for Tc-SC as proposed by Byron [14]. However, this model structure could not be reconciled with the whole of the data used herein (see **Discussion**).

Model Parameter Estimation

Regression of model parameters, regardless of model structure, was performed sequentially as follows. Model parameters were estimated using nonlinear least-squares regression (via *lsqnonlin* in MATLAB, ©2013, The MathWorks, Natick, MA) between model predictions and experimental data. The experimental design allowed for sequential estimation of the MCC and absorption rate parameters as follows:

1. The parameters that govern MCC (k_{LT} and FFCA) were fit to the Tc-SC retention data.
2. The regressed MCC parameters were then fixed, and the absorption rate parameters (k_{DB} and k_{LB}) were fit to the absorption curve.
3. Parameter uncertainty was calculated using the *nlparci* function in MATLAB (©2013, The MathWorks, Natick, MA) to obtain confidence intervals on all model parameters.

Model Analysis

The assumptions above were tested individually, and in combination, for appropriateness using the Akaike Information Criterion (AIC). Akaike [21] originally proposed that model appropriateness could be assessed according to the equation:

$$AIC = (-2)ln(maximum\ likelihood) + 2k \qquad (6)$$

Where a Gaussian distribution represents the maximum likelihood of the data and k is the number of free parameters in the model. Thus, the model with the least value of AIC is deemed most appropriate in terms of model fit and parsimony. Yamaoka and colleagues [27] further elaborated on this information criterion by proposing that for a process with Gaussian error the AIC can found from the equation:

$$AIC = Nln(\sum_{i=1}^{N}((\hat{y}_i) - y_i)^2/N) + 2k \qquad (7)$$

Where $\hat{y}_i$ is the model fit and y_i is the data value at the ith image of our N = 80n set because there are 80 images per patient and n patients per study group.

In Vitro Assessment of Ciliary Activation

We developed an *in vitro* imaging assay to measure the fraction of the epithelium that has functional MCC in order to test our hypotheses that FFCA is decreased in CF and that hydration can recruit areas of otherwise non-functional cilia. Fully differentiated human bronchial epithelial (HBE) cell cultures were viewed using a phase-contrast objective (Nikon Eclipse TI). These cultures were derived from lungs removed at the time of lung transplantation and prepared using previously described methods approved by the University of Pittsburgh IRB [28]. A series of 10 images was taken of each culture that allowed for the determination of the change in pixel intensity between successive images in the stack. Ciliary beat can be observed under these conditions and is characterized by a change in light intensity measured by the camera. This change in light intensity can be translated to a change in pixel intensity in the images obtained when placed in sequence to form a movie of ciliary motion (see Figure S2 and Video S1). The average change in pixel intensity of all cultures was determined in both CF lines (n = 6) and a non-CF line. Average changes in the intensity of each pixel from 12 untreated cultures from the non-CF line were measured and the average change in intensity over all pixels was used as a baseline measurement of functional ciliary movement. Pixels in each stack with average change in intensity greater than the non-CF baseline were said to have functional ciliary movement. To test the effect of osmotic agents, 5 μL of either isotonic (300 mOsm) or hypertonic (600 mOsm) saline was added to the apical surface of cells prior to imaging (see Table S2 for data). To test for saturating effects of hydration, we sequentially added Dulbecco's Modified Eagle Medium (DMEM) from the basolateral bath to the apical surface of the cultures as follows: 10 μL of DMEM was added to the apical surface of the cells from the basolateral bath before the cells were imaged, and an additional 10 μL of basolateral DMEM was added to the apical surface prior to a second, identical, imaging routine (see Table S3 for data).

Supporting Information

Figure S1 Shown is the initial posterior frame of a Tc-SC imaging series. The dotted outline of the right lung is a tracing of the outline of the lung as it appears in a transmission scan. The filled in blue rectangle is the *C* ROI. The remaining lung ROI represents *P*.

Figure S2 A pseudo-color image of non-CF HBE cells under 10× enhancement is shown. The viewing frame is identical to that in Video S1. Darker (more blue) regions show areas with lower average change in pixel intensity during Video S1 whereas lighter (more yellow) regions show areas with higher average change. In combination with Video S1 we show that regions that display little visible movement are more blue, and the regions with visible motion, particularly the hurricane regions, are more yellow.

Table S1 Raw Tc-SC and In-DTPA counts in whole lung ROI and central lung ROI over the length of imaging.

Table S2 FFCA in CF HBE cells is shown at baseline compared to a 5 ul addition of either isotonic or hypotonic saline.

Table S3 FFCA in CF HBE cells is shown at baseline, after one 10 ul addition of basolateral DMEM, and after a second, sequential addition of basolateral DMEM.

Video S1 A video of ciliary motion in non-CF HBE cells under 10× phase-contrast enhancement is shown. The viewing frame is identical to that in Figure S2. Three hurricane type regions of ciliary motion are visible in the field of view. In combination with Figure S2 we show that regions that display little visible movement have lower average change in pixel intensity, and the regions with visible motion, particularly the hurricane regions, have higher average change in pixel intensity.

Acknowledgments

The authors would like to thank Li Ang Zhang for his assistance in code development and Stefanie Brown for her assistance in maintaining the HBE cell lines used in this work.

Author Contributions

Conceived and designed the experiments: MRM TEC LWL MMM RSP. Performed the experiments: MRM TEC LWL. Analyzed the data: MRM TEC LWL MMM RSP. Contributed reagents/materials/analysis tools: MRM TEC LWL MMM JMP RSP. Wrote the paper: MRM TEC LWL MMM JMP RSP. Designed software used in analysis: MRM LWL MMM. Obtained permission for use of cell line: MMM JMP. Obtained informed consent of patients: MMM JMP.

References

1. O'Reilly R, Elphick HE (2013) Development, clinical utility, and place of ivacaftor in the treatment of cystic fibrosis. Drug Design, Development and Therapy 7: 929–37.
2. Boucher RC (2007) Cystic fibrosis: a disease of vulnerability to airway surface dehydration. Trends in Molecular Medicine 13: 231–40.
3. Corcoran TE, Thomas KM, Myerburg MM, Muthukrishnan A, Weber L, et al. (2010) Absorptive clearance of DTPA as an aerosol-based biomarker in the cystic fibrosis airway. The European Respiratory Journal 35: 781–6.
4. Donaldson SH, Bennett WD, Zeman KL, Knowles MR, Tarran R, et al. (2006) Mucus clearance and lung function in cystic fibrosis with hypertonic saline. The New England Journal of Medicine 354: 241–50.
5. Elkins MR, Robinson M, Rose BR, Harbour C, Moriarty CP, et al. (2006) A controlled trial of long-term inhaled hypertonic saline in patients with cystic fibrosis. New England Journal of Medicine 354: 229–240.
6. Accurso FJ, Rowe SM, Clancy J, Boyle MP, Dunitz JM, et al. (2010) Effect of vx-770 in persons with cystic fibrosis and the g551d-cftr mutation. New England Journal of Medicine 363: 1991–2003.
7. Bennett WD, Ilowite JS (1989) Dual pathway clearance of 99mtc-dtpa from the bronchial mucosa1~3. The American review of respiratory disease 139: 1132.
8. Ilowite JS, Bennett WD, Sheetz MS, Groth ML, Nierman DM (1989) Permeability of the bronchial mucosa to 99mtc-dtpa in asthma. American Review of Respiratory Disease 139: 1139–1143.
9. Corcoran TE, Thomas KM, Brown S, Myerburg MM, Locke LW, et al. (2013) Liquid hyper-absorption as a cause of increased DTPA clearance in the cystic fibrosis airway. EJNMMI research 3: 14.
10. Locke L, Myerburg M, Markovetz M, Parker R, Weber L, et al. (2014) Quantitative Imaging of Airway Liquid Absorption in Cystic Fibrosis. European Respiratory Journal: In Press.
11. Eckford PDW, Li C, Ramjeesingh M, Bear CE (2012) Cystic fibrosis transmembrane conductance regulator (CFTR) potentiator VX-770 (ivacaftor) opens the defective channel gate of mutant CFTR in a phosphorylation-dependent but ATP-independent manner. The Journal of Biological Chemistry 287: 36639–49.
12. Van Goor F, Hadida S, Grootenhuis PDJ, Burton B, Stack JH, et al. (2011) Correction of the F508del-CFTR protein processing defect *in vitro* by the investigational drug VX-809. Proceedings of the National Academy of Sciences of the United States of America 108: 18843–8.
13. Byron P, Patton J (1994) Drug delivery via the respiratory tract. Journal of Aerosol medicine 7: 49–75.
14. Sakagami M, Byron PR, Venitz J, Rypacek F (2002) Solute disposition in the rat lung *in vivo* and *in vitro*: determining regional absorption kinetics in the presence of mucociliary escalator. Journal of Pharmaceutical Sciences 91: 594–604.
15. Sakagami M (2006) In vivo, *in vitro* and ex vivo models to assess pulmonary absorption and disposition of inhaled therapeutics for systemic delivery. Advanced Drug Delivery Reviews 58: 1030–60.
16. Weber B, Hochhaus G (2013) A pharmacokinetic simulation tool for inhaled corticosteroids. The AAPS Journal 15: 159–71.
17. Sturm R (2012) An advanced stochastic model for mucociliary particle clearance in cystic fibrosis lungs. Journal of Thoracic Disease 4: 48–57.
18. Biddiscombe MF, Meah SN, Underwood SR, Usmani OS (2011) Comparing lung regions of interest in gamma scintigraphy for assessing inhaled therapeutic aerosol deposition. Journal of aerosol medicine and pulmonary drug delivery 24: 165–173.
19. Donaldson SH, Corcoran TE, Laube BL, Bennett WD (2007) Mucociliary clearance as an outcome measure for cystic fibrosis clinical research. Proceedings of the American Thoracic Society 4: 399–405.
20. Newman S, Bennett WD, Biddiscombe M, Devadason SG, Dolovich MB, et al. (2012) Standardization of techniques for using planar (2d) imaging for aerosol deposition assessment of orally inhaled products. Journal of aerosol medicine and pulmonary drug delivery 25: S–10.
21. Akaike H (1974) A new look at the statistical model identification. Automatic Control, IEEE Transactions on 19: 716–723.
22. Raue A, Kreutz C, Maiwald T, Bachmann J, Schilling M, et al. (2009) Structural and practical identifiability analysis of partially observed dynamical models by exploiting the profile likelihood. Bioinformatics (Oxford, England) 25: 1923–9.
23. Hoegger MJ, Fischer AJ, McMenimen JD, Ostedgaard LS, Tucker AJ, et al. (2014) Impaired mucus detachment disrupts mucociliary transport in a piglet model of cystic fibrosis. Science 345: 818–822.
24. Boucher R (2004) New concepts of the pathogenesis of cystic fibrosis lung disease. European Respiratory Journal 23: 146–158.
25. Regnis Ja, Robinson M, Bailey DL, Cook P, Hooper P, et al. (1994) Mucociliary clearance in patients with cystic fibrosis and in normal subjects. American Journal of Respiratory and Critical Care Medicine 150: 66–71.
26. Robinson M, Eberl S, Tomlinson C, Daviskas E, Regnis J, et al. (2000) Regional mucociliary clearance in patients with cystic fibrosis. Journal of Aerosol Medicine 13: 73–86.
27. Yamaoka K, Nakagawa T, Uno T (1978) Application of Akaike's information criterion (AIC) in the evaluation of linear pharmacokinetic equations. Journal of Pharmacokinetics and Biopharmaceutics 6: 165–75.
28. Myerburg MM, Harvey PR, Heidrich EM, Pilewski JM, Butterworth MB (2010) Acute regulation of the epithelial sodium channel in airway epithelia by proteases and trafficking. American Journal of Respiratory Cell and Molecular Biology 43: 712–9.

Permissions

All chapters in this book were first published in PLOS ONE, by The Public Library of Science; hereby published with permission under the Creative Commons Attribution License or equivalent. Every chapter published in this book has been scrutinized by our experts. Their significance has been extensively debated. The topics covered herein carry significant findings which will fuel the growth of the discipline. They may even be implemented as practical applications or may be referred to as a beginning point for another development.

The contributors of this book come from diverse backgrounds, making this book a truly international effort. This book will bring forth new frontiers with its revolutionizing research information and detailed analysis of the nascent developments around the world.

We would like to thank all the contributing authors for lending their expertise to make the book truly unique. They have played a crucial role in the development of this book. Without their invaluable contributions this book wouldn't have been possible. They have made vital efforts to compile up to date information on the varied aspects of this subject to make this book a valuable addition to the collection of many professionals and students.

This book was conceptualized with the vision of imparting up-to-date information and advanced data in this field. To ensure the same, a matchless editorial board was set up. Every individual on the board went through rigorous rounds of assessment to prove their worth. After which they invested a large part of their time researching and compiling the most relevant data for our readers.

The editorial board has been involved in producing this book since its inception. They have spent rigorous hours researching and exploring the diverse topics which have resulted in the successful publishing of this book. They have passed on their knowledge of decades through this book. To expedite this challenging task, the publisher supported the team at every step. A small team of assistant editors was also appointed to further simplify the editing procedure and attain best results for the readers.

Apart from the editorial board, the designing team has also invested a significant amount of their time in understanding the subject and creating the most relevant covers. They scrutinized every image to scout for the most suitable representation of the subject and create an appropriate cover for the book.

The publishing team has been an ardent support to the editorial, designing and production team. Their endless efforts to recruit the best for this project, has resulted in the accomplishment of this book. They are a veteran in the field of academics and their pool of knowledge is as vast as their experience in printing. Their expertise and guidance has proved useful at every step. Their uncompromising quality standards have made this book an exceptional effort. Their encouragement from time to time has been an inspiration for everyone.

The publisher and the editorial board hope that this book will prove to be a valuable piece of knowledge for researchers, students, practitioners and scholars across the globe.

List of Contributors

Dieter Böning, Angela Littschwager, Matthias Hütler and Ralph Beneke
Institut für Sportmedizin, Charité - Universitätsmedizin Berlin, Berlin, Germany

Doris Staab
Klinik für Pädiatrische Pneumologie und Immunologie, Charité - Universitätsmedizin Berlin, Berlin, Germany

Hannah K. Bayes and Tom J. Evans
Institute of Infection, Immunology and Inflammation, College of Medical, Veterinary and Life Sciences, University of Glasgow, Glasgow, United Kingdom

Stephen Bicknell and Gordon MacGregor
West of Scotland Cystic Fibrosis Centre, Gartnavel General Hospital, Glasgow, United Kingdom

Eugenia Bruzzese, Valeria Raia, Sara Viscovo, Riccardo Scotto, Vittoria Buccigrossi, Andrea Lo Vecchio, Eliana Ruberto and Alfredo Guarino
Department of Translational Medical Science, Section of Pediatrics, University Federico II, Naples, Italy

Maria Luisa Callegari, Susanna Ferrari and Lorenzo Morelli
Centro Ricerche Biotecnologiche, Università Cattolica del Sacro Cuore, Cremona, Italy

Laurie-Anne Payet, Caroline Norez, Sandra Mirval, Frédéric Becq, Clarisse Vandebrouck and Thierry Ferreira
Signalisation et Transports Ioniques Membranaires, ERL CNRS 7368, Université de Poitiers, Poitiers, France

Linette Kadri
Ecologie et Biologie des Interactions, UMR CNRS 7267, Université de Poitiers, Poitiers, France

Sébastien Giraud
Service de Biochimie, CHU Poitiers, Poitiers, France
Inserm U1082, Poitiers, France
Faculté de Médecine et de Pharmacie Université de Poitiers, Poitiers

Christophe Jayle
Service de Chirurgie Cardiothoracique, CHU Poitiers, Poitiers, France

Yong-hua Gao, Wei-jie Guan., Gang Xu, Yan Tang, Yang Gao, Zhi-ya Lin, Zhi-min Lin, Nan-shan Zhong and Rong-chang Chen
State Key Laboratory of Respiratory Diseases, National Clinical Research Center for Respiratory Disease, Guangzhou Institute of Respiratory Diseases, The First Affiliated Hospital of Guangzhou Medical University, Guangzhou, Guangdong, China

Natalia Molenda, Katarina Urbanova, Nelly Weiser, Kristina Kusche-Vihrog and Hermann Schillers
Institute of Physiology II, University of Münster, Münster, Germany

Dorothee Günzel
Institute of Clinical Physiology, Charité Campus Benjamin Franklin, Berlin, Germany

Celia N. Sanchez-Dominguez, Maria del C. Villalobos-Torres, Augusto Rojas-Martinez, Herminia G. Martinez-Rodriguez, Hugo A. Barrera-Saldaña and Rocio Ortiz-Lopez
Departamento de Bioquimica y Medicina Molecular, Facultad de Medicina, Universidad Autonoma de Nuevo Leon, Monterrey, Nuevo Leon, Mexico

Miguel A. Reyes-Lopez
Laboratorio de Medicina de Conservacion, Centro de Biotecnologia Genomica, Instituto Politecnico Nacional, Reynosa, Tamaulipas, Mexico

Adriana Bustamante
Clinica de Fibrosis Quistica, Centro de Prevencion y Rehabilitacion de Enfermedades Pulmonares Cronicas (CEPREP), Facultad de Medicina y Hospital Universitario "Dr. Jose Eleuterio Gonzalez", Universidad Autónoma de Nuevo Leon, Monterrey, Nuevo Leon, Mexico

Ricardo M. Cerda-Flores
Facultad de Enfermeria, Universidad Autonoma de Nuevo Leon, Monterrey, Nuevo Leon, Mexico

Hugo L. Gallardo-Blanco
Departamento de Genetica, Facultad de Medicina, Universidad Autonoma de Nuevo Leon, Monterrey, Nuevo Leon, Mexico

Augusto Rojas-Martinez and Rocio Ortiz-Lopez
Centro de Investigacion y Desarrollo en Ciencias de la Salud, Universidad Autonoma de Nuevo Leon, Monterrey, Nuevo Leon, Mexico

Ewa Ziętkięwicz, Ewa Rutkięwicz, Barbara Klimek, Katarzyna Voelkel and Michał Witt
Department of Molecular and Clinical Genetics, Institute of Human Genetics, Polish Academy of Sciences, Poznan, Poland

Andrzej Pogorzelski
Department of Pneumology and Cystic Fibrosis, Institute of Tuberculosis and Lung Diseases, Rabka, Poland

Michał Witt
International Institute of Molecular and Cell Biology, Warsaw, Poland

Katherine L. Tuggle, Susan E. Birket, Jeong Hong, Li Ping Tang, James A. Fortenberry, Ming Du, David M. Bedwell, Steven M. Rowe, Eric J. Sorscher and Michelle V. Fanucchi
Gregory Fleming James Cystic Fibrosis Research Center, University of Alabama at Birmingham, Birmingham, Alabama, United States of America

Katherine L. Tuggle
Department of Environmental Health Sciences, School of Public Health, University of Alabama at Birmingham, Birmingham, Alabama, United States of America

Susan E. Birket, Steven M. Rowe and Eric J. Sorscher
Department of Medicine, University of Alabama at Birmingham, Birmingham, Alabama, United States of America

Xiaoxia Cui, Joe Warren, Lara Reid, Andre Chambers, Diana Ji and Kevin Gamber
SAGE Labs, Inc., St. Louis, Missouri, United States of America

Jeong Hong
Department of Cell, Developmental, and Integrative Biology, University of Alabama at Birmingham, Birmingham, Alabama, United States of America

Kengyeh K. Chu and Guillermo Tearney
Wellman Center for Photomedicine, Harvard Medical School, Massachusetts General Hospital, Boston, Massachusetts, United States of America

Kengyeh K. Chu
Department of Dermatology, Massachusetts General Hospital, Boston, Massachusetts, United States of America

Guillermo Tearney
Animal Resources Program, Office of the Vice President for Research, University of Alabama at Birmingham, Birmingham, Alabama, United States of America

Ming Du and Joan M. Cadillac
Animal Resources Program, Office of the Vice President for Research, University of Alabama at Birmingham, Birmingham, Alabama, United States of America

David M. Bedwell
Department of Microbiology, University of Alabama at Birmingham, Birmingham, Alabama, United States of America

Jessica E. Char, Marlene H. Wolfe, Hyung-ju Cho, Il-Ho Park, Jin Hyeok Jeong and Eric Frisbee
Cystic Fibrosis Research Laboratory, Stanford University, Stanford, California, United States of America

Colleen Dunn, Zoe Davies, Carlos Milla, Richard B. Moss and Jeffrey J. Wine
Department of Pediatrics, Stanford University School of Medicine, Stanford, California, United States of America

Ewart A. C. Thomas and Jeffrey J. Wine
Department of Psychology, Stanford University, Stanford, California, United States of America

Joanne Armstead, Julie Morris and David W. Denning
National Aspergillosis Centre, University Hospital South Manchester, The University of Manchester and Manchester Academic Health Science Centre, Manchester, United Kingdom

Kaivon Assani and Benjamin T. Kopp
Center for Microbial Pathogenesis, The Research Institute at Nationwide Children's Hospital, Columbus, Ohio, United States of America

Mia F. Tazi and Amal O. Amer
Department of Microbial Infection and Immunity and the Department of Internal Medicine, The Ohio State University, Columbus, Ohio, United States of America

Benjamin T. Kopp
Section of Pediatric Pulmonology, Nationwide Children's Hospital, Columbus, Ohio, United States of America

Nathalie Benz, Sophie Le Hir, Mathieu Kerbiriou, Marie-Laure Calvez, Pascal Trouvé and Claude Férec
Institut National de la Santé et de la Recherche Médicale, UMR1078, Brest, France

Nathalie Benz
Association Gaetan Saleun, Brest, France

Sophie Le Hir and Claude Férec
C.H.U. Brest, Hôpital Morvan, Laboratoire de Génétique Moléculaire, Brest, France

Caroline Norez and Frédéric Becq
Institut de Physiologie et Biologie Cellulaires, Centre national de la recherche scientifique FRE 3511, Université de Poitiers, Poitiers, France

Mathieu Kerbiriou, Marie-Laure Calvez and Claude Férec
Université de Bretagne Occidentale, Faculté de Médecine et des sciences de la santé, Brest, France

Claude Férec
Etablissement Français du Sang - Bretagne, Brest, France

Giovanna Tomaiuolo, Sergio Caserta, Antonio Carciati and Stefano Guido
Dipartimento di Ingegneria Chimica, dei Materiali e della Produzione Industriale, Università di Napoli Federico II, Napoli, Italy

Giovanna Tomaiuolo, Sergio Caserta and Stefano Guido
CEINGE-Advanced Biotechnologies, Napoli, Italy

Antonio Sasso
Dipartimento di Fisica, Università di Napoli Federico II, Complesso Universitario M.S. Angelo, Napoli, Italy

Vincenzo Carnovale and Pasquale Abete
Dipartimento di Scienze mediche Traslazionali - Unità di Fibrosi Cistica dell'adulto, Università di Napoli Federico II, Napoli, Italy

Anne-Laure Michon, Estelle Jumas-Bilak, Brigitte Lamy and Hélène Marchandin
UMR 5119 ECOSYM, Equipe Pathogènes et Environnements, U.F.R. des Sciences Pharmaceutiques et Biologiques, Universite´ Montpellier

Anne-Laure Michon, Brigitte Lamy and Hélène Marchandin
Laboratoire de Bactériologie, Hôpital Arnaud de Villeneuve, Centre Hospitalier Régional Universitaire de Montpellier, Montpellier, France

Estelle Jumas-Bilak
Laboratoire d'Hygiène hospitalière, Centre Hospitalier Régional Universitaire de Montpellier, Montpellier, France

Raphaël Chiron
Centre de Ressources et de Compétences pour la Mucoviscidose, Hôpital Arnaud de Villeneuve, Centre Hospitalier Régional Universitaire de Montpellier, Montpellier, France

Liudmila Cebotaru and Daniele Rapino
Department of Ophthalmology, School of Medicine, The Johns Hopkins University, Baltimore, Maryland, United States of America

Liudmila Cebotaru and Daniele Rapino and William B. Guggino
Department of Physiology, School of Medicine, The Johns Hopkins University, Baltimore, Maryland, United States of America

Valeriu Cebotaru
Department of Medicine, School of Medicine, The Johns Hopkins University, Baltimore, Maryland, United States of America

Bruna Mendes Lourenço, Kauê Machado Costa and Manoel da Silva Filho
Institute of Biological Sciences, Federal University of Pará, Belém, Pará, Brazil

Bruna Mendes Lourenço
João de Barros Barreto University Hospital, Federal University of Pará, Belém, Pará, Brazil

Daniel J. Smith, Scott C. Bell and David W. Reid
Department of Thoracic Medicine, The Prince Charles Hospital, Brisbane, Queensland, Australia

Daniel J. Smith, Scott C. Bell and David W. Reid
School of Medicine, University of Queensland, Brisbane, Queensland, Australia

Geoffrey R. Hill
Bone Marrow Transplant Laboratory, QIMR Berghofer Medical Research Institute, Brisbane, Queensland, Australia

Daniel J. Smith and David W. Reid
Infection and Inflammation Laboratory, QIMR Berghofer Medical Research Institute, Brisbane, Queensland, Australia

Scott C. Bell
Queensland Children's Medical Research Institute, Royal Children's Hospital, Brisbane, Queensland, Australia

James E. A. Zlosnik, Paul Y. Mori, Derek To, James Leung, Trevor J. Hird and David P. Speert
Centre for Understanding and Preventing Infection in Children, Department of Pediatrics, Faculty of Medicine, University of British Columbia, Vancouver, British Columbia, Canada

Markus Wettstein
Physiotherapy Institute, Inselspital, Bern University Hospital and University of Bern, Bern, Switzerland

Lorenz Radlinger
Bern University of Applied Sciences, Health, Bern, Switzerland

Thomas Riedel
Paediatric and Neonatal Intensive Care Medicine, Department of Paediatrics, Inselspital, Bern University Children's Hospital and University of Bern, Bern, Switzerland

Ludovic Jeanson, Serge Amselem and Estelle Escudier
Service de Génétique et Embryologie Médicales, Unité Mixte de Recherche_Scientifique 933, Institut National de la Santé et de la Recherche Médicale, Université Pierreet Marie Curie - Paris 6, and Assistance Publique - Hôpitaux de Paris, Hôpital Armand Trousseau, Paris, France

Ludovic Jeanson, Ida Chiara Guerrera, Cerina Chhuon and Aleksander Edelman
Unité_1151, Institut National de la Santé et de la Recherche Médicale, Université Paris Descartes, Paris, France

Ida Chiara Guerrera, Cerina Chhuon and Aleksander Edelman
Plateau Proteome Necker, Structure Fédérative de Recherche de Necker, Université Paris Descartes, Paris, France

Jean-François Papon, Patricia Zadigue and André Coste
Unité Mixte de Recherche_Scientifique 855, Institut National de la Santé et de la Recherche Médicale, Université Paris

Jean-François Papon, Virginie Prulière-Escabasse and André Coste
Service d'Otorhinolaryngologie et de chirurgie cervico-faciale, Assistance Publique - Hô pitaux de Paris, Hôpital inter-communal et Groupe Hospitalier Henri Mondor-Albert Chenevier, Créteil, France

Judy M. Bradley
Institute of Nursing and Health Research, University of Ulster, Ulster, Northern Ireland

Paul Koker and Qiqi Deng
Boehringer Ingelheim Pharmaceuticals Inc, Ridgefield, Connecticut, United States of America

Petra Moroni-Zentgraf
Boehringer Ingelheim Pharma GmbH and Co KG, Ingelheim, Germany

Felix Ratjen
The Hospital for Sick Children, Toronto, Ontario, Canada

David E. Geller
Florida State University College of Medicine, Orlando, Florida, United States of America

J. Stuart Elborn
Centre for Infection and Immunity, Queen's University Belfast, Belfast, Northern Ireland

Matthew R. Markovetz, Timothy E. Corcoran and Robert S. Parker
Department of Chemical and Petroleum Engineering, Swanson School of Engineering, University of Pittsburgh, Pittsburgh, PA, United States of America

Timothy E. Corcoran, Landon W. Locke, Michael M. Myerburg and Joseph M. Pilewski
Pulmonary Allergy and Critical Care Medicine, University of Pittsburgh, Pittsburgh, PA, United States of America

Robert S. Parker
McGowan Institute of Regenerative Medicine, University of Pittsburgh, Pittsburgh, PA, United States of America
Clinical Research, Investigation, and Systems Modeling of Acute Illness (CRISMA) Laboratories, University of Pittsburgh, Pittsburgh, PA, United States of America
University of Pittsburgh Cancer Institute, University of Pittsburgh, Pittsburgh, PA, United States of America

Timothy E. Corcoran
Department of Bioengineering, Swanson School of Engineering, University of Pittsburgh, Pittsburgh, PA, United States of America

Index